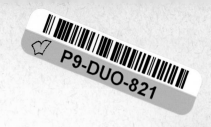

PROGRESS IN BRAIN RESEARCH
VOLUME 45
PERSPECTIVES IN BRAIN RESEARCH

PROGRESS IN BRAIN RESEARCH

ADVISORY BOARD

PROGRESS IN BRAIN RESEARCH

VOLUME 45

PERSPECTIVES IN
BRAIN RESEARCH

Proceedings of the 9th International Summer School of Brain Research,
Organized by the Netherlands Central Institute for Brain Research, Amsterdam,
and held at the Royal Netherlands Academy of Arts and Sciences at Amsterdam,
The Netherlands on July 28 — August 1, 1975

EDITED BY

M. A. CORNER

AND

D. F. SWAAB

(J. Sels Assistant Editor)

Netherlands Central Institute for Brain Research,
IJdijk 28, Amsterdam (The Netherlands)

ELSEVIER SCIENTIFIC PUBLISHING COMPANY

AMSTERDAM/NEW YORK/OXFORD

1976

PUBLISHED BY:
ELSEVIER/NORTH-HOLLAND BIOMEDICAL PRESS
335 JAN VAN GALENSTRAAT, P.O. BOX 211
AMSTERDAM, THE NETHERLANDS

SOLE DISTRIBUTOR FOR THE U.S.A. AND CANADA:
ELSEVIER/NORTH-HOLLAND INC.
52 VANDERBILT AVENUE
NEW YORK, N.Y. 10017, U.S.A.

Library of Congress Cataloging in Publication Data

International Summer School of Brain Research,
    9th, Amsterdam, 1975.
    Perspectives in brain research.

    (Program in brain research ; v. 45)
    Includes index.
    1. Brain--Congresses. I. Corner, M. A.
II. Swaab, D. F. III. Amsterdam. Nederlands
Centraal Instituut voor Hersenonderzoek. IV. Title.
V. Series: [DNLM: 1. Brain--Congresses.
2. Research--Congresses. Wl PR667J v. 45 / WL20
I614 1975p]
QP376.P7 vol. 45   599'.01'88 ' 76-49820
ISBN 0-444-41457-6

WITH 176 ILLUSTRATIONS AND 22 TABLES

List of Contributors

J. ARIËNS KAPPERS, Netherlands Central Institute for Brain Research, Amsterdam, The Netherlands.

G.P. BAERENDS, Zoological Laboratory, University of Groningen, Groningen, The Netherlands.

R. BALÁZS, Medical Research Council, Developmental Neurobiology Unit, Carshalton, Surrey, Great Britain.

P. BARTS, Institute of Medical Physics TNO, Utrecht, The Netherlands.

B. BOHUS, Rudolf Magnus Institute for Pharmacology, University of Utrecht, Utrecht, The Netherlands.

V. BRAITENBERG, Max-Planck-Institute for Biological Cybernetics, Tübingen, G.F.R.

W. BURR, Institute of Medical Physics TNO, Utrecht, The Netherlands.

M.A. CORNER, Netherlands Central Institute for Brain Research, Amsterdam, The Netherlands.

O. CREUTZFELDT, Max-Planck-Institute for Biophysical Chemistry, Dept. of Neurobiology, Göttingen, G.F.R.

G.S. DAWES, The Nuffield Institute for Medical Research, University of Oxford, Oxford, Great Britain.

R.M. GAZE, National Institute for Medical Research, London, Great Britain.

W.H. GISPEN, Rudolf Magnus Institute for Pharmacology, University of Utrecht, Utrecht, The Netherlands.

E.G. GRAY, University College London, Dept. of Anatomy, London, Great Britain.

E. van HEUSDEN, Institute of Medical Physics TNO, Utrecht, The Netherlands.

R.A. HOPE, National Institute for Medical Research, London, Great Britain.

H. HYDÉN, University of Göteborg, Institute of Neurobiology, Göteborg, Sweden.

R. LEVI-MONTALCINI, Lab. of Cell Biology, Rome, Italy and Dept. of Biology, Washington University, St. Louis, Mo., U.S.A.

F.H. LOPES DA SILVA, Institute of Medical Physics TNO, Utrecht, The Netherlands.

J. OLDS, California Institute of Technology, Division of Biology, Pasadena, Calif., U.S.A.

B.T. PICKERING, University of Bristol, Dept. of Anatomy, Bristol, Great Britain.

J.S. ROBINSON, The Nuffield Institute for Medical Research, University of Oxford, Oxford, Great Britain.

S.P.R. ROSE, The Open University, Brain Research Group, Milton Keynes, Bucks., Great Britain.

A. van ROTTERDAM, Institute of Medical Physics TNO, Utrecht, The Netherlands.

B. SCHARRER, Albert Einstein College of Medicine, Dept. of Anatomy, Bronx, N.Y., U.S.A.

J. SCHERRER, University of Paris, Medical Faculty, Pitié Salpêtrière, Lab. of Physiology, Paris, France.

R.W. SPERRY, California Institute of Technology, Division of Biology, Pasadena, Calif., U.S.A.

W. STORM VAN LEEUWEN, University Hospital Utrecht, Dept. of Clinical Neurophysiology, Utrecht, The Netherlands.

L. SVENNERHOLM, University of Göteborg, Dept. of Neurochemistry, Psychiatric Research Centre, Göteborg, Sweden.

I. URBAN, Rudolf Magnus Institute for Pharmacology, University of Utrecht, Utrecht, The Netherlands.

H. VAN DER LOOS, University of Lausanne, Medical Faculty, Institute of Normal Anatomy, Lausanne, Switzerland.

P.D. WALL, University College London, Cerebral Functions Research Group, Dept. of Anatomy, London, Great Britain.

P.A. WEISS, Rockefeller University, New York, N.Y., U.S.A.

vi

V.P. WHITTAKER, Max-Planck-Institute for Biophysical Chemistry, Dept. of Neuro-chemistry, Göttingen, G.F.R.

D. de WIED, Rudolf Magnus Institute for Pharmacology, University of Utrecht, Utrecht, The Netherlands.

TJ.B. van WIMERSMA GREIDANUS, Rudolf Magnus Institute for Pharmacology, University of Utrecht, Utrecht, The Netherlands.

J.Z. YOUNG, University College London, Dept. of Anatomy, London, Great Britain.

Introduction

"Perspectives in Brain Research" was the theme of the 9th in a series of International Summer Schools organized by the Netherlands Central Institute for Brain Research in Amsterdam. The series was started in the early 1960s on the initiative of Dr. J.P. Schadé, shortly after the assumption of the directorate of the Institute by Dr. J. Ariëns Kappers, until then Professor of Anatomy at the University of Groningen. The fact that Prof. Ariëns Kappers was a close relative of C.U. Ariëns Kappers, the founder and first director of the same institute, lent a unique flavor to the occasion of his retirement in the Summer of 1975. It seemed to us, therefore, that there existed a certain appropriateness for choosing a more general theme than had been the case in previous Summer Schools: one that would complete a cycle, as it were, by pausing to consider where the outstanding unsolved questions in experimental neurobiology now lie, almost 70 years after Prof. Ariëns Kappers' initiative in stimulating basic research in this field.

Such an assessment was all the more appropriate at this time, since the Brain Research Institute was itself deeply engaged in re-evaluating its own research activities in terms of a collaborative multidisciplinary approach. An explosive growth in the previous decade had left the Institute in possession of material, as well as theoretical, facilities necessary for handling the challenges posed by the study of the nervous system. What was still needed was a well-founded consideration of the direction(s) in which a concerted effort could best be made. Little did any of us anticipate then that a special poignancy was soon to be added to the occasion of the second Prof. Ariëns Kappers' retirement: a ministerial decision to terminate the very existence of the institution which the first Prof. Ariëns Kappers had created so many years before. The cycle was indeed to be completed, but with a vengeance! This danger since seems to have been averted by a hairsbreadth, for which we warmly thank our scientific colleagues throughout the world — whose overwhelming response against this decision last year proved to have played a decisive part in persuading the Dutch parliament to reconsider the liquidation order.

As regards the present volume, we started out by trying to have represented as many as possible of the areas deemed to be of major importance for neuroscience research in the coming years. In addition to the gaps which are undoubtedly present in this conception owing to our own limitations of imagination, there are also some unavoidable lacunae resulting from our failure to have approached in time all the potential contributions for each of the desired topics. The coverage was of course in practise still further thinned by the human impossibility of adequately covering any of the assigned themes within the limited time and space available. Nevertheless, we hope that the missing intellectual fare will only have caused the mesh of the proferred "net" of ideas to become somewhat less fine, without rupturing its overall structural integrity.

The material is presented under five main headings, each of which is subdivided into four chapters. Twenty distinguished investigators present their ideas about the direction their fields are (or ought to be) moving; in many cases the authors' own most recent findings themselves vividly illustrate the power of the research proposals being made. Starting from those molecular processes in nervous tissue which are most closely related to the chemistry of living cells in general, we progress to a detailed consideration of a more specialized biochemical mechanism: neuronal production of hormones and responses to them, in turn. The subject of nervous systems as information-processing networks is then arbitrarily subdivided into a part dealing with morphological, and another concerning physiological organization, before winding up the main body of the book with a section treating the biological raison d'être of all these masterpieces of natural design: their own perpetuation (and ultimately evolution) through the generation of motor activities adapted to the exigencies of environmental challenges.

In the introductory section of the book Prof. Weiss presents an extensive survey of the many basic challenges still remaining to neuroscience research, putting the spotlight on a number of persistent problems, some of which in fact touch the mysteries of life processes in general. Prof. Young then offers us an assessment of some methodological problems inherent in the strategy of looking to "simpler" living forms for suitable models of more general biological phenomena. At the end of the volume the reader is treated to two attempts to look beyond elemental brain processes and structural entities, into a qualitatively distinct domain: the integrated functioning of this most complicated of all organ systems. We are most fortunate here in having two experimental neurologists of the stature of Profs. Creutzfeldt and Sperry to take on the perhaps thankless task of trying to conceptualize the immense difficulties even in usefully formulating such questions for scientific purposes.

Before concluding, it is worthwhile mentioning that one cannot but be struck by the frequency with which classic problems from *developmental* neurobiology — e.g., "plasticity" in its many guises, "tropisms" and trophic interactions among nerve cells — keep popping up, far exceeding the emphasis which we had allocated to ontogeny when planning the symposium. This fact only underscores our own conviction at the Amsterdam Institute that brain maturation and adaptation, and the host of factors which regulate their course and expression throughout the life cycle, constitute perhaps the most imminently fruitful source of current research possibilities. Both C.U. Ariëns Kappers and his co-worker (and eventual successor) S.T. Bok, were already convinced on this point in their own time, so that the developmental approach to the nervous system is in fact a research tradition of long standing at the "Brain Institute".

Acknowledgements

We are pleased to acknowledge the generous financial support given to the Summer School by all of the following:

Ahrin B.V.
B.V. Metaalindustrie v/h Beyer & Eggelaar
Brunschwig Chemie B.V.
Ciba-Geigy B.V.
Eiga B.V., Medische Instrumenten-handel
Elmekanic B.V.
European Training Programme in Brain and Behaviour Research
Gist-Brocades N.V.
Hoffmann-La Roche B.V.
Hope Farms B.V.
C.H. van den Houten Fund
IBM Nederland N.V.

'A. de Jong T.H.' B.V.
Laméris Instrumenten B.V.
L.K.B.-Produkten B.V.
Ministry of Education and Science
Van Oortmerssen B.V. Wetenschappelijke Instrumenten
Simac Electronics B.V.
Organon Nederland B.V.
Philips-Duphar B.V.
Dr. Saal van Zwanenberg Foundation
Schering Nederland B.V.
Shell Nederland B.V.
P.M. Tamson B.V.
World Federation of Neurology

The editors would also like to acknowledge the following publishers, and all the authors involved, for their cooperation in allowing the reproduction of figures originally appearing in their own publications.

Academic Press, for two figures in the article of Lopes da Silva et al. (from *Progr. theoret. Biol.*, 2, 1972); for Fig. 8 of Olds (from *Pleasure, Reward, Preference*, 1973, Ch. 2) and Fig. 5 of Baerends (from *Fish Physiology, Vol. 6*, 1971); Acta Paediatrica Scandinavica, for Fig. 4 (from *Acta paediat. (Uppsala),* 63, 1974) and Fig. 6 of Svennerholm (from *Acta paediat. (Uppsala),* 64, 1975); American Association for the Advancement of Science, for Fig. 8 of Van der Loos (from *Science*, 179 (1973) 395–398) and Fig. 31 of Weiss (from *Science*, 167 (1970) 979–980); American Physiological Society, for Fig. 9 of Olds (from *J. Neurophysiol.*, 36, 1973); Arch. ital. Biol., for Fig. 5 of Levi-Montalcini (from *Arch. ital. Biol.*, 113, 1975); E.J. Brill (Publishers), for Figs. 3, 6 and 7 of Baerends (from *Behaviour*, Suppl. 17, 1970); Cambridge University Press, for Fig. 1 of Dawes and Robinson (from *Foetal and Neonatal Physiology*, 1973); Cold Spring Harbor Symposia on Quantitative Biology, for various portions of text and figures in Whittaker (from *Cold Spr. Harb. Symp. quant. Biol.*, Vol. 40, 1975); Federation of American Societies for Experimental Biology, for Table VI of Svennerholm (from *Fed. Proc.*, 32, 1973); Macmillan Journals Ltd., for Table III of Svennerholm (from *Nature (Lond.)*, 257, 1975); National Academy of Sciences, for Fig. 9 (from *Proc. nat. Acad. Sci. (Wash.)*, 67, 1970) and Fig. 5 of Hydén (from *Proc. nat. Acad. Sci. (Wash.)*, 71, 1974); *Neurobiology* for Figs. 2, 3 and 4 (from *Neurobiology*, 4, 1974) and Fig. 8 of Hydén (from *Neurobiology*, 5, 1975); Neuroscience Research Program, for

Fig. 1 of Gray (from *Neurosci. Res. Prog. Bull.*, 6, 1968); New York Academy of Sciences, for Fig. 6 of Pickering (from *Ann. N.Y. Acad. Sci.*, 248, 1975); Raven Press, for Figs. 2, 3, 4 and 7 of Olds (from *Biological Foundations of Psychiatry*, 1976). Rockefeller University Press, for Fig. 2 of Gray (from *J. Cell Biol.*, 46, 1970); J. Saunders Co., for Fig. 2 of Svennerholm (from *Med. Clin. N. Amer.*, 53, 1969); Springer-Verlag, for Fig. 8 of Whittaker (from *J. neural. Trans.*, Suppl. XII, 39, 1974) and Fig. 5 of Pickering (from *Cell Tiss. Res.*, 156, 1975); and University of Chicago Press, for Fig. 3 of Weiss (from *Genetic Neurobiology*, 1950).

Contents

SESSION I

PROLOGUE

A Glance at Some Problems Facing Brain Research Today

J. ARIËNS KAPPERS

Netherlands Central Institute for Brain Research,
Amsterdam (The Netherlands)

The present volume contains the proceedings of the Ninth Summer School of Brain Research of our Institute, held from July 28–August 1, 1975 at the Royal Netherlands Academy of Arts and Sciences, Amsterdam, and organized by Drs. Corner and Swaab. I am deeply grateful to them for devoting so much of their time and energy in performing this complicated task, but which, in addition, could never have been accomplished so well without the invaluable help of Miss Sels.

The general topic chosen was: "Perspectives in Brain Research", which means that recently acquired knowledge in certain aspects of neurobiology will be presented, with the emphasis being upon future research possibilities. That only some of the many interesting neurobiological subjects will be dealt with during this meeting is of course unavoidable for practical reasons.

The choice of the general topic has perhaps not been entirely gratuitous: perspectives, being vistas and possibilities of future development, are for a large part projections from what has been going on in the past. For me, personally then, officially participating for the last time in an International Summer School, the continuation of past activities into times still to come becomes an especially appropriate theme. For the institute too, this is a natural moment for reflection upon its future course, and I suppose that all this has been at the back of the mind of the organizers.

During the 45 years comprising my active research life, and especially after World War II, the neurosciences have made an astonishing and most dramatic progress. I vividly remember the words of the grand old man of Dutch neurohistology, Professor Boeke from Utrecht, in summarizing the proceedings of the first meeting of neurobiologists (1955). He gave expression to his amazement and admiration that so much new and integrated knowledge had been gathered in such a relatively short time, and that so much had been contributed to the solution of problems on which he had worked during a life-time. He ended by stating that he hoped that not all problems would find their final solution in the end and that it would remain possible to wonder and accept wonders. I do not think that the people present at this meeting live in the expectation that very soon we will know all that there is to know about the brain. On the contrary, modern workers are more conscious than ever of the intricacy of the problems involved in the study of living matter, and especially of nervous tissue. They are very much aware that the solution of one problem inevitably opens up many more questions which deserve to be solved. Moreover, I am not of the opinion that even exhaustive knowledge of the facts, and of their structural and functional interrelationships, would ever necessarily preclude our wonderment that these facts and relationships indeed exist — even if one were to accept the somewhat naïve hypothesis that the cosmos, including man, has evolved entirely due to chance processes.

I would like to dwell shortly here on some problems which are a natural consequence of the rapid progress made in the neurosciences. The wide field of neurobiology has now been more or less split up in many super-specializations. This differentiation is inevitable and necessary, but also offers its own problems. Ever larger numbers of neuroscientists produce an ever faster growing number of papers, published in ever increasing numbers of journals. Therefore, it has become very difficult for young research workers, not to mention old ones, to get even an idea of what is going on in every region of this broad field. For those scientists who desire to integrate the knowledge obtained by workers in a variety of related fields into their own thinking, and whose mind is more inclined to synthesis than to particularization, the struggle is often fierce. Time to read and think is scarce, the more so when the research worker has also to be a teacher, an organizer or an administrator. As a result, scientists are now in the habit of scarcely reading papers published earlier than at most 15 years ago, even when these are highly relevant to their current investigation. The consequence is that facts, known for a long time, sometimes are not used in new work because they are entirely unknown to the young research worker. Several times it has struck me that scientific discoveries made long ago were "discovered" again and presented as new findings!

Another very recent problem related to the rapid advancement of the neurosciences on the one hand, and the development of general affairs in this world on the other, is that young scientists in the developing countries rightly want to be introduced to the latest knowledge and technical methods in the field of neurobiology. Here gaps have to be filled quickly and thoroughly, often without optimal knowledge of basic facts. Much earlier knowledge and interpretation of facts have become obsolete, however, while not all facts are of fundamental importance — especially when practical application of neuroscience is what is wanted most. Some of these problems can therefore be solved by good courses in neurobiology in which basic facts are blended with recent discoveries. Organizations like the International Brain Research Organization and the World Health Organization, to mention only two, are very much aware of this important task and do whatever is possible in view of restrictions on manpower and money.

Looking back at the many years I was involved in the study of the nervous system I feel that I cannot be grateful enough for living during a period in which I was able to do research more or less freely. Times are rapidly changing, however, and there is an increasing tendency to curtail the further development of basic scientific research. There is a certain distrust of the community of pure scientists insofar as their activities do not lead immediately to some kind of tangible, practical result. More often than in earlier times, science as such is considered to be a financial and social luxury, rather than a cultural activity of the utmost importance. This is in some way related to the fact that society has become very much secularized and materialistic to the virtual exclusion of all other values. Such an attitude also has its potential merits in view of the material living conditions of so many people who are still in want of the most basic necessities, without which cultural activities are quite impossible. However, the distaste and misunderstanding of values other than the most crass materialistic ones, shown by vast numbers of people living in relatively prosperous conditions, is not only alarming but in the end also devastating for society itself. In the not too distant future, the position of the pure scientist may become socially as difficult as that of the artist, who may sometimes be financially supported by the government but is basically regarded to be somewhat queer in the head, because he is not primarily concerned with the improvement of his own material circumstances or with that of others. Creativity and detachment from material conditions are unfortunately not very popular in modern society. There seems also to be a fear of independent men having ideas which do not readily jibe with current temporary mass opinions and prejudices — with the spectre of the return to an age of authoritarian dogmatism.

In recent times the government has been taking over more and more the financial support and control of scientific research which, among other things, means that both politicians and an ever growing bureaucracy become involved. Given the fact that, in addition, most governments now have less money available than in recent years, it is inevitable that pure scientific research is being looked at in a more critical way and that the cry is for practical applications and results — and on short notice! Promises of better living conditions of the sort readily understood by the majority of people is the only way in which the public will "buy" the large expenditures required for the support of the sciences. Much wisdom and self restraint will indeed be needed on the part of the government and its advisory institutions to guarantee that some degree of freedom to perform purely scientific work will be maintained. I am not too optimistic in this respect*, but I am also aware that part of the trouble to be expected is due to the attitude of some scientists shown in the past: their lack of organization, self sufficiency, pettiness, egotism, competition instead of cooperation, craving for power, and, sometimes, their lack of interest in social conditions different from their own and lack of real contact with workers in other regions of society. It is also true that money can be wasted in scientific research by bad planning or by tackling problems which are no longer problems at all, or by starting research which has already shown good development in other laboratories.

---

* This astonishingly prophetic remark was made exactly one month before the government's announcement to economize by closing down the Netherlands Central Institute for Brain Research, the very institute from which Professor Kappers was retiring as director! An appeal to the international scientific community (see Neurosci. Lett., 1 (1975) 191) brought in hundreds of protest letters to the Dutch Ministry of Sciences and Education, which contributed greatly to the subsequent unanimous decision of the Parliament to reconsider the whole closure issue.

The Editors

Neurobiology in Statu Nascendi

PAUL A. WEISS

Rockefeller University, New York, N.Y. (U.S.A.)

INTRODUCTION

My 55 years in neurobiological research have passed through an age of scientific evolution comparable, perhaps, to the span between the age of the Meistersinger craftsmen and today's mass production industries. In retrospect, the advances in what we have learned seem phenomenal. But I am more impressed by how much more we have come to realize of what we do not know; namely, how wide the gap still is between our detailed acquaintance with the *elements* of structure and activity of the neural fabric and our true understanding of the integral function of the nervous system. Too many keystones are in fact still missing. As most of my own exploratory treks have ended at just such gaps, I shall inaugurate this exercise on "Perspectives in Brain Research" with a sampling of how far away my enquiries — all products of hunches, logic, or sheer accident — have still remained from giving me even an inkling of how the organism works in such a harmonious (and surely not machine-like) coordinated whole.

In 1918, when I started my neurobiological studies, embryology itself was still in its embryonic stage. For instance, despite Ross Harrison's proof in vitro (1907, 1910) that each nerve fiber was a discrete sprout from a single cell, contentions that the neuronal network was a continuous web — a syncytium — lingered on. Moreover, aside from static descriptions, information about how the cell strip on top of the embryo, called the "neural tube", managed to form the orderly sequence of all the parts of the brain — eye, spinal cord, ganglia, etc. — was wholly rudimentary. Cover terms kept obscuring ignorance and created the fiction that the formative processes were plain and simple. Yet, as my first picture (Fig. 1) shows, quite the opposite is true: they are manifold and intricately interwoven in steps of increasing complexity from the embryo up to the mature nervous system. The manner of the operations of the various arrows are mostly still undefined, except for one fact: they are definitely not microprecisely pretimed for the exact moment of mutual interactions. And, despite that degree of chronological latitude, they still end up as a reasonably typical total product: a human brain with a minimum of 10^{11} nerve cells (Weiss, 1973) with only such a miniscule discrepancy in behavior as that between a genius and an imbecile.

8

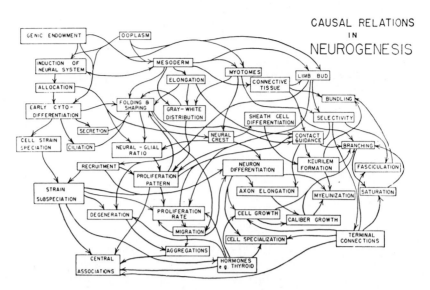

Fig. 1. Major interdependencies of developmental events in neurogenesis from germ (top) to functional brain (bottom).

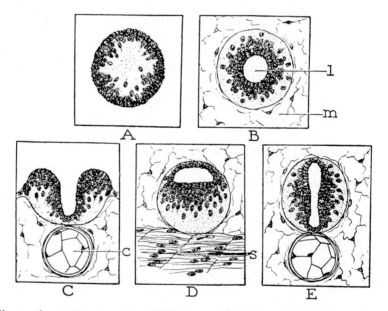

Fig. 2. Shape of neural tube under different conditions (from Holtfreter, 1934). A: solid neural mass developed in explantation: nuclei of gray matter crowded near the surface; white matter in the interior. B: neural tube surrounded by mesenchyme: shape cylindrical with central lumen; nuclei massed at the inner (free) surface. C: asyntaxia dorsalis (failure of the tube to close); thinning of the floor of the tube in contact with the notochord; gray matter along the free surface. D: neural tube underlain by musculature; lumen eccentric at far side; white matter at near side. E: neural tube underlain by notochord; normal appearance: slit-shaped lumen, oriented towards notochord. Abbreviations: 1, lumen; m, mesenchyme; c, notochord; s, segmented musculature.

Although the stepwise diversification which the embryonic nerve tube thus undergoes is again sheltered under the single term "differentiation", its facets are far more numerous and diverse: they include changes of chemical constitution, reactivity, structure, shape, affinity, motility, and so forth — of cells as well as of cell groups — and all of them are in interactive interdependence, mutually and with their surroundings.

One simple set of experiments by Holtfreter (1934) might serve as an example (Fig. 2). It shows the different configurations assumed by a cluster of embryonic nerve cells in vitro when they are wholly surrounded by either liquid (top left) or mesenchyme (top right), or in unequal surroundings (lower row from left to right), with liquid above and notochord below (Fig. 2C), or mesenchyme above and musculature below (Fig. 2D), or mesenchyme above and notochord below (Fig. 2E). And the orderly interplay between not only these five, but many more complements, is relevant to the morphogenetic orderliness of the rudimental architecture of the spinal cord. Going on further from here would only lead us into a pathless jungle of ignorance.

PROGRAMMING OF DEVELOPING NERVE CELLS

Thus far I have only touched upon crudely visible criteria. Much less is known about how the billions of neurons acquire those intrinsic characteristics that define their later functional idioms. Some seem to be preprogrammed at an early stage, others seem to gain specifications secondarily from their surroundings or contacts, and still others remain consistently pluripotent.

Briefly, two examples from the meager list available: Fig. 3 (from Hamburger and Levi-Montalcini, 1950) shows three successive stages of the spinal cord of 4-, 5- and 8-day-old chick embryos. On the left (A), the neuroblasts in the longitudinal columns are uniformly distributed; later (B) some cell mass in the thoracic region (th) is seen to migrate toward the cord axis to form the nucleus of Terni, and gradually the cervical cell columns (C) show some degeneration. Yet, whether this parcellation is autonomous or cued by some correspondingly segmented features of the body, is quite unknown.

Far more conclusive evidence that early preprogramming of neurons is a fact is manifested by Mauthner cells of amphibian larvae, a pair of single neurons in the medulla, distinctive by their giant sizes and destined for some sensory function in aquatic life. According to Stefanelli (1950), a small fragment of future medulla of an egg in neurulation, explanted into a neutral medium, will still give rise to a singular giant Mauthner cell amidst a mass of conventionally small-sized neurons. But aside from its gigantism, this peculiar cell also seems pre-endowed with the potential for its specific future reactivity. The evidence is the following. According to Weiss and Rossetti (1951), the larva of *Xenopus* grows conspicuously for about a month, and so do its two Mauthner cells. Thyroid secretion then supervenes and transforms the larva into the metamorphosed frog, which continues to grow. But while the other brain cells likewise keep enlarging, the two Mauthner cells shrink down to indistinctiveness. No external intervention such as amputating the tail, transecting the long Mauthner fibers, etc., has any effect. Yet, when we implanted a thyroid source

10

precociously (see Kollros, 1943) into the 4th ventricle, the Mauthner cells promptly lost size amidst all the other fast-growing neurons. Since control implants of parotid gland pieces had no effect, we must conclude that the selective reactivity to thyroid must have been latent in that cell long before its call came. The facts are there. But the when, where and how a neuron receives such anticipatory specifications still eludes our comprehension.

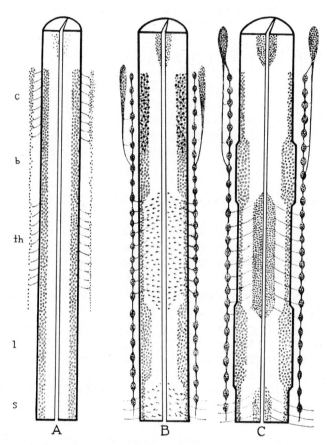

Fig. 3. Diagrammatic frontal sections of the spinal cord of chick embryos of age 4 days (A), 5 days (B) and 8 days (C), showing the regionally differing formation of the motor columns from a morphologically rather uniform condition. In B, degeneration of cells in the cervical region (c, black circles), and centripetal emigration of cells in the thoracic (th) and sacral (s) regions have set in, resulting in the distribution shown in C. (From Hamburger and Levi-Montalcini, 1950.)

A little bit more has become known about the way the individual nerve cells interlace into networks that intercommunicate with each other and with the non-nervous tissues with which they are to correspond. In many minds, the simile of a telephone system and its laying down still prevails. All my space allows me to do here is to pinpoint some complications of that old-fashioned simplicity, amplified by Gasser (1937) into the dogma (p. 171) that "admittedly the nervous system can be understood only as it is operating as a whole, but it is equally true that an insight into its working can be gained only by a detailed analysis of its parts". This was in turn based upon the verdict: "the phenomena taking place in the CNS could be explained without the assumption of any properties which could not be experimentally identified in peripheral nerve".

My question to the future is: how can anyone be so apodictic before we have exhausted our knowledge about those elementary fiber connections and what they can do and, even more so, what they cannot do?

Let me turn for a moment to this last problem. I have already referred to Harrison's proof (1907, 1910) that nerve fibers (axons, dendrites) are simply filamentous extensions of the cytoplasm of the neuronal cell body. From his studies on fibroblast cells, Harrison also inferred that the tips of these extensions are mechanically guided along fibrous structures in their surroundings. Invited to his Yale laboratory, I not only confirmed, but expanded this concept (Weiss, 1934), leading to the principle of "contact guidance" (Weiss,

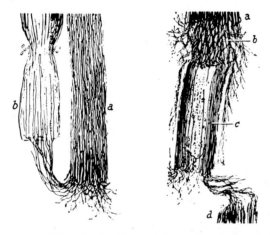

Fig. 4. Regenerating nerve fibers having, in part, formed "bridges" between proximal stumps (a; c) and dislocated distal stumps (recurrent, b; laterally displaced, d). (From Cajal, 1928.)

1941d). But this was not at all compatible with Ramón y Cajal's (1928) presumption of *chemotactic attraction* between neural tissues across considerable distances. When Cajal faced the proximal end of a nerve stump, capable of regeneration, with the end of a slightly displaced stump of a degenerating nerve (Fig. 4), he noted a preferential (though not absolute) diversion of the outgrowing regenerates towards the degenerating entrance; he ascribed this to a chemotactic attraction of the growing fiber tips by emissions from the blind end.

That observation was right but its interpretation wrong. The main error came from the common habit to consider all white spaces on an illustration as a physical vacuum in contrast to the structural entities made conspicuous by proper stains or other means. Let me refer to my counter-evidence (Weiss, 1952, 1955). Cajal's experiment is easy to reproduce in tissue culture, even between two degenerating nerve stumps containing no regenerating nerve fibers (Fig. 5). You note the straight bridge of outgrowing fibroblasts and Schwann cells that has formed between the two ends. If nerve sprouts had been present

12

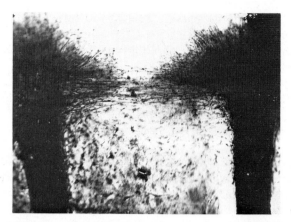

Fig. 5. "Bridge" of Schwann cells grown out in 4.5 days in vitro between the ends of two adult rat nerve trunks explanted after 17 days of Wallerian degeneration.

to grow out, they would of course by "contact guidance" have used that fibrous connection. The explanation was that cell proliferation at a wound causes a dehydration of the local connective tissue. The resulting local shrinkage of the matrix at the two contracting spots yields a connecting stress pattern over which the cells then move. If they were attracted by massive chemical emissions from the two exits, they would obviously have stayed at home, where the concentration gradients have their peaks.

To clinch the disclaimer for chemotactic guidance of neural sprouts toward distant goals, I add just two experiments out of many: (1) in Fig. 6 a bundle of outgrowing nerve fibers (from a spinal ganglion) in tissue culture pass the open end of a degenerating nerve stump without any inclination to enter it; (2) in Fig. 7, the proximal nerve stump (P) of an adult rat has been inserted into the stem of a bifurcated piece of artery (a), one of whose branches (t) had been

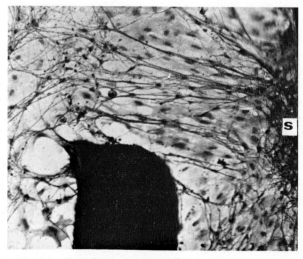

Fig. 6. Neurons growing out from spinal ganglion (s) in plasma clot in vitro, passing around the open end of degenerating nerve stump (lower left).

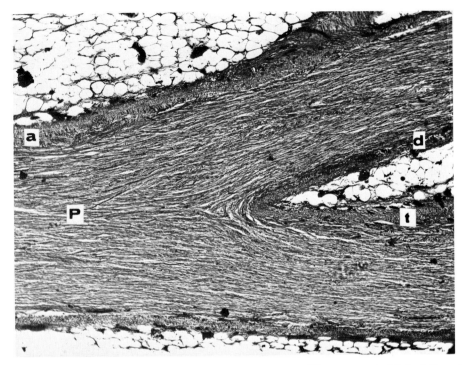

Fig. 7. Adult nerve fiber bundle from proximal stump (P), regenerated into bifurcated channel, one branch (t) ending blind, the other (d) leading to the open end of a degenerating nerve.

tied off distally while the other (d) leads into a distal nerve stump. Yet both branches have been equally invaded and repleted with regenerating fibers without any bias.

Having discounted simple chemotaxis (Weiss and Taylor, 1944), let me then return to "contact guidance". Most cell types cannot swim and need a substrate along which to advance — an interface or some other structure, either fibrous, as in Fig. 8, or grooved, as in Fig. 9, which shows connective tissue cells on smooth glass rodlets in A and on a scored glass plate in B. To proceed one step further, this principle of road structure building is being utilized in the workshops of the cells themselves. As I have pointed out before, in rectifying Cajal's experiment, *proliferating* cell groups (like open nerve ends) which are enmeshed in a fiber net contract the surrounding fabric concentrically as in Fig. 10. Where there are *two* such centers at a distance, the two-sided tensions acting upon the fibers in-between stretch the latter along the connecting line, thus forming a direct straight pathway for the outgrowing nerve fibers and cells to follow blindly from one point to the other. Fig. 11 shows such a cell bridge connection formed without any external intervention between *three* spinal ganglia, spaced apart in a thin blood plasma clot.

Up to that point, I had tended to consider the guidance of cells and nerve fibers as being essentially a simple mechanical process, involving adhesive and axially deforming forces, but *indiscriminately*. Once again, this conclusion

14

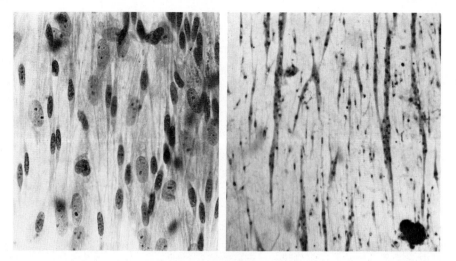

Fig. 8. Connective tissue cells assuming longitudinal orientation along submicroscopic fibrin fibrils in stretched plasma clot.

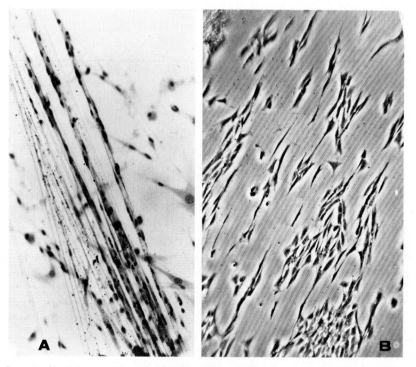

Fig. 9. Longitudinal orientation of cells along glass fibers (A) and rills of scored glass plate (B).

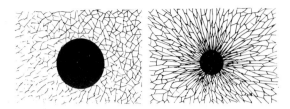

Fig. 10. Left: tissue fragment (black area) freshly explanted in fibrous clot of blood plasma. Right: after 3 days, dehydratizing exudates from the rapidly proliferating cells have markedly reduced the water content of the surrounding fibrous network yielding a much greater local diminution of the surrounding region than is compensated by the reproducing cell mass, thus resulting in the concentric shrinkage of the whole site.

proved to be far too simple. We soon found that in their primary outgrowth into the periphery, even pioneer fibers seemed to choose different routes, depending on whether they came from motor or sensory roots (Taylor, 1944). Furthermore, fibers growing out subsequently clearly tended to apply themselves to the surfaces of their corresponding type of predecessor (Fig. 12), a phenomenon I called "selective fasciculation" (Weiss, 1941d, 1955). Now, since there is a further selectivity between sensory and motor fiber classes in that either type (regardless of the course over which it arrived at its destination) is accepted for synaptic junctions only by a matching type of end organ (Weiss and Edds, 1945), an added provision is superimposed over the initial and less determinate contact guidance. Only in muscle does any cell seem to accept any motor fiber (Weiss and Hoag, 1946); sensory fibers will be discussed later.

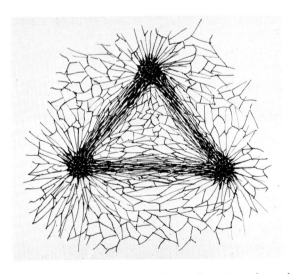

Fig. 11. Diagrammatic reproduction of triangular cell pattern formed between 3 spinal ganglia in thin plasma clot.

16

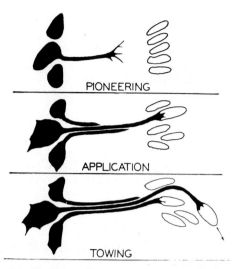

Fig. 12. Three phases in development of nerves (diagrammatic). Top: pioneering phase (free fiber tip advances into surroundings). Middle: application phase (pioneering tip has become attached to peripheral cell, younger tips apply themselves to course of older ones). Bottom: towing phase (shift of peripheral cell produces corresponding displacement of attached nerve fiber).

DEVELOPMENT OF FUNCTIONAL ORGANIZATION

The foregoing general principles were only dimly known when I discovered in 1922 that in the *functional* activation of the musculature actually every *individual* muscle is called into action as a discrete individual entity, just as if called by its name. There are about 40 of these in an amphibian limb, each with its personal specificity, so that this obviously also calls for a corresponding diversity in the centers. Logically, one would want to explain this — and many have done so — by conceding specific preprogramming, not only to classes of neurons but also to each individual nerve cell, endowing every one with the capacity of somehow finding its predestined effector or receptor ending. I kept on testing this assumption experimentally (see Weiss, 1936) and all tests turned out to be disavowals of this conjecture. This proved positively that the coordinated response of peripheral effectors is definitely *not* the result of some point-for-point selective laying of telephone wire connections from sender to receiver. This negative statement seems indisputable, but a positive explanation does not yet lie within the limited repertory of present-day neurobiological theory or knowledge (see Weiss, 1975a).

Let me just briefly restate the crucial facets of the phenomenon, as a challenge for the future. The diagram of Fig. 13 represents conventional ideas about a coordinated movement of a forelimb during ambulation. Comparing the CNS with the conductor of an orchestra let us choose only 4 out of the 40 instruments (that is, muscles) engaged in yielding the intended melody: an elbow flexor (F), a shoulder abductor (B), an elbow extensor (E), and a shoulder adductor (D). Such an orderly F–B–E–D sequence (Fig. 13, L) has variously

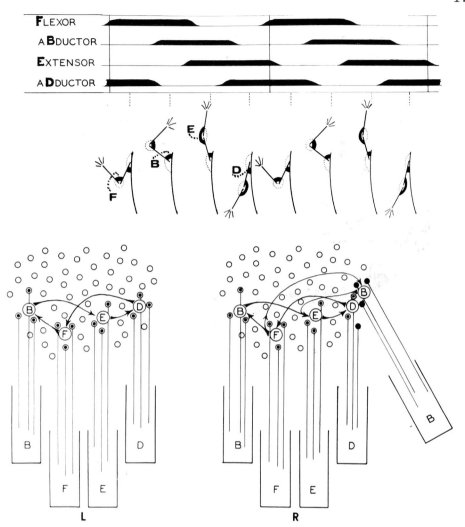

Fig. 13. Diagram of participation of 4 forelimb muscles in coordinated ambulation of amphibian larva. L, in normal limb; R, after adding a supernumerary transplant. Explanation in text.

been pictured either as empirical fixation by trial and error of successful sequences or by somehow predetermined chains of "reflex arcs" (see Weiss, 1941b, c, 1950b). Evidently, these simplistic visions could not survive my experimental demonstration (Fig. 13, R) that any duplicate instrument I had added to the orchestra, let us say another muscle B, would unfailingly respond exactly together with its normal namesake B in the animal's own leg despite having been arbitrarily positioned in a, biologically speaking, absurd and useless place. And this reference to a single test muscle applies to every other muscle in the set of 40 in a whole limb graft. In fact, the results were the same if more than one, indeed up to 3, supernumerary legs were grafted to the brachial region. Hypotheses neither of complete "relearning" nor complete "rewiring"

18

seemed to fit the facts. Why should a totally useless extra limb be brought to ape what its normal prototype nearby is carrying out sensibly?

One had to conclude that the CNS deals with the individual muscles through individually distinctive modalities — "myotypically" for short — with no regard to functional appropriateness; a sort of communication through strictly personal signals. But just *how*, remains another one of the great riddles — real, though highly discomforting to those craving for final answers today. Therefore, the haze that still beclouds references to "myotypic" response is not too surprising. Perhaps a few restatements of the safely established facts might help to clear some of the fog. I realize that many past mis-statements and misinterpretations in the literature can be traced to a lack of acquaintance with the detailed cinematographic and anatomical analysis of one of our key witnesses, the notable 6-legged frog (Verzár and Weiss, 1930; Weiss, 1931) and particularly my 4 lengthy reports of 1937a-d — pardonable omissions in an age of literary mass production.

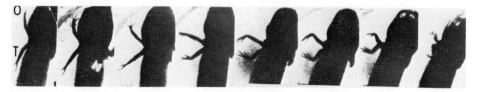

Fig. 14. Eight frames from a continuous film strip of forelimb ambulatory movements in myotypic symmetry between the original left limb (O) and the nearby, inversely symmetrical grafted right limb (T).

So, let us take a look at least at one crucial example: a right limb, T, grafted next to a left limb, O (Fig. 14), both sharing the left brachial plexus. The musculatures of two such limbs are of course exact mirror images of each other. Thus, on the myotypic principle, all movements of the two should be synchronous as well as visually and functionally mirroring each other in their inverse symmetry. And so they did precisely, at all times, for the rest of the animal's life (Weiss, 1937a).

Several potential "explanations" thus far proposed can be dispensed with because of their derivation, either from overly one-sided experimental methods or from disconcern with individual muscles, in favor of lumping them simply into "flexors" and "extensors" (much like lumping cats and horses together, in contrast to fishes and frogs, as representatives of land-living and water-living groups, respectively, without any further discrimination).

Bypassing such innocent self-deceptions, two kinds of "explanations" deserve serious attention: (1) that some afferent sensory information from a transplanted muscle provided the centers with a correct cue of the new arrival's name for appropriate central coupling with its corresponding namesake; or (2) that the centers of individual muscles sent out new regenerating nerve branches of appropriate single-muscle specificity to find and operate the corresponding endings in the grafted mass. Both of these conjectures could be conclusively dispelled in the following fashion. (1) The myotypical phenomenon occurs just the same in transplants with a completely deafferented nerve supply (Weiss,

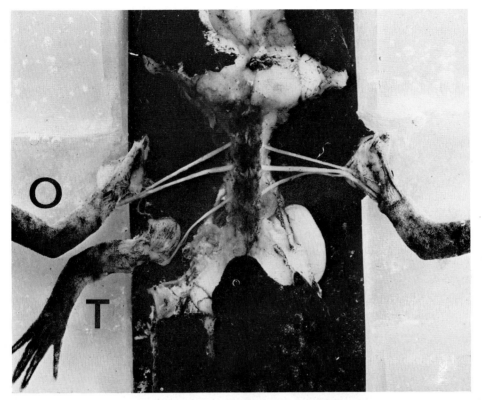

Fig. 15. Nerve supply of pair of inverse forelimbs, original left arm (O) and transplanted right arm (T), 3 months postoperative, with the standard, myotypically correct, i.e., mirror-image function. Of the 3 major nerves of the brachial plexus (III, IV, V), III and IV had been left with O, while V had been assigned to T at the time of operation. Note lack of any perceptible size difference between the left plexus supplying two legs and its opposite side with a single limb.

1937c); (2) the intimation of a fresh regenerative nerve supply being sent from the cord to innervate an extra limb is factually fully nullified (Weiss, 1937b, 1975a), as will be documented in the following figures. Fig. 15 shows an animal as in the preceding Fig. 14 with a right limb grafted 3 months previously to the left side and innervated by the left 5th brachial root.

As you will note, the nerve roots leaving the cord on the extra-legged side have not enlarged over those of the opposite control side. The numerical count (Fig. 16) not only confirms this, but also shows that the grafted leg contains, nonetheless, about as many nerve fibers as does its normal neighbor as a result of considerable fiber branching in the peripheral stretch. This has been typical for all the numerous cases canvassed in detail. Since, on an average there are no more than 4 motor fiber branches available for each muscle, the contention that each of these distal branches would be prefitted for its own preassigned muscle individual becomes untenable. In further support, I present the next picture (Fig. 17) of a graft deliberately given its whole nerve supply from a small branch of the forearm flexor bundle and yet reacting with its full

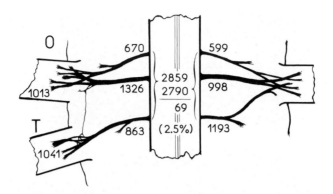

Fig. 16. Bilateral numerical count of myelinated fibers in serial cross-sections of the nerve plexuses illustrated in Fig. 15.

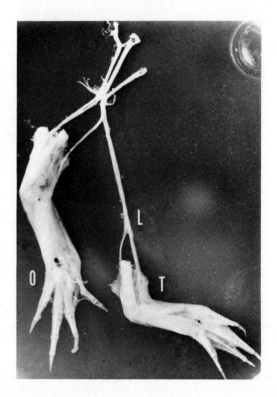

Fig. 17. Dissection of left shoulder plexus, 6 months after transplantation of supernumerary left forelimb (T) to left shoulder region and supplying graft with the mesial (flexor) branch of the nervus brachialis longus inferior, cut at the elbow level of O and transposed to base of T. (Prior to photography, the proximal parts of both upper arms were cut off to reveal the distal nerve distribution.) Note that the *mesial* flexor nerve inserted into T has bifurcated into a *superior* (extensor) and an *inferior* (flexor) branch.

complement of muscles "myotypically" with its normal neighbor, who had furnished that donor nerve.

In conclusion, the muscle-specific response occurs without the generation of new neurons for supernumerary muscles, and the innervation of the latter is non-selective. I insist on keeping the conclusion on that level of definiteness, with all further "explanations" having no claim to certainty. I myself had thus logically inferred that each muscle, according to its protein specificity would "modulate" the end of its reinnervating nerve branch, which would pass on that module up into the cord so that only messages of correspondingly conformant coding would be responded to. However, my *basic* attitude has remained one of skeptic uncertainty (see Weiss, 1975a), far more so than one finds expressed in less broadly informed discussions of the problem.

Just to add a brief annex regarding the *afferent* (sensory) sector: I could demonstrate that the same principle of central ⇋ peripheral correspondence prevailed there as in the selectivity of *"myotatic reflexes"*. In the presence of multiple synonymous muscles, the stretching of one given muscle would be answered by the contraction of all other muscles of the same name (Verzár and Weiss, 1930). Later, transplantations of eyes to the ear region proved that touch to the cornea of the graft would evoke the lid-closure reflex of the untouched normal eye on the same side (Weiss, 1942). Sensory identification by the centers thus matched experiences on the motor side of communication.

A great upsurge of that interest, started with the experimental eye reversals by my former student, Roger Sperry (1943, 1963), and expanded by Gaze (1970) and a great many others, led to the conclusion (originally rather pat but later softened) that transected and regenerating fibers of the optic nerve will "find" their original sites upon arrival at the tectal region, so that an essentially correct retina-to-tectum projection would be re-established. Here again was the story of a nerve fiber supposedly being able to "find its proper place". Unfortunately, since no secondary listening-in device was available as in our muscle experiments, some relevant questions must be left unanswered. But there is one very relevant problem that cannot be passed off. Even granting preordained guidance of each optic nerve fiber from its origin in the retinal ganglion cell to its predestined tectal respondent, thus projecting the *innermost* (ganglionic) layer of the retina upon the brain, just how does the *ganglionic* layer itself receive an equally matching, point-for-point, correctly stereotyped and topographically corresponding projection of the primary (and *outermost* positioned) layer of the *visual receptor* cells, which register the image of the outer world in the first place? The latter are not connected by direct radial point-to-point transmitters with the inner ganglion cells at all. On the contrary, they are separated from the latter by two networks of horizontal, amply branched interlayers (amacrines and bipolars), through which point excitations from the visual layer have been shown to be dispersed laterally over ranges of up to 1 sq. mm. How does the mosaic of ganglion cells then, in its turn, resurrect from the scatter of those interlayers the correctly patterned visual image to be passed on only *thereafter* to the brain? Should not this latter question be conceded precedence over any hurried answers about how that "thereafter" process is being managed? I am raising this puzzling question merely as a random sample of our state of scientific "statu nascendi", or, in translation, "embryonic immaturity".

As for the broader concept of selective terminal connections, one should remember that limbs grafted to *flank* segments in amphibians are readily innervated by intercostal nerves, and do move. Yet, they yield only uncoordinated twitching. They evidently received no coordinated limb messages from that level of the cord, just bioelectric "noise" instead of patterned musical scores. At any rate, primary selective connectivity finds little support in such experiences. So, let us not forget that it is biology that is in statu nascendi, not nature, and let us listen to what nature tries to tell our often prejudiced minds.

This leads me to our ancient habit of identifying reality with tangibility, visibility and audibility — all confined to the limited range of human capacities. Man then designed instruments trying to bring nature's phenomena within that range. If he failed, he coined new words to substitute for knowledge. But deep down in us that devilish habit still reigns. To the microscopist "only seeing is believing" or, worse, "not seeing is not believing", have long been the unspoken ground rules, not always realizing that "whether or not" can never test the real presence or absence of an object, but only reveal the resolving power of a tool. Electron microscopy is not altogether free from this attitude several orders of magnitude down from light microscopic resolution. Similarly, selective staining of nerve fibers (for instance, with silver), which marks them adequately and conspicuously, has soon led to viewing them as free agents in a sort of vacuum, especially when printed black on the white background of a textbook page. Only recently has their coat of sheath cells gained again in status, and even the physical continuity of a whole ganglion or brain system is no longer considered as functionally irrelevant.

If we are still too ignorant about the operation of a nervous *system*, as distinct from a sheer *sum* of neuronal units, the blame goes simply to our lack of attention to the former. Again, by sheer accident, I found a striking example (Weiss, 1940, 1941c, 1950a). I transplanted sections of the spinal cord or of brain parts of larval or fully mature urodele amphibians into the very loose tissue of their dorsal fin, and added a limb graft to signal any functional activity if functional neural connections between the two grafts were to occur, which they did. My operative method had opened a connecting tunnel between the two grafts, which in combination with later fasciculation served as a pathway for the nerve fibers growing out from the central fragment, and landing in the muscles of the grafted limb (Fig. 18). Note that the central fragment had been thoroughly disorganized, deliberately or accidentally, either by mincing or by extensive cell degeneration. Much of the neuron source that innervated the grafted limbs was thus in the "central gray", lacking motoneurons.

Here follows a brief sketch of the unexpected results. First, anatomically: the fasciculated nerve connection had always formed a single perfectly cylindrical cord, with a few glial cells and a rather dense "ground substance", set off by a membrane from the surrounding loose connective tissue bed. An occasional glial cell mitosis shows well the close packing of the nerve fibers in the bundle. The constitution of this central nerve is morphologically quite different from an ordinary peripheral nerve. Even more odd were its functional effects upon the grafted limb at the other end, which showed intermittent series of motor spasms often resembling epileptic seizures. Thus, we were faced here with a most elementary manifestation of a disorganized primitive piece of CNS on an attached set of muscles, hardly attributable at all to "reflex chains".

The marked dependence of the seizures on the metabolic and ionic environment (Desmedt, 1954) deserves the further pursuit of these experiments, but perhaps the most significant key to progress lies in the differences between motor responses to fragments of different brain parts (Corner, 1964): Medulla oblongata produced discharges at rather regular intervals of about

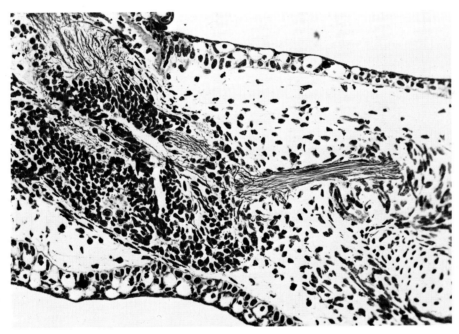

Fig. 18. Nerve connection between deplant of minced cord and limb (cartilage visible in lower right corner).

1 sec; midbrain yielded only tonic contractures without clonic reactions and forebrain had no effect at all. Finally, the most relevant observation was this: when a length of spinal cord was given *two* limbs to innervate, one facing the front and the other the rear end of the central fragment, both limbs displayed seizures always at the same time and of essentially *identical patterns*. Evidently, the whole cord fragment acted *in unison*. After later transecting such a grafted unit, that correspondence between front and rear leg activities ceased, each one continuing to operate spontaneously but independently; gradually the severed cord pieces became reconnected by a bridge of regenerated nerve fibers, but, although some excitatory interaction between the reconnected central fragments was restored, there was never a sign of resumption of the former unified control over both limbs. We learn from this loss that an *integral* CNS

portion has properties and faculties far beyond what we would have expected from the *isolated* knowledge of a network of interconnected wires alone. And wherein would that superiority of the whole over a mere addition of all the parts lie? This is another great challenge for the future.

DYNAMIC NATURE OF NERVE CELLS

I now pass on to my most unexpected shock to any residual complacency regarding standard dogmas. This was the haphazard discovery that neurons are by no means the rigid, stationary and durable fixtures for which we once had taken them, but are in fact highly unstable and reproductively active cellular units of our tissues (Weiss, 1944; Weiss and Hiscoe, 1948; Weiss, 1969, 1974). Although I originally named the phenomenon "axonal", or more generally "neuroplasmic flow", advancing knowledge has surely called for further terminological refinement. The fact that a fixed nerve preparation, or its image

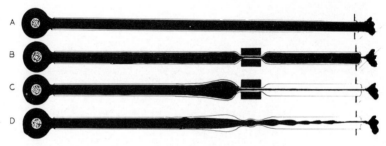

Fig. 19. Schematic diagram of effect of moderate local constriction (without disruption) of mature nerve fiber. A: initial size. B: state immediately after application of contractile ring. C: same fiber in resulting steady state. D: shortly after removal of "bottleneck".

on a book page, looks the same year after year has certainly contributed to our picture of constancy and immutability. Our vagueness of language has added further to it. The term "growth" was usually connected with cell proliferation, so that the cessation of nerve cell divisions (about postpartum in man) meant stoppage of protoplasmic reproduction. However, there is continued cell growth without mitotic division. Nevertheless, even the regenerative sprouting of an adult neuron was generally viewed as the reactivation of a dormant embryonic faculty rather than as a sign of a continuously on-going process of *growth*. In order to avoid a resurgence of such interpretations, I shall confine the following remarks to fully mature nerves, leaving out, as being partly misleading, all work on embryonic or regenerating neurons. Even so, space allows only the most condensed of reviews.

The story starts in 1942 during my direction of a comprehensive program on nerve repair in war victims. I had some success in replacing nerve suturing by means of tubular splicing of the severed stumps, by cuffs of live arteries (see Weiss, 1944). This led to studying the effects of an arterial sleeve on intact nerves, as is illustrated schematically in Fig. 19. Any constriction of the nerve caliber passed itself on to the nerve fibers contained in it, and soon yielded a cumulative bulging of neuroplasm at the proximal side of the stricture, with a corresponding caliber reduction at the far sides of the same axons. This damming up in front of a constriction of neuroplasm indicated a constant outflow of substance from the central cell body which, when handicapped in its flow, would pile up in front of the obstruction, with the material progressing only in proportion to the bottleneck available for transit. Removal

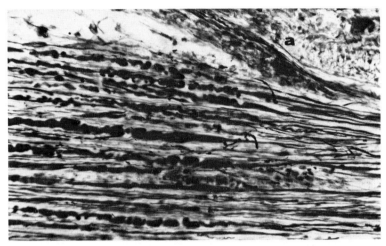

Fig. 20. "Damming" of axoplasm at proximal end of "bottleneck" (narrowed arterial cuff, a), 4 weeks postoperative. Note the sudden diminution of caliber and straightness of the constricted portion of fibers.

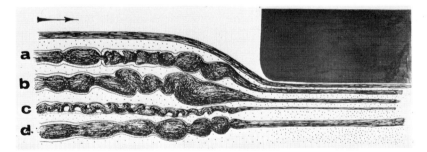

Fig. 21. Major configurations of "dammed" parts of axons such as in preceding figure. a: telescoping. b: meandering and bulging. c: curling and crinkling (of thin fibers). d: beading.

of the constriction many months later immediately released the piled up intracellular mass, which then advanced freely at an average rate of about 1 mm/day (Weiss and Cavanaugh, 1959). More exact studies (Figs. 20 and 21) proved the bulgings, spiralings and bunchings in front of a constriction to be deformations and distortions of relatively solid columns (Weiss, 1972a) arising from the resistance to the advance of an oversized mass through a locally undersized channel lumen. Electron microscopic pictures of such areas showed the whole axonal microstructure of filaments, tubules, etc., to have been subject to the same stress-produced disfigurations.

26

The combined evidence assembled from time-lapse motion pictures of living fibers, electron microscopy, technical (rheological) studies of the driving forces and radiographic measurements of isotope markers (Weiss, 1959, 1961, 1963, 1971a, b, 1974) have confirmed that the movement thus far discussed is not a convection of fluid within a stable stationary axon, but a continuous cellulifugal shift of the whole axon at the well-nigh universal rate of about 1 μm/min (about 1 mm/day). This is the progress that should be termed "axonal flow proper", because it refers to the whole axonal body as in a state of continuous outgrowth from the neuronal cell body, much as a hair grows out from its follicle. In addition to this growth process, increasing evidence has accumulated for an extensive traffic of liquids, and even small particles, *within* the axon at much higher convection rates (up to > 100 times faster). In contradistinction to the slow *"axonal flow"*, this fast transfer would better be called *"transport"* (McEwen and Grafstein, 1968; Ochs, 1972).

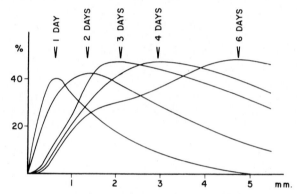

Fig. 22. Percentage daily progress of newly produced radioactively marked axonal protein along the optic nerve from its exit from the eye bulb to the brain.

Both studies have gained greatly by the introduction of radioactive marking techniques. Although we had used it first to measure liquid flow between nerve fibers (Weiss et al., 1945), major advances came first with the radioautographic labeling of fresh protein synthesis by means of tritiated amino acids (Droz and Leblond, 1963). We succeeded in confining the application of such radioactive markers to circumscribed neuron sources, such as the retina for the optic nerve (Weiss and Taylor, 1965) and the nostrils for the olfactory nerve (Weiss and Holland, 1967). A small drop of tritiated leucine injected into the eye bulb was incorporated selectively into the retinal ganglion cells, and could be identified thereafter as a component of newly formed protein in the optic nerve axons. Its peak of concentration shifted, as seen in the tracings (Fig. 22), about 1 mm along the nerve fibers each day. The progressive broadening of the crest is presumably an index of some intra-axonal content passing down still faster, as I mentioned earlier.

A similar marking of freshly synthesized protein in cells of origin of the olfactory axons in one nostril (Fig. 23), leaving the opposite nostril unmarked for control, has brought the further advantage of tracing the exact course of

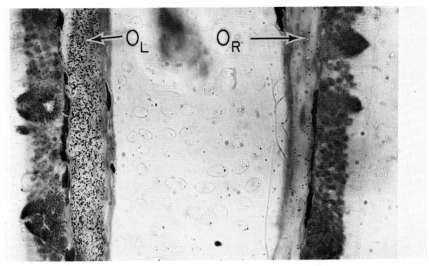

Fig. 23. Radioautogram of longitudinal section of nasal septum of toad, two weeks after radioactively labeling the proteins in the left nostril. Note the high radioactivity (silver grains) advanced toward the brain in the left olfactory nerve (O_L) in contrast to the blankness of its unlabeled control nerve on the right (O_R).

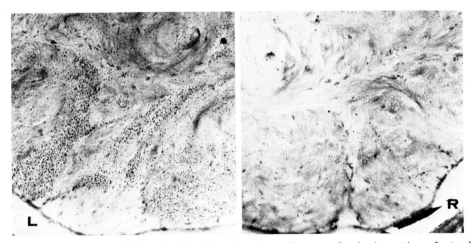

Fig. 24. Symmetrical left (L) and right (R) sectors from the same forebrain section of a toad, 11 days after labeling of the left nostril as in Fig. 23, showing the various radioactive olfactory bundles flaring out after their entrance into the brain with strict confinement to the left half.

the marked fibers after their entry into the brain. Fig. 24 shows both halves of the same forebrain section of such a preparation, revealing distinctly on the marked side the pattern of distribution of the fiber bundles to their first central synaptic endings. This has initiated a wholly new method of anatomical tracking down central connections in fully intact living brains. Far more punctilious still is the labeling technique lately introduced by Kreutzberg and Schubert (1973), of microinjecting the radioactive marker directly into a single nerve cell, thus allowing one to trace the course of a single neuron amidst its unlabeled companions. This marker could even be combined, using a triple microinjector, with an electric stimulating and recording device so as to make possible the study of relations between excitation and rate of protein synthesis, and the like.

Without going any further into the wide range of experiences and applications of the phenomenon of axonal flow, let me add just a brief sample from the large stock of motion picture records of live mature fibers which have helped in the explorations; for here, actually, "seeing *is* believing" (Weiss, 1972b). In rough terms, the story is this: like a factory, each neuronal cell body keeps reproducing its complement of proteins and derivative macro-molecules at daily renewal rates of up to 100% (Lasek, 1970; Miani, 1964). The new products are then partly used for replacements in the cell body and its dendrites, but the most conspicuous disposal is the surplus extrusion into the periphery, both to replenish the internal losses and to carry products for export (enzymes, transmitters, trophic substances, etc.) to their distant destinations. The driving mechanism for the convection consists of peristaltic pulse waves passing down the axonal surface at intervals of 20–30 min at the indicated rate of about 1 μm/min (see Weiss, 1972b; Biondi et al., 1972).

Many of the axonal organelles are carried along by the axonal flow, indicating that they are continuously reproduced in the cell body and dissipated at the end of the line. For the neurotubules, their origin and passive convection in the axon seems reasonably certain (Weiss and Mayr, 1971b), but their fate at the end is speculative. On the other hand, the destiny of mitochondria is less dubious (Weiss and Pillai, 1965), the rate of their proximodistal travel is the same as that of axoplasm, suggesting that they likewise are carried along passively by its flow, although the possibility of some limited capacity for local self-propagation should not be discounted.

Interestingly, however, when mitochondria are halted in their proximodistal advance, they dissolve within a few days at the obstacle point. Fig. 25 shows

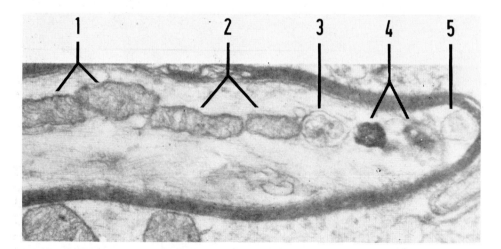

Fig. 25. Progressive decomposition of mitochondria (from left to right) after their consecutive arrival in blind pocket of constricted axon.

the "death history" of a column of mitochondria sequentially trapped in a "blind alley". The most recent arrivals (1) are perfectly normal, while their predecessors in front show signs of progressive decay, from at first slight vacuolization (2), then internal destructuring (3), chemical dissolution into a lipid (heavily osmiophilic) mass (4), to finally a clear blister (5) (presumably of phospholipids). The same events are observed in mitochondria bunched up in front of bottlenecks due to constrictions. Logically then, one should expect it to happen regularly at the end of the line of every axon, which is its ending. And looking for it at neuromuscular junctions, there it was (Weiss and Mayr, 1971a). Fig. 26 shows a myoneural junction of a mouse. You recognize the

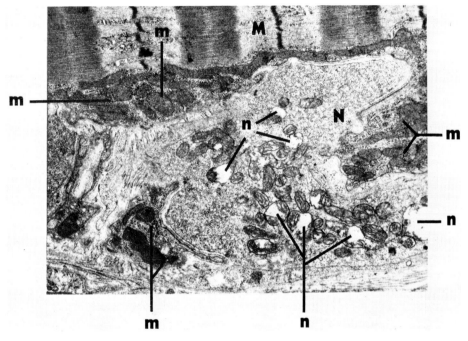

Fig. 26. Terminal decomposition of mitochondria in nerve terminal at motor end plate. M, muscle fiber; m, fully intact mitochondria in muscular tissue; n, degenerating mitochondria in neuronal ending (N). (Yet mitochondria are still fully intact in same axon a fraction of a millimeter further proximally.)

muscular portion (M) with all its own mitochondria (m) perfectly normal in shape and structure, in contrast to those in the *nerve ending* (N) which show various degrees of vacuolization and breakdown (n).

My prime conclusion drawn from the experiences with axonal flow had been that the protein factory of the neuron lies in the nucleated part — the perikaryon. This contention became shaky when counter-evidence was brought up, indicating some protein to be produced in the nerve endings. This left the whole story somewhat in the dark until, alerted by (1) the mitochondrial data just presented; (2) the reports that mitochondria contain an endogenous equipment of DNA, RNA and necessary accessories to produce their own proteins and enzymes; and (3), putting (1) and (2) together, I deduced that the distal protein production previously reported might simply be the work of the mitochondrial factory equipment that spills from its decomposing carriers into the synaptosomal space. The test (Weiss and Mayr, 1971a) was easy and conclusive. We cut 3 equal pieces from a series of adult nerves and put them into a standard medium to start Wallerian degeneration, during which mitochondria tend to gather at the two transected ends (see Zelená, 1969). We then measured separately the protein productivity of the content of each 1-mm fraction. Twice as much protein is produced within the first millimeter near each original cut than in the intermediate region. However, when we preceded the protein test by a brief submersion of the nerve in *chloramphenicol* (a specific inhibitor of mitochondrial protein formation), although the whole protein yield was reduced, the reduction was greater near the cut ends — where the density of mitochondria was highest. It would be desirable, of course, to have corresponding results available from intact living nerves, but the analogy is close enough at least to strongly suggest an explanation for the second, peripheral, source of certain proteins in neurons.

My having given a relatively extensive treatment here of the phenomenon of axonal flow is explained by its great disparity from past concepts of the nervous system. So many favored neurobiological views may now have to be reviewed, opening new vistas from the most elementary basic and familiar textbook versions up to almost inconceivably diverse prospects of novel practical approaches to problems of neurology, neuropathology, pharmacology, neurosurgery and even psychiatry. Another challenge for the future to really *search* (as against just "re-search").

You might ask why I have said so little about *intra-axonal transport.* The answer is that, in contrast to axonal growth, we know so little about how it works. None of the proposed conjectures seem to fit (for a brief early comment, see Weiss, 1969). For macromolecules, or larger particles up to several tens of nanometers in size, to race down the fiber at a rate of $1\ \mu m/sec$ is quite a puzzle in terms of rheological physics. Imaginative *neurotubular* mechanisms have been postulated but they fall down when sizes, frictions, fluid resistance, etc., are taken into account. To be realistic, let us face the problem on a truly tough object: the chromatophores in fish (Fig. 27).

Melanin granules, several hundred nanometers in diameter, lying dispersed in the radial arms of their cell, will, on the impact of a drop of adrenaline, race toward the nuclear center at the same rate as the fast transport in axons, that is, about $1\ \mu m/second$ (or even faster) without contact with microtubules (Green, 1968). Therefore, let me infer that studies on *neural* transport alone are not necessarily the road to success. However, though the translatory mechanism remains unknown, even the descriptive demonstration of intra-axonal pathways for traffic from center to periphery (and in some cases also in reverse) has been one of the most prosperous byproducts of the general principle that the neuron is not static, but rather is in constant mobile action. The rest is again for the future; impatient speculations have been aired (some even by myself) but most of them do not conform to the little we yet know about microrheology and transport mechanisms in biological systems.

I will intersperse here a pertinent example from my own laboratory (Grover, 1966) (Fig. 28): Collagen, the fibrous protein of connective tissue, forms the firm ropes of tendons by assembling several thousand parallel polymerized

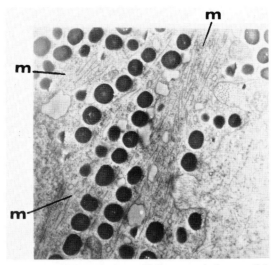

Fig. 27. Chromatophores on fish scale in rapid linear rush from cell branches toward nuclear center upon adrenaline stimulus. Electron micrograph with microtubules (m) well evident.

molecules in linear bundles of about 50 nm in diameter. The compacted strands show a regular periodicity of 64 nm marked by darker cross bands, the clustered layers of polar side chains. Note how a minute amount of metal dye (e.g., uranyl nitrate), introduced at a tiny spot spreads along the fiber bundles, not evenly but in saltatory accumulations at the polar bands, and at velocities many times faster than by ordinary diffusion. Electrically neutral particles, e.g.

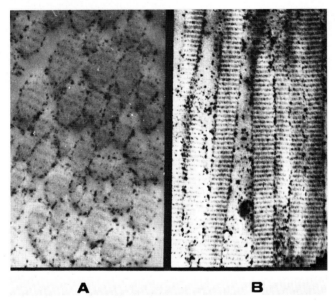

Fig. 28. Electron micrographs of collagen fibers of tendon after uranilnitrate point-source injection. A: oblique section. B: longitudinal section. Note gathering of the metallic stain at interface between fiber and ground substance as well as at the dark cross bands (periodicity of 64 nm).

32

colloidal gold or some neutral viruses, spread instead much at random. This electrical transport mechanism has apparently not yet been taken into consideration.

Now that we have stepped down to the ultramicroscopic dimensions, in which electron microscopy has brought so many revelations, some words on the reliability of its "seeing is believing" principle might be appropriate. Good sections of an axon (Fig. 29) show neurotubules, about 22 nm across, which are clearly defined; I mentioned earlier their advance with the axonal flow. They are *real* structures, but it is questionable whether this last criterion of reality is applicable to the mass of fibrillar units named "neurofilaments"

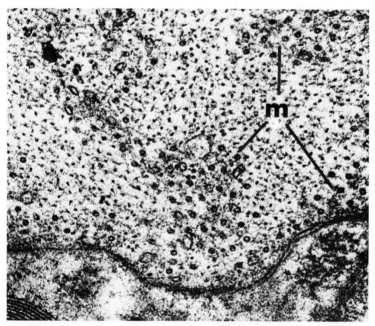

Fig. 29. Electron micrograph of neuronal cross-section with clusters of neurotubules (m) and matrix with "neurofilaments".

(about 8 nm wide) which fill the cross-section. The question arose from the rather conspicuous regularity of their distribution, all "filaments" assuming apparently equally sized domains. Once again, we turned to mathematics (Weiss and Mayr, 1971c), measuring the quite variable cross-sectional areas along the course of a single axon, then counting the number of filaments in those sections, and plotting the data in Fig. 30. To our amazement, the ratio of filament number to the corresponding cross-sectional area was *constant* along the whole length, and above all, the curves were linear, passed through the zero point, and had the same angle for all three different nerves.

This all looked like a non-biological artifact, to which rather recent studies in the ceramic industries seemed to offer an explanatory basis. In a sample experiment (Gerdes et al., 1970) of so-called "eutectic laminal flow", a mixture of powdered 15% tungsten and 85% neutral uranium oxide was melted, and the melt let flow down an inclined plate in order to congeal. Electron micrographic

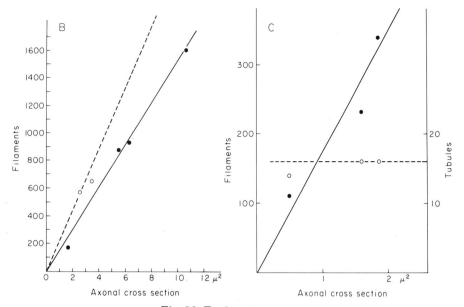

Fig. 30. Explanation in text.

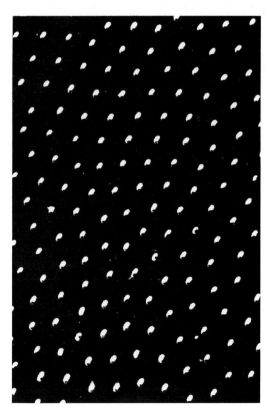

Fig. 31. Eutectic laminal flow pattern. Explanation in text. (From Gerdes et al., 1970.)

sections through the melted mass (Fig. 31) revealed that in the process uniform aggregates of filaments of tungsten had sorted themselves out within the neutral matrix, so as to form by self-segregation the lattice pattern shown in the picture. Our mathematical characteristics of the "neurofilament" patterns in axons strongly suggest that a similar process of orderly self-segregation, between dispersed filamentous elements and a common ground substance, takes place in the axonal matrix during the artifactual physicochemical transformations intervening between the living condition and the actual electron microscopic observation. I myself had for a long time taken the physical entity and continuity of neurofilaments for granted, either as structural supports or excitatory guide lines. Now all of this probably has to be given up as spurious. What is structurally fixed in a microscopic or electron microscopic preparation, separated from the living state by several steps of artificial interventions, can only be accepted as a potential clue to backward inferences about a momentary (dynamic) structural condition of the living system, but never as a true copy. Remember that prior to the introduction of glutaraldehyde fixation, neurotubules had remained "invisible", yet should one have denied their "existence"? Our experience with the neurofilaments now presents itself as a phenomenon in exactly the reverse sense.

A similar spirit of deliberative caution seems to be indicated for all of our extrapolations from fixed specimens to the dynamics of the living system or even for tests of the living state using solely a single recording device or method (in the hope of being able to "explain" retroactively the context of a *whole* organized phenomenon from those linear snap-shots). This cautionary attitude has made me, the more I have come to learn from such single-track excursions, to become more aware of the immenseness of our residual ignorance. For me, this applies also to the "understanding"* of the *dynamics* of the nervous system, despite the dramatically rapid advances in its study. I feel that in its "statu nascendi", full birth of the neurosciences may not be very far off, and may well yield a vigorous and harmoniously built infant. I doubt, however, whether a smug complacency with the present developmental state of the "fetus" will be enough to enable its successful delivery to surmount the dangers of a still-birth.

I have simply presented sets of data, many much younger than the groundrock on which our present neurobiology rests. I fully realize their prospects for continued differentiation, maturation, disavowal and deletion — and, ultimately, oblivion. This is the way of life itself, and it has always been the source and the course of any science that is alive — curious, alert, fearless of facing the unknown. It looks for questions never yet solved, or even recognized, instead of trying to deduce its questions mainly from answers already well established. "Established", or merely accepted? Adopted through validation, or simply seeming plausible? To clarify my point, let me just throw out haphazardly two almost trivial questions, yet rarely asked and never answered.

(1) What is the life expectancy of a synaptic ending? Are synapses permanent for life or subject to replacement? One need only remember the

---

* Which is far above sheer "knowledge" (Weiss, 1975b).

gustatory papillae on the tongue, the sensory receptor cells of which are continually being shed and replaced, which imposes on the neuronal endings incessantly new terminal connections.

(2) How can we be sure that the *simple* electrochemical conception of excitation and inhibition, as well as impulse conduction in nerve fibers, is really all that simple? Is it surprising that, as long as we ask nerves only "electric" questions without coded patterns, we must expect equally *unpatterned* "electric" answers? After all, an ordinary black and white photographic plate reproduces only differences of light intensity, no colors. Could we not visualize homologous series of macromolecular chains passing on, selectively, specifically configurated messages (electric *patterns*) which would be conformingly received by attuned receptors? After all, a radio receiver responds to a musical emission with beautifully patterned sound, but to "static" only with flickers of *noise*.

Here then is my concluding message to the young generation, to whose hands and minds the future of neurobiology (in statu nascendi) will be entrusted: walk more through the wilds of nature, and drive less over preformed and congested superhighways. Help in the maturation of a harmoniously constituted, well-coordinated system of knowledge and ideas, known as neurobiology. With your help this branch of science may well be destined to emerge as the greatest spur to human rational progress through the benefits accruing from *understanding* both the *potential might* of our own powerful instrument of rationality — the brain— as well as its *natural limitations.*

ACKNOWLEDGEMENTS

All illustrations whose author is not specifically identified by name are products of the laboratories of the author of the present paper, jointly with his collaborators, many of which are listed in the citation of literature referring to the respective topics. It is my sincere wish, however, to express my deep gratitude to all of them for their effective, dedicated and faithful collaboration — to them as well as to the many institutions and Foundations who over the years have given generous support to my work program.

REFERENCES

Biondi, R., Levy, M. and Weiss, P. (1972) An engineering study of the peristaltic drive of axonal flow. *Proc. nat. Acad. Sci. (Wash.)*, 69: 1732–1736.

Cajal, S. Ramón y (1928) *Degeneration and Regeneration of the Nervous System.* Translated and edited by R.M. May, Oxford University Press.

Corner, M. (1964) Localization of capacities for functional development in the neural plate of *Xenopus laevis. J. comp. Neurol.*, 123: 243–255.

Desmedt, J. (1954) Paroxystic activity of deplanted nerve centers in Amphibia, as influenced by the ionic environment. *Proc. Soc. exp. Biol. (N.Y.)*, 85: 491–494.

Droz, B. and Leblond, C. (1963) Axon migration of proteins in the central-nervous system and peripheral nerves as shown by radioautography. *J. comp. Neurol.*, 121: 325–346.

Gasser, H.S. (1937) The control of excitation in the nervous system. *Harvey Lect.*, 32: 169–193.

Gaze, R. (1970) *The Formation of Nerve Connections. A Consideration of Neural Specificity Modulation and Comparable Phenomena.* Academic Press, New York.

Gerdes, R., Chapman, A. and Clark, G. (1970) Refractory oxide-metal composites: scanning electron microscopy and X-ray diffraction of uranium dioxide-tungsten. *Science,* 167: 979–980.

Green, L. (1968) Mechanism of movements of granules in melanocytes of *Fundulus heroclitus. Proc. nat. Acad. Sci. (Wash.),* 59: 1179–1186.

Grover, N. (1966) Anisometric transport of ions and particles in anisotropic tissue spaces. *Biophysics J.,* 6: 71–85.

Hamburger, V. and Levi-Montalcini, R. (1950) Some aspects of neuroembryology. In *Genetic Neurology,* P. Weiss (Ed.), Univ. of Chicago Press, Chicago, Ill., pp. 128–160.

Harrison, R. (1907) Observations on the living developing nerve fiber. *Anat. Rec.,* 1: 116–118.

Harrison, R. (1910) The outgrowth of the nerve fiber as a mode of protoplasmic movement. *J. exp. Zool.,* 9: 787–848.

Holtfreter, J. (1934) Formative Reize in der Embryonalentwicklung der Amphibien, dargestellt an Explantationsversuchen. *Arch. exp. Zellforsch.,* 15: 281–301.

Kollros, J. (1943) Experimental studies on the development of the corneal reflex in Amphibia. II. Localized maturation of the reflex mechanism effected by thyroxin-agar implants into the hindbrain. *Physiol. Zool.,* 16: 269–279.

Kreutzberg, G. and Schubert, P. (1973) Neuronal activity and axonal flow. In *Metabolic Regulation and Functional Activity in the Central Nervous System,* H. Herken and E. Genazzani (Eds.), Springer, Berlin, pp. 84–93.

Lasek, R. (1970) Protein transport in neurons. In *International Reviews in Neurobiology, Vol. 13,* C. Pfeiffer and J. Smythies (Eds.), Academic Press, New York, pp. 289–324.

McEwen, B. and Grafstein, B. (1968) Fast and slow components in axonal transport of protein. *J. Cell Biol.,* 38: 494–508.

Miani, N. (1964) Proximo-distal movement of phospholipid in the axoplasm of the intact and regenerating neurons. In *Mechanisms of Neural Regeneration, Progr. Brain Res., Vol. 13,* M. Singer and J. Schadé (Eds.), Elsevier, Amsterdam, pp. 115–126.

Ochs, S. (1972) Rate of fast axoplasmic transport in mammalian nerve fibers. *J. Physiol. (Lond.),* 227: 627–645.

Sperry, R. (1943) Visuomotor coordination in the newt (*Triturus viridescens*) after regeneration of the optic nerve. *J. comp. Neurol.,* 79: 33–55.

Sperry, R. (1963) Chemoaffinity in the orderly growth of nerve fiber patterns and connections. *Proc. nat. Acad. Sci. (Wash.),* 50: 703–710.

Stefanelli, A. (1950) Studies on the development of Mauthner's cell. In *Genetic Neurology,* P. Weiss (Ed.), University of Chicago Press, Chicago, Ill., pp. 210–211.

Taylor, A. (1944) Selectivity of nerve fibers from the dorsal and ventral roots in the development of the frog limb. *J. exp. Zool.,* 96: 159–185.

Verzár, F. and Weiss, P. (1930) Untersuchungen über das Phänomen der identischen Bewegungsfunktion mehrfacher benachbarter Extremitäten. *Pflügers Arch. ges. Physiol.,* 223: 671–684.

Weiss, P. (1931) Die Nervenversorgung der überzähligen Extremitäten an dem von Verzár und Weiss in Bd. 223 dieser Zeitschrift beschriebenden hypermelen Frosch. *Pflügers Arch. ges. Physiol.,* 228; 486–497.

Weiss, P. (1934) In vitro experiments on the factors determining the course of the outgrowing nerve fiber. *J. exp. Zool.,* 68: 393–448.

Weiss, P. (1936) Selectivity controlling the central-peripheral relations in the nervous system. *Biol. Rev.,* 11: 494–531.

Weiss, P. (1937a) Further experimental investigations on the phenomenon of homologous response in transplanted amphibian limbs. I. Functional observations. *J. comp. Neurol.,* 66: 181–209.

Weiss, P. (1937b) Further experimental investigations on the phenomenon of homologous response in transplanted amphibian limbs. II. Nerve regeneration and the innervation of transplanted limbs. *J. comp. Neurol.,* 66: 481–535.

Weiss, P. (1937c) Further experimental investigations on the phenomenon of homologous response in transplanted amphibian limbs. III. Homologous response in the absence of sensory innervation. *J. comp. Neurol.*, 66: 537–548.

Weiss, P. (1937d) Further experimental investigations on the phenomenon of homologous response in transplanted amphibian limbs. IV. Reverse locomotion after the interchange of right and left limbs. *J. comp. Neurol.*, 67: 269–315.

Weiss, P. (1940) Functional properties of isolated spinal cord grafts in larval amphibians. *Proc. Soc. exp. Biol. (N.Y.)*, 44: 350–352.

Weiss, P. (1941a) Further experiments with deplanted and deranged nerve centers in amphibians. *Proc. Soc. exp. Biol. (N.Y.)*, 46: 14–15.

Weiss, P. (1941b) Does sensory control play a constructive role in the development of motor coordination? *Schweiz. med. Wschr.*, 71: 591–595.

Weiss, P. (1941c) Self-differentiation of the basic patterns of coordination. *Comp. Psychol. Monogr.*, 17: 1–96.

Weiss, P. (1941d) Nerve patterns: the mechanics of nerve growth. *Growth*, 5: 163–203.

Weiss, P. (1942) Lid-closure reflex from eyes transplanted to atypical locations in *Triturus torosus*: evidence of a peripheral origin of sensory specificity. *J. comp. Neurol.*, 77: 131–169.

Weiss, P. (1944) The technology of nerve regeneration: a review. Sutureless tubulation and related methods of nerve repair. *J. Neurosurg.*, 1: 400–450.

Weiss, P. (1945) Experiments on cell and axon orientation in vitro: the role of colloidal exudates in tissue organization. *J. exp. Zool.*, 100: 353–386.

Weiss, P. (1950a) The deplantation of fragments of nervous system in amphibians. I. Central reorganization and the formation of nerves. *J. exp. Zool.*, 113: 397–461.

Weiss, P. (1950b) Central versus peripheral factors in the development of coordination. *Proc. Ass. Res. nerv. ment. Dis.*, 30: 3–23.

Weiss, P. (1952) "Attraction fields" between growing tissue cultures. *Science*, 115: 293–295.

Weiss, P. (1955) Nervous system (neurogenesis). In *Analysis of Development*, B.H. Willier, P. Weiss and V. Hamburger (Eds.), Saunders, Philadelphia, Pa., pp. 346–401.

Weiss, P. (1959) Evidence by isotope tracers of perpetual replacement of mature nerve fibers from their cell bodies. *Science*, 129: 1290.

Weiss, P. (1961) The concept of perpetual neuronal growth and proximo-distal substance convection. In *Regional Neurochemistry*, S.S. Kety and J. Elkes (Eds.), Pergamon Press, Oxford, pp. 220–242.

Weiss, P. (1963) Self-renewal and proximo-distal convection in nerve fibers. In *The Effect of Use and Disuse on Neuromuscular Functions*, E. Guttman (Ed.), Czechoslovak Akad. of Sciences, Prague, pp. 171–183.

Weiss, P. (1969) Neuronal dynamics and neuroplasmic ("axonal") flow. In *Cellular Dynamics and the Neuron, Symp. Int. Soc. for Cell Biol., Vol. 8*, S.H. Barondes (Ed.), Academic Press, New York, pp. 3–34.

Weiss, P. (1972a) Neuronal dynamics and axonal flow. V. The semisolid state of the moving axonal column. *Proc. nat. Acad. Sci. (Wash.)*, 68: 620–623.

Weiss, P. (1972b) Neuronal dynamics and axonal flow. VI. Axonal peristalsis. *Proc. nat. Acad. Sci. (Wash.)*, 69: 1309–1312.

Weiss, P. (1973) *The Science of Life: The Living System — A System for Living.* Futura Publ. Co., Mt. Kisco, New York, 137 pp.

Weiss, P. (1974) Dynamics and mechanics of neuroplasmic flow. In *Dynamics of Degeneration and Growth in Neurons*, K. Fuxe, L. Olson and Y. Zotterman (Eds.), Pergamon Press, Oxford, pp. 203–213.

Weiss, P. (1975a) Neural specificity: fifty years of vagaries. In *The Neurosciences: Paths of Discovery*, F. Worden, J. Swazey and G. Adelman (Eds.), M.I.T. Press, Cambridge, Mass., pp. 77–100.

Weiss, P. (Ed.) (1975b) *Knowledge in Search of Understanding: The Frensham Papers.* Futura Publ. Co., Mt. Kisco, New York, 278 pp.

Weiss, P. and Cavanaugh, M. (1959) Further evidence of perpetual growth of nerve fibers: recovery of fiber diameter after the release of prolonged constrictions. *J. exp. Zool.*, 142: 461–473.

38

Weiss, P. and Edds, M., Jr. (1945) Sensory-motor nerve crosses in the rat. *J. Neurophysiol.*, 8: 173–193.

Weiss, P. and Hiscoe, H. (1948) Experiments on the mechanisms of nerve growth. *J. exp. Zool.*, 107: 315–395.

Weiss, P. and Hoag, M. (1946) Competitive reinnervation of rat muscles by their own and foreign nerves. *J. Neurophysiol.*, 9: 413–418.

Weiss, P. and Holland, Y. (1967) Neuronal dynamics and axonal flow. II. The olfactory nerve as model test object. *Proc. nat. Acad. Sci. (Wash.)*, 57: 258–264.

Weiss, P. and Mayr, M. (1971a) Neuronal organelles in neuroplasmic ("axonal") flow. I. Mitochondria. *Acta neuropath. (Berl.)*, Suppl. V: 187—197.

Weiss, P. and Mayr, M. (1971b) Neuronal organelles in neuroplasmic ("axonal") flow. II. Neurotubules. *Acta neuropath. (Berl.)*, Suppl. V: 198–206.

Weiss, P. and Mayr, M. (1971c) Organelles in neuroplasmic ("axonal") flow. III. Neurofilaments. *Proc. nat. Acad. Sci. (Wash.)*, 68: 846–850.

Weiss, P. and Pillai, A. (1965) Convection and fate of mitochondria in nerve fibers: axonal flow as vehicle. *Proc. nat. Acad. Sci. (Wash.)*, 54: 48–56.

Weiss, P. and Rossetti, F. (1951) Growth responses of opposite sign among different neuron types exposed to thyroid hormone. *Proc. nat. Acad. Sci. (Wash.)*, 37: 540–556.

Weiss, P. and Taylor, A. (1944). Further experimental evidence against "neurotropism" in nerve regeneration. *J. exp. Zool.*, 95: 233–257.

Weiss, P. and Taylor, A.C. (1965) Synthesis and flow of neuroplasm: a progress report. *Science*, 148: 669–670.

Zelená, J. (1969) Bidirectional movements of mitochondria along axons of an isolated nerve segment. *Z. Zellforsch.*, 92: 186–196.

Are Invertebrate Nervous Systems Good Models for the Functional Organization of the Brain?

J. Z. YOUNG

Department of Anatomy, University College, London (Great Britain)

This question raises at once the problem of what it is that we want to know about nervous systems. It is easy enough to specify some of the immediate questions that are under investigation — say, about nerve impulses or synaptic transmitters. But if we are looking at longer perspectives we have to ask how these current questions are related to the whole history of studies of the nervous system and of biology in general, and even of philosophy. Fashions of research develop for reasons that may be extrinsic to the real interests of the subject as a part of human knowledge. Study of the nervous system in this century has been greatly influenced by the development of artificial means of human communication, from telegraphy and telephoning onwards to television. The technical aids developed for these purposes have determined both the practical and theoretical developments of the study of nervous conduction in the last 50 years. More recently cybernetics has invaded neurology (and vice versa). Still more recently, the possibilities of the analysis of small quantities of material opened up by chromatography have revolutionized the biochemistry of synaptic studies.

Such links with various technologies are of course fundamental for research in biology, but they may also divert attention from important topics for which they cannot be used and from other paths of enquiry that might be profitable. The many things that we should like to know about the nervous system could perhaps be summarized in the question: "How does it compute the responses that maintain life" and, in particular, "How does it perform the more complex computations such as those that go on in our own brains". We need to find materials and techniques that will allow the study of masses of nervous tissue, as well as the units of which they are composed.

It might seem at first that for answering such questions the brains of invertebrates are not very suitable. Almost by definition they are very different from our own. For instance, the differences of scale between ourselves and the insects mean that very different principles are in some respects involved in the organization of their lives. It seems absurd to some people to look for the secrets of the human brain in the organization of the eyes of flies such as *Drosophila* or water fleas like *Daphnia*. In fact, precisely the contrary is the case. From the history of biology it is very clear that, in spite of such differences of scale and habits, the great problems have begun to yield solutions only when they have been simplified by the use of suitable animal material. We could quote many examples for the nervous system, but perhaps the best is the knowledge of the nature of the nerve impulse, which was suspected from the study of the nerves of vertebrates but enormously deepened by the use of invertebrate nerves, such as those of crustaceans and squids (Katz, 1966).

Biologists have found over and over again that the study of simpler organisms has revealed principles applicable to all animals. The genetic code is the same from bacteria to man, and nerve impulses and synaptic transmitters are very similar in all animals. It might seem that this strategy would not be as likely to apply to the study of higher nervous functions, especially those that we like to think are peculiarly well developed in ourselves. It is probable that such an attitude will prove to be only another piece of anthropocentric arrogance. There are signs that even the most intricate problems of the nervous system will find some large parts of their solutions in invertebrate systems.

The central difficulty in the study of the nervous system arises from the method of coding that it adopts. Each item of information is, in the main, carried in a distinct channel. An enormous number of channels is thus involved, and the problem is to discover how signals passing along so many different paths cooperate to produce behavior. Thomas Young suggested as early as 1801 that color discrimination involved passing signals along 3 different channels. Helmholtz and Müller confirmed this, and developed the doctrine of specific nerve energies. But how are we to study the way in which the information in many channels is brought together? Obviously it is important to know the nature of the nerve signals themselves (nerve impulses) and for this, as has been said, invertebrate nerves have already provided most of the information. Next we need to know how the signals are decoded and enabled to cooperate at the synapses. Here too the problems of synaptic integration that are involved have already been greatly helped by work on large cells of invertebrates, including gastropod and cephalopod molluscs, insects and crustacea. There is undoubtedly very much more that can be done with these large cells to elucidate the biophysical and biochemical characteristics of synaptic processes. Perhaps these systems with few cells are *too* simple, it might be said. But they allow us to find out many things that we could not know if we did not have access to both sides of a synapse, as for instance in the stellate ganglion of squids (Miledi, 1967).

Yet however much we discover about simple nervous systems, the really difficult problems appear when we try to study how thousands of cells cooperate. There are clear signs that invertebrates can help very much with these problems too. There are many stages of complexity between *Aplysia* and man, after all, and what we find in the brain of Diptera or Hymenoptera or Cephalopoda provides us with different levels of complexity, each of them helpful in finding the solution to the problem.

Questions about the functional interaction of neurons in part resolve themselves into how the connections in the nervous system came to be made in the first place, and here invertebrates are likely to be most helpful indeed. We need to know what parts of the pattern are determined by heredity, and for this the rapid reproduction and known genetics of *Drosophila* are proving most helpful (Quinn et al., 1974). In all these questions the problem is to find something simple enough to start with — we cannot attack the great problem of the mammalian nervous system head-on. If we could understand how specific connections come to be made in animals with a fixed number of cells, such as nematode worms, we should already be much further along.

The actual method of outgrowth of fibers and how they find their "correct" connection lies very close to the heart of the question. The connections of the cells of a fly's eye show an astonishingly detailed pattern, whose development can be a model for many other animals (Braitenberg, 1967). The details of such systems require the resolution of electron microscopy, and this is helped by the choice of suitably *small* systems such as have been found in the eyes of *Daphnia*, where the outgrowing nerve fibers can be reconstructed (Lopresti et al., 1973).

The understanding of complex brain patterns depends upon finding the principles that control not only development but also later changes in connectivity. These later changes include those involved in adaptive response and regeneration, and culminate in those that produce learned behavior. To study these we need parts of the nervous system that show various degrees of patterning. The displays of color shown by an octopus have proved to be very suitable for the study of pattern regeneration. The colors are produced by chromatophores operated by muscles and controlled by nerves. After nerve section the denervated skin no longer plays any part in the displays, but there can be complete regeneration (Sanders and Young, 1974). If the lesion is severe, however, regeneration shows various deficiencies from which we can learn much about the conditions that enable regenerating fibers to return to make correct connections.

Invertebrates provide a great range of patterns of innervation, both central and peripheral. They provide us with an enormous set of natural experiments. We cannot (yet) make complicated nervous systems to test our theories, but we can make use of the great variety of them that has been evolved to meet different environments.

Thus, when we come to the most difficult question of all — the nature of memory changes — we can make use of the fact that each type of animal has a memory system suited to a different way of life. From the features that are common to all of them we should be able to learn the principles that are involved in storage of the memory record.

It would be absurd to pretend that we have yet gone very far with this method — but no other one has told us much about memory either. Study of the higher centers of invertebrate brains has only just begun, but already we can see something of the possibilities. In the octopus brain there are two clearly distinct memory systems, one for vision and one for touch. Each contains a similar set of 4 lobes. From a study of their patterns of connectivity and the results of removing them, we learn not only what they do but also principles that may apply to all memory systems (see Sanders, 1975). For instance, what is learned with one arm can be performed by the other seven, and we know something of how this is achieved. Such generalization must be a feature of many (or all) memory systems, and the octopus is particularly well suited to study it.

An even more general principle is the control of the *level* of action by higher nervous centers. In a multichannel system it is essential that only the appropriate channels shall operate at any moment, while the others must be suppressed. Means for ensuring this inhibition can be seen in various invertebrates. In *Octopus* there are in each of the two memory systems lobes with masses of microneurons, amacrine cells whose axons do not leave the lobe. There is evidence that at least part of their general effect is to regulate the level of excitation, so that learned decisions are performed correctly and unwanted operations are suppressed (Young, 1964). We do not know how these effects are produced, but the cephalopod molluscs should be ideal for the study of the biophysics and biochemistry of these microneurons, as they have already been for the study of giant neurons, their impulses and their synapses. Moreover, similar collections of small cells also occur in those arthropods that learn well (especially the Hymenoptera) and indeed even in the more active polychaete worms (*Nereis*). The point is that these invertebrates may provide the material that we need for a study of some of the highest parts of the nervous system, for it is not too much to say that in some respects these regulations of the level of action, especially by inhibition, are similar to those performed by our latest evolutionary development, the frontal lobes.

REFERENCES

Braitenberg, V.B. (1967) Patterns of projection in the visual system of the fly. I. Retina-lamina projections. *Exp. Brain Res.*, 3: 271–298.

Katz, B. (1966) *Nerve, Mucle and Synapse*, McGraw Hill, New York.

Lopresti, V., Macagno, E.R. and Levinthal, C. (1973) Structure and development of neuronal connections in isogenic organisms: cellular interactions in the development of the optic lamina of *Daphnia. Proc. nat. Acad. Sci. (Wash.)*, 70: 433–437.

Miledi, R. (1967) Spontaneous synaptic potentials and quantal release of transmitter in the stellate ganglion of the squid. *J. Physiol. (Lond.)*, 192: 379–406.

Quinn, W.G., Harris, W.A. and Benzers, S. (1974) Conditioned behavior in *Drosophila melanogaster. Proc. nat. Acad. Sci. (Wash.)*, 71: 708—712.

Sanders, G.D. (1975) The cephalopods. In *Invertebrate Learning III*, W.C. Corning, J.A. Dyal and A.O.D. Willows (Eds.), Plenum Press, New York.

Sanders, G.D. and Young, J.Z. (1974) Reappearance of specific colour patterns after nerve regeneration in *Octopus. Proc. roy. Soc. B*, 186: 1–11.

Young, J.Z. (1964) *A Model of the Brain*, Clarendon Press, Oxford.

SESSION II

BRAIN AS A TISSUE

Tissue Fractionation Methods in Brain Research

V.P. WHITTAKER

Max-Planck-Institut für biophysikalische Chemie, Göttingen (G.F.R.)

INTRODUCTION

Beginning with the work of Bensley and Hoerr (1934) on the isolation of mitochondria from liver cells, but largely pioneered by Claude and his distinguished pupils at the Rockefeller Institute (reviewed by Porter and Novikoff, 1974), cell fractionation techniques have developed into one of the most powerful tools of modern cell biology, and have led to the generalization that the various functions of the cell are localized in specific subcellular structures. At first sight, the brain, with its wide variety of cell types and complex structure, seems a highly unfavorable tissue to which to apply these techniques. However, starting with the isolation of detached presynaptic nerve terminals (Whittaker, 1960; Gray and Whittaker, 1960, 1962) — later called synaptosomes (Whittaker et al., 1964) — it became apparent that, in nervous tissue too, cell fractionation techniques had an important contribution to make to an understanding of the molecular architecture of the nervous system. It is almost true to say that there is now no component of nervous tissue that cannot be isolated by cell fractionation techniques in a reasonably pure form.

Cell fractionation techniques were initially mainly concerned with the isolation of cell organelles from cells whose plasma and cytoplasmic membranes were broken by the application of liquid shear forces in a suitable medium, non-ionic to prevent clumping and iso-osmotic with the cell sap to prevent osmotic damage. The separation of the various organelles into relatively pure fractions was found to be accomplished most expediously and efficiently by centrifugation, using moving boundary ("differential centrifuging") or density gradient (isopycnic or rate sedimentation) techniques in continuous or step gradients. The theoretical and experimental basis for this technique was initially due to Svedberg (see Svedberg and Pedersen, 1940); its development was greatly aided by the invention, by Pickels and coworkers (see Bauer and Pickels, 1940) of more compact ultracentrifuges with aluminum rotors which eventually led to the first generally available analytical and preparative ultracentrifuges. In more recent times it has been realized that basically similar techniques can be used to isolate, on the one hand, intact cells or even multicellular complexes from tissues and, on the other hand, pure membrane fragments of defined morphological origins which may be components of more complex subcellular structures, and which serve as the starting point for the isolation of specific structural and functional membrane proteins. For this broader range of fractionation techniques, the term tissue rather than cell fractionation is preferred.

In Table I some examples of the structures that can be isolated from nervous tissue by these techniques are given.

Of primary importance is the method selected for tissue disruption (column 2). When this involves gentle dispersion by teasing the tissue through nylon bolting of decreasing mesh size, perhaps after initial softening by incubation with enzymes such as trypsin, whole neuronal perikarya are detached from their dendrites and axons and can be centrifugally separated on

TABLE I

SCOPE OF TISSUE FRACTIONATION METHODS

Structure isolated — example	How isolated
MULTICELLULAR COMPLEXES —	
capillary beds	Gentle dispersion
CELL BODIES — of neurons and glia	Gentle dispersion or hand homogenization
SUBCELLULAR STRUCTURES	
Large complexes — cerebellar glomerulae	Hand homogenization
Smaller complexes — synaptosomes	Mechanical homogenization
Cell organelles — nuclei, mitochondria, lysosomes	Mechanical homogenization
Cell membrane fragments — dendritic and glial fragments, axonal fragments (myelin)*, vesicles derived from plasma and cytomembranes (microsomes)	Mechanical homogenization
Suborganelles — outer and inner mito- chondrial membranes, synaptic vesicles, synaptosome "ghosts", postsynaptic membranes**	*Osmotic shock
Membrane proteins — receptor for acetylcholine, other structural and functional membrane components	**Detergents, molecular exclusion and affinity chromatography

a sucrose-Ficoll density gradient from tissue debris, capillaries and astrocytes (Rose, pp. 67–82 in this volume). High molecular weight polymers, such as the polysaccharide Ficoll, may help to stabilize plasma membranes, as well as provide osmotically inactive solutes of considerable density. Very little is known about the effect of mild liquid shear on arrays of cells and it is conceivable that multicellular complexes (such as the "barrels" of Van der Loos, pp. 259–278 in this volume) could be isolated from cortical tissue. So far, the only multicellular complexes to be isolated from the brain are large fragments of capillary bed (Joó, personal communication, 1974); kidney glomerulae (Cook and Pickering, 1959) are an example from another type of tissue.

In the direction of subcellular complexes, the recent bulk isolation of cerebellar glomerulae (Balázs et al., 1975) — a complex subcellular structure consisting of the nerve terminal of a mossy fiber surrounded by torn-off granule cell dendrites and Golgi-type II nerve terminals, and encapsulated in a glial sheath — illustrates the effect of mild liquid shear, as applied by a hand-operated "homogenizer", to a specific area of the CNS. Such structures are somewhat more complex than the mossy fiber synaptosomes isolated by previous workers using more intense shear forces (Israël and Whittaker, 1965; Lemkey-Johnson and Larramendi, 1968; del Cerro et al., 1969) generated by motor-driven homogenizers.

One limitation inherent in many cellular or subcellular functions prepared from the brain is that they consist of elements derived from many different types of cells. Thus synaptosome preparations derived from cerebral cortex contain detached terminals from neurons utilizing many different transmitters. We have sought to overcome this difficulty by looking for simpler systems; as far as the cholinergic neuron is concerned, the electromotor system of the *Torpedo* has provided an hypertrophied model cholinergic system, all parts of which (cell bodies, axons and nerve terminals) are readily accessible and present in a large quantity. The remainder of this article will illustrate the potentialities of tissue fractionation techniques by describing recent work from my department on this system.

THE ELECTROMOTOR SYSTEM OF *TORPEDO:* A MODEL CHOLINERGIC SYSTEM

General description of the electromotor system

Elasmobranch fish belonging to the world-wide family of Torpedinidae possess large paired electric organs (Fig. 1A), one on each side of the head. These organs consist of stacks of flattened electrocytes, packed together in a honeycomb-like array. The electrocytes are derived embryologically from muscle (Fritsch, 1890) and possess a profuse innervation on their under surfaces. The nerve terminals (Fig. 1D) resemble those in muscle except that the synaptic vesicles, which are present in high concentration in the presynaptic terminal cytoplasm, are somewhat larger than in mammalian muscle, mean diameter 84 ± 4 S.E.M. (57) nm (Sheridan et al., 1966) compared with 45 ± 2 S.E.M. (406) nm (Andersson-Cedergren, 1959). As at the neuromuscular junction, transmission is cholinergic (Feldberg and Fessard, 1942), and these electric organs are among the richest of any animal tissue in acetylcholine. Choline acetyltransferase is also present in abundance. The postsynaptic membranes are rich in acetylcholinesterase and in a protein with the properties expected of a recognition-site in a nicotinic postsynaptic cholinoceptive receptor (for reviews see Heilbronn, 1975 and Raftery et al., 1975). The discharge of the organ, measured in air, reaches 25-35 V, and consists of the summated postsynaptic potentials of the synchronously stimulated electrocytes (Grundfest, 1957).

The cell bodies of the electromotor nerves innervating the electric organ are located in prominent paired lobes (Fig. 1A-C) on the dorsal surface of the brain stem. These are homologous with the hypoglossal nuclei of other vertebrates,

48

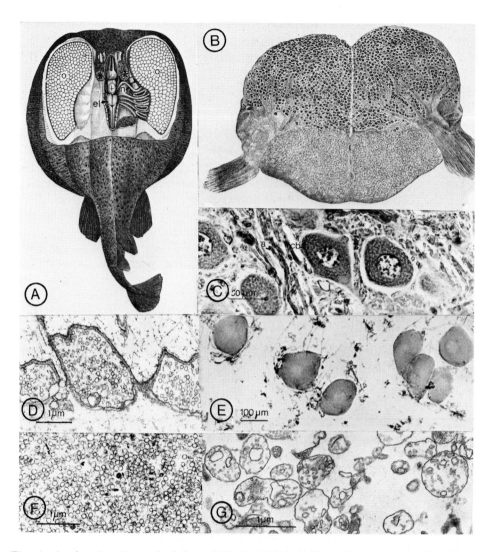

Fig. 1. A: drawing (retouched from Fritsch, 1890) of *Torpedo marmorata* showing (el)
electric lobes containing the cells of origin of the cholinergic electromotor neurons, (n)
electromotor nerve trunks and (o) electric organ. B: cross-section of the brain stem showing
the lobe (above) and command nucleus (below). C: enlargement of a paraffin section of the
lobe tissue showing (a) axons and (cb) cell bodies of the electromotor neurons. D: electron
microscopic cross-section of an electroplaque cell, showing ventral, innervated face with
electromotor nerve terminals. E: isolated electromotor perikarya obtained from hand-
homogenized electric lobe tissue by density gradient centrifuging (fraction c in Fig. 2a). F:
fraction (peak b in Fig. 4) rich in bound acetylcholine and synaptic vesicles obtained from a
cytoplasmic extract of comminuted electric organ by zonal centrifuging. G: synaptosomes
prepared from homogenized electric organ by density gradient centrifuging (fraction A_4 in
Fig. 2b).

but are greatly hypertrophied, weighing 200-400 mg in adult fish. The cell bodies are large (about 120 μm in diameter) and have several unusual characteristics. They are tightly packed in the lobe, being separated from each other only by thin sheets of glial material and without synapses. Their dendrites are few and thin but form numerous synapses whose presynaptic component derives from the neurons of the command nucleus below the electric lobes. Their axons pass out as 4 large myelinated nerve bundles on each side of the head to the electric organs. Their nuclei are large (about 40 μm in diameter) and usually have only one well-defined nucleolus, but two nucleoli are not uncommon. Their cytoplasm is unusually full of smooth-surfaced endoplasmic reticulum and vesicles of varying sizes, many of them the size of synaptic vesicles. The electromotor cells are not cholinoceptive, but the transmitter utilized by the command neurons has not yet been identified. ·

The electromotor system is thus an excellent one with which to study cholinergic mechanisms, particularly at the biochemical level, and may make a contribution to our understanding of the cholinergic system equivalent to that which another simple, hypertrophied system, the adrenal medullary cell, has made to adrenergic neurochemistry. In this section an account is given of some recent studies of this system made in our laboratory; for a fuller account, see other recent reviews by Whittaker and Zimmermann, 1976 and Dowdall et al., 1976, from which parts of this article have been abstracted.

Isolation of electromotor perikarya

If electric lobe tissue is dispersed by mild liquid shear (12-20 up- and down-strokes in a hand-operated loosely fitting homogenizer) in 1·5–1·8 M

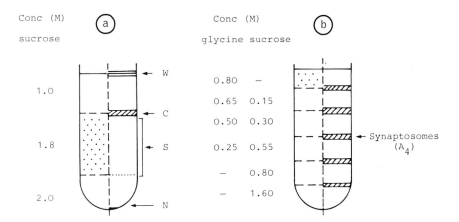

Fig. 2. Separation of (a) electromotor perikarya and (b) synaptosomes derived from electromotor terminals of *Torpedo marmorata*. The left hand side of each diagram shows the appearance of the tube before and the right hand side the appearance of the tube after centrifuging at (a) $10^6 \times g \times 30$ min and (b) $68,000 \times g \times 120$ min. In (a) the perikaryal fraction (C) sediments below a white pellicle (W) of axonal, dendritic and glial fragments and above a pellet of nuclei, N. The region S consists of the cytoplasmic contents and membranes of broken cells. In (b) the synaptosomes mainly sediment at the interface between 0·5 M glycine–0·3 M sucrose and 0·25 M glycine–0·55 M sucrose.

50

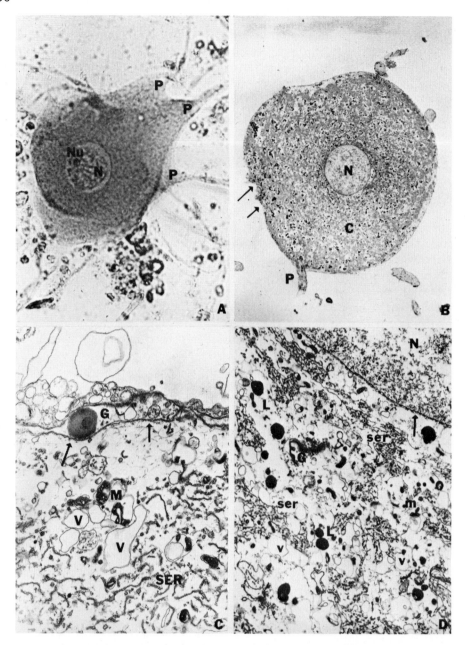

Fig. 3. A: phase contrast micrograph of an unfixed isolated electric lobe neuron from the cell body fraction of the sucrose gradient system. A spherical nucleus (N) and nucleolus (Nu) along with numerous neuronal processes (P) are present. x 450. B: light micrograph of an isolated electric lobe neuron processed for electron microscopy following sucrose gradient centrifugation. The integrity of the cell appears well maintained with a relatively homogenous cytoplasmic (C) and nuclear (N) component. The nuclear membrane remains intact whereas some ruptures have occurred along the plasma membrane (arrows). A stump of a neuronal process (P) still remains. Toluidine blue-stained 1 μm section. x 450. C: electron micrograph of the plasma membrane (arrows) and adjacent cytoplasm of an electric lobe neuron following sucrose gradient centrifugation. A glial element (G) remains adhered

sucrose, a large proportion of the electromotor perikarya, shorn of their dendrites and axons, survive intact and can be recovered by a simple density gradient procedure (Fig. 2) (Whittaker, 1975; Fiore and Whittaker, 1975; Whittaker et al., 1976). The cell fraction is free from major contamination; the cells appear to be well conserved, with most of their processes reduced to stumps (Figs. 1E and 3A, B). In the electron microscope (Fig. 3C, D) the plasma membrane is often largely intact (with areas still covered with thin sheets of glia), the cytoplasm retains its content of Golgi membranes and vesicles, and the nuclear membrane is well conserved. The yield of cells using dispersion in $1.8\ M$ sucrose is high: 249 ± 26 S.E.M. (10) /mg of tissue. The volume of a cell of $125\ \mu$m diameter is 1 nl; thus, if the tissue consisted *entirely* of cells of density 1.0, there would be 1000 cells/mg; the actual value might well be a half or a third of this. Fritsch (1890), counting axons and assuming one cell per axon, came up with the figure of 60,000 cells per lobe; for a mean paired lobe weight of 417 ± 25 S.E.M. (26) mg this is about 288 cells/mg.

There is much evidence from mammalian studies that cholinergic neurons contain the main components of the cholinergic system (acetylcholine, choline acetyltransferase and acetylcholinesterase) throughout their length. The electromotor neurons are no exception. Our isolated cell preparation contains appreciable amounts of all 3 components (Table II column 6, Table IV). Choline acetyltransferase and acetylcholinesterase are well localized in the cell body fraction (C), but appreciable amounts of acetylcholine are also recovered from the subnatant sucrose (S); in view of the presence of acetylcholinesterase in the preparation this must be bound — perhaps vesicular — acetylcholine, but the presence of vesicles in this fraction has yet to be established. The cytoplasmic marker lactate dehydrogenase is present in the cell body fraction but also in considerable amounts in the subnatant (S) fraction, indicating that this contains soluble cytoplasm, which is no doubt released during homogenization from broken glia, axons, dendrites and electromotor perikarya.

Measurements of enzyme occlusion showed that both choline acetyltransferase and lactate dehydrogenase were considerably occluded in the cell preparation (62 and 52% respectively); other evidence that a considerable proportion of the cells are sealed is that respiration in glucose is not markedly stimulated by the addition of the mitochondrial substrate succinate. By contrast, disrupted cells, in which mitochondria are freely accessible to substrates, utilize succinate but show little ability to metabolize glucose.

---

to the perikaryon. Mitochondria (M), clear vacuoles (V) and individual segments of smooth endoplasmic reticulum (SER) are distributed throughout the cytoplasm. ×15,750. D: interior of an electric lobe neuron showing nucleus (N) and nuclear membrane (arrow) along with mitochondria (m), vacuoles (v), smooth endoplasmic reticulum (ser), Golgi (G), and structures tentatively identified as lysosomes (L). × 10,800. (Results from Whittaker et al., 1976.)

TABLE II

DISTRIBUTION OF PROTEIN, ACETYLCHOLINE AND ENZYMES IN CELL FRACTIONS FROM THE ELECTRIC LOBES OF TORPEDO

Values are means ± range (two experiments) or S.E.M. (3 or more experiments)/g of tissue. Enzyme occlusion is measured as the difference between the activity in iso-osmotic reaction mixtures with and without the addition of detergent to disrupt cell membranes expressed as a percentage of total activity (i.e., that measured in the presence of detergent).

Component	Units	No. of experiments	Dispersion (units/g)	Distribution (as % of recovered) in*				Recovery (%)
				W	C	S	N	
Protein	mg	7	88·5 ± 23·6	9 ± 4	62 ± 9	26 ± 6	3 ± 1	89 ± 19
Acetylcholine	nmol	5	9·0 ± 4·4	10 ± 5	46 ± 5	36 ± 103	<8 ± 5	83 ± 22
Acetylcholinesterase	μmol/min	5	4·6 ± 2·2	1 ± 1	88 ± 2	11 ± 2	0 ± 0	102 ± 41
Choline acetyltransferase	nmol/min	6	311 ± 102	5 ± 5	70 ± 10	23 ± 5	2 ± 1	102 ± 21
(% occlusion)		2	(62 ± 8)	—	(62 ± 3)	—	—	—
Lactate dehydrogenase	μmol/min	4	26·0 ± 2·8	13 ± 9	32 ± 8	52 ± 7	3 ± 2	103 ± 24
(% occlusion)		4	(21 ± 2)	(60 ± 37)	(52 ± 12)	(12 ± 2)	(9 ± 9)	—

* W = white pellet of axonal, dendrite and glial fragments, C = perikaryal fraction, S = cytoplasm and broken cell membranes and N = nuclei (see Fig. 2).

Isolation of synaptosomes

The electric organ is highly collagenous, conventional mechanical homogenization is difficult and, unlike cerebral cortex, few synaptosomes are formed (Sheridan et al., 1966). Recently, however, synaptosomes (Fig. 1G) have been isolated in our laboratory from homogenized electric organ (Zimmermann and Dowdall, 1975a) in low yield, but high purity, by submitting the much less collagenous electric organ of juvenile fish to conventional homogenization, or by homogenizing the tissue of adult specimens after a very brief period of comminution in a blender, and then separating the synaptosomes on a density gradient (Fig. 2). Such synaptosomes have an extremely high acetylcholine

TABLE III

ACETYLCHOLINE CONTENT OF CHOLINERGIC SYNAPTOSOMES

Species, tissue	Acetylcholine content of synaptosome fraction (nmol/mg of protein)	Reference
Guinea pig, cerebral cortex	0·29	Barker et al., 1972
theoretical, for cholinergic synaptosomes*	31	see footnote
Squid, optic ganglia**	13·5	Dowdall and Whittaker, 1973
Torpedo, electric organ	41	Dowdall and Zimmermann, 1976

*Calculated on assumptions that guinea pig cerebral cortical homogenates contain (per g) 90 mg of protein, 15 nmol of acetylcholine (Barker et al., 1972) and $3·88 \times 10^{11}$ synaptosomes of mean radius of 0·56 μm (Clementi et al., 1966) of which 15% are cholinergic (Whittaker and Sheridan, 1965), and that the protein content of synaptosomes is the same as that of whole tissue.
**Calculated from results given in the reference.

concentration (Table III), even higher than that estimated for pure cholinergic synaptosomes from guinea pig brain. They are also rich in the high affinity choline uptake system (known to be specific for cholinergic terminals) in acetylcholinesterase and in choline acetyltransferase (Table IV). Comparisons of the concentrations of these components in the terminals and cell bodies can now be made, and it is clear that on a protein weight basis the terminal is richer in all of them than the cell body. This is consistent with the notion that the terminal is a region of very active transmitter storage and metabolism, and is a receiving area for components of the acetylcholine system manufactured by the cell body and transported thither by axonal flow.

Interestingly, neither cell bodies nor terminals have detectable amounts of the receptor protein (Dowdall, Heilbronn and Elfman, unpublished observations, 1975).

54

TABLE IV

COMPARISON OF THE COMPOSITION OF ISOLATED ELECTROMOTOR PERIKARYA
AND TERMINALS

| Component | Units | Activity (units/mg of protein) | | |
		Synaptosomes	Perikarya	Ratio
Lactate dehydrogenase	μmol/min	0·54	0·17	3·13
Acetylcholine	nmol	40·8	3·44	11·9
Choline acetyltransferase	nmol/min	15·0	4·03	3·72
Acetylcholinesterase	μmol/min	1·08	0·08	13·5
Choline uptake*	pmol/min**	139	6·21	22·3

* High affinity system; K_{T_H} = 2 μM at 24 $^{\circ}$C (synaptosomes) or 4 μM at 20 $^{\circ}$C (cells).
** V_{max} at 24 $^{\circ}$C (synaptosomes) or 20 $^{\circ}$C (cells).

Isolation of synaptic vesicles

The comminution of electric tissue normally leads to the rupture of
practically all the nerve terminals and the release of the synaptic vesicles. For
the relatively large scale preparation of synaptic vesicles we have found the best
and most rapid method of comminution to be crushing the tissue after
rendering it brittle by freezing in liquid nitrogen. The coarse powder so
obtained is then extracted with iso-osmotic saline, and the cytoplasmic extract
freed from larger particles by centrifuging at moderate g values.

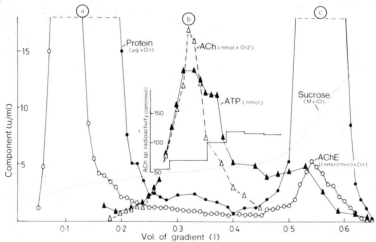

Fig. 4. Distribution of protein, acetylcholinesterase, acetylcholine and ATP in a density
gradient after centrifugal separation of 50 ml of a cytoplasmic extract derived from 50 g of
Torpedo mamorata electric organ in a zonal rotor. Note the presence of (a) solubilized
acetylcholinesterase and much soluble protein in an initial peak, (b) the presence of ATP and
acetylcholine in an intermediate peak identified morphologically as a peak of synaptic
vesicles and (c) particle-bound acetylcholinesterase in a third peak of membrane fragments
derived, in part, from postsynaptic membranes. The ACh/ATP ratio falls significantly on the
"dense" side of the isolated vesicle peak; this region is very radioactive if a pulse of
radiolabeled precursor is injected before the tissue is homogenized. (From Zimmermann and
Baker, 1975 (insert) and unpublished results of Ohsawa.)

Fig. 4 shows the results of centrifuging such a cytoplasmic extract of crushed, frozen electric organ into a density gradient using a 650 ml capacity zonal rotor. Three main peaks are apparent: a peak (SP) containing soluble cytoplasmic components, including (though not shown) lactate dehydrogenase, choline acetyltransferase, nucleotides (including ATP) and (shown) the soluble fraction of acetylcholinesterase; a second peak (VP) (see Fig. 1F) rich in vesicles, acetylcholine and also a second, vesicular fraction of ATP (Whittaker et al., 1972a, b; Dowdall et al., 1974), distinguishable from the ATP in fraction SP by its immunity to the hydrolytic action of a mixture of apyrase and

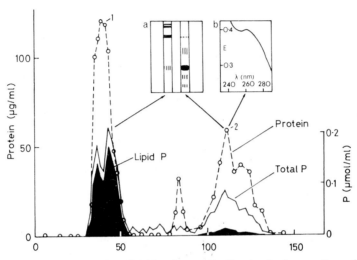

Fig. 5. Gel filtration, on Sephadex G-200, of osmotically shocked synaptic vesicles isolated from *Torpedo marmorata* electromotor synapses. Main diagram: vesicle protein (circles and broken line) appears in two main fractions, a void volume high-molecular-weight, membrane-bound fraction rich in phosphorus (continuous line) which is mainly lipid phosphorus (black profile), and a low-molecular-weight fraction rich in non-lipid phosphorus, identified, on the basis of its UV absorption (insert b), as nucleotide. On disc gel electrophoresis in SDS (insert a) the membrane-bound protein is found to comprise 3 main components (insert a, left diagram) whereas the soluble protein (presumably derived from the core) consists of only one main component (insert a, right) further identified as an acidic protein rich in glutamate, aspartate and serine residues (Whittaker et al., 1974). A small, phosphorus poor, intermediate peak has been identified as contaminating soluble cytoplasmic protein.

myokinase; and a third peak (MP) rich in membrane-bound acetylcholinesterase and containing numerous vesicular membrane fragments, probably derived from both the pre- and postsynaptic sides of the synapse. Numerous experiments have shown that the differences in the acetylcholine:ATP ratio across the peak are not due to experimental error; the vesicle population is intrinsically heterogeneous, and this heterogeneity is expressed by the width of the vesicle peak and variations in the acetylcholine:ATP ratio, and also by the acetylcholine content per vesicle across it. On stimulation, the vesicles of median density and highest acetylcholine:ATP ratio are the first to disappear (Zimmermann and Whittaker, 1974a).

Hypo-osmotic disruption of vesicles, followed by gel filtration on Sephadex G-200 (Fig. 5) (Whittaker et al., 1974), enables the vesicle proteins to be separated into two groups; one of these, seen to consist of 3 main (fairly high molecular weight) components when separated on disc gel electrophoresis (Fig. 5, insert a, left), comes through the void volume of the gel in association with lipid; the other, seen on gel electrophoresis to consist (Fig. 5, insert a, right) of one main low (approximately 10,000) molecular weight component (vesiculin), is associated with non-lipid (presumably necleotide) phosphorus, since it has a strong absorption at 260 nm (Fig. 5, insert b); this nucleotide phosphorus is believed to be derived from the vesicular ATP.

TABLE V

ACETYLCHOLINE CONTENT OF SYNAPTIC VESICLES FROM *TORPEDO*

Values relate to peak acetylcholine fractions and are means ± range (2) or S.D. (3 or more experiments; number of experiments in parentheses).

| | | Acetylcholine content | | |
Condition*	Fraction**	(nmol/mg of protein***)	(molecules/ vesicle) (x 10^{-3})	Reference
FT	ZVP	423 ± 162(4)	—	Nagy et al. (1975)
NA	ZVP	566 ± 144(4)	108 ± 29†(2)	Whittaker et al. (1972b)
A	ZVP	2310 ± 1110(6)	—	Zimmermann and Whittaker (1974a)
NA'	ZVP	4802 ± 1258(3)	—	
A	ZVP	4393 ± 1587(4)	78	Ohsawa et al. 1976
A	GVP	12,250 ± 2250(2)	90 ± 4(2)	

* FT, frozen tissue from fish anesthetized with Tricaine methosulfate before killing; NA, no anesthetic; NA', no anesthetic, brain rapidly crushed; A, anesthetized before killing.
** ZVP, zonal rotor peak as in Fig. 4 (peak b); GVP, synaptic vesicles free from soluble and membrane protein contamination by passing ZVP through a column of porous glass beads (pore size, 300 nm).
*** The higher results in the later experiments are mainly due to more effective removal of soluble protein contamination and reduced loss of vesicular acetylcholine during the intial preparatory stages.
† Vesicles counted after tagging with a known number of polystyrene beads and negative staining. Since counting techniques are not affected by contamination the most recent results are similar to the earlier ones.

So far we have not been successful in obtaining antibodies to vesiculin, but the vesicle membrane proteins have proved antigenic (Ulmar and Whittaker, 1974a, b), and have enabled us to determine the presence of vesicular membrane protein in the electromotor cell bodies and axons which accumulates in the latter above a ligature. Recent studies (Nagy et al., 1975; Ohsawa et al., 1975) have shown that residual soluble protein and larger membrane contamination, present in the vesicle peak obtained by zonal centrifuging, can be removed by filtration through columns of porous glass beads (pore size approximately 300 nm). Larger membrane fragments are excluded by the glass and pass out in the void volume; vesicles are then readily separated from soluble protein by making use of their large difference in elution volume. A method has been devised (Ohsawa et al., 1976) for counting the vesicles based on electron microscopy of the vesicles that adhere to a known area of filter after passage of a known volume of vesicle suspension, and in this way the number of acetylcholine molecules has been calculated to be about 90,000 (Table V). The detailed stoichiometry and lipid composition of the vesicles is now being worked out.

Effect of stimulation on vesicle yield and composition

Stimulation in vivo (Zimmermann and Whittaker, 1974a) at 5 Hz for up to 20,000 stimuli via the electric lobe (Fig. 6) causes a marked diminution in the

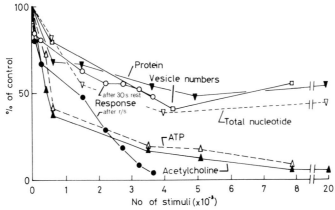

Fig. 6. Effect of stimulating the electromotor synapses of the *Torpedo* in vivo through electrodes placed on the electric lobe on vesicle numbers (□) as determined from micrographs of biopsy samples of organ, synaptic vesicle protein (▼), total nucleotide (▽), ATP (△) and acetylcholine (▲) determined in vesicles isolated from the organ after different periods of stimulation. Results are expressed as percentages of those from an unstimulated control organ denervated just before the experiment. Also included is the electrical response of the organ to repetitive stimulation at 5 Hz (●) and that following recovery for 30 sec (○). Responses are expressed as a percentage of the initial value. Note that short-term recovery appears to be limited by the proportion of vesicles surviving stimulation. (Results from Zimmermann and Whittaker, 1974a, b.)

response of the organ ($< 1\%$ of initial) and depletion of vesicle numbers, which can be detected morphologically in biopsy samples, and also in the fall in the yield of isolated vesicles. Such vesicles are, on average, depleted of both acetylcholine and ATP, but their vesiculin and adenine nucleotide contents remain normal. Presumably, however, the vesiculin, ATP and acetylcholine of the vesicles which have disappeared have been released; direct evidence for the release of ATP as well as acetylcholine at the neuromuscular junction has recently been obtained (Silinsky, 1975). Morphological studies provide evidence for massive exocytosis of vesicles, with a consequent increase in the surface area of the external presynaptic membrane. However, it is difficult to bring about complete ($> 70\%$) depletion in vesicle numbers or ($> 90\%$) in transmitter content.

58

Recovery appears to take place in 3 stages. In *stage 1* there is a rapid recovery (within minutes) of the response of the organ to single test shocks: this is shown by the empty circles in Fig. 6. This recovery appears to be limited by the *store of remaining vesicles* (note coincidence of limit of electro-physiological response and amount of vesicle protein left in the tissue) but the amount of vesicular acetylcholine and ATP remains low. *Stage 2* of recovery, in which the organ recovers its response completely to single shocks, is accompanied by a *return of vesicle numbers to normal* and takes place in hours (8–24 hr) rather than minutes. However, the organ remains abnormally fatigable (see Fig. 7, dotted line), i.e., its response to repetitive stimulation declines abnormally rapidly. At this stage of recovery, vesicular acetylcholine and ATP remain extremely low. *Stage 3*, or complete recovery, takes days (3–8

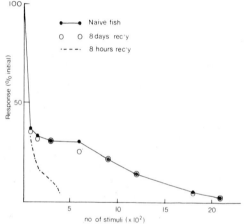

Fig. 7. Response of organ to repetitive stimulation at 5 Hz of the electromotor system through the electric lobes (a) initially (filled circles), (b) after 8 hr recovery (broken line) and (c) after 8 days recovery (open circles). Note that after 8 hr the organ has recovered its responsiveness to an initial stimulus, but is abnormally fatigable (as measured by the smaller number of stimuli required to produce a state of exhaustion (response < 1% of initial).
Temperature of fish during recovery was $12°C$. (Unpublished results of Zimmermann.)

days or more at $12°C$) rather than hours and is accompanied by the return to normal, first of vesicular acetylcholine and then of vesicular ATP. Fig. 7 (open circles) shows the recovery of normal fatigability, and Fig. 8 summarizes the time course of return to normal of (upper traces) responsiveness to single and repetitive stimuli and of (lower traces) vesicle numbers, acetylcholine and ATP. During the period of the reappearance of "empty" vesicles (1–2 days) repetitive restimulation of the organ causes depletion of vesicles without, as we have seen, normal responsiveness of the postsynaptic membrane; thus vesicle exocytosis in response to stimulation does not depend on normal levels of transmitter.

Other recent studies (Zimmermann and Dowdall, 1975b) indicate that in addition to the massive exocytosis observed under conditions of repetitive stimulation to exhaustion, transient exocytosis occurs. If organs in vitro are stimulated at a low rate (e.g., 0·1 Hz), vesicle reformation and reloading can apparently more easily keep pace with stimulation; the "shoulder" apparent in the response of the organ and in the levels of vesicular acetylcholine and ATP in Figs. 6 and 7 is much shallower and more prolonged (> 6 hr). If, during prolonged (6 hr) stimulation at such low rates, dextran is perfused through the organ, the dextran is taken up by about 80% of the vesicles as shown both by morphological observation on whole tissue and by isolation of the vesicles; this shows that at some time during stimulation, 80% of the vesicle interiors have been in communication with the extracellular space.

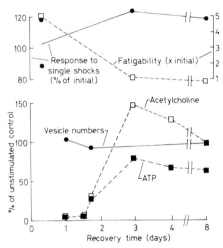

Fig. 8. Time course of recovery, in an organ stimulated to exhaustion, of (bottom diagram) vesicle numbers (●), vesicular ATP (■), vesicular acetylcholine (□) and (upper diagram) responsiveness to single shocks (●) and fatigability (□). The fatigability is measured as the reciprocal of the number of pulses required to reduce the response of the organ to 1% of initial and is plotted relative to the initial fatigability of the organ. Note that whereas responsiveness to single shocks returns to normal *pari passu* with vesicle numbers (and may thereafter become supernormal), fatigability only returns to normal as vesicular acetylcholine and ATP recover. Temperature of fish during recovery was $12°C$. (Results from Whittaker et al., 1975.)

False transmitters in the cholinergic system

False transmitters may be defined as structural analogues of a natural transmitter which are stored by presynaptic nerve terminals and released on stimulation. If the structural analogue has, as is often the case, a smaller action on the postsynaptic receptors than the natural agonist, but a comparable affinity for them, it will exert a competitive blocking action. Such false transmitters have provided, in the adrenergic field, good evidence (for review see Smith, 1972) that for a substance to be released from an adrenergic terminal on stimulation it must first be taken up into the synaptic vesicles.

It has recently been found that certain analogues of choline, notably N-methyl-N-hydroxyethylpyrrolidinium (PCh) iodide, are readily taken up by cholinergic nerve terminals and acetylated (Barker and Mittag, 1974; Barker et

60

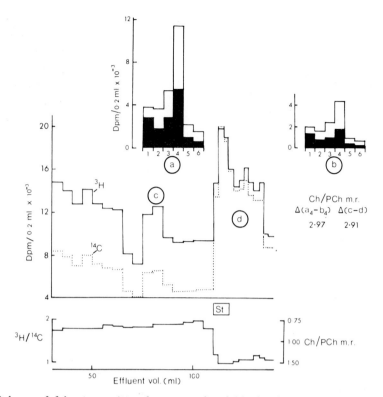

Fig. 9. Release of false transmitter from a perfused block of innervated electric organ in vitro. Main diagram: level of ^{3}H and ^{14}C due, respectively, to N-methyl-N-hydroxy-ethylpyrrolidinium (PCh) and choline (Ch) in effluent from a perfused tissue block (c) before stimulation and (d) during and following stimulation at 5 Hz for 10 min. The tracing below shows the change in the ratio of ^{3}H to ^{14}C and the molar ratio (m.r.) of choline to PCh calculated from it. Before (a) and after (b) stimulation vesicles were isolated from tissue samples by density gradient centrifuging and ^{3}H (white blocks) and ^{14}C (black blocks) were determined in the gradient. The highest radioactivity was associated with the vesicles (fraction 4). From comparisons of c and d and fraction 4 of a and b (a_4, b_4) the molar ratio of the bases lost from the tissue [Δ(c−d)] or the vesicles [Δ(a_4−b_4)] as a result of stimulation can be calculated. The two ratios show good agreement (insert table). (Results of Zimmermann and Dowdall, 1975b.)

al., 1974, 1975). The acetate ester of this base has now been found to be a false transmitter at the electromotor synapse (Zimmermann and Dowdall, 1975a, b). A typical experiment is shown in Fig. 9. A block of electric tissue comprising the territory of a single electromotor nerve trunk was perfused with ^{14}C-labeled choline and ^{3}H-labeled PCh while low frequency stimulation (0.1 Hz) was applied through the nerve to promote uptake of transmitter into vesicles. Paraoxon was added to block cholinesterases. The tissue block was then perfused with choline and PCh-free medium for 3 hr to wash out isotopes. Hemicholinium-3 was added to the perfusion medium to block reuptake. The final stages of this wash-out are seen as section c of Fig. 9.

On stimulating the organ at 5 Hz, there was an increased output of *both* isotopes indicating that both [^{14}C]choline and [^{3}H]PCh were being released. Extraction of the bases by a liquid ion-exchange technique followed by chromatography showed that the additional amounts of the bases appearing in the perfusate as a result of stimulation were in the form of the acetate esters. The molecular ratio choline:PCh of the extra amounts of base appearing as a result of stimulation $[\Delta(c-d)]$ was found to be 2·91, or 3·79 if calculated as the basis of the acetate esters released (the latter figure is less reliable due to the additional manipulations involved in extraction and separation of the bases). Vesicles were isolated from the tissue blocks (a) just before and (b) just after stimulation. As is seen in Fig. 9a and b, the isolated vesicles (localized in fraction 4 of the density gradient) contained both isotopes, but there was less in the vesicle fraction isolated *after* stimulation than before. By comparing these two vesicle fractions it was possible to calculate the molar ratio of the bases lost from the vesicles disappearing as a result of stimulation $[\Delta(a_4-b_4)]$: the result is 2·97. Thus the results as a whole are entirely consistent with the view that released transmitter (true or false) comes from the vesicle fraction.

A difficulty with experiments in which radioactive choline alone is used to label the transmitter pools as a preliminary to identifying the source of released transmitter (Chakrin and Whittaker, 1969; Potter, 1970; Collier, 1969; Chakrin et al., 1972; Dunant et al., 1972) is that, if the vesicle population is metabolically heterogeneous (and there is now direct evidence that it is: Zimmermann and Baker, 1975), the specific radioactivity of a homogenate or an isolated vesicle fraction does not necessarily reflect the specific radioactivity of that portion of the vesicle pool that is involved in release. The use of two labeled bases, as in the experimental design just described, avoids this difficulty and enables the pool directly involved in transmitter release to be identified.

DISCUSSION

The work described in the previous section will have served to illustrate the wide range of neuronal structures, from perikarya 100 μm or more in diameter to synaptic vesicles one thousand times smaller, that can be isolated by present-day tissue fractionation techniques, and how by applying these techniques to physiological preparations in different functional states (resting, stimulated and recovered) specific processes, such as the mechanism of transmitter storage and release, can be better understood in molecular terms.

The work on the electromotor synapse of *Torpedo* has, in fact, provided convincing additional evidence for the role of synaptic vesicles in transmitter storage and release in a cholinergic system. It now seems clear that synaptic vesicles in cholinergic nerve terminals undergo two kinds of exocytosis: (1) transient exocytosis, which can be detected by high molecular weight markers which are normally incapable of crossing the presynaptic plasma membrane, and (2) full exocytosis in which vesicle contents are lost in toto and the membrane — at least for a while — fuses with, and forms part of, an extended plasma membrane. Our morphological observations with the electromotor synapse are paralleled by similar observations on the mammalian or amphibian neuromuscular junctions by other workers. Thus Heuser and Reese (1973), Ceccarelli et al. (1972, 1973) and Ceccarelli and Hurlbut (1975) have shown that horseradish peroxidase is readily taken up into vesicles upon stimulation, whereas depletion of vesicles by fusion with the external membrane has also been demonstrated upon prolonged stimulation (Korneliusson, 1972; Ceccarelli et al., 1972; Heuser and Reese, 1973) or treatment with Black Widow spider venom (Clark et al., 1972) or lanthanum (Heuser and Miledi, 1971). In the absence of toxic agents, vesicles readily reform locally, and this is independent of their transmitter content as measured by Black Widow spider venom-induced release of miniature potentials (Ceccarelli and Hurlbut, 1975).

The dual advantage of the electromotor system of *Torpedo* is: firstly, that the processes of vesicle reformation and reloading are slower than in muscle, and can thus be more easily dissociated; and, secondly, that vesicles can be isolated from the tissue and their content of exocytosis-markers and transmitter determined directly. These techniques have shown that vesicles undergoing transient exocytosis retain their capacity to store transmitter whereas vesicles reformed after extensive "full" exocytosis has taken place are largely empty. Since restoration of normal transmitter levels is a slow process with a time-scale comparable to that of axonal flow it is likely that vesicles reformed after "full" exocytosis are not competent to store transmitter and may have to return to the cell body for reprocessing. Such vesicles may have to be replaced by vesicles freshly synthesized in the cell body and conveyed to the terminal by axonal flow. A fuller understanding of vesicle synthesis and translocation is needed, and seems to be attainable by application of the techniques described in this review.

REFERENCES

Andersson-Cedergren, E. (1959) Ultrastructure of motor end plate and sarcoplasmic components of mouse skeletal muscle fiber as revealed by three-dimensional reconstructions from serial sections. *J. Ultrastruct. Res.*, Suppl. 1.

Balázs, R., Hajós, F., Johnson, A.L., Reynierse, G.L.A., Tapia, R. and Wilkin, G.P. (1975) Subcellular fractionation of rat cerebellum: an electron microscopic and biochemical investigation. III. Isolation of large fragments of the cerebellar glomeruli. *Brain Res.*, 86: 17–30.

Barker, L.A. and Mittag, T.W. (1974) Comparative studies of substrate and inhibitors of choline transport and choline acetyltransferase. *J. Pharmacol.*, 192: 86–94.

Barker, L.A., Dowdall, M.J. and Whittaker, V.P. (1972) Choline metabolism in the cerebral cortex of guinea pigs: stable-bound acetylcholine. *Biochem. J.*, 130: 1063–1080.

Barker, L.A., Dowdall, M.J., Vickers, G.R. and Mittag, T.W. (1974) High affinity choline transport: uptake and metabolism of choline and pyrrolcholine by synaptosomes from the optic lobe of squid (*Loligo pealii*). *Biol. Bull.*, 147: 468 (abstract).

Barker, L.A., Dowdall, M.J. and Mittag, T.W. (1975) Comparative studies on synaptosomes: high affinity uptake and acetylation of [^{3}H]choline and [^{3}H]N-methyl-N-hydroxy-ethylpyrrolidinium by squid optic lobe synaptosomes. *Brain Res.*, 86: 434–438.

Bauer, J.H. und Pickels, E.G. (1940) Hochgeschwindigkeits-Ultrazentrifuge mit Luftturbine-antrieb. In *Die Ultrazentrifuge, Handbuch der Kolloidwiss.*, Vol. 7, Th. Svedberg and K.O. Pedersen (Eds.), Steinkopff, Dresden, pp. 167–189.

Bensley, R.R. and Hoerr, N. (1934) Studies on cell structure by the freeze-drying method. VI. The preparation and properties of mitochondria. *Anat. Rec.*, 60: 449–455.

Ceccarelli, B. and Hurlbut, W.P. (1975) The effects of prolonged repetitive stimulation in hemicholinum on the frog neuromuscular junction. *J. Physiol. (Lond.)*, 247: 163–188.

Ceccarelli, B., Hurlbut, W.P. and Mauro, A. (1972) Depletion of vesicles from frog neuromuscular junction by prolonged tetanic stimulation. *J. Cell Biol.*, 54: 30–38.

Ceccarelli, B., Hurlbut, W.P. and Mauro, A. (1973) Turnover of transmitter and synaptic vesicles at the frog neuromuscular junction. *J. Cell Biol.*, 57: 499–524.

Chakrin, L.W. and Whittaker, V.P. (1969) The subcellular distribution of [N-Me-^{3}H]acetylcholine synthesized by brain in vivo. *Biochem. J.*, 118: 97–107.

Chakrin, L.W., Marchbanks, R.M., Mitchell, J.F. and Whittaker, V.P. (1972) The origin of the acetylcholine released from the surface of the cortex. *J. Neurochem.*, 19: 2727–2736.

Clark, A.W., Hurlbut, W.P. and Mauro, A. (1972) Changes in the fine structure of the neuromuscular junction of the frog caused by black widow spider venom. *J. Cell Biol.*, 52: 1–14.

Clementi, F., Whittaker, V.P. and Sheridan, M.N. (1966) The yield of synaptosomes from the cerebral cortex of guinea pigs estimated by a polystyrene bead "tagging" procedure. *Z. Zellforsch.*, 72: 126–138.

Collier, B. (1969) The preferential release of newly synthesized transmitter by a sympathetic ganglion. *J. Physiol. (Lond.)*, 205: 341–352.

Cook, W.F. and Pickering, G.W. (1959) The location of renin in the rabbit kidney. *J. Physiol. (Lond.)*, 149: 526–536.

del Cerro, M.P., Snider, R.S. and Oster, M.L. (1969) Subcellular fractions of adult and developing rat cerebellum. *Exp. Brain Res.*, 8: 311–320.

Dowdall, M.J. and Whittaker, V.P. (1973) Comparative studies in synaptosome formation: the preparation of synaptosomes from the head ganglion of the squid, *Loligo pealii. J. Neurochem.*, 20: 921–935.

Dowdall, M.J. and Zimmermann, H. (1976) Purification and properties of peripheral cholinergic synaptosomes from the electric organ of *Torpedo.* In preparation.

Dowdall, M.J., Boyne, A.F. and Whittaker, V.P. (1974) Adenosine triphosphatase: a constituent of cholinergic synaptic vesicles. *Biochem. J.*, 140: 1–12.

Dowdall, M.J., Fox, G., Wächtler, K., Whittaker, V.P. and Zimmermann, H. (1976) Recent studies on the comparative biochemistry of the cholinergic neuron. *Cold Spr. Harb. Symp. quant. Biol.*, 40: 65–81.

Dunant, Y., Gautron, J., Israël, M., Lesbats, B. et Manaranche, R. (1972) Les compartiments d'acétylcholine de l'organe électrique de la torpille et leur modifications par la stimulation. *J. Neurochem.*, 19: 1987–2020.

Feldberg, W. and Fessard, A. (1942) The cholinergic nature of the nerves to the electric organ of the Torpedo (*Torpedo marmorata*). *J. Physiol. (Lond.)*, 101: 200–215.

Fiore, L. and Whittaker, V.P. (1975) Isolation of cell bodies of cholinergic neurones from the electric lobe of *Torpedo marmorata. Abstr. 5th Int. Meet. Int. Soc. Neurochem.*, Barcelona, p. 130.

Fritsch, G. (1890) *Die elektrischen Fische. Zweite Abteilung. Die Torpedineen*, von Veit, Leipzig.

Gray, E.G. and Whittaker, V.P. (1960) The isolation of synaptic vesicles from the central nervous system. *J. Physiol. (Lond.)*, 153: 35–37P.

Gray, E.G. and Whittaker, V.P. (1962) The isolation of nerve endings from brain: an electron-microscope study of cell fragments derived by homogenization and centrifugation. *J. Anat. (Lond.)*, 96: 79–88.

Grundfest, H. (1957) The mechanisms of discharge of the electric organs in relation to general and comparative electrophysiology. *Progr. Biophys.*, 7: 1–85.

Heilbronn, E. (1975) Biochemistry of cholinergic receptors. In *Cholinergic Mechanisms*, P.G. Waser (Ed.), Raven Press, New York, pp. 343–364.

Heuser, J. and Miledi, R. (1971) The effect of lanthanum ions on function and structure of frog neuromuscular junction. *Proc. roy. Soc. B*, 179: 247–260.

Heuser, J.E. and Reese, T.S. (1973) Evidence for recycling of synaptic vesicle membrane during transmitter release at the frog neuromuscular junction. *J. Cell Biol.*, 57: 315–344.

Israël, M. and Whittaker, V.P. (1965) The isolation of mossy-fibre endings from the granular layers of the cerebellar cortex. *Experientia (Basel)*, 21: 325–326.

Korneliusson, H. (1972) Ultrastructure of normal and stimulated motor endplates. *Z. Zellforsch.*, 130: 28–57.

64

Lemkey-Johnson, N. and Larramendi, L.M.H. (1968) The separation and identification of fractions of non-myelinated axons from the cerebellum of the cat. *Exp. Brain Res.*, 5: 326–340.

Nagy, A., Baker, R.R., Morris, S.J. and Whittaker, V.P. (1976) The preparation and characterization of synaptic vesicles of high purity. *Brain Res.*, 109: 285–309.

Ohsawa, K., Dowe, G.H.C., Morris, S.J. and Whittaker, V.P. (1976) Preparation of ultra-pure synaptic vesicles from the electric organ of *Torpedo marmorata* by porous glass bead chromatography and estimation of their acetylcholine content. *Exp. Brain Res.*, 24: 19.

Porter, K.R. and Novikoff, A.B. (1974) The 1974 Nobel Prize for physiology and medicine. *Science*, 186: 516–520.

Potter, L.T. (1970) Synthesis storage and release of [^{14}C]acetylcholine in isolated rat diaphram muscles. *J. Physiol. (Lond.)*, 206: 145–166.

Raftery, M.A., Bode, J., Vandlen, R., Chao, Y., Deutsch, J., Duguid, J.R., Reed, K. and Moody, T. (1975) Characterization of an acetylcholine receptor. In *Biochemistry of Sensory Functions*, L. Jaenicke (Ed.), Springer Verlag, Berlin, pp. 541–563.

Sheridan, M.N., Whittaker, V.P. and Israël, M. (1966) The subcellular fractionation of the electric organ of *Torpedo*. *Z. Zellforsch.*, 74: 291–307.

Silinsky, E.M. (1975) On the association between transmitter secretion and the release of adenine nucleotides from mammalian motor nerve terminals. *J. Physiol. (Lond.)*, 247: 145–162.

Smith, A.D. (1972) Cellular control of the uptake, storage and release of noradrenaline in sympathetic nerves. *Biochem. Soc. Symp.*, 36: 103–131.

Svedberg, Th. und Pedersen, K.O. (Eds.) (1940) *Die Ultrazentrifuge, Handbuch der Kolloidwiss.*, Vol. 7, Steinkopff, Dresden.

Ulmar, G. and Whittaker V.P. (1974a) Immunological approach to the characterization of cholinergic vesicular protein. *J. Neurochem.*, 22: 451–454.

Ulmar, G. and Whittaker, V.P. (1974b) Immunohistochemical localization and immuno-electrophoresis of cholinergic synaptic vesicle protein constituents from the *Torpedo*. *Brain Res.*, 71: 155–159.

Whittaker, V.P. (1960) The binding of neurohormones by subcellular particles of brain tissue. In *Regional Neurochemistry: The Regional Chemistry, Physiology and Pharmacology of the Nervous System, Proc. 4th Int. Neurochem. Symp. Varenna*, S.S. Kety and J. Elkers (Eds.), Pergamon, London, pp. 259–263.

Whittaker, V.P. (1975) Aspects of the biochemistry of cholinergic transmission in *Torpedo* and *Loligo*. In *Biochemistry of Sensory Functions*, L. Jaenicke (Ed.), Springer Verlag, Berlin, pp. 515–534.

Whittaker, V.P. and Sheridan, M.N. (1965) The morphology and acetylcholine content of cerebral cortical synaptic vesicles. *J. Neurochem.*, 12: 363–372.

Whittaker, V.P. and Zimmermann, H. (1976) The innervation of the electric organ of Torpedinidae: a model cholinergic system. In *Biochemical Perspectives in Marine Biology, Vol. 3*, D.C. Malins and J.R. Sargent (Eds.), Academic Press, London, pp. 253–302.

Whittaker, V.P., Michaelson, I.A. and Kirkland, R.J.A. (1964) The separation of synaptic vesicles from nerve-ending particles ("synaptosomes"). *Biochem. J.*, 90: 293–303.

Whittaker, V.P., Dowdall, M.J. and Boyne, A.F. (1972a) The storage and release of acetylcholine by cholinergic nerve terminals: recent results with non-mammalian preparations. *Biochem. Soc. Symp.*, 36: 49–68.

Whittaker, V.P., Essman, W.B. and Dowe, G.H.C. (1972b) The isolation of pure cholinergic synaptic vesicles from the electric organs of elasmobranch fish of the family Torpedinidae. *Biochem. J.*, 128: 833–846.

Whittaker, V.P., Dowdall, M.J., Dowe, G.H C., Facino, R.M. and Scotto, J. (1974) Proteins of cholinergic synaptic vesicles from the electric organ of *Torpedo*: characterization of a low-molecular-weight acidic protein. *Brain Res.*, 75: 115–131.

Whittaker, V.P., Zimmermann, H. and Dowdall, M.J. (1975) The biochemistry of cholinergic synapses as exemplified by the electric organ of *Torpedo*. *J. Neural. Trans.*, Suppl. 12: 39–60.

Whittaker, V.P., Fox, G. and Fiore, L. (1976) Isolation of the perikarya of the cholinergic electromotor neurones of *Torpedo marmorata. Exp. Brain Res.*, 25: 22.

Zimmermann, H. and Baker, R.R. (1975) Separation of a small pool of highly labelled vesicular components after electrical stimulation of the *Torpedo* electric organ. *Pflügers Arch. ges. Physiol.*, 359 (Suppl.): 163.

Zimmermann, H. and Dowdall, M.J. (1975a) Synthesis, vesicular uptake and release of a cholinergic false transmitter. *Abstract 5th Int. Meet. Int. Soc. Neurochem.*, Barcelona. Exp. Brain Res., 23: Suppl. 225.

Zimmermann, H. and Dowdall, M.J. (1975b) Uptake and release of low- and high-molecular-weight substances from cholinergic vesicles. *Abstract First Europ. Neurosci. Meet.*, Munich, p. 225.

Zimmermann, H. and Whittaker, V.P. (1974a) Effect of electrical stimulation on the yield and composition of synaptic vesicles from the cholinergic synapses of the electric organ of *Torpedo:* a combined biochemical, electrophysiological and morphological study. *J. Neurochem.*, 22: 435–450.

Zimmermann, H. and Whittaker, V.P. (1974b) Different recovery rates of the electro-physiological, biochemical and morphological parameters in the cholinergic synapses of the *Torpedo* electric organ after stimulation. *J. Neurochem.*, 22: 1109–1114.

Functional Biochemistry
of Neurons and Glial Cells

S.P.R. ROSE

Brain Research Group, Open University, Walton Hall, Milton Keynes
(Great Britain)

INTRODUCTION

The title of the present paper is so broad that it could contain virtually every aspect of our biochemical knowledge of brain activity. What I will discuss, however, will be much more restricted, as biochemistry's ignorance concerning the metabolic and structural — let alone functional — interrelationships between neurons and their surrounding cellular milieu remains profound. I do not even propose to attempt to review systematically what knowledge we have. I have tried (as have others) to do this elsewhere (e.g., Johnston and Roots, 1970; Rose, 1972, 1975; Hamberger and Sellström, 1975). Instead it seems to me more fitting to discuss here some particular problems and methods which our laboratory is developing.

Our aim is to describe the biochemical dynamics of neuronal/glial interactions in the adult brain, and to relate these both to those genetic and developmental pathways through which they arise and by which they are determined, and also to the capacity of the brain as a system to make transient and longer-term plastic responses to changed environmental circumstances. Thus throughout our work we are concerned not so much with static structures as with flux and process. Our approach over the last decade — now adopted in a considerable number of laboratories — has been that of the separation and preparation, on a relatively large scale, of neuronal and glial cell fractions, from developing and adult brain regions, in conditions which enable their metabolism, in vivo or in vitro, to be followed.

The basic method has been derived, with only minor modifications, from that first published 10 years ago (Rose, 1965, 1967) and will not be described in detail. Essentially, brain tissue is mechanically disaggregated into an isotonic, buffered Ficoll-containing medium and subjected to density gradient centrifugation. Four fractions are recovered, of which two principally concern us here; a glial cell-enriched fraction, containing some 10–20% of the starting tissue protein, which we call B, or *neuropil*, and a neuronal cell body-enriched fraction, C, containing some 5–10% of the starting protein. These and the other fractions can be collected and further subfractionated — for example into subcellular fractions, or into individual protein components by gel or chromatographic methods.

Enzymes or structural substances present in the cell fractions can be compared, and cellular metabolism studied in vitro, or separation may follow in vivo administration of isotopes. Such techniques have enabled us to report on, for instance, the neuronal concentration of lysosomal enzymes (Sinha and Rose, 1972), and the compartmentation of glucose and amino acid metabolism (Rose, 1970). I do not propose to review this work in detail, but merely to make here the point that interpretation of data derived from cell fractions in terms of properties of the in vivo system demands circumspection. First, it must be remembered that in the intact tissue the cell body fractions whose metabolism is being studied represent only a few per cent of the total tissue volume, the rest being composed of processes, synaptic junctions, capillaries, endothelial cells — and extracellular space (Blinkov and Glezer, 1968; Rose, 1972). Second, cell fractions may give misleading results because of the presence of contaminants and of cell damage, sometimes adversely affecting one cell type differentially. The precautions which enable these problems to be, if not circumvented, then at least minimized, have been reviewed elsewhere (Rose, 1972, 1975); the crucial points are that comparisons should always be between cell fractions derived from the same gradient; and that recovery studies and light microscopic examination of the fractions and/or marker enzyme assay, for instance of β-galactosidase for neurons and carbonic anhydrase for glia, should be routinely carried out. It is regrettable how often one still reads papers reporting results for which these precautions have been omitted.

With this background, I would like to describe briefly 4 recent developments from our laboratory, the first two still primarily at the methodological stage and the others revealing an important aspect of metabolic interaction between neurons and glia and its sensitivity to changes in the environment of the organism.

ISOLATION OF CELL FRACTIONS FROM THE DEVELOPING BRAIN

We have known for several years that our cell isolation method works well only with relatively adult brain tissue: in rats, above about 3 weeks of age. Below this age, little or no glial material can be obtained. This is partly because in the young rat there is, of course, very much less neuropil present, and partly because the cells appear to change their properties on the gradient with age, perhaps as a function of their changing lipid content. We have, therefore (A Sinha, L. Sinha, Spears and Rose, unpublished; Sinha et al., 1975), developed a modified gradient system from which neuronal and neuropil fractions can be obtained from forebrain (cortex) of rats from just neonatal to 21 days and older. In this procedure, the tissue is disaggregated by chopping in a buffered medium containing 8% Ficoll and polyvinylpyrrolidone, passing through successively finer nylon meshes, and finally filtering through a 40 μm stainless steel mesh. The gradient system is still a two-stage one, as for the adult system, but its composition is changed, the bottom layer consisting of 1.7 M sucrose, above which is 30% Ficoll. Centrifugation is for 30 min at 13,000 × g. This procedure yields a neuropil fraction at the 8%–30% Ficoll interface in which

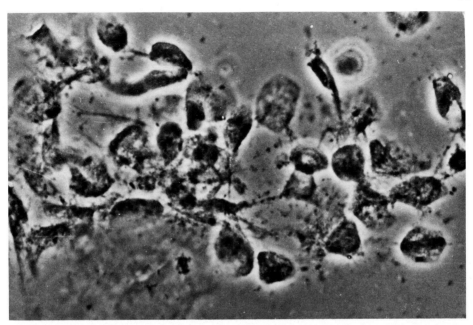

Fig. 1. Unfixed neuronal perikarya and neuroblasts from 1-day-old rat forebrain. Phase contrast, × 1500.

TABLE I

PROTEIN, DNA AND RNA RATIOS IN NEURON AND GLIAL ENRICHED FRACTIONS FROM CEREBRAL CORTEX IN DIFFERENT AGED RATS

Each gradient was derived from 3–6 rat brains of the stated ages (day of birth is day 0) as starting material, and each ratio is the mean of the 14 determinations not differing by more than ± 10% S.E.M. (From Sinha et al., 1975.) The elevation in RNA/DNA ratio in both cell types at day 10 is significant ($P < 0.01$).

	Age (days)				
	2	5	10	15	20
Neurons					
RNA/DNA	2·4	2·8	6·9	7·1	9·4
Protein/DNA	2·6	2·6	2·7	3·2	3·3
Neuropil					
RNA/DNA	11·3	8·2	20·6	21·7	13·1
Protein/DNA	2·1	3·5	4·4	3·2	4·4

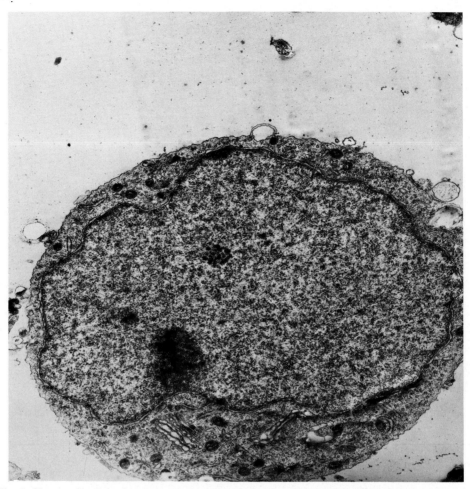

Fig. 2. Neuronal cell body observed in initial tissue suspension after disruption of 1-day-old rat forebrain. The suspension was fixed with 1.5% aqueous gluturaldehyde for 30 min, centrifuged at 10,000 revs/min for 5 min and postfixed in osmium tetroxide for 1 hr. Pellets were embedded in durcurpan, sectioned on a Reichert OM U 3 ultramicrotome and strained with uranyl acetate and lead citrate. × 15,000.

78% of the identifiable cell bodies are glial, and a neuronal fraction at the 30% Ficoll–sucrose interface in which 80% of the identifiable cells are neuronal. The criteria for this identification have been discussed elsewhere (Sinha and Rose, 1971). Fig. 1 shows a field of unfixed, isolated neurons from 1-day-old rat forebrain viewed under phase contrast; Fig. 2 is an electron micrograph of a single immature neuron showing well preserved morphology, including an external cell membrane and organized cytoplasmic structure. For comparison purposes a similar cell, as it appears in a sectioned tissue block, is presented in Fig. 3. The electron microscopic appearance of these cells is better than we have yet been able to achieve with material from adult cortex, and we have been able to use the neuronal and neuropil fractions to follow the ontogeny of RNA and protein metabolism, both in vivo and in vitro. Some data on protein, DNA and RNA levels during development are presented in Table I.

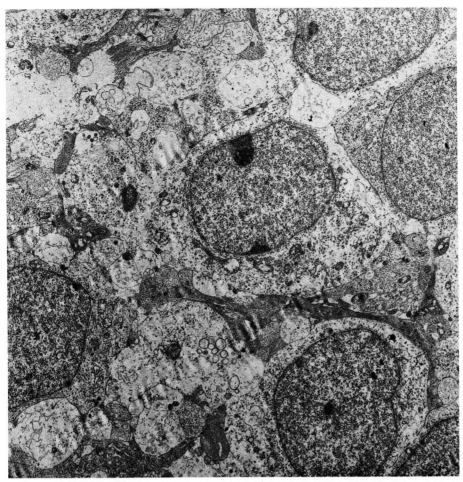

Fig. 3. A tissue block from 1-day-old rat forebrain was sliced into 1 mm pieces, fixed, embedded and stained as in the caption to Fig. 2. × 10,000.

ISOLATION OF CEREBELLAR CELL TYPES

The unique organization of the cerebellum, with its distinctive neuronal types and well-defined wiring diagram, has over the past few years begun to make it a favored preparation for both physiological and biochemical study (e.g., Eccles et al., 1967). What is more, the existence of a series of neurologically mutant mouse strains in which there seems to be a very specific defect in cellular ontogeny in the cerebellum, associated with characteristic behavioral abnormalities (the Weaver, Staggerer, Reeler etc. strains), also suggests that the availability of homogeneous preparations of particular cell types, derived from normal and mutant cerebellar tissue at different stages during development, could represent a powerful contribution to the elucidation of key features of cerebellar specificity. Making use of a novel technique in which cell separation is based largely on size, rather than on mass or density:

the unit gravity sedimentation method, Cohen, Dutton and Currie, working in collaboration with Balázs at the M.R.C. laboratories at Carshalton, Great Britain, have developed a method for the preparation, in adequate amounts for biochemical analysis, of isolated cell fractions. This includes a cerebellar Purkinje cell fraction either from normal rat or mouse, or from mutant mouse.

The procedure involves chopping the cerebellum into 400 μm slices and dispersing the tissue blocks in a Krebs-Ringer-bicarbonate buffer containing bovine serum albumin and glucose in the presence of low (0.025% w/v) trypsin concentrations at 37° C for 15 min. At the end of this period a trypsin inhibitor is added and the tissue further dissociated by incubation in a Ca^{2+}- and Mg^{2+}-free medium in the presence of EDTA and of DNAse to prevent clumping. The dissociated perikarya are pelleted at about $50 \times g$ for 5 min through a bovine serum albumin cushion, after which they can be further sedimented through the unit gravity chamber for size separation (Cohen et al., 1973, 1974; Dutton et al., 1975a, b). The cells have been shown to be viable in vitro, and aspects of their protein and glycoprotein metabolism, in vivo and in vitro, have begun to be studied.

PROTEIN SYNTHESIS IN NEURONS AND NEUROPIL

I turn now to the main biochemical theme I wish to discuss, that of protein synthesis in neurons and glia. It has been long suspected, on the basis both of histochemical observation of the rich ribosomal content of cortical neurons (e.g., Palay and Chan-Palay, 1972) and of autoradiographic results (e.g., Droz and Koenig, 1970), that the predominant portion of the rapid protein synthesis known to occur even in the adult brain is neuronally located, and for the last few years work in both our laboratory and that of Hamberger in Göteborg has been directed towards a study of protein metabolism in isolated neurons and neuropil. Polyacrylamide gel fractionations of even crude neuronal and neuropil soluble and insoluble protein fractions reveal, scarcely surprisingly, the presence of characteristically different protein bands in the two cell types (e.g., Packman et al., 1971; Sinha, Rose and Sinha, unpublished). In vitro labeled amino acids are incorporated into neuronal protein at rates of between 2 and 6 times higher than into neuropil, depending on the precursor and incubation conditions (Blomstrand and Hamberger, 1969; Tiplady and Rose, 1971). Similarly, if a 30 min or 1 hr pulse of intraperitoneally injected [^{3}H]lysine is given in vivo and the cell fractions subsequently separated, the specific radioactivity of neuronal proteins is up to 1.8 times that of the neuropil proteins (Rose and Sinha, 1974a).

However, when we followed up these observations by extending the time course of radioactive labeling in vivo from 1 hr to 4 hr or more, the picture changed. Whereas at 1 hr neuronal protein specific radioactivity was higher than neuropil, by 4 hr it had fallen substantially, whilst neuropil incorporation continued to rise. The net result was that at 4 hr neuronal specific radioactivity was some 40% of that of neuropil, and, furthermore, extending the in vivo incorporation period as far as 192 hr was without further effect on the *ratio* of neuronal to neuropil incorporation, although in absolute terms both fell slightly over the period. This phenomenon was not specific to the precursor used, as it could also be found with $[^{14}C]$phenylalanine.

These results suggested to us that there is present in the neuronal fraction a protein component which, incorporating label rapidly at early times after injection of precursor, subsequently disappears from the perikaryon. A simple calculation shows that this cannot merely represent turnover since, if we assume that incorporation of labeled lysine proceeds 1.5 times faster in neurons than in glia, and that the two cell types comprise similar proportions of total tissue protein, then a 25% decline in neuronal specific radioactivity between 1 hr and 4 hr after administration of label should produce a 17% decline in whole cortex specific radioactivity. However, this does not occur; instead there is a 24% *increase*. It seems likely that the decline therefore represents the transport of labeled material from the cell body to a compartment which is separated from the perikaryon during the cell fractionation procedure. It is of interest to go back at this point to the autoradiographic evidence of Droz and Koenig (1970). They observed a similar phenomenon with $[^{3}H]$leucine as precursor: intense labeling of the perikaryon at short times after injection of precursor, followed by a relative decline, compatible with, in their words: "a transfer of protein from the nerve cell bodies into regions made up with nerve cell processes". Further, the data of Blomstrand and Hamberger (1969) and of Babitch et al. (1975) support this interpretation.

Two general questions follow: what more can one say about the nature of the protein fraction which interests us, identified, as it is, purely on the basis of kinetic analysis; and to where, in the neuropil, does the label migrate?

Concerning the first question, we have two relevant pieces of information. By homogenizing the neuronal and neuropil fractions after isolation and separating into soluble and particulate components, we have concluded that the rapidly labeling and transported component is particulate rather than soluble. We then substituted $[^{3}H]$fucose, a glycoprotein precursor, for $[^{3}H]$lysine in the intraperitoneal injection. Table II shows that the incorporation of labeled fucose into neuronal and neuropil fractions follows a similar pattern to that for labeled lysine; a neuronal/neuropil incorporation ratio of 1.37 after 1 hr of incorporation had fallen by 4 hr to 0.77. Thus the time course of fucose labeling suggests that the rapidly labeling and transported neuronal protein fraction includes glycoprotein.

Concerning the fate of the migrating label, the fact that neuropil specific radioactivity continues to rise over the 4 hr period suggests that we may be observing a migration of labeled protein from the neuronal perikarya to the neuropil. The neuropil fraction contains glial cells and also dendritic and axonal processes and synaptosomes. We have made a variety of experiments which together enable us to suggest which of these compartments might be the recipient of the neuronal protein. To rule out the synaptosomes we performed a standard subcellular fractionation using 1 hr and 4 hr in vivo lysine-labeled cerebral cortex homogenates. As expected from the earlier work of Barondes (1968) there was no net accumulation of radioactivity in the synaptosomes over the 4 hr period. Thus this compartment can be eliminated as recipient. We then attempted to perform a "chase" experiment, pulse labeling the tissue in vivo for 1 hr with $[^{3}H]$lysine, then taking cortex slices and incubating them in vitro with [14C]lysine for a further 1 hr. In this type of experiment, over the hour of in vitro incubation new 14C-labeled protein is being synthesized whilst previously labeled [3H]protein is turning over, undergoing metabolism or transport. At the end of the in vitro incubation, slices are fractionated into neuronal and neuropil fractions in the usual way and the 3H/14C ratio in the fractions determined. The results showed that during the in vitro incubation period considerable incorporation of 14C occurred in all fractions, but that there was a disproportionate loss of already synthesized highly 3H-labeled protein from the slice to the medium. High specific radioactivity protein was thus leaking out of the neurons during incubation, although it was not being reaccumulated in the neuropil fraction under these in vitro conditions.

TABLE II

[3H]FUCOSE INCORPORATION INTO NEURONAL AND NEUROPIL FRACTIONS

[3H]Fucose was injected intraperitoneally into rats, the animals killed 1 or 4 hr later, cortex fractionated into neurons and neuropil, and the cell fractions precipitated with TCA, washed and counted. Results are means ± S.E.M. of 12 determinations. The decline in neuronal specific radioactivity, and the elevation in neuropil, is significant ($P < 0.001$). (Fucose data are from Rose and Sinha, unpublished. Data in last row, from a separate set of experiments with [3H]lysine precursor, are from Rose and Sinha, 1974a.)

Fraction	Specific radioactivity (disint./min/ mg protein)	
	1 hr	4 hr
Suspension	602 ± 47	583 ± 43
Neuron	535 ± 37	386 ± 36
Neuropil	440 ± 31	587 ± 108
Neuron/neuropil	1.37 ± 0.12	0.77 ± 0.11
Neuron/neuropil ([3H]Lysine precursor)	1.38 ± 0.20	0.42 ± 0.04

We next examined the effect of two substances which interfere with protein synthesis and distribution: cycloheximide, which is an inhibitor of protein synthesis, and colchicine, which is without overall effect on protein synthesis but is known to inhibit axonal transport. We predicted that in the presence of cycloheximide transport of prelabeled protein would still occur and thus over a 4 hr period the neuronal/neuropil incorporation ratio should be *lower* than that of saline controls. On the other hand, with colchicine to block axonal transport, if this was the mechanism of migration, then the neuronal/neuropil incorporation ratio at 4 hr should be *higher* than in controls. Animals were injected with [3H]lysine intraperitoneally; 15 min later either cycloheximide (approximately 6 mg/kg) or saline was also injected, and animals killed after a further 45 or 225 min and neuronal and neuropil fractions prepared. The cycloheximide dose was enough to inhibit more than 90% of protein synthesis in whole cortex for up to 4 hr. The results of this series of experiments (Table III) show that neuronal protein incorporation seems more sensitive to cycloheximide than that of neuropil, so that the residual neuronal/neuropil incorporation ratio, even at 1 hr, was only 0.64 and did not change much in the period to 4 hr. This pattern of results was more complex than we had predicted and does not permit a simple interpretation — the differential sensitivity of a fraction of neuronal protein synthesis to cycloheximide, however, is certainly an interesting observation.

TABLE III

EFFECT OF CYCLOHEXIMIDE ON [^{3}H]LYSINE INCORPORATION IN NEURONS AND NEUROPIL

Rats were injected intraperitoneally with [^{3}H]lysine, followed after 15 min with cycloheximide (6 mg/kg) or saline, and killed after a further 45 or 225 min. Neuronal and neuropil fractions were prepared, precipitated with TCA and counted. Results are expressed here as incorporation in cycloheximide-injected animals as a percentage of saline controls at 1 or 4 hr of incorporation, and are means of 12 determinations not differing by more than ± 15%. Note the differential sensitivity of neuronal protein synthesis. (Rose and Sinha, unpublished.)

Fraction	$\dfrac{Cycloheximide\ incorporation}{Saline\ incorporation}$ × 100	
	1 hr	*4 hr*
Suspension	42·0	57·5
A (debris etc.)	36·7	63·0
B (neuropil)	40·5	49·5
C (neurons)	15·1	34·0
D (nuclei etc.)	32·4	46·3
Neuron/neuropil (cycloheximide)	0·64	0·53
Neuron/neuropil (saline)	1·96	0·73

The effect of injecting colchicine at 35 μg/kg, a dose sufficient to block axonal transport for many hours, but without effect on the overall [^{3}H]lysine incorporation rate, is shown in Table IV. In this experiment the inhibitor was injected 1 hr prior to the isotope, and we expected to find neuronal protein synthesis unimpaired whilst, if axonal transport was blocked, there would be a steady rise of specific radioactivity of neuronal protein over the 1 to 4 hr period, instead of the fall found in the absence of the inhibitor. The results of Table IV show a slightly more complex picture; the specific radioactivity of neuronal protein at 1 hr was lower in the presence of colchicine than in the saline controls, even though in the total brain suspension no inhibitory effect could be detected. Once again, therefore, it appears as if a fraction of neuronal protein synthesis is differentially sensitive to an added drug. However, if incorporation into the cell fractions in the presence of colchicine is compared, at 1 hr and 4 hr, with that into controls, it can be seen that our more simple-minded prediction is fulfilled. Between 1 hr and 4 hr the overall specific radioactivity of the total cell suspension, in the presence or absence of colchicine, rises some 20%. In the absence of colchicine, neuronal specific radioactivity falls slightly, whilst that of neuropil rises markedly. In the presence of colchicine, neuronal specific radioactivity rises by 40%, whilst the rise in neuropil specific radioactivity is markedly reduced.

TABLE IV

EFFECT OF COLCHICINE ON [^{3}H]LYSINE INCORPORATION IN NEURONS AND NEUROPIL

Rats were injected (35 μg/kg) with colchicine or saline intraperitoneally. After 1 hr [^{3}H]lysine was injected and animals killed after a further 1 or 4 hr. Neuronal and neuropil fractions were prepared, precipitated with TCA and counted. Results are expressed here as (incorporation at 4 hr/incorporation at 1 hr) x 100, and are the means of 12 determinations not differing by more than ± 15%. Note the accumulation of radioactivity in neurons for colchicine-injected animals at 4 hr compared to the saline controls. In these experiments colchicine was without effect on overall protein incorporation in the whole cell suspension (incorporation + colchicine/incorporation + saline at 1 hr, 103%, at 4 hr, 101%). (Rose and Sinha, unpublished.)

| | (Incorporation at 4 hr/incorporation at 1 hr) x 100 | |
	Saline	Colchicine
Suspension	123	120
Neurons	94	140
Neuropil	260	135

We conclude, therefore, from these studies that synthesis of the rapidly labeling neuronal protein fraction whose fate we have been following is especially sensitive to the effects of cycloheximide and of colchicine, and that its transport from the neuronal perikaryon is inhibited by colchicine. If blocking of axonal flow is the only effect of colchicine, the rapidly labeling component must indeed be part of the axonally transported protein under normal circumstances and, presumably, over the 4 hr period of our analysis will still be present in axons, not yet having measurably accumulated at the synapse. We have no evidence that neuronally synthesized protein accumulates in the glial cells.

EFFECTS OF SENSORY DEPRIVATION AND STIMULATION ON NEURONAL PROTEIN SYNTHESIS

The final example I want to give of our current work on neuronal/glial biochemical interrelations moves us firmly into the field of function. Up till now I have been discussing what we may describe as "normal" neuronal biochemistry, without reference to what must be one of our major long-term goals, the cellular description of the mechanisms of neuronal plasticity. For several years now we have, alongside our cellular studies, been examining the effects of modifying the environment of the organism on such neurochemical parameters as RNA and protein synthesis and levels of activity of transmitter enzymes (for review, see Rose et al., 1976). In these experiments we have been studying the biochemical sequelae of learning (using the chick imprinting system: Horn et al., 1973) and of visual deprivation and stimulation in the young rat. In the latter system we have shown that 50 days of dark-rearing followed by visual stimulation results in a transient elevation of incorporation of amino acids into a number of protein fractions in the visual cortex, lateral geniculate and retina (Richardson and Rose, 1973); the elevation is maximal between 1 and 3 hr after onset of light stimulation and, in the whole visual cortex, is of the order of 20–30% above the level in control animals maintained in the dark. It was an obvious question to ask whether the elevation in incorporation was confined to one cell type, or was a more general effect. Fractionation of visual cortex in the dark-reared and subsequently light-exposed animals, after 1 hr of incorporation showed that the elevation in incorporation is an entirely neuronal phenomenon (Rose et al., 1973). The neuropil fraction is thus being unaffected by light-exposure following dark-rearing.

This cellular specificity was very exciting to us. The observation became still more intriguing when we looked at the results in terms of the neuronal/neuropil incorporation ratio. For a 60 min pulse of $[^3H]$lysine, whereas in the normally reared animal an incorporation ratio of up to 2.0 would be observed, the ratio in the dark-reared rat visual cortex was only 0.6, while in the 1 hr-light-exposed rat it rose to around 1.0. The ratio after 1 hr in the dark-reared animals was thus close to that observed after a 4 hr pulse in the normal animals. Was this because dark-rearing suppressed the rapidly labeling fraction? If so, then prolonging the pulse length in the dark-reared animals should be without effect on the ratio. If, on the other hand, there is a general suppression of incorporation into visual cortex neuronal protein in the dark-reared animals, then increasing the pulse length to 4 hr should result in a reduction of the neuronal/neuropil ratio by some 70%, to about 0.2.

Table V shows the results of an experiment to test this possibility. By contrast with normally reared littermate controls, in the visual cortex of the dark-reared animals there was no change in the neuronal/neuropil incorporation ratio at either 4 hr or 24 hr as compared with 1 hr. At 4 hr the ratio was the same as that at 1 hr, whereas in the normals the ratio at 4 hr was 26% of that at 1 hr. As a consequence of this, whereas at 1 hr the incorporation rate in dark-reared animals was only 54% of that in normally reared animals, by 4 hr

TABLE V

NEURONAL/NEUROPIL INCORPORATION RATIO WITH [³H]LYSINE PRECURSOR IN NORMAL AND DARK-REARED ANIMALS FOLLOWING PULSE-LABELING

[³H]Lysine was injected intraperitoneally into 50-day-old, dark-reared rats and littermate controls reared in a 12 hr light/dark animal house cycle. Dark-reared animals were replaced in the dark for the period of incorporation. One hour later animals were killed and neuronal and neuropil fractions from visual and motor cortex regions prepared, precipitated with TCA and counted. The number of animals used for each measure with the dark-reared animals were: visual cortex: 1 hr, 8; 4 hr, 7; 24 hr, 5 and motor cortex 6. Data represent means ± S.E.M. in each case. Differences in ratios between 1 and 4 or 24 hr are significant ($P < 0.001$) for normal animals but not for visual cortex in dark-reared animals. Differences between neuronal and neuropil specific activities (depression) in visual cortex in dark-reared animals is significant ($P < 0.01$) at all times. Difference (elevation) in dark-reared motor cortex is significant at the 0.05 level. (From Rose and Sinha, 1974b.)

Specific radioactivity (disint./min/mg protein)

	Normal Ratio	Dark-reared (visual cortex)			Dark-reared (motor cortex)		
		Neuronal	Neuropil	Ratio	Neuronal	Neuropil	Ratio
1 hr	1·28 ± 0·18	3074 ± 186	5090 ± 420	0·69 ± 0·03	4954 ± 356	4266 ± 239	1·27 ± 0·07
4 hr	0.33 ± 0.04	4405 ± 427	5859 ± 453	0.75 ± 0.03	—	—	—
24 hr	0.44 ± 0.06	4365 ± 677	6186 ± 625	0.70 ± 0.05	—	—	—

the figure has risen to 227%. On the other hand, in the frontal (motor) cortex region, where no elevation in protein incorporation occurs when dark-reared animals are exposed to the light, the neuronal/neuropil incorporation ratio at 1 hr was almost exactly the normal level. Further fractionation showed that, as with the rapidly labeled fraction in neurons from normal animals, the fraction whose labeling is suppressed in dark-reared animals and enhanced when the dark-reared animals are exposed to light belongs to the particulate (water-insoluble) proteins of the neurons.

These results are consistent with the hypothesis that incorporation into the rapidly labeling insoluble protein fraction present in cortical neurons in normally reared animals is specifically suppressed in the visual but not the motor cortex of dark-reared rats. It is relevant to the interpretation of these data to note that elevations in incorporation of orotic acid into RNA have also been found in the visual cortex of dark-reared and subsequently light-exposed rats in an analogous experimental situation to ours (Dewar et al., 1973). This would suggest that for the rapidly labeling neuronal protein fraction to be synthesized, new messenger RNA may be involved.

CONCLUSION AND SUMMARY

This paper is a report of work in progress, part of an ongoing attempt to describe the dynamic state of cerebral cellular metabolism. It is based on a particular methodology, the bulk separation of fractions containing purified, viable populations of a specific cellular type. We have satisfied ourselves of the relative high degree of biochemical integrity and purity of the fractions which we can obtain, and have begun to describe some of the ways in which metabolism is compartmented between the cell types. In relation to protein metabolism in general, we believe that we have been able to identify a neuronally synthesized particulate glycoprotein fraction which is probably axonally transported. We have shown that the synthesis of this fraction is (rather) specifically sensitive not merely to inhibitors of protein synthesis and axonal flow, but also to the environmental circumstances of the organism. We have proposed elsewhere (Rose, 1974; Rose et al., 1976) that neuronal and glial metabolism is *state-dependent*, that is, it fluctuates with the changing environmental circumstances of the organism. The dynamic biochemical interactions between the neuronal perikaryon, its processes and synapses, and the surrounding glial cells are presumably, at the cellular level, correlates of neuronal functional plasticity at the physiological level, and thus of altered behavior at the organismic level.

ACKNOWLEDGEMENTS

This paper draws on the work of and discussions with all the members of the Brain Research Group at the Open University, but in particular Arun Sinha,

Layla Sinha, Dave Spears, Gary Dutton, Jim Cohen and Neil Currie. I thank all of them, especially for their agreement to my drawing on some still unpublished work.

Grants from the Medical Research Council and Science Research Council are also gratefully acknowledged.

REFERENCES

Babitch, J.A. Blomstrand, C. and Hamberger A. (1975) Amino acid incorporation into neurons and glia of guinea pigs with experimental allergic encephalomyelitis. *Brain Res.*, 86: 459–467.

Barondes, S. (1968) Further studies of the transport of protein to nerve endings. *J. Neurochem.*, 15: 343–350.

Blinkov, S.M. and Glezer, I.I. (1968) *The Human Brain in Figures and Tables.* Plenum Press, New York.

Blomstrand, C. and Hamberger, A. (1969) Protein turnover in cell-enriched fractions from rabbit brain. *J. Neurochem.*, 16: 1401–1407.

Cohen, J. Mareš, V. and Lodin, Z. (1973) DNA content of purified preparations of mouse Purkinje neurons isolated by a velocity sedimentation technique. *J. Neurochem.*, 20: 651–657.

Cohen, J., Dutton, G.R., Wilkin, G.P., Wilson, J.E. and Balázs, R.A. (1974) Preparation of viable cell perikarya from developing rat cerebellum with preservation of a high degree of morphological integrity. *J. Neurochem.*, 23: 899–902.

Dewar, A.J., Reading, H.W. and Winterburn, A.K. (1973) RNA metabolism in the cortex of newly weaned rats following first exposure to light. *Life Sci.*, 13: 565–573.

Droz, B. and Koenig, H.L. (1970) Localization of protein metabolism in neurons. In *Protein Metabolism of the Nervous System*, A. Lajtha (Ed.), Plenum Press, New York, pp. 93–108.

Dutton, G.R., Cohen, J. and Currie, D.N. (1975a) Some properties of viable perikarya from weaver and litter-mate cerebella. *Trans. Amer. Soc. Neurochem.*, 6: 97.

Dutton, G.R., Cohen, J. and Wilkin, G.P. (1975b) In vivo incorporation of labeled fucose and glucosamine into glycoproteins from cerebellar neuronal perikarya and nerve endings. *Trans. Amer. Soc. Neurochem.*, 6: 98.

Eccles, J.C., Ito, M. and Szentagothai, J. (1967) *The Cerebellum as a Neuronal Machine.* Springer, New York.

Hamberger, A. and Sellström, A. (1975) Techniques for separation of neurons and glia and their application to metabolic studies. In *Metabolic Compartmentation and Neurotransmitters*, S. Berl, D.D. Clark and D. Schneider (Eds.), Plenum, New York, pp. 145–166.

Horn, G., Rose, S.P.R. and Bateson, P.P.G. (1973) Experience and plasticity in the nervous system. *Science,* 181: 506–514.

Johnston, P.V. and Roots, B.I. (1970) Neuronal and glial perikarya preparations: an appraisal of present methods. *Int. Rev. Cytol.*, 29: 265–295.

Packman, P.M., Blomstrand, C. and Hamberger, A. (1971) Disc electrophoresis separation of proteins in neuronal, glial and subcellular fractions from cerebral cortex. *J. Neurochem.*, 18: 1–9.

Palay, S.L. and Chan-Palay, V. (1972) In *Metabolic Compartmentation in the Brain*, R. Balázs and J.E. Cremer (Eds.), Macmillan, London, pp. 187–208.

Richardson, K. and Rose, S.P.R. (1973) Differential incorporation of ^{3}H-lysine into visual cortex protein fractions during first exposure to light. *J. Neurochem.*, 21: 531–537.

Rose, S.P.R. (1965) Preparation of enriched fractions of isolated metabolically active neuronal cells. *Nature (Lond.)*, 208: 621–622.

Rose, S.P.R. (1967) Preparation of enriched fractions from cerebral cortex containing isolated, metabolically active neuronal and glial cells. *Biochem. J.*, 102: 33–43.

Rose, S.P.R. (1970) The compartmentation of glutamate and its metabolites in fractions of neuronal cell bodies and neuropil studied by intraventricular injection of U-^{14}C glutamate. *J. Neurochem.*, 17: 809–816.

Rose, S.P.R. (1972) Cellular compartmentation of metabolism in the brain. In *Metabolic Compartmentation in the Brain*, R. Balázs and J.E. Cremer (Eds.), Macmillan, London, pp. 287–304.

Rose, S.P.R. (1974) Neuronal protein synthesis and environmental stimulation: state dependent and longer term effects. *Trans. biochem. Soc.*, 2: 30–33.

Rose, S.P.R. (1975) Cellular compartmentation of brain metabolism and its functional significance. *Int. J. neurosci. Res.*, 1: 19–30.

Rose, S.P.R. and Sinha A.K. (1974a) Incorporation of amino acids into proteins in neuronal and neuropil fractions of rat cerebral cortex: presence of a rapidly labeling neuronal fraction. *J. Neurochem.*, 23: 1055–1076.

Rose, S.P.R. and Sinha, A.K. (1974b) Incorporation of ^{3}H-lysine into a rapidly labelling neuronal protein fraction in visual cortex is suppressed in dark-reared rats. *Life Sci.*, 15: 223–230.

Rose, S.P.R. and Sinha, A.K. (1976) Rapidly labeling and exported neuronal protein; ^{3}H-fucose as a precursor and effects of cycloheximide and colchicine. *J. Neurochem.*, in press.

Rose, S.P.R., Sinha, A.K. and Broomhead, S. (1973) Precursor incorporation into cortical protein during first exposure of rats to light: cellular localisation of effects. *J. Neurochem.*, 21: 539–546.

Rose, S.P.R., Hambley, J. and Haywood, J. (1976) Neurochemical approaches to learning and memory. In *Neural Approaches to Learning and Memory*, E. Bennett and M.R. Rosenzweig (Eds.), M.I.T. Press, Cambridge, Mass., in press.

Sinha, A.K. and Rose, S.P.R. (1971) Bulk separation of neurons and glia: a comparison of techniques. *Brain Res.*, 33: 205–217.

Sinha, A.K. and Rose, S.P.R. (1972) Compartmentation of lysosomes in neurons and neuropil; and a new neuronal marker. *Brain Res.*, 39: 181–196.

Sinha, A.K., Rose, S.P.R. and Sinha, L. (1975) Separation of neuronal and neuropil fractions from developing rat cerebral cortex. *Trans. biochem. Soc.*, 3: 97–98.

Tiplady, B. and Rose, S.P.R. (1971) Amino acid incorporation into protein in neuronal cell body and neuropil fractions in vitro. *J. Neurochem.*, 18: 549–558.

DISCUSSION

R. BALÁZS: It would be worthwhile to spend a little time about one question which is very relevant, and basic to other conclusions that you can draw from isolated cell populations: that is, the *integrity* of the preparations. Unfortunately, in most of the preparations that have been used up till now, the cells were gravely damaged; cell membranes are torn apart, most of the mitochondria are small or completely lost. What is remaining from the cell structure is only the nucleus and the cytoplasm. Even in our most recent preparations, which are very much better than most of the preparations which are presently available, we are not able to get from adult animals a sufficient yield of good cells in order to do reasonable biochemical work. And I should like to put up a plea here, and that is that one should always get electron microscopic low magnification pictures in order to appreciate what properties the preparations have, because what you really can see is also a question of how long you look. Until we have got reasonable preparations where the integrity is preserved, it is very difficult to put *any* interpretation at all on the biochemical data.

S.P.R. ROSE: Of course, all the concern about the morphological integrity of cell preparations is quite right — this is a point we have repeatedly emphasized. The problem has always been that the biochemical data was compatible with intact cells, the morphological data less so. We have always had good evidence for biochemical integrity of the cells. We feel now that in fact a lot of the bad morphology was due to the inadequacy of the electron microscopic techniques! A great deal depends on the exact conditions under which you *maintain* the preparations for electron microscopy, under which you *fix* them, under which you *observe* them, and so on. George Gray's experience with albumin would bear out the problem of finding structures by means of the electron microscope, even though they may be there at the biochemical level.

V.P. WHITTAKER: I agree with you, because our own first electron micrographs of cells from the electric layer of the *Torpedo* were just terrible, but they got better and better as E.M. techniques have improved. There is, I think, a great deal that we still do not know about the best way of fixing isolated structures for E.M., without the support that you get in a whole tissue block from the surrounding structures. For the isolation of neuronal and glial cell bodies we are using Hamberger's techniques. Whereas the synaptosome preparations are very reproducible, the cell body preparations are sometimes good but sometimes quite bad. So just because you get a bad result it does not mean that the whole preparation is bad: it may just be that the particular technique is bad. Dr. Hamberger admits that in his own laboratory, where they are very experienced in making these preparations, about 50% of the preparations are not what they would call really good (while the other 50% are really excellent preparations). So there is an intrinsic variability, and we can only hope to find out in the future what the tricks are.

S.P.R. ROSE: I think you are right: there is a fair bit of "noise" in the system, though I believe we do a good bit better than 50/50. Hamberger's technique is very similar to ours and we get variation in our system as well. That was why I emphasized the need for routine screening and routine use of either light microscopy or enzyme markers.

Plastic Changes of Neurons During Acquisition of New Behavior as a Problem of Protein Differentiation

H. HYDÉN

Institute of Neurobiology, Göteborg (Sweden)

THOUGHTS ON THE PROBLEM

Fifteen years of research on biochemical brain correlates to learning and long-term memory have not given any key answers as to how the brain stores information in long-term memories and retrieves them at will. Nor has it become clear how electrical phenomena are related to molecular and structural cell processes. Central in all studies on learning are qualitative brain cell changes, not quantitative ones. The latter seem to occur as a function of most sensory and motor stimuli, and of chemical effects. On the other hand, the knowledge now available delineates some neurobiological problems which are basic in the complex problem of behavior.

Brain cells are chiefly of two kinds, neurons and glia. Results from recent years tell that these two cell types take part in a dual collaboration. There exists a close metabolic and functional relationship between neurons and glia, but it is not known which substances are exchanged between these cells. This is one promising line of research which has now been taken up in several laboratories, not that new facts from the last 15 years are lacking (Svaetichin et al., 1961; Hydén, 1967).

Another promising field has been opened by immunochemical approaches. In 1961, Mihailović and Janković presented evidence that antiserum prepared against the caudate nucleus, when injected there abolished the electrical activity of this brain region (Mihailović and Janković, 1961). Mihailović and Hydén (1969) sampled glia surrounding the perikarya of large Deiters' neurons; such glial protein extracts were injected into guinea pigs and antiserum prepared both to the glia and to Deiters' neurons. The distribution of glial and neuronal antigens were then studied. With the rapid advance of immunological techniques, it can be expected that specific substances and their effect on brain cells will soon be studied by such approaches (Levine and Moore, 1965). This would open the possibility of negating or accepting concepts of "memory macromolecules". Uptake, turnover and blocking of cellular constituents would give a tentative answer to such questions. At present, there is no evidence that a macromolecule can store information in its interior which can be experienced at retrieval as a psychic memory.

Many behavioral studies which aim at biochemical correlates of learning do not fulfil necessary requirements. The type of learning test is a crucial and often neglected part of the experiment. The rat has been a favorite, and is an ecologically and socially successful animal (Barnett, 1963). It is my conviction that, in order to give a characteristic response, the rat learning test should be of the type image-driven behavior: rather difficult to solve and modelled on behavior in natural environments. The jumping to a shelf when shocked by electricity, or pressing of a lever, which have been frequent tests in "biochemical psychobiology" are poor choices. Comparison with active control animals is mandatory. These animals are placed in the test environment but do not learn, since the arrangements are made at random. Cage animals are unsuitable as controls in learning experiments since simply visiting the learning quarter is enough to produce certain biochemical brain cell changes (Hydén et al., 1974).

The other requirement is localization of analysis in the complex brain structure. The result obtained by, for example, a quantitative biochemical determination performed on whole brain of a trained animal seems to be next to worthless. Qualitative glial and neuronal analysis of molecular events in defined parts of the brain seems a logical goal in behavioral research. In 1965 antiserum was prepared against a brain-specific protein, called S100 (Levine and Moore, 1965). This marked the beginning of a series of studies of brain-specific proteins by immunological procedures (Schneider et al., 1973).

For the specific problem of learning and behavior, my view is that studies of membrane antigens of both neurons and glia will help to reveal mechanisms for identification of stimuli both from the exterior and the interior environment. Most of the knowledge about membrane antigens stems from blood cells, notably lymphocytes and erythrocytes (Singer and Nicolson, 1972). The new data have led to the view of the cell membrane as a plastic structure, housing receptors and antigens which move laterally in the plane of the membrane and have a considerable turnover of such protein governed by stimuli from the environment on the active genes of the cell. It is unlikely that membrane antigens of neurons and glia have the same behavior as those of lymphocytes. As will be discussed in this article, neuronal membrane antigens seem to be a product of cellular differentiation. At least one of them, the S100 protein, does not move laterally in the plane of the membrane but is more stable. An interesting question is whether neurons have a pattern of membrane antigens which characterize classes of different neurons functionally. The conformational state of such antigens can therefore be expected to constitute an important field of future research. Besides brain-specific proteins, peptides with hormonal effects have already proved to be of prime importance in the establishment of a new behavior, and are dealt with by de Wied in this volume (Chapter 11, p. 181).

Analysis of events during learning will certainly require analysis of system changes in the brain. This approach has been used long ago in electrophysiological studies of behavior (Adey, 1967, 1970; Adey et al., 1963). In experiments on cats and monkeys, Adey et al. found, for example, the occurrence of long trains of theta waves in the hippocampus which was correlated with the acquisition and performance of learned tasks and attention to cues during training. The theta train had the characteristics of a single frequency. Concomitantly, a theta rhythm without pacemaking characteristics appeared in subthalamus, midbrain and visual cortex. How the activities are regulated by the different centers and the information — previously stored or new — is processed is not well known. The hippocampal theta waves, however, originate between the basal and apical dendrites of pyramidal cells which in their turn are affected by activities from the septal nucleus via the dorsal fornix.

In addition, data obtained will give more pertinent information about the mechanism in the open hierarchic brain when the result is treated under the general systems theory (von Bertalanffy, 1968).

The term "open hierarchic" as regards interrelationships between brain areas emphasizes that knowledge about properties of single molecules or substances alone can elucidate organized systems like the brain. Still, however, the mathematical treatment of dynamic hierarchic orders is only in its beginning..

MODERN BIOCHEMICAL APPROACHES

This paper will discuss plastic changes in brain cells during acquisition of a new behavior from two aspects:

(1) protein changes as relative specific changes in defined brain areas of trained animals versus those of active controls, and

(2) as a problem of protein differentiation in the nerve cell plasma membrane and synapses. The proteins involved, S100 and 14-3-2 (Moore, 1973; Calissano, 1973), are two of the brain-specific proteins. The discussion will not deal with qualitative RNA changes in brain cells. The reader is referred to articles by Hydén (1973) and by Shashoua (1974).

All biological systems are served by subsystems which have restricted degrees of freedom in their functions. Such a subsystem will be discussed as a cooperative mechanism which is formed during the early postnatal period by differentiation of the nerve cell membranes including synapses. Cooperativity means that the system of macromolecules and ultrastructures act together and switch from one state to another and that the new state may persist.

The system involved is:

(1) actin-like filaments under the nerve cell membrane in the form of a continuous network;

(2) S100 protein bound to some areas of the membrane and the postsynaptic areas, and

(3) Ca^{2+} as a trigger of the mechanism. Ca^{2+} is increased as a function of training and gives rise to conformational changes in the two mentioned proteins. This is assumed to lead to a modulation of the membrane.

The observations which form the basis of the hypothesis to be presented have been made on isolated nerve cells which are sampled by free hand isolation technique. Fig. 1 shows 3 isolated nerve cells from the brain stem surrounding a collection of glial cells in the middle. Such cells respire well in a suitable medium, show a membrane potential of up to 70 mV and phosphorylate and incorporate amino acids (Hillman and Hydén, 1965a and b).

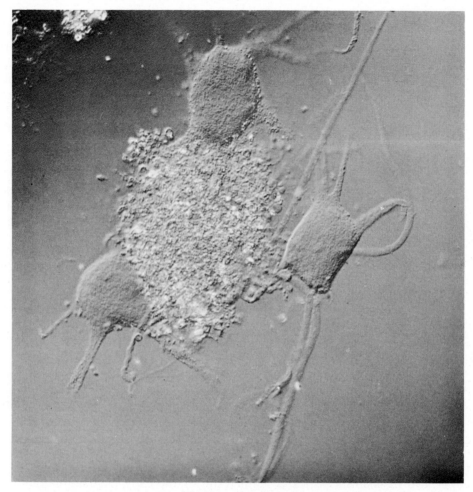

Fig. 1. Free nerve cells isolated by free hand dissection from the brain stem. The nerve cells are surrounding a collection of glial cells.

From a biochemical point of view it is a well-defined system with respect to the type of nerve cells, or to glial versus nerve cells. A number of microchemical methods now exist for the analysis of 10^{-7}–10^{10} g samples which represents material from 20–30 isolated nerve cell bodies. Recent methods include quantitative immunoelectrophoresis and microcomplement fixation.

A cooperative mechanism for modulating the synapse and the cell membrane

(a) The existence of a membrane-associated network in neurons

The first component of the mechanism consists of a network of protein microfilaments which is localized under and close to the nerve cell plasma membrane. The filaments are attached to the subsynaptic structures and are thus membrane-associated. This membrane net can be observed in ultra-thin membrane preparations made by free hand microsurgery of isolated nerve cells

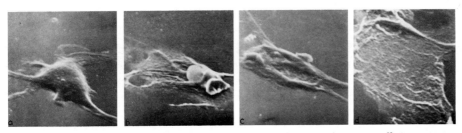

Fig. 2. a–d demonstrate free hand microdissection of isolated nerve cell to prepare a 100–300 nm thick nerve cell membrane. Note the remaining nucleus like a tennis ball in b. (From Hansson and Hydén, 1974.)

(Hansson and Hydén, 1974). Fig. 2a–d demonstrates through the scanning electron microscope how the membrane preparation is obtained. The nerve cell, freed from glia, is cut open by a stainless steel microknife. The nucleus and the cell content are then removed. Note the exposed nucleus, like a tennis ball, in Fig. 2b. The membrane preparation is finally made thin (Fig. 2d) by removing material close to the membrane with a micropipette ejecting fluid, usually 0·15 M sucrose. The final preparation varies in thickness, from 10 to 50 nm up to compilations of electron dense cytoplasm. The preparations are fixed for 1 min with 1% uranyl acetate in water, pH 4·4, rinsed and air-dried. They are then scanned in a transmission electron microscope. At high resolution (Fig. 3) a continuous network of coiled 7 nm filaments can be seen all over the cell surface and extending into the dendrites. Each 7 nm filament is composed by two 2 nm unit filaments coiled around each other with a spacing of 9 nm. The

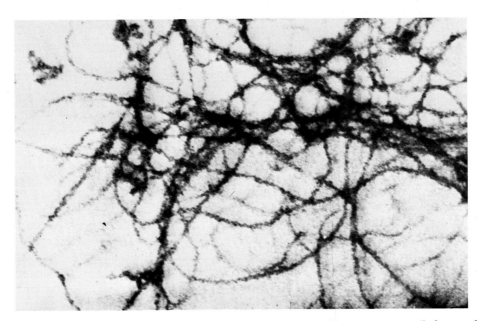

Fig. 3. The membrane-associated network of 2 nm diameter filaments, two coiled around each other. The network is continuous, the filaments contain actin-like protein and are also intimately associated with postsynaptic webs of synapses. (From Hansson and Hydén, 1974.)

filaments are insoluble in water and salt solutions but are destroyed by pronase and trypsin. They do not contain DNA or RNA but probably have some carbohydrates. Of the tested divalent ions only Ca^{2+} causes the filaments all through the network to uncoil (Fig. 4). As a sign of this structural change, a shift of the fluorescence towards longer wave lengths could be observed following the addition of Ca^{2+} when membrane preparations were stained with aniline naphthalene sulfonate. A second significant reaction was obtained by adding heavy meromyocin to glycerinated cell membrane preparations, which· gave a characteristic dressing of the filaments with arrow heads. This reaction was obliterated by ATP treatment prior to treatment with heavy meromyocin. Cytochalasine B and colchicine did not destroy the filaments.

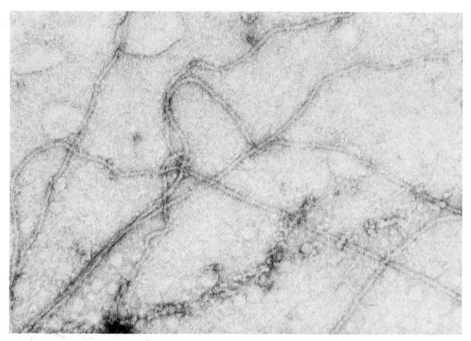

Fig. 4. Addition of 2 mM Ca^{2+} uncoils the filaments of the network shown in Fig. 3. (From Hansson and Hydén, 1974.)

A detailed study of the membrane preparations revealed the important fact that the filaments of the network pass the cell membrane and adhere to the postsynaptic structure. This was also confirmed in an electron microscope study of the network in sectioned cell material. Fragments of the filaments within the dimension of the cell section could clearly be seen entangled with the postsynaptic rim (Metuzals and Mushynski, 1974).

Thus, close to the inner side of the nerve cell membrane there is a continuous ultrastructural network of actin-like protein filaments, attached to the synapses and depending on Ca^{2+} for their state of coiling. The filaments proceed into the dendrites. Fig. 5 gives a schematic picture of the 2 nm coiled filaments of the network at a synapse.

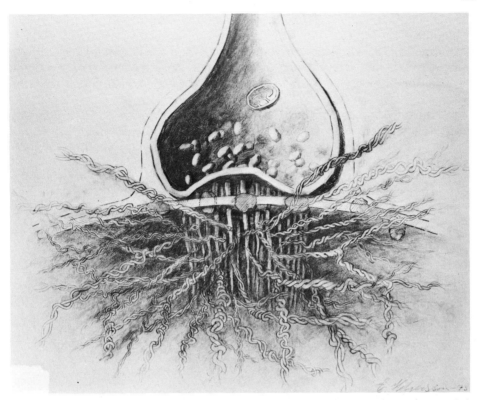

Fig. 5. Schematic picture of a synapse and part of the plasma nerve cell membrane and the protein microfilaments which form a network and are intimately connected to the postsynaptic web. (From Hydén, 1974.)

A confirmation of the presence of protein filaments with a diameter of 2 nm is presented by Röhlich (1975).

(b) Membrane-bound S100 protein with heterogeneous distribution

The second component of the proposed cooperative mechanism is membrane-bound, brain-specific S100 protein. The S100 is an acidic protein with a molecular weight of 21,000 and consists of 3 subunits with slight differences in the primary composition (Moore, 1973; Calissano, 1973). S100 binds to antiserum against S100 from man to invertebrates. It is mainly a glial protein and can be produced by glial cells, but is also present in neuronal nuclei (Haglid et al., 1974, 1975b; Hydén and Rönnbäck, 1975a, b; Hansson et al., 1975). The main part of S100 is soluble both in water and saturated ammonium sulfate, from which latter property is derived its name S100. However, approximately 12% of the neuronal, and 5% of the glial S100 is not soluble in water or salt solutions but rather in n-pentanol. This fraction is membrane-bound (Haglid et al., 1975a).

An adult rat brain contains 120 μg of S100/g wet weight. A characteristic of the S100 molecule is that, when it binds Ca^{2+} it undergoes a conformational change with partial unfolding along with unmasking of tryptophan and two SH

90

groups, and this change may remain stable after removal of Ca^{2+}. The S100 has 8 binding sites for Ca^{2+}, of which 3 have an association constant of $10^{-6} M$ (Calissano, 1973). Different nerve cell types were used: Purkinje cells, Deiters' cells, cells of the descending mesencephalic Vth nucleus, the hypoglossal nucleus, the hippocampus, the thalamus, spinal ganglion cells and anterior horn cells.

We used monospecific anti-S100 antiserum conjugated with fluorescein to study the distribution of S100 over the neuronal surface. The basis of this

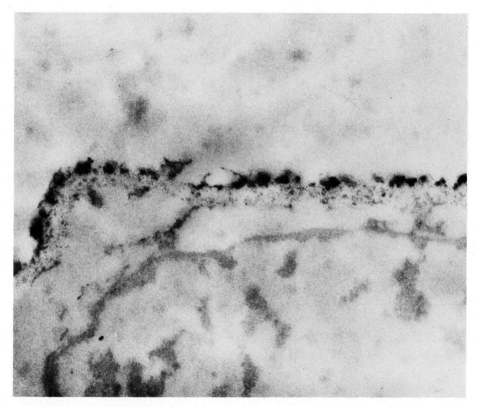

Fig. 6. Section through a nerve cell treated with peroxidase-conjugated antiserum against S100 and photographed in the electron microscope. The dark precipitates on or in the nerve cell membrane demonstrate the presence of S100. (From Hansson et al., 1975.)

study was a technique to sample nerve cells, including part of their dendrites, without damaging the plasma membrane (Hydén and Rönnbäck, 1975a, b). The essence of the technique is not to touch the cells with the microtools used, or let them adhere temporarily to a glass surface. The specificity of the antiserum was checked by immunodiffusion, microcomplement fixation, and SDS electrophoresis. Direct as well as indirect labeling of the isolated cells was used (Hydén and Rönnbäck, 1975a). Proper controls of various types included antiserum to S100 repeatedly absorbed with S100, extraction by n-pentanol, F_{ab} fragments of anti-S100 antiserum, and concanavalin A.

In a separate study, sections through isolated nerve cells were incubated in peroxidase-conjugated antiserum against S100. In Fig. 6 the dense precipitation

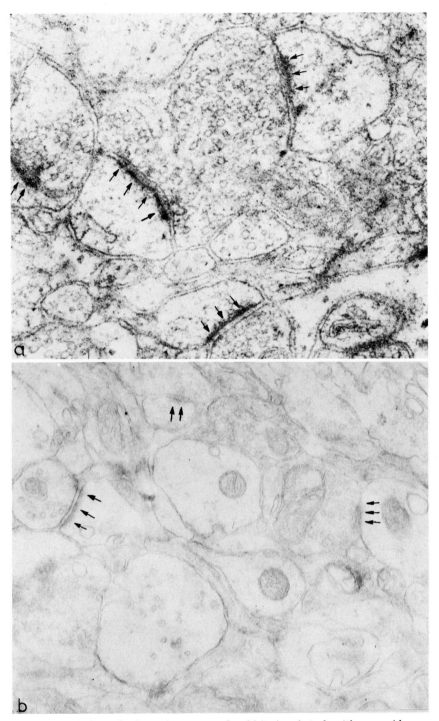

Fig. 7. a: section through frontal cortex of rabbit incubated with peroxidase-coupled antiserum against S100. Note the dark precipitation in the postsynaptic area indicated by arrows. b: control sections where peroxidase-coupled antiserum against S100 absorbed several times by S100 has been used. (From Haglid et al., 1975.)

92

on/in the plasma membrane demonstrates the presence of S100 (Hansson et al., 1975). The reaction did not become positive in all membrane areas. Using tissue sections it became clear that especially the postsynaptic area contained a high concentration of the S100 protein (Haglid et al., 1974) (Fig. 7). The specific fluorescence of the neuronal surface has a characteristic distribution. In small (15–20 μm diameter) nerve cells the fluorescence is seen as an irregular ring around the equator when focussed. This can be expected from the geometry of the cells and the optics. On large nerve cells with a volume of up to 150,000 cu. μm, larger areas of the plasma membrane can be observed. The specific fluorescence is heterogeneously distributed, and is frequently collected over one cell pole including its dendrites (Fig. 8). Note that the surface fluorescence of the cell in Fig. 8b partly covers the non-fluorescent nucleus seen inside the cell. S100 is present also on dendrites and the axon. The last observation was made on pseudo-unipolar trigeminal nerve cells. The polar

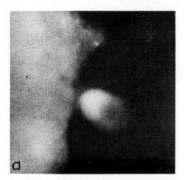 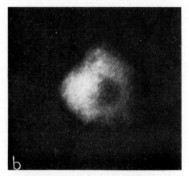

Fig. 8. a and b: two isolated fresh Deiters' nerve cells from rabbit incubated with fluorescein-labeled antiserum against S100 and photographed in a fluorescence microscope. The specific fluorescence of S100 is heterogeneously distributed and localized in the plasma membrane and at one of the poles. The nucleus is not stained since the plasma membrane prohibits entry of the antibody molecule. Note in b that the surface fluorescence is partly covering the nucleus. (From Hydén and Rönnbäck, 1975c.)

distribution of the membrane fluorescence became more distinct when cells were incubated in F_{ab} fragments conjugated with fluorescein of anti-S100 antiserum. Membrane preparations were made from nerve cells with specific S100 fluorescence and, when spread out, showed fluorescence only over the part corresponding to its polar distribution. If the plasma membrane is intact, antibodies cannot penetrate into the cells and the nucleus remains non-fluorescent and dark. If, intentionally, the membrane is damaged, the antiserum enters the cell interior and the nucleus immediately becomes fluorescent. Treatment with n-pentanol (which removes non-soluble S100) prior to antiserum incubation will prevent a positive reaction for S100.

These observations together with *control tests* (e.g., antiserum against S100 absorbed with S100 repeatedly, or, such antiserum where the antibodies were removed by S100 insolubilized on Sepharose) demonstrate that membrane fluorescence of nerve cells with fluorescein-conjugated anti-S100 antiserum is due to membrane-bound S100 protein. Is this polar localization of the antigen S100 to the nerve cell membrane an analogue to the cap formation in lymphocytes? The answer is no. If a receptor immunoglobulin on a lymphocyte membrane binds a fluorescein-labeled anti-immunoglobulin at room temperature, fluorescent patches form rapidly over the cell surface, followed by a fluorescent cap formation at one pole. The cap will be endocytosed or discarded (Singer and Nicolson, 1972). The cap formation is dependent on cellular metabolism and inhibited by antimetabolites. We therefore incubated nerve cells in sodium azide, cyanides, dinitrophenol, cycloheximide and at low temperature, but this made no difference to the distribution of the S100, nor does the membrane protein disappear by endocytosis.

The ontogeny of the membrane S100 is characteristic, furthermore. It does not appear until 2–3 weeks postnatally in the rat and rabbit (Hydén and Rönnbäck, 1975a, b) which species are very immature at birth. In the guinea pig, on the other hand, which is quite mature right from birth, the heterogeneous membrane S100 is already present from that time. The conclusion is that in nerve cells the S100 protein is a membrane constituent, and often has a distribution over one pole of the cell with a high concentration especially in the postsynaptic area. The presence of this protein in the membrane seems to be a consequence of cellular differentiation.

Calcium increase in hippocampus during training

The third component of the cooperative mechanism is Ca^{2+}. During training for a new behavior, the amount of Ca^{2+} increases in the hippocampus (Haljamäe and Lange, 1972; Table I). There was no increase of H_2O, Na^+ or K^+. Therefore, a changed circulatory condition in the area can be excluded as a cause of the calcium increase. This increase of Ca^{2+} causes part of the S100 to undergo conformational changes which lead to a more rapid electrophoretic mobility of one fraction of S100 (Hydén and Lange, 1972).

A hypothetical mechanism for modulating synapses by the interaction of two Ca^{2+}-dependent proteins, the actin-like network and the S100 protein of the plasma membrane

The basis of the hypothesis is that the S100 protein differentiates the plasma membrane into a polar area rich in S100, and the remaining area lacking S100. The plasma membrane would thus have a certain complexity in S100 pattern, with consequences for the synapses within this area. S100 binds Ca^{2+} with high affinity in at least two binding sites, the binding curve having a sigmoid form (Calissano, 1973). By binding Ca^{2+}, the S100 undergoes a conformational change which may become stable.

The conformational state of membrane and synapses would be controlled, according to the model, by interaction of the membrane protein network with Ca^{2+} with different results in areas rich or poor in membrane S100. In areas rich in S100, the network filaments would not be able to compete with S100 for Ca^{2+}. They would remain coiled and exert a tension on the membrane and synapses, which in such a state are proposed to be difficult to activate.

In membrane areas lacking S100, on the other hand, the network filaments can bind Ca^{2+} and then uncoil. This would result in an expansion effect on the membrane and its synapses. The synaptic clefts would become tight, and

94

TABLE I

WATER, POTASSIUM, SODIUM AND CALCIUM CONTENTS OF SAMPLES FROM THE CA3 REGION IN THE
HIPPOCAMPUS FROM THE TWO BRAIN HALVES OF CONTROL RATS AND TRAINED RATS

Electrolyte values both on wet weight and dry weight bases. n, number of CA3 areas; m, number of animals, S.E.M., values from the n individual measurements. Test of significance based on the average value from each animal (17 d.f.)

	H_2O (%)	Potassium (mEq./100 g)		Sodium (mEq./100 g)		Calcium (mg/100 g)	
		Dry weight	Wet weight	Dry weight	Wet weight	Dry weight	Wet weight
Control (n = 18) (m = 9)	81·1	51·20	10·17	20·43	3·87	37·0	7·36
S.E.M. ±	0·4	1·60	0·38	0·35	0·07	1·9	0·27
Trained (n = 20) (m = 10)	81·0	50·42	9·99	20·04	4·04	44·0*	8·04**
S.E.M. ±	0·5	1·50	0·34	0·43	0·10	1·8	0·19

* $P < 0.001$ vs. control (17 d.f.).
** $P < 0.05$ vs. control (17 d.f.).

membrane and synapses consequently easier to activate (Kornguth, 1974). A similar S100 pattern and state of modulation can in principle be shared by numerous neurons in different brain loci. The actin-like network may also control the mobility and transport of substances along the plasma membrane.

A pertinent problem is how Ca^{2+} may increase and be released in localized areas. Adey and Rees (1975) have found that very weak electrical signals with field gradients of only $2.5 \mu V/cm$ can release calcium. It may be that Ca^{2+} is the mediator of exterior or inner stimuli which are transduced into remaining molecular changes of brain cells.

OTHER OBSERVATIONS IMPLICATING THE S100 PROTEIN IN NEURAL FUNCTION

There are several empirical reasons why S100 protein can be discussed in basic functional contexts. On training to reverse handedness in rats, the amount of soluble S100 increases in hippocampal nerve cells by 20% and the incorporation of labeled precursors increases by 300%; part of S100 protein undergoes a conformational change (Hydén and Lange, 1970).

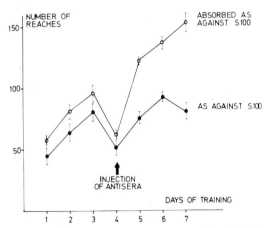

Fig. 9. The effect of injection of 60 μl x 2 of antiserum against S100 intraventricularly in rats trained to reverse handedness. A group of rats was trained for 3 days with 2 sessions of 25 min per day. On the 4th day the antiserum or antiserum against S100 absorbed with S100 were injected intraventricularly. The training was continued for 3 more days as described. Rats injected with antiserum against S100 showed a deflection of the learning curve. (From Hydén and Lange, 1970.)

An increase of the S100 protein during learning in itself does not make this substance a causal factor in behavior: it may be an unspecific response. If it were possible, however, to influence behavior by interfering with the membrane-bound S100, this protein would take on another importance. In order to study this question, a group of rats were trained for 4 days, 2 x 25 min/day, to reverse handedness. (For a discussion of this behavioral test, see Hydén and Lange, 1970.) On day 4, highly specific antiserum against the

S100 was injected intraventricularly, 60 μl × 2 per rat. On further training the learning curve became deflected, which was not the case with any of the various types of control (Fig. 9). We were able to demonstrate that the antiserum in this experiment succeeded in reaching the hippocampal and adjacent cells. This indicates that the membrane-bound S100 protein takes part in some still unknown way in processes taking place during learning.

SOME SYSTEM CHANGES IN BRAIN DURING TRAINING

When animals are trained to learn a new behavior a wave of protein activity traverses the brain (i.e., increased amounts and incorporation of amino acids into defined protein fractions are found as a function of training and time). We have used reverse-handedness training in carrying out complicated movements such as paw and arm precision movements monitored by vision and cerebellar-cortical activity. Rats which used the preferred paw to perform the same task, and which received the same amount of reward served as controls. Table II demonstrates that the incorporation of label into the unseparated, soluble protein increased in the hippocampus, but decreased initially in several cortical and other areas during training. With increasing training and time these values reversed (Hydén and Lange, 1972).

TABLE II

RELATIVE SPECIFIC ACTIVITIES OF 8 DIFFERENT BRAIN AREAS OF CONTROLS AND RATS TRAINED TO REVERSE HANDEDNESS

Training was for 2 × 25 min/day during 4 + 2 + 2 days with 14 days intermission between the 3 training periods; 9 control rats, 12 trained rats. Control values as averages for the whole training period.

Brain area	Training			Control
	4 days	6 days	8 days	
Cortex	0·40 ± 0·01	0·51 ± 0·02	0·53 ± 0·02	1·40 ± 0·15
Thalamus, nucl. dorsomed.	0·28 ± 0·01	0·35 ± 0·02	0·39 ± 0·03	0·95 ± 0·15
Entorhinalis	0·25 ± 0·002	0·32 ± 0·01	0·46 ± 0·02	0·84 ± 0·02
Septum	0·19 ± 0·004	0·29 ± 0·01	0·26 ± 0·01	0·78 ± 0·12
Corp. mam.	0·39 ± 0·02	0·48 ± 0·04	0·43 ± 0·04	0·87 ± 0·09
Nucl. dentatus	0·39 ± 0·02	0·34 ± 0·01	0·41 ± 0·03	0·81 ± 0·03
Hippocampus	0·69 ± 0·04	0·38 ± 0·03	0·47 ± 0·03	0·75 ± 0·06
Formatio ret.	0·32 ± 0·01	0·36 ± 0·03	0·52 ± 0·03	0·90 ± 0·03

The fractions containing the 14-3-2 brain-specific protein in the CA3 region (the main integrating center) of the hippocampus likewise respond with a significant increase in amount and incorporation of [3]- and [14C]valine and leucine during training to reverse handedness (Hydén and Lange, 1968, 1972; Haglid et al., 1975). A specificity of this response is indicated by 3 observations: (1) overtraining does not result in an increase of 14-3-2 synthesis; (2) a re-reversal after one month back to the original paw in the handedness test does do so — the learning curve indicates that the animals respond to the re-reversal training as to a new task (Hydén and Lange, 1972); and (3) in the last-mentioned studies there was no change observed in the values of overall brain cell protein between learning animals and control. This also indicates a specificity of the 14-3-2 protein response in the hippocampal cells. It may be pertinent to quote Penfield (1952): "Without hippocampus the recording of current experience by man is impossible". The same can apparently be said for other species. In the rat for instance, the hippocampus collects information about the spatial relationship between objects in the environment and controls acquisition and retrieval of important information. As is exemplified, the molecular changes in hippocampus during the establishment of a new behavior are conspicuous. Hippocampal damage impairs the animal's capacity to learn an intelligent behavior.

CONCLUSIONS AND SUMMARY

Differentiation of neurons during learning

When animals are trained to acquire a new behavior, brain system changes occur in terms of protein increase and incorporation of labeled amino acids into protein. This response dominates in the CA3 region of the hippocampus. The incorporation values of hippocampal cells vary inversely compared to cortical areas during the first part of training to acquire a new behavior. The involvement of brain-specific protein, especially of S100, is documented by the observations of:

(1) increase in amount of S100 and precursor incorporation early during training as compared to controls;

(2) interruption of the learning process following uptake of antibodies against S100 by the membrane-bound S100;

(3) lack of cellular protein response at overtraining;

(4) occurrence of cellular protein response at re-reversal training; and

(5) response of the brain-specific protein fractions but not of the total protein.

The hypothesis is that the neuronal membrane including postsynaptic areas is differentiated by the S100 protein. It would be dependent for its conformational state on Ca^{2+}, and this characteristic is shared by the actin-like filaments of the membrane-associated network. The plastic changes during learning would thus be a continuous molecular and structural differentiation of neurons.

The relationship in time between protein increase and precursor incorporation in the different brain loci might be the effect of the diffusion of small molecules (for example peptides) which are released either by glia or neurons.

REFERENCES

Adey, W.R. (1967) Intrinsic organization of cerebral tissue in alerting, orienting and discriminative responses. In *The Neurosciences*, G.C. Quarton, T. Melnechuk and F.O. Schmitt (Eds.), The Rockefeller University Press, New York, pp. 615–633.

98

Adey, W.R. (1970) Spontaneous electrical brain rhythms accompanying learned responses. In *The Neurosciences Second Study Program*, F.O. Schmitt (Ed.), The Rockefeller University Press, New York, pp. 224–243.

Adey, W.R. and Rees, D.A. (1975) Evidence for cooperative mechanisms in the susceptibility of cerebral tissue to environmental and intrinsic electric fields. In *Functional Linkage in Biomolecular Systems*, F.O. Schmitt, D.M. Schneider and D.M. Crothers (Eds.), Raven Press, New York.

Adey, W.R., Kado, R.T., Didio, J. and Schindler, W.J. (1963) Impedance changes in cerebral tissue accompanying a learned, discriminative performance in the cat. *Exp. Neurol.*, 7: 259–281.

Barnett, S.A. (1963) *The Rat. A Study in Behaviour*. Aldine Publ., New York.

Bertalanffy, L. von (1968) *General System Theory: Foundations, Development, Applications*. Braziller, New York.

Calissano, P. (1973) Specific properties of brain specific protein S100. In *Proteins of the Nervous System*, D.J. Schneider, R.H. Angeletti, R.A. Bradshaw, A. Grasso and B.W. Moore (Eds.), Raven Press, New York, pp. 13–26.

Haglid, K.G., Hamberger, A., Hansson, H.-A., Hydén, H., Persson, L. and Rönnbäck, L. (1974) S100 protein in synapses of the central nervous system. *Nature (Lond.)*, 251: 532–534.

Haglid, K.G., Hamberger, A., Hansson, H.-A., Hydén, H., Persson, L. and Rönnbäck, L. (1975a) *J. Neurol. Sci.*, in press.

Haglid, K.G., Hansson, H.-A. and Rönnbäck, L. (1975b) S100 in the central nervous system of rat, rabbit and guinea pig during postnatal development. *Brain Res.*, in press.

Haljamäe, H. and Lange, P.W. (1972) Calcium content and conformational change of S100 protein in the hippocampus during training. *Brain Res.*, 38: 131–142.

Hansson, H.-A. and Hydén, H. (1974) A membrane-associated network of protein filaments in nerve cells. *Neurobiology*, 4: 364–375.

Hansson, H.-A., Hydén, H. and Rönnbäck, L. (1975) Localization of the S100 protein in isolated nerve cells by immunoelectron-microscopy. *Brain Res.*, 93: 349–352.

Hillman, H. and Hydén, H. (1965a) Membrane potentials in isolated neurons in vitro from Deiters' nucleus of rabbit. *J. Physiol. (Lond.)*, 177: 398–410.

Hillman, H. and Hydén, H. (1965b) Characteristics of the ATP-ase activity of isolated neurons of rabbit. *Histochemie*, 4: 446–450.

Hydén, H. (1967) RNA in brain cells. In *The Neurosciences*, G.C. Quarton, T. Melnechuk and F.O. Schmitt (Eds.), The Rockefeller University Press, New York, pp. 248–266.

Hydén, H. (1973) Changes in brain protein during learning. Nerve cells and their glia: relationship and differences. RNA changes in brain cells during change in behaviour and function. In *Macromolecules and Behaviour*, G.B. Ansell and P.B. Bradley (Eds.), MacMillan, London, pp. 3–75.

Hydén, H. (1974) A calcium-dependent mechanism for synapse and nerve cell membrane modulation. *Proc. nat. Acad. Sci. (Wash.)*, 71: 2965–2968.

Hydén, H. and Lange, P.W. (1968) Protein synthesis in the hippocampal pyramidal cells of rats during a behavioral test. *Science*, 159: 1370–1373.

Hydén, H. and Lange, P.W. (1970) S100 brain protein: correlation with behaviour. *Proc. nat. Acad. Sci. (Wash.)*, 67: 1959–1966.

Hydén, H. and Lange, P.W. (1972) Protein synthesis in hippocampal nerve cells during re-reversal of handedness in rats. *Brain Res.*, 45: 314–317.

Hydén, H. and Rönnbäck, L. (1975a) Membrane-bound S100 protein on nerve cells and its distribution. *Brain Res.*, 100: 615–628.

Hydén, H. and Rönnbäck, L. (1975b) The brain specific S100 protein on neuronal cell membranes. Accepted for publication, *J. neurol. Sci.*

Hydén, H. and Rönnbäck, L. (1975c) S100 on isolated neurons and glial cells from rat, rabbit and guinea pig during early postnatal development. *Neurobiology*, 5: 291–302.

Hydén, H., Lange, P., Mihailović, L. and Petrović-Minić, B. (1974) Changes of RNA base composition in nerve cells of monkeys subjected to visual discrimination and delayed alternation performance. *Brain Res.*, 65: 215–230.

Kornguth, S.S. (1974) The synapse: a perspective from in situ and in vitro studies. *Rev. Neurosci.*, 1: 63–114.

Levine, S. and Moore, B.W. (1965) Structural relatedness of a vertebrate brain acidic protein as measured immunochemically. *Neurosci. Res. Progr. Bull.*, 3: 18–22.

Metuzals, J. and Mushynski, W.E. (1974) Electron microscope and experimental investigations of the neurofilamentous network in Deiters' neurons. Relationship with the cell surface and nuclear pores. *J. Cell Biol.*, 6: 701–722.

Mihailović, L. and Hydén. H. (1969) On antigenic differences between nerve cells and glia. *Brain Res.*, 16: 243–256.

Mihailović, L. and Janković, B.D. (1961) Effects of intraventricularly injected anti-N. caudatus antibody on the electrical activity of the cat brain. *Nature (Lond.)*, 192: 665–666.

Moore, B.W. (1973) Brain specific proteins. In *Proteins of the Nervous System*, D.J. Schneider, R.H. Angeletti, R.A. Bradshaw, A. Grasso and B.W. Moore (Eds.), Raven Press, New York, pp. 1–12.

Penfield, W. (1952) Memory mechanisms. *Arch. Neurol. Psychiat. (Chic.)*, 67: 178–191.

Röhlich, P. (1975) Membrane-associated actin filament in the cortical cytoplasm of the rat mast cell. *Exp. Cell Res.*, 93: 293–298.

Schneider, D.J., Angeletti, R.H., Bradshaw. R.A., Grasso, A. and Moore, B.W. (Eds.) (1973) *Proteins of the Nervous System,* Raven Press, New York.

Shashoua, V.E. (1974) RNA metabolism in the brain. *Int. Rev. Neurobiol.*, 16: 183–221.

Singer, S.J. and Nicolson, G.L. (1972) The fluid mosaic model of the structure of cell membrane. *Science*, 175: 720–731.

Svaetichin, G., Laufer, M., Mitarai, G., Fatechand, R., Vallecalle, E. and Villegas, J. (1961) Glia control of neuronal networks and receptors. In *Neurophysiologie und Psychophysik des visuellen Systems*, R. Jung and H. Kornhuber (Eds.), Springer-Verlag, Berlin, pp. 445–456.

DISCUSSION

S.P.R. ROSE: In those very interesting experiments in which you injected S100 antiserum, could you explain why the changes are very specific to the behavioral situation that you are studying? If S100 is modulating the synaptic connectivity in many places, then one should expect many behavioral effects of such an antiserum.

H. HYDÉN: Yes indeed. But we do not inject the antibody in the entire brain. We inject it in the lateral ventricle, severing very slightly the ependyma layer, so the antiserum will diffuse into the hippocampus and related fields. The antiserum probably affects the glia. We have also observed that antiserum against S100, if injected, adheres to those parts of the nerve cell membrane which contain S100, including the postsynaptic plate in which the concentration of S100 is high. In the rat, an intact hippocampus is indispensable both for the formation of long-term memory (if the task is sufficiently difficult), retrieval and for information about spatial relationship in the environment, underlying, for example, the acquisition of three-dimensional maps by the rat. All these modalities could be expected to be influenced by the S100 antiserum. As I pointed out we measured a distinct effect on reversal, but observed no other motor or sensory alterations.

J. OLDS: How do you decide when an animal is learning? An animal is learning all the time, and you present him then with a special learning situation where he is learning what you want him to learn, and you say: the learning has started. Now it has always seemed to me that an animal has a right to learn when he chooses, and it is very hard to decide when he is learning, and when he is not. Added to that point is the question of how you distinguish between something that is just correlated to the activity of the hippocampus and something that is correlated to a modification in the hippocampus. It has long been known in rat psychology that hippocampal lesions make reversal difficult. And in experiments in our laboratory we have recorded from hippocampus and cortex during reversal, and found that hippocampus consolidates the extinction of the old response, which must come first, for neocortex consolidates the acquisition of the new response which comes second. And it seemed that the two activities were occurring in that successive order. So your protein could be correlated just with the activity and not with the modification.

H. HYDÉN: An animal is presumably learning all the time. Of the new and important material presented, the hippocampus and related parts of the limbic system help to decide what should be processed and transformed into long-term memory. In our case, the animals are permitted during several days to be familiar with the test box. They sniff around and even snooze in the box. On the day of the test we do not press the animal to begin to take food pills out of the tube with the non-preferred paw. The tube with food pills is simply presented. The rat can begin to take food out of it whenever it likes. It has the right to choose when to begin to learn and that usually does not take many minutes. The 25 min allotted has proven to be a sufficiently long period. I completely agree with you that one should let animals learn when they want to learn. This idea formed the basis of the handedness experiment when we began with it 12 years ago. We record the number of successful reaches within the 25 min and compare the result with that of control rats. The controls are animals which use the *preferred* paw to retrieve food pills and exert approximately as many reaches as the learning rats and get the same amount of reward. The result is of course based on this comparison. Your second question was if the S100 protein could be correlated with the activity of the hippocampus and not with the modification introduced by the S100 antiserum. In a *difficult* instrumental learning test, an intact hippocampus is indispensable. If therefore a blocking in the hippocampus of the glial, membrane and synaptic S100 by S100 antiserum prohibits further acquisition, this result can be related to at least one of the S100 functions removed in the experiment and modifying the hippocampal cells.

E.G. GRAY: If S100 is indeed related to learning situations, would spinal cord neurons not have any S100?

H. HYDÉN: They have S100, but not as much membrane-bound as the brain cells.

E.G. GRAY: How do the spinal cord neurons then learn?

H. HYDÉN: Spinal cord neurons differentiate and I suppose the end result is "a change by use", which means the state left after acquisition by experience.

H. VAN DER LOOS: Can you explain how a long thin microfiber that is coiled, can suddenly uncoil?

H. HYDÉN: Well, this is a general phenomenon in cells. Chromosomes are a good example. They measure 0·8−1·0 nm, and we are dealing with 2 nm fibers.

Molecular Neuropathology

LARS SVENNERHOLM

Department of Neurochemistry, Psychiatric Research Centre, University of Göteborg, Göteborg (Sweden)

HISTORICAL INTRODUCTION

The chronicle of molecular neuropathology began almost 100 years ago, when the British ophthalmologist, Warren Tay, in 1881 described a child in his care who had a red spot in the eye and severe muscular weakness. Later, in 1887, the American neurologist, Bernard Sachs, published the first description of the pathology of the disease, after having studied 19 children from several families. Nine years later, Sachs (1896) concluded that this was a hereditary degenerative disease caused by a lipid disturbance, since the neurons were engorged with lipid material. It was not until almost 50 years later that the nature of the stored lipid was recognized by Erwin Klenk (1939/1940). This may seem astonishing, since as early as 1884 Thudicum had published the structure of an allied glycolipid, the cerebroside. But all the important advances made in the last decade of the 19th century were focused into the background and forgotten when the wave of psychoanalysis swept over Europe. In 1942, Klenk coined the name ganglioside for the lipid which he had a few years earlier found to be increased in Tay-Sachs disease. Klenk assumed that there was only one brain ganglioside, but using a chromatographic method, I found that the gangliosides constituted several related acidic glycolipids (Svennerholm, 1956). In Tay-Sachs disease there was only one ganglioside that was increased in amount. It had a high galactosamine concentration. This finding led me to postulate the lack of an enzyme which splits off the hexosamine in the catabolism of gangliosides (Svennerholm, 1957). It took a further 5 years to isolate the Tay-Sachs ganglioside and to show that it contained a terminal N-acetylgalactosamine, and that it differed from the normal major mono-sialoganglioside by its lack of the terminal galactose (Svennerholm, 1962; Fig. 1).

Using an enzymatic method elaborated by Robinson and Stirling (1968) for the separation of human hexosaminidases in spleen, Okada and O'Brien (1969) showed that hexosaminidase A was lacking in the classical Tay-Sachs disease. O'Brien et al. (1970) then devised a simplified fluorometric assay for the estimation of both hexosaminidases in serum from controls, patients and obligate heterozygotes. No overlapping occurred, and that very year the first pregnancy was monitored in a family in which the mother had previously borne

$$Gal\beta1\rightarrow3GalNAc\beta1\rightarrow4Gal\beta1\rightarrow4Glc1\rightarrow1Ceramide$$

GM1

$$3$$
$$\uparrow$$
$$\alpha2.NeuNAc$$

$$GalNAc\beta1\rightarrow4Gal\beta1\rightarrow4Glc1\rightarrow1Ceramide$$

GM2

$$3$$
$$\uparrow$$
$$\alpha2NeuNAc$$

Fig. 1. The chemical structure of the major monosialoganglioside GM1 and the Tay-Sachs ganglioside GM2.

a child with Tay-Sachs disease (Schneck et al., 1970). Since then more than 100 pregnancies at risk have been monitored in Tay-Sachs families.

Tay-Sachs disease has been a model not only for all the other storage diseases but also for other inherited diseases, because (a) it was the first to be detected, (b) it is the most common early fatal disease in a certain population (Askhenazi Jews), and (c) it can be prevented by prenatal diagnosis in pregnancies at risk. This short history of the progress in our knowledge about Tay-Sachs disease may be used as a guide in the investigation of any inherited disease.

(1) Careful clinical examination, including anamnesis, examination of all organs, particularly the nervous system, examination of the patient's state, laboratory examination of blood, urine and cerebrospinal fluid and X-ray examination.

(2) Determination of the mode of genetic transmission.

(3) Pathological-anatomical examination, including electron microscopy and histochemistry.

(4) Isolation and chemical characterization of the accumulated substance(s).

(5) Elucidation of the enzymic lesion with various substrates and determination of enzyme kinetics.

(6) Examination with simple, specific assay procedures for pre- and postnatal diagnosis of affected individuals, and postnatal detection of carriers.

THE NUMBER OF INHERITED METABOLIC DISEASES

McKusick (1971) has published a catalogue of Mendelian characteristics of man in which he lists more than 1850 genetically known and uncertain genetic diseases reported up to 1971. The number of known genetic diseases is shown in Table I. It is evident that particularly the number of recessive autosomal diseases increased between 1958 and 1971. The biochemical disorder is known in about 200 diseases, mainly autosomal recessive diseases, but also in a small number of sex-linked diseases. In about 30 of these diseases, the prenatal diagnosis has been performed, and today it would be technically possible to perform it in a further 30. The inherited metabolic diseases are generally rare and their average rate of prevalence is usually less than 1:10,000.

It has often been discussed whether it is not a wasteful use of time and money to diagnose and try to find a form of treatment of the individuals with inherited diseases. It is true that each disease by itself is rare, but there are many such diseases, and their combined frequency is appreciably high.

TABLE I

THE NUMBER OF SIMPLY INHERITED (MENDELIAN) GENETIC DISEASES

	1958	1971
Autosomal dominant	285	430
Autosomal recessive	89	380
X-linked	38	86

DIAGNOSIS OF INHERITED DISEASES

The diagnosis of the inherited diseases can be made at 4 levels in the biological chain between genotype and phenotype (Fig. 2). Diagnosis at the fourth clinical level is generally too late to help the patient. I am only aware of two diseases (galactosemia and maple syrup disease) in which the clinical diagnosis can be made and dietary treatment started before the results of the early postnatal screening are obtained. A diagnosis can also be made at the other end of the chain, namely at the level of the gene, which is done by cytogenetic methods. This is an important laboratory service, since Down's syndrome is at present the most common single cause of mental retardation. But screening at this level for point mutations, which occur in the inherited metabolic disorders, is not yet possible.

Screening for inherited metabolic disorders must be performed at the level of the primary gene product, the enzyme, or at the substrate-product level. For a low molecular weight compound, it is often possible to give effective treatment once the nature of the metabolite has been diagnosed. By the introduction of

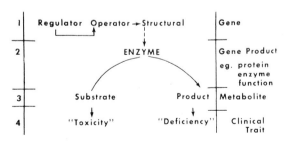

Fig. 2. Phenotypic levels at which screening for the effect of a mutation might be undertaken. (From Scriver, 1969.)

chromatographic methods in clinical medicine, the identification of minute amounts of metabolites has also been possible. Screening of body fluids for amino acid disturbances since the early fifties has led to the discovery of a rapidly increasing number of previously unknown amino acid diseases. The detection of many new diseases with a disturbed carbohydrate metabolism is another example of the tremendous importance of partition chromatography on paper or thin-layer plates for the detection of new inherited metabolic diseases. Another chromatographic procedure, gas-liquid chromatography, seems to be of still greater importance. In all diseases with a disturbed organic acid metabolism, which present themselves to the clinician as cases of unexplained metabolic acidosis, gas-liquid chromatography is the method of choice. But also most other low molecular weight metabolites and a large number of complex lipids and oligosaccharides can be converted to volatile compounds which can be analyzed by gas-liquid chromatography. The discriminative power of gas-liquid chromatography can be enhanced by the use of capillary columns, and in combination with mass spectrometry, it should be possible to increase its possibilities of differentiating and recognizing 800 compounds normally occurring in the human body (Eldjarn et al., 1975). A disturbance of low molecular weight compounds can be diagnosed in body fluid, but complex biological substances, such as lipids, proteins, and polysaccharides, often occur only in low concentrations, and the analyses must therefore be performed on tissue specimens from the appropriate organ. In the diagnosis of the neurolipidoses we use not only brain tissue but also liver and lymph nodes.

THE LYSOSOMAL STORAGE

When the metabolism of a complex biological compound is disturbed, the enzymic lesions affect the degradation of the substance which occurs in the lysosomes of the cells. Blockage of the biosynthesis of an important biological substance will generally lead to a non-viable fetus. A lesion of the catabolic enzyme will lead to an early serious accumulation of its substrate in the lysosome. When the fetus cannot metabolize a low molecular weight compound, the mother's enzyme system might be capable of metabolizing it for the fetus, provided that the substance can pass across the placenta. No significant degradation by the mother's enzyme system may occur when the substance should be degraded in the fetal lysosomes. Since the rate of metabolism, both of the biosynthesis and of the degradation, is higher during fetal life than at any other time, a considerable accumulation will occur in the lysosomes during early intrauterine life, which has been amply demonstrated in aborted fetuses (Schneck et al., 1972; Brady et al., 1971b; O'Brien et al., 1971; Ellis et al., 1973). It is widely assumed that the clinical symptoms in the storage diseases (Fig. 3) will occur when the lysosomes are so enlarged that the enormous lysosomal accumulation of gangliosides in GM1- and GM2-gangliosidoses will lead to serious impairment of the neuronal function. But the mechanism is not the same in all diseases. In Krabbe disease there is a primary lesion of cerebroside β-galactosidase, but there is no generalized storage of

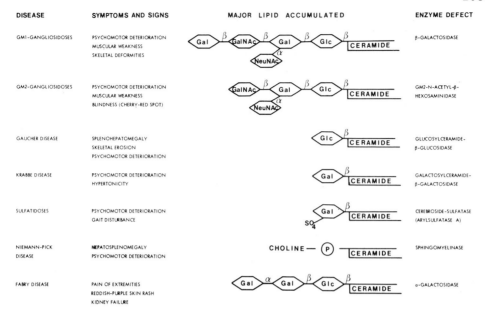

Fig. 3. Major features of the lipid storage diseases.

cerebrosides in the nervous system or any other organs of the body. Instead the brain content of cerebroside (galactosylceramide) is severely diminished (Fig. 4). We have recently been able to resolve this paradox (Vanier and Svennerholm, 1975), by showing that the level of psychosine (galacto-sylsphingosine) is increased 100-fold in cerebral and cerebellar tissue of patients with Krabbe disease. Psychosine is the lyso-compound of cerebrosides and, like all other lyso compounds, it is strongly cytotoxic (Taketomi and Nishimura, 1964; Miyatake and Suzuki, 1972). We suggest that psychosine is normally formed as a biochemical aberration in the oligodendroglial cells, but is immediately transported to the lysosome and degraded. Because of the enzymic lesion, this cannot occur in Krabbe disease: psychosine will

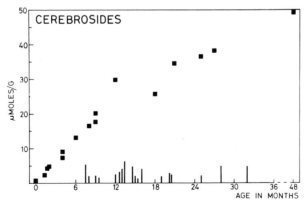

Fig. 4. Concentration of cerebrosides in cerebral white matter of normal infants (■) and of patients with Krabbe disease (columns). (From Vanier and Svennerholm, 1974.)

accumulate, and the function of the oligodendroglial cells will be impaired. There will be a delay in the myelinization early in development and myelin will cease to form altogether at the age of 2–4 months.

THE ENZYMIC LESION

It was formerly assumed that the mutation of the gene occurred only in a few sites, but this has since been refuted by investigations on human inherited abnormalities and polymorphism of plasma proteins, hemoglobin and red cell enzymes. For example, the rate of discovery of inherited variations in human glucose-6-phosphate dehydrogenase has been exponential in the past decade (Childs, 1967). The number of mutant variants of the enzymes involved in the inherited metabolic diseases is probably also very large, but it is more difficult

TABLE II

GM1-GANGLIOSIDOSES

Phenotype		Stored substance	β-Galactosidase activity % of controls	
			Mu-β-Gal*	GM1
Type I	Infantile		<2	<2
Type II	Juvenile		<5	<5
Type III	Juvenile	Glycolipids, glycopeptides, oligo-	10–20	10–20
Type IV	Adult	saccharides with a terminal galactose	5–10	5–10
Type V	Infantile Swedish form	in α,β-linkage to N-acetylgalactos- amine or N-acetylglucosamine	10–15	10–15
Type VI	Juvenile Swedish form		10–15	10–15

*4-Methylumbelliferyl (MU)-β-galactoside.

to assess this number, since it is very seldom possible to isolate an enzyme in a sufficiently pure form to characterize it as a protein. We must therefore study its functional properties instead. This can be done by analysis of the affected enzyme with different substrates and different concentrations (determination of K_m). The number of mutants can also be determined from the number of phenotypes for a disease and by cell hybridization. GM1-gangliosidosis can be used as an example. Until recently only two forms were known (Table II) in which there was no difference in the enzymic activity when tested with synthetic substrate and GM1-ganglioside. Type I differs from Type II by a much more extensive involvement of the skeleton and viscera. The lysosomal storage in extraneural organs in Type I patients does not consist of gangliosides, but of glycoproteins and oligosaccharides with a terminal galactose residue (Fig. 5). One might well imagine that it would be possible to differentiate between the two forms by an enzymic assay if the accumulated oligo-saccharides were used as substrates. Type III and Type IV have considerable residual enzymic activity, besides which these two forms also run a slower clinical course.

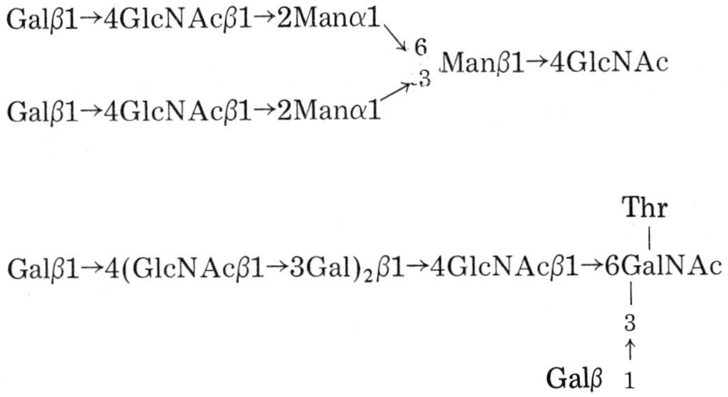

$$\text{Gal}\beta1\rightarrow4\text{GlcNAc}\beta1\rightarrow2\text{Man}\alpha1}$$
$$_6\searrow$$
$$\text{Man}\beta1\rightarrow4\text{GlcNAc}$$
$$_3\nearrow$$
$$\text{Gal}\beta1\rightarrow4\text{GlcNAc}\beta1\rightarrow2\text{Man}\alpha1}$$

$$\begin{array}{c}\text{Thr}\\|\\\text{Gal}\beta1\rightarrow4(\text{GlcNAc}\beta1\rightarrow3\text{Gal})_2\beta1\rightarrow4\text{GlcNAc}\beta1\rightarrow6\text{GalNAc}\\|\\3\\\uparrow\\\text{Gal}\beta\ 1\end{array}$$

Fig. 5. The chemical structures of two oligosaccharides stored in GM1-gangliosidosis. (From Tsay et al., 1975 and Wolfe et al., 1974.)

In cell hybridization studies Galjaard et al. (1975), by fusion of Type I cells with Type IV cells, have shown much higher activities in 50% of the hybridized nuclear cells after fusion than in any of the parental cells before fusion (Table III). This shows a genetic complementation and a restoration of the β-galactosidase activity, which suggests that the lesion is located in two different cistrons and that the enzyme is composed of at least two different polypeptide chains. In the two Swedish forms the remaining β-galactosidase activity is high also when determined with GM1-ganglioside as substrate. We still have no explanation for the rapid fatal course of the disease, but one can guess that some hitherto unknown cytotoxic compound accumulates in these two types.

The prototype of all inherited diseases, Tay-Sachs disease, is still an enzymatic mystery. N-acetyl-β-hexosaminidase hydrolyzes N-acetyl-β-galactosamine and N-acetyl-β-glucosamine residues from the non-reducing terminal of various substrates. The enzyme of human tissues can be separated

TABLE III

β-GALACTOSIDASE ASSAYS USING NATURAL AND SYNTHETIC SUBSTRATES IN SOMATIC CELL HYBRIDS OF DIFFERENT GM1-GANGLIOSIDOSIS VARIANTS

	Enzyme activity (nmol/hr/mg protein)	
	GM1-β-galactosidase	4-MU-β-galactosidase
Type I x Type I	3·5	1·8
Type II x Type II	4·3	4·0
Type IV x Type IV	10·5	13·4
Type I x Type II	< 1	< 1
Type I x Type IV	44·1	38·6
Type I x Type IV*	99·8	75·3
Control	193·8	246·7

* After fusion cells have been grown on medium with 10% fetal calf serum, that has been treated with alkali (pH 10.7) during 3 hr at 37°C to destroy enzyme activity in the medium. (After Galjaard et al., 1975.)

into two major components A and B (Robinson and Stirling, 1968). Okada and O'Brien (1969) demonstrated in the classical form of Tay-Sachs disease that there was a deficiency of hexosaminidase A, the determination of which has since been used in the diagnosis of hundreds of cases of Tay-Sachs disease and the identification of thousands of carriers of the condition. More pregnancies have been monitored in Tay-Sachs families by the assay of hexosaminidase A in cultivated amnion cells than in any other inherited disease. But it has not yet been possible to show that hexosaminidase A can hydrolyze GM2-ganglioside under proper kinetic conditions.

It is widely believed that neutral glycolipids such as the trihexoside, GA2, the asialo derivative of GM2-ganglioside and the tetrahexoside, globoside, can be hydrolyzed by component A and B, but that GM2-ganglioside can be hydrolyzed only by component A (Sandhoff and Wässle, 1971; Wenger et al., 1972). This assumption explains the ganglioside and glycolipid pattern in Tay-Sachs disease (Svennerholm, 1962; Eeg-Olofsson et al., 1966; Öhman et al., 1971), and in Sandhoff-Jatzkewitz variant form in which both hexosaminidase

TABLE IV

GM2-GANGLIOSIDOSES, TAY-SACHS DISEASE

Type	Form	Stored substance	Enzyme defect
I	Sandhoff variant	GM2, GA2, globoside	Hexosaminidase A and B lacking
II	Classical Tay-Sachs	GM2	Hexosaminidase A lacking
III	Atypical Tay-Sachs	GM2	Hexosaminidase A and B normal
IV	Juvenile	GM2	Hexosaminidase A partially reduced

A and B are deficient (Sandhoff et al., 1968; Table IV). But it cannot explain why there is an accumulation of GM2-ganglioside in patients with juvenile GM2-gangliosidosis but not in carriers of Tay-Sachs disease who have a similar, partial deficiency of hexosaminidase A. Suzuki and Suzuki (1970) postulated that only a subcomponent of hexosaminidase A was responsible for the degradation of GM2-ganglioside and that this component was deficient in juvenile GM2-gangliosidosis. This hypothesis would also explain the so-called AB variant of GM2-gangliosidosis in which both A and B hexosaminidase components, determined by artificial substrates, appear to be normal and yet there occurs an accumulation of GM2-ganglioside (Sandhoff et al., 1971). In a recent paper, Bach and Suzuki (1975) claim that only the most acidic subfraction of human liver hexosaminidase A hydrolyzes GM2-ganglioside. This is incompatible with the earlier finding by Tallman et al. (1974) that both hexosaminidase A and B of human placenta hydrolyzed GM2-ganglioside. However, both research groups found that the enzymic action on GM2-ganglioside was less than 1:1000 of that on the neutral glycolipids, which in its turn was less than 1:1000 of that on synthetic substrate. These studies demonstrate how urgent it is to find the appropriate conditions for the assay of GM2-ganglioside β-hexosaminidase activity and the risks of using only synthetic substrates in the diagnosis of neurolipidoses.

EXPRESSION OF ENZYMIC LESION

Clinical symptoms of storage disease will generally occur when lysosomal accumulation is so large as to impair cellular function. The factor which determines the time of onset of symptoms is mainly the degree of enzymic defect. In the lipidoses, various forms are known with different times of onset: infantile, juvenile and/or adult forms. In general, the specific enzyme is lowest in the infantile form and highest in the adult form, while the juvenile form has an intermediate value for remaining enzymic activity. The enzymic defect is generalized and can be demonstrated in most tissues and tissue fluids, but the lysosomal accumulation will produce symptoms referable only to the organs

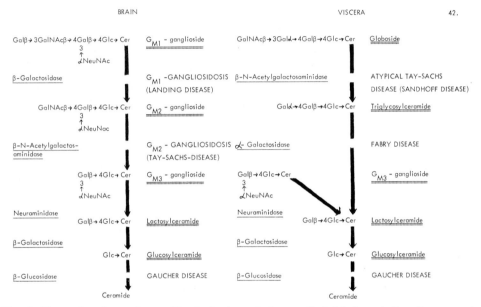

Fig. 6. The major glucosylceramides in brain and viscera, their biodegradation, the enzymic lesion and the name of the lipid storage disease.

which have to handle comparatively large amounts of substrate for the deficient enzyme (Fig. 6). It is for this reason that the clinical signs of ganglioside storage are confined to the nervous tissue in GM1- and GM2-gangliosidoses, although the increase of the respective gangliosides can be much higher in liver, for example, than in brain (Öhman et al., 1971). It is also for this reason there will be no sign of early psychomotor deterioration in Fabry disease.

The phenotypic expression in Gaucher disease is much more complicated and has been an intellectual challenge to the physician and the neurobiologist. The precursor of the stored glucocerebrosides in the brain is, in the infantile form, mainly the brain ganglioside, which is evident from their ceramide composition. The glucocerebrosides of the spleen and liver have two possible precursors: the globoside of the erythrocytes or the lactosylceramide of the leukocytes. The fatty acid pattern of the glucocerebroside stored in the liver and spleen suggests that at least 75% of the cerebroside is derived from leukocytic glycolipids. The turnover of gangliosides in human brain is fast only during fetal life and the first 6 postnatal months, after which time the daily lysosomal formation of glucocerebroside is low. When, in patients with Gaucher disease, the remaining cerebroside β-glucosidase activity almost suffices to hydrolyze the glucocerebroside derived from the brain gangliosides during fetal life and early postnatal months, the level of glucocerebroside in brain will be raised, but there will be only discrete histological signs of storage of lysosomal glucocerebroside. The cerebroside β-glucosidase of extraneural organs is unable to hydrolyze all glucocerebrosides in any form of Gaucher disease and a lysosomal storage in reticulohistiocytic cells will start early in fetal life and will continue at an undiminished rate throughout life, since the formation of leukocytes, in contrast with other cells, does not decrease with age. The spleen is the organ of predilection for storage of cerebrosides and it increases steadily in size and hypersplenism develops. When splenectomy has to be performed the operation is followed by a rise in the plasma level of cerebrosides and an increased storage of cerebrosides in the skeleton, which manifests itself by erosions of the long bones, pelvis and spine (Hillborg and Svennerholm, 1960) as well as in the nervous system, the last leading to neurological symptoms (Herrlin and Hillborg, 1962). The blood vessels of the cerebellum and basal ganglia are surrounded by a large number of Gaucher cells containing cerebrosides of white blood cell type, which indicates that they have been transported into the brain (Sourander and Svennerholm, in preparation).

The time of onset of symptoms depends also on the functional importance of an organ. A lysosomal storage in the neurons will lead to early symptoms because of the specialized function of the nervous system. The first symptoms will also be those of the central nervous system since the development of the brain starts earlier and proceeds faster than that of other organs.

SUBSTRATES FOR THE ENZYMIC ASSAY OF NEUROLIPIDOSES

Dr. Henri Hers in Louvain, who created the concept of inborn lysosomal disease for the lysosomal storage diseases (Hers, 1965), assumed that the lysosomal hydrolases had a low degree of specificity and furthermore were not specific for particular substrates, but had only specificity for certain linkages. He therefore considered synthetic substrates to be the most suitable for the diagnoses of inborn lysosomal diseases. Later experience has shown that of the 7 neurolipidoses listed, Krabbe and Niemann-Pick diseases can be diagnosed only with the natural specific substrate for the enzyme, that many cases of juvenile and adult Gaucher disease have normal β-glucosidase activity with synthetic substrates, that GM2-gangliosidosis of the classical Tay-Sachs form in Ashkenazi Jews can be diagnosed with synthetic substrates, while natural substrate seems to be desirable in variant forms. For the remaining 3 diseases — GM1-gangliosidosis, sulfatidosis and Fabry disease — natural substrate does not seem to be necessary. It is my opinion that natural substrate should be used in every new index case and, when natural substrates are used for the assay, they should always be labeled. Gatt and coworkers (Gatt, 1967) used unlabeled substrates for the elucidation of the catabolic pathways of gangliosides and neutral glycolipids, but it is important to point out that these assay methods cannot be used for quantitative estimations. It is also relatively simple to make labeled substrates for the assay of enzymes affected in the neurolipidoses. Four of the 7 substrates (Table V) have a terminal galactose or galactosamine residue which can be labeled by oxidation with galactose oxidase and subsequent reduction with tritiated sodium borohydride (Radin, 1972). Glucosylceramide (Brady et al., 1965) and sphingomyelin (Stoffel et al., 1971) can be prepared from natural substances by semisynthesis, and sulfatides are prepared by injection of radioactive sulfate into the brain of 15–20-day-old rats and isolation of the sulfatide after 24 hr.

TABLE V

LABELED SPHINGOGLYCOLIPIDS PREPARED BY GALACTOSE OXIDASE TREATMENT OF NATIVE SUBSTRATES AND SUBSEQUENT REDUCTION BY TRITIATED (*) SODIUM BOROHYDRIDE

Substrate	Disease
Ceramide(1←1)β*Gal	Krabbe
Ceramide(1←1)βGlc(4←1)βGal(4←1)α*Gal	Fabry
Ceramide(1←1)βGlc(4←1)βGal(4←1)β*GalNAc	Tay-Sachs

Ceramide(1←1)βGlc(4←1)βGal(4←1)β*GalNAc
     |
    NeuNAc	

Ceramide(1←1)βGlc(4←1)βGal(4←1)β GalNAc(3←1)β*Gal	GM1-gangliosidosis

Ceramide(1←1)βGlc(4←1)βGal(4←1)βGalNAc(3←1)β*Gal
     |
    NeuNAc	

DIAGNOSES OF NEUROLIPIDOSES IN THE INDEX CASES

The aim of the investigation of all inherited metabolic diseases is to obtain an early diagnosis. When treatment is possible, such as in the amino acid diseases, it should be started as soon as possible. In general, no treatment is available in the neurolipidoses, but an early diagnosis can help the family to seek prenatal diagnosis during a subsequent pregnancy, or at least result in prompt genetic counseling to the family. The biochemical diagnoses should include identification of the stored substances and determination of the enzymic lesion. Niemann-Pick and Gaucher diseases can be diagnosed by examination of a biopsy specimen of the liver or a lymph node and Fabry disease and sulfatidosis, by lipid estimation of urinary sediment. GM1- and GM2-gangliosidosis, like Krabbe disease, require brain biopsy which should not be performed until late in the disease. Enzymic assay should be performed on isolated leukocytes with natural and synthetic substrates, and the activity should be related to a marker enzyme (β-galactosidase or β-hexosaminidase). The enzymic assay is preferably also performed on cultured skin fibroblasts and white cells. The cultured cells should then be stored in a cell bank for later analysis. The final and complete examination is performed on autopsy material from the nervous system and several other organs. In a case of neurolipidosis it is equally important to analyze extraneural visceral organs as well as the nervous system, since the changes can be more pronounced and specific in the extraneural organs than in brain. A storage process in the brain, like an inflammation, can lead to early death of the ectodermal cells specific for the nervous system and replacement of them by cells of mesenchymal origin. These mesenchymal cells have a glycolipid pattern completely different from that of the nervous system and their fatty acid patterns in both glycolipids and phosphoglycerides reflect better that of extraneural organs, rather than of brain (Eto and Suzuki, 1971; Vanier and Svennerholm, 1974, 1975). It is therefore essential that the neurochemical examinations are combined with careful pathoanatomical investigations. The enzymic defect of the index case should be assayed in several organs with both natural and synthetic substrates. If the affected enzyme has any residual measurable activity the K_m value should always be determined. Material should be placed in an airtight polythene film bag and stored preferably at −60 to −80° C.

DETECTION OF CARRIERS

When a case of an inherited disease has been diagnosed, all the family members should be invited to participate in a screening for the affected enzyme. But the costs of a general screening, both tangible and intangible, are considerable and must be weighed against the resulting benefits to individuals and to society. The benefits are economic as well as humanitarian. It has been argued that the carrier screening of Ashkenazi Jews is economically justifiable (O'Brien, 1972b). I will not dispute the estimated costs, but I think it would not be possible to keep the costs so low for public screening of another larger population. Brady et al. (1971a) suggested the use of automated serum enzyme assays for large scale screening for heterozygous carriers of lipid storage diseases which, in combination with intrauterine diagnosis, could lead to the preventive control of such disorders. It is true that serum can be used for screening of carriers of Tay-Sachs disease, but a positive test has always to be confirmed by the analysis of white cells or cultured fibroblasts. Carrier values for Tay-Sachs disease will be found in all women after the third gestational month as well as if a person is affected by an infection or degenerative disease (O'Brien, 1972a). The number of carriers that will be missed by serum screening is not known. Serum has also been tried for screening of carriers of sulfatidosis (Beratis et al., 1973) but the serum assay was not a reliable method for identifying heterozygous subjects. Suzuki and Suzuki (1971) have found serum to be the most reliable source for carrier detection in Krabbe disease but we could not confirm it (Svennerholm et al., 1975). In the other neurolipidoses serum has not been used for detection of carriers. Thus it is obvious that at present mass screening for the neurolipidoses on serum is not technically possible.

Carrier diagnosis can be carried out on leukocytes or on cultured fibroblasts. Kaback and Leonard (1972) suggested that the diagnosis should be performed on cultured skin fibroblasts. The activities of lysosomal hydrolases vary widely, however. Many studies have been undertaken on the fluctuations in the activity of lysosomal enzymes in cultured fibroblasts (Beutler et al., 1971; Milunsky et al., 1972; Okada et al., 1971) but it has not been possible to manage them yet. In a recent report Galjaard et al. (1974b) stated that cultured skin fibroblasts cannot be used for heterozygote screening for the lysosomal storage diseases. White blood cell preparations were first used by Brady et al. (1971a) for the detection of heterozygous carriers of Gaucher disease, Niemann-Pick disease and Fabry disease with radioactive natural substrates. However, their claim that artificial substrates may be used with confidence for detecting carriers for all lipid storage diseases except Niemann-Pick disease and Krabbe disease is wrong and not based on experimental results. For example, about 50% of our cases of

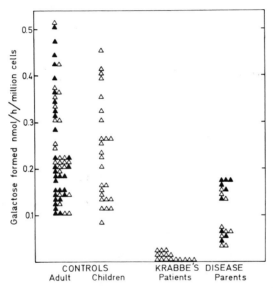

Fig. 7. Galactosylceramide β-galactosidase activities in leukocytes of children with Krabbe disease and of their parents. $\triangle$, adult females and children, $\blacktriangle$, adult males. (From Svennerholm et al., 1975.)

juvenile and adult Gaucher disease were missed with synthetic substrates. In our laboratory we have been using white blood cells and specific natural substrates for carrier detection of the common neurolipidoses. The obligate carriers had significantly lower values than the controls and significantly higher values than the affected children in GM1-gangliosidosis and Gaucher disease, but it was not possible to diagnose carriers of Krabbe disease, the most common form of the lipidoses in Scandinavia (Svennerholm et al., 1975; Fig. 7).

ENZYME THERAPY IN LYSOSOMAL STORAGE DISEASE

The principles of enzyme replacement treatment of lysosomal storage disease are based mainly on the premise that the lysosomal apparatus of the cell can take up enzyme from extracellular fluid by means of endocytosis. The blood-brain barrier seems to prevent the enzymes from reaching the central nervous system. Of the lipidoses, only Fabry disease and the juvenile and the adult form of Gaucher disease are not accompanied by any significant primary storage of lipids in the central nervous system, and they should theoretically be likely candidates for enzyme replacement therapy. This can be achieved by transplantation of a healthy organ which should serve as a continuous source of endogenous enzyme in the body. Kidney transplantation has been carried out on at least 8 patients with Fabry disease. Philippart (1973) reported clinical and pathological improvement 14 and 30 months after transplantation in his two patients. Also Desnick et al. (1973) reported such improvement in two patients. Tager and coworkers (Rietra et al., 1974) are critical to their reports and conclude that there is no indication for kidney transplantation in patients

TABLE VI

THERAPEUTIC POSSIBILITIES

Enzyme replacement

(A) Organ transplantation
(B) Parenteral administration of purified enzymes
    (1) human preparations
    (2) animal sources
    (3) encapsulated enzyme in biodegradable microspherules
    (4) percolation of blood or plasma over stably bound enzyme

Activation of mutated enzyme by antibody activation of enzyme by allosteric factors genetic engineering
(A) Administration of DNA
    (1) transducing viruses
(B) Hybridization and replacement of patient's cells

(from Brady, 1973)

with Fabry disease for purposes other than correction of the uremia. We tried spleen transplantation in a patient with juvenile Gaucher disease (Groth et al., 1971). The patient reacted intensely to the graft, and there was no clinical or laboratory evidence that the course of the disease was improved by the transplantation.

Parenteral administration of purified human enzyme preparations have been tried in a large number of diseases. The only good source for adequate amounts of pure enzyme seems to be the human placenta, but the costs of such treatment seem to be very high. The annual cost for the treatment of one case of Pompe disease was recently estimated to be one million French francs (Dr. Charles Merieux, personal communication) if the purification should continue to a product which did not give rise to immunological complications.

We found spleen transplantation not to produce the desired result in Gaucher disease, but Brady et al. (1975) reported very promising results in two cases by placental glucocerebrosidase therapy. After, respectively, a single and two injections of purified glucocerebrosidase two patients with adult Gaucher disease were said to get clearance of liver glucocerebrosides in amounts corresponding to the daily accumulation of cerebrosides during 4 and 13 years, respectively. The report can be seriously criticized because all calculations are based on a single biopsy before, and a second 24 h after, the therapy. In summary, injections of the missing enzyme is an extremely expensive method which seems to be of little benefit in the neurolipidoses.

Another mode for the enzyme replacement may be to lower the level of accumulated lipid in the blood by extracorporeal circulation over an immobilized enzyme capable of hydrolyzing the lipid. A different approach (Table VI) is activation of the mutant enzyme either by antibodies or by allosteric factors (Arora and Radin, 1972). No practical result has yet been proven. Finally, the possibility of genetic engineering has caused considerable excitement in some investigators. I can only feel anxiety and I hope that the rigorous standards that have been adopted by the National Academy of Science committee for the research in cloning of recombinant DNA molecules will be maintained in the future.

INDICATIONS FOR AMNIOCENTIC SCREENING FOR INHERITED DISEASES

(1) The high risk group of couples consists of those who already have a child with a fatal recessive disease such as one of the 7 neurolipidoses. The risk of their subsequent children having the disease is 1:4, and few Swedish parents will take that risk. When pregnant the mother will ask for abortion unless the fetus can be demonstrated to be normal. In this case one can say that amniocentesis is performed to avoid abortion of a healthy child. The small risk which the procedure involves is acceptable both to the parent and the physician. For society the cost of prenatal examination is small compared with the costs for the care of a diseased child.

(2) The second high risk group are parents who have been shown to be carriers of a fatal disease. We screen all persons under 35 years of age who are related to an index case of neurolipidoses. Since they are often living in isolates in the north we have detected many families in which both spouses were found to be carriers before they have got an affected child. The indications for amniocentic screening is the same as for the first group.

(3) The moderate risk group: the mother is a carrier but the father refuses carrier screening or is unknown. Further, relatives of families in which a child has been born with fatal inherited disease, but in which carrier screening is not yet possible. Krabbe disease is an example of such a disorder, and it is the most common neurolipidosis in Scandinavia.

PRENATAL DIAGNOSIS

The standard procedure is transabdominal amniocentesis performed from the 14th to the 16th week, with withdrawal of 10–20 ml of amniotic fluid. The cells are centrifuged off and cultured for 3–4 weeks before the biochemical

116

assay with radioactive, specific or unspecific synthetic substrate is performed. By application of microtechniques (Niermeijer et al., 1974) it has been possible to reduce the culture period to 12–14 days after amniocentesis. Uncultured cells and amniotic fluid have also been used in order to shorten the waiting period for the mother. It is a general experience that amniotic fluid can be used for the detection of fetuses affected with GM1- and GM2-gangliosidoses, Fabry disease and sulfatidoses, but cultured cells should always be used for confirming the diagnosis. Carrier values for an affected fetus can be due to contamination of the amniotic fluid with mother's blood, but I am not aware of any case in which the fluid has shown that the fetus has been affected, but where cultured cells have shown only carrier or normal values. It therefore seems possible to perform abortion directly after the amniocentesis, if the fluid shows the fetus to be affected. In my opinion there is a greater risk of finding values for an affected fetus, although the fetus is healthy, when uncultured cells are used. Many of the uncultured cells are dead and they have very little or no enzymic activity. Such cells constitute a large portion when amniocentesis is performed late in the pregnancy. The fluctuations of the levels of enzymic activity of lysosomal hydrolases with time in culture as found for cultured fibroblasts were also the same as those for amniotic fluid cells (Butterworth et al., 1973; Sutherland et al., 1974; Galjaard et al., 1974b). It is our experience, however, that in typical cases of each of the lipidoses, an affected fetus can safely be demonstrated if the following precautions are taken.

(1) Cells from a fetus at risk should always be cultured together with cells from control cases in the same medium. When possible, cells from the index case should also be analyzed at the same time as the cultured amniotic fluid cells. We also often include cultured cells from one of the two parents.

(2) Synthetic substrate should be used only when it has been demonstrated to give adequate results for the index case and the two obligate carriers (the parents).

TABLE VII

TISSUE CULTURE VARIABLES AFFECTING ENZYME ACTIVITY

(1) Cell density
(2) Stage of culture: confluent or not
(3) Type of medium
(4) Cell type
(5) Cell age
(6) Site of origin

(3) Many factors determine the activity of the cultured cells (Table VII) and the culture conditions should be standardized, particularly the culture period and the time after confluency when the cells are harvested.

(4) The enzymic activity should be expressed not only in relation to cell number or total protein, but also in relation to a marker enzyme (β-galactosidase or N-acetyl-β-glucosaminidase).

(5) The analyses should be performed in a biochemical laboratory with experience from enzymatic work and lipid biochemistry.

PROSPECTS FOR THE FUTURE

The recent advances in the diagnoses of inherited metabolic diseases have made it possible to monitor a pregnancy with prenatal diagnosis. So far, a prenatal diagnosis has been made in some 30 different diseases, and methods have been developed for the diagnoses of a further 30. In principle, any protein-based Mendelian disorder, in which the biochemical lesion is known and expressed in the amniotic cells, or which is associated with a distinctive marker substance, should be detectable in utero. This is a medical achievement with extensive consequences. The enzymic assay with synthetic substrate is also very simple to carry out even by a person without any basic knowledge of enzyme kinetics. In fact, the simplicity of enzymic tests has increased the risk for misdiagnoses since prenatal diagnosis of a certain disease is performed in many laboratories in quite a few countries although the frequency of the disease is very low. In many laboratories no relevant control material has been run, and the ranges for normals and obligate carriers are not known. Mistakes have been made in the past, and there is a risk that this will continue as long as each laboratory gets so little experience because of the large numbers of laboratories that wish to perform the tests. The presently positive attitude of the general public and the medical profession to prenatal diagnoses may well become negative because of this.

Prenatal diagnosis has hitherto been too glamorous. The period of easily gained success seems to be over, and it is time to make prenatal diagnosis of inherited metabolic diseases a general medical routine method. The prenatal diagnosis of inherited diseases should in the future be organized on a regional basis. The number of laboratories for each group of diseases should be small until more experience has been gained. In a center receiving a large number of cases to be analyzed the whole biochemical spectrum of each disorder could be studied. Such a center would also be in a much better position to evaluate new technical advances, develop new methods, and to study large control materials. As for the neurolipidoses, it is a common opinion among neurochemists that all prenatal examinations for the neurolipidoses should be performed with specific natural substrates, and synthetic substrates should be accepted only if it has been shown in the index case that the synthetic substrate is feasible in the family being studied. From a technical point of view, the fact that the prenatal diagnosis will take 3–4 weeks and that the abortion cannot be performed before the 20th week offers no difficulties, but the anxiety of the mother who is waiting for the result may be a serious problem. Therefore, micromethods of the type suggested by Galjaard et al (1974a) should be elaborated for natural substrates.

I think that we should not have exaggerated visions of future molecular neuropathology in the form of mass screening for lethal genes, of genetic engineering, or of enzyme replacement therapy of genetic diseases affecting mainly the nervous system. The costs of such programs would be very high when compared with the benefits. In a world in which 500 million children are suffering from malnutrition which can lead to mental retardation, it cannot be acceptable that the medical profession of the rich countries elaborate costly sophisticated programs in molecular neuropathology. I feel therefore that our major aim should be to prevent in high risk families the birth of children with a fatal inherited disease.

ACKNOWLEDGEMENT

The author's own work presented in this review has been performed with grants (project No. 3X-627) from the Swedish Medical Research Council.

REFERENCES

Arora, R.C. and Radin, N.S. (1972) Stimulation in vitro of galactocerebroside galactosidase by N-decanoyl-2-amino-2-methylpropanol. *Lipids*, 7: 56–59.

Bach, G. and Suzuki, K. (1975) Heterogeneity of human hepatic N-acetyl-β-D-hexosaminidase A activity toward natural glycosphingolipid substrates. *J. biol. Chem.*, 250: 1328–1332.

Beratis, N.G., Aron, A.M. and Hirschhorn, K. (1973) Metachromatic leukodystrophy: detection in serum. *J. Pediat.*, 83: 824–827.

Beutler, E., Kuhl, W., Teplitz, R. and Nadler, H. (1971) β-Glucosidase activity in fibroblasts from homozygotes and heterozygotes for Gaucher's disease. *Amer. J. hum. Genet.*, 23: 62–66.

Brady, R.O. (1973) The abnormal biochemistry of inherited disorders of lipid metabolism. *Fed. Proc.*, 32: 1660–1667.

Brady, R.O., Kanfer, J. and Shapiro, D. (1965). The metabolism of glucocerebrosides. I. Purification and properties of a glucocerebroside-cleaving enzyme from spleen tissue. *J. biol. Chem.*, 240: 39–43.

Brady, R.O., Pentchev, P.G. and Gal, A.E. (1975) Investigations in enzyme replacement therapy in lipid storage diseases. *Fed. Proc.*, 34: 1310–1315.

Brady, R.O., Johnson, W.G. and Uhlendorf, B.W. (1971a) Identification of heterozygous carriers of lipid storage diseases. *Amer. J. Med.*, 51: 423–431.

Brady, R.O., Uhlendorf, B.W. and Jacobson, C.B. (1971b) Fabry's disease: antenatal detection. *Science*, 172: 174–175.

Butterworth, J., Sutherland, G.R., Broadhead, D.M. and Bain, A.D. (1973) Lysosomal enzyme levels in human amniotic fluid cells in tissue culture. I. α-Glucosidase and β-glucosidase. *Life Sci.*, 13: 713–722.

Butterworth, G. Sutherland, G.R., Broadhead, D.M. and Bain, A.D. (1974a) Effect of serum concentration, type of culture medium and pH on the lysosomal enzyme activity of cultured human amniotic fluid cells. *Clin. chim. Acta*, 53: 239–246.

Butterworth, J., Sutherland, G.R., Broadhead, D.M. and Bain, A.D. (1974b) Lysosomal enzyme levels in human amniotic fluid cells in tissue culture. III. β-Glucuronidase, N-acetyl-β-D-glucosaminidase, α-mannosidase and acid phosphatase. *Clin. Genet.*, 5: 356–362.

Childs, B. (1967) Genetics and child development. *Amer. J. Dis. Child.*, 114: 464–469.

Desnick, R.J., Allen, K.Y., Simmons, R.L., Woods, J.E., Andersson, C.F., Najarian, J.S. and Krivit, W. (1973) Fabry disease: correction of the enzymatic deficiency by renal transplantation. In *Enzyme Therapy in Genetic Diseases, Birth Defects: Original Article Series, Vol. IX, No. 2*, D. Bergsma (Ed.), Williams and Wilkins, Baltimore, Md., pp. 88–95.

Eeg-Olofsson, O., Kristensson, K., Sourander, P. and Svennerholm, L. (1966) Tay-Sachs disease. A generalized metabolic disorder. *Acta paediat. scand.*, 55: 546–562.

Eldjarn, L., Jellum, E. and Stokke, O. (1975) Inborn errors of metabolism — a challenge to the clinical chemist. *Clin. Chem.*, 21: 63–66.

Ellis, W.G., Schneider, E.L., McCulloch, I.R., Suzuki, K. and Epstein, C.J. (1973) Fetal globoid cell leukodystrophy (Krabbe disease). *Arch. Neurol. (Chic.)*, 29: 253–257.

Eto, Y. and Suzuki, K. (1971) Brain spingolipids in Krabbe's globoid cell leukodystrophy. *J. Neurochem.*, 18: 503–511.

Galjaard, H., Hoogeveen, A., Keijzer, W., de Wit-Verbeck, E. and Vlek-Not, C. (1974a) The use of quantitative cytochemical analysis in rapid prenatal detection and somatic cell genetic studies of metabolic diseases. *Histochem. J.*, 6: 491–509.

Galjaard, H., Reuser, A.J.J., Henkels-Dully, M.J., Hoogeveen, A., Keijzer, W., de Wit-Verbeek, H.A. and Niermeijer, M.F. (1974b). Genetic heterogeneity and variation of lysosomal enzyme activities in cultured human cells. In *Enzyme Therapy in Lysosomal Storage Diseases*, J.M. Tager, G.J.M. Hooghwinkel and W.Th. Daems (Eds.), North-Holland Publishing Co., Amsterdam, pp. 35–51.

Galjaard, H., Hoogeveen, A., Keyzer, W., de Wit-Verbeek, H.A., Reuser, A.J.J., Ho, M. W. and Robinson, D. (1975) Genetic heterogeneity in different variants of GM1-gangliosidosis studied by β-galactosidase assays in (single) somatic hybrid cells. *Nature (Lond.)*, 257: 60–62.

Gatt, S. (1967) Comparison of four enzymes from brain which hydrolyze sphingolipids. In *Inborn Disorders of Sphingolipid Metabolism*, S. Aronson and B.W. Volk (Eds.), Pergamon Press, Oxford, pp. 261–266.

Groth, C.G., Hagenfeldt, L., Dreborg, S., Löfström, B., Öckerman, P.A., Samuelsson, K., Svennerholm, L., Werner, B. and Westberg, G. (1971) Splenic transplantation in a case of Gaucher's disease. *Lancet*, i: 1260–1264.

Herrlin, K.M. and Hillborg, P.O. (1962) Neurological signs of a juvenile form of Gaucher's disease. *Acta paediat. scand.*, 51: 137.

Hers, H.G. (1965) Inborn lysosomal diseases. *Gastroenterology*, 48: 625–633.

Hillborg, P.O. and Svennerholm, L. (1960) Blood level of cerebrosides in Gaucher's disease. *Acta paediat. scand.*, 49: 707–710.

Kaback, M.M. and Leonard, C.O. (1972) Control studies in the antenatal diagnosis of human genetic-metabolic disorders. In *Early Diagnosis of Human Genetic Defects*, M. Harris (Ed.), U.S. Government Printing Office, Washington D.C., pp. 169–178.

Klenk, E. (1939/1940) Beiträge zur Chemie der Lipoidosen I. Niemann-Pick'sche Krankheit und amaurotische Idiotie. *Hoppe-Seyler's Z. physiol. Chem.*, 262: 128–143.

Klenk, E. (1942) Über die Ganglioside, eine neue Gruppe von Zuckerhaltigen Gehirnlipoiden. *Hoppe-Seyler's Z. physiol. Chem.*, 273: 76–86.

McKusick, V.A. (1971) *Mendelian Inheritance in Man: Catalogs of Autosomal Dominant, Recessive, and X-Linked Phenotypes*, 3rd ed.,Johns Hopkins Press, Baltimore, Md.

Milunsky, A., Spielvogel, C. and Kanfer, J.N. (1972) Lysomal enzyme variations in cultured normal skin fibroblasts. *Life Sci.*, 11: 1101–1107.

Miyatake, T. and Suzuki, K. (1972) Globoid cell leukodystrophy: additional deficiency of psychosine galactosidase. *Biochem. biophys. Res. Commun.*, 48: 538–543.

Navon, R., Padeh, B. and Adam, A. (1973) Apparent deficiency of hexosaminidase A in healthy members of a family with Tay-Sachs disease. *Amer. J. hum. Genet.*, 25: 287–293.

Niermeijer, M.F., Fortuin, J.J.H., Koster, J.F., Jahodova, M. and Galjaard, H. (1974) Prenatal diagnosis of some lysosomal storage diseases. In *Enzyme Therapy in Lysosomal Storage Diseases*, J.M. Tager, G.J.M. Hooghwinkel and W.Th. Daems (Eds.), North Holland/American Elsevier, Amsterdam, pp. 25–33.

O'Brien, J.S. (1972a) Ganglioside storage diseases. *Advanc. hum. Genet.*, 3: 39–98.

O'Brien, J.S. (1972b) In *Early Diagnosis of Human Genetic Defects*, M. Harris (Ed.), U.S. Government Printing Office, Washington D.C., pp. 62–65.

O'Brien, J.S., Okada, S., Chen, A. and Fillerup, D.L. (1970) Tay-Sachs disease: detection of heterozygotes and homozygotes by serum hexosaminidase assay. *New Engl. J. Med.*, 283: 15–20.

O'Brien, J.S., Okada, S., Fillerup, D.L., Veath, M.L., Adornato, B., Brenner, P.H. and Leroy, G. (1971) Tay-Sachs disease: prenatal diagnosis, *Science*, 172: 61–64.

120

Öhman, R., Eklund, H. and Svennerholm, L. (1971) The diagnosis of Tay-Sachs disease. *Acta paediat. Scand.*, 60: 399–406.

Okada, S. and O'Brien, J.S. (1969) Tay-Sachs disease: generalized absence of beta-D-N-acetylhexosaminidase component. *Science*, 165: 698–700.

Okada, S., Veath, M.L., Leroy, J. and O'Brien, J.S. (1971) Ganglioside GM2 storage diseases: hexosaminidase deficiencies in cultured fibroblasts. *Amer. J. hum. Genet.*, 23: 55–61.

Philippart, M. (1973) Fabry disease: kidney transplantation as an enzyme replacement technic. In *Enzyme Therapy in Genetic Diseases, Birth Defects: Original Article Series, Vol. IX, No. 2*, D. Bergsma (Ed.), Williams and Wilkins, Baltimore, Md., pp. 81–87.

Radin, N.S. (1972) Labeled galactosylceramide and lactosylceramide. In *Methods in Enzymology, Vol. 28B*, S.P. Colowick and N.O. Kaplan (Eds.), Academic Press, New York, pp. 300–306.

Rietra, P.J.G.M., van den Bergh, F.A.J.T.M. and Tager, J.M. (1974) Recent developments in enzyme replacement therapy of lysosomal storage disease. In *Enzyme Therapy in Lysosomal Storage Diseases*, J.M. Tager, G.J.M. Hooghwinkel and W.Th. Daems (Eds.), North-Holland/American Elsevier, Amsterdam, pp. 53–79.

Ryan, C.A., Lee, Y.S. and Nadler, H.L. (1972) Effect of culture conditions on enzyme activities in cultivated human fibroblasts. *Exp. Cell Res.*, 71: 388–392.

Robinson, D. and Stirling, J.L. (1968) N-Acetyl-β-D-glucosaminidases in human spleen. *Biochem. J.*, 107: 321–327.

Sachs, B. (1887) On arrested cerebral development with special reference to its cortical pathology. *J. nerv. ment. Dis.*, 14: 541–553.

Sachs, B. (1896) A family form of idiocy generally fatal, associated with early blindness. *J. nerv. ment. Dis.*, 21: 475–479.

Sandhoff, K. und Wässle, W. (1971) Anreicherung und Charakterisierung zweier Formen der menschlichen N-acetyl-D-hexosaminidase. *Hoppe-Seyler's Z. physiol. Chem.*, 352: 1119–1133.

Sandhoff, K., Andreae, U. and Jatzkewitz, H. (1968) Deficient hexosaminidase activity in an exceptional case of Tay-Sachs disease with additional storage of kidney globoside in visceral organs. *Life Sci.*, 7: 283.

Sandhoff, K., Harzer, K., Wässle, W. and Jatzkewitz, H. (1971) Enzyme alterations and lipid storage in three variants of Tay-Sachs disease. *J. Neurochem.*, 18: 2469–2489.

Schneck, L., Valenti, C., Amsterdam, D., Friedland, J., Adachi, M. and Volk, B.W. (1970) Prenatal diagnosis of Tay-Sachs disease. *Lancet*, i: 582–584.

Schneck, L., Adachi, M. and Volk, B.W. (1972) Fetal aspects of Tay-Sachs disease. *Pediatrics*, 49: 342–351.

Scriver, C.R. (1969) Treatment of inherited disease: realized and potential. *Med. Clin. N. Amer.*, 53: 941–963.

Sourander, P. and Svennerholm, L. The storage of glycosylceramide in brain tissue in cases of infantile and juvenile Gaucher disease. In preparation.

Stoffel, W., Lekim, D. and Tschung, T.S. (1971) A simple chemical method for labelling phosphatidylcholine and sphingomyelin in the choline moiety. *Hoppe-Seyler's Z. physiol. Chem.*, 352: 1058–1064.

Sutherland, G.R., Butterworth, J., Bradhead, D.M. and Bain, A.D. (1974) Lysosomal enzyme levels in human amniotic fluid cells in tissue culture. II. α-Galactosidase, β-galactosidase and α-arabinosidase. *Clin. Genet.*, 5: 351–355.

Suzuki, Y. and Suzuki, K. (1970) Partial deficiency of hexosaminidase component A in juvenile G_{M2}-gangliosidosis. *Neurology (Minneap.)*, 20: 848–851.

Suzuki, Y. and Suzuki, K. (1971) Krabbe's globoid cell leukodystrophy: deficiency of galactocerebrosidase in serum, leucocytes and fibroblasts. *Science*, 171: 73–75.

Svennerholm, L. (1956) Composition of gangliosides from human brain. *Nature (Lond.)*, 177: 524–525.

Svennerholm, L. (1957) The nature of the gangliosides in Tay-Sachs' disease. In *Cerebral Lipidoses*, J.N. Cumings (Ed.), Blackwell, Oxford, pp. 139–145.

Svennerholm, L. (1962) The chemical structure of normal human brain and Tay-Sachs ganglioside. *Biochem. biophys. Res. Commun.*, 9: 436–441.

Svennerholm, L., Håkansson, G. and Vanier, M.T. (1975) Chemical pathology of Krabbe's disease. IV. Studies of galactosylceramide and lactosylceramide-β-galactosidases in brain, white blood cells and amniotic fluid cells. *Acta paediat. scand.*, 64: 649–656.

Taketomi, T. and Nishimura, K. (1964) Physiological activity of psychosine. *Jap. J. exp. Med.*, 34: 255–265.

Tallman, J.F., Brady, R.O., Quirk, J.M., Villalba, M. and Gal, A.E. (1974) Isolation and relationship of human hexosaminidases. *J. biol. Chem.*, 249: 3489–3499.

Tay, W.A. (1881) Symmetrical changes in the region of the yellow spot in each eye of an infant. *Trans. ophthal. Soc. U.K.*, 1: 55–57.

Tondeur, M., Vamos-Hurvitz, E., Mockel-Pohl, S., Dereume, J.P., Cremer, N. and Loeb, H. (1971) Clinical, biochemical and ultrastructural studies in a case of chondrodystrophy presenting the I-cell phenotype in tissue culture. *J. Pediat.*, 79: 366–378.

Thudichum, J.L.W. (1884) *A Treatise on the Chemical Constitution of the Brain.* Ballière, Tindall and Cox, London.

Tsay, G.C., Dawson, G. and Li, Y.T. (1975) Structure of the glycopeptide storage material in GM1-gangliosidosis. *Biochim. biophys. Acta (Amst.)*, 385: 305–311.

Vanier, M.T. and Svennerholm, L. (1974) Chemical pathology of Krabbe's disease. I. Lipid composition and fatty acid patterns of phosphoglycerides in brain. *Acta paediat. scand.*, 63: 494–500.

Vanier, M.T. and Svennerholm, L. (1975) Chemical pathology of Krabbe's disease. III. Ceramide-hexosides and gangliosides in brain. *Acta paediat. scand.*, 64: 641–648.

Vidgoff, J., Buist, N.R.M. and O'Brien, J.S. (1973) Absence of N-acetyl-D-hexosaminidase A activity in a healthy woman. *Amer. J. hum. Genet.*, 25: 372–381.

Wenger, D.A., Okada, S. and O'Brien, J.S. (1972) Studies on the substrate specificity of hexosaminidase A and B from liver. *Arch. Biochem.*, 153: 116–129.

Winick, M., Brasel, J.A. and Rosso, P. (1972) Nutrition and cell growth. In *Nutrition and Development*, M. Winick (Ed.), Wiley, New York, pp. 49–97.

Wolfe, L.S., Senior, R.G. and Ng Ying Kin, N.M. (1974) The structures of oligosaccharides accumulating in the liver of GM1-gangliosidosis, type I. *J. biol. Chem.*, 249: 1828–1838.

DISCUSSION

H. VAN DER LOOS: Dr. Svennerholm, you said that cerebrosides, or a particular cerebroside is accumulated in the cerebellum and not in the cerebrum. Is there a particular attraction of the cerebellum for cerebrosides, or could this predilection have something to do with the vascularization pattern? Also, I wonder whether you can take your samples from smaller areas than just from the cerebellum, for instance from specific pieces of cerebellum; and from regions projecting to cerebellum, such as inferior olive, lateral cuneate nucleus, column of Clarke, pontine nuclei, etc., and see how in these regions the accumulation compares with, for example, the thalamus, a region projecting not only to cerebellum but also to cerebral cortex?

L. SVENNERHOLM: I am not aware of any major chemical difference between the cerebral cortex and the cerebellum or the basal ganglia. I assume that the brain barrier function is less developed in the cerebellum and the basal ganglia than in the cerebral cortex, or that there is a big difference in the vascularization of cerebellar cortex, since the concentration of extraneuronal glucocerebrosides was found to be 10–20 times higher in cerebellar than in cerebral cortex.

E.G. GRAY: One difference that I can think of, is that there is quite a large amount of myelin in the cerebral cortex, while there is practically no myelin in the cerebellar cortex apart from the deeper parts of the granule layer.

L. SVENNERHOLM: I have mostly mentioned the cerebellar cortex, but the accumulation of extraneural glucocerebrosides was also at least 10 times higher in cerebellar white matter than in cerebral white matter. I should also have mentioned that the extraneuronal glucocerebrosides have no metabolic relationship to the galactocerebrosides of myelin.

H. STEFFEN: Are there already any possibilities of synthesizing the lacking enzymes?

L. SVENNERHOLM: No, but it is rather easy to isolate an active enzyme preparation from a good source such as human placenta. But it is expensive to purify the enzymes to such an extent that they will not cause any toxic reaction of the patient. In addition, in most of the inherited diseases there is an early fetal affection of the central nervous system, and in these disorders the substitution therapy will fail. In some other diseases with lysosomal storage there is no primary affection of the nervous system and these diseases seem to be possible candidates for enzyme replacement therapy, e.g. Pompe disease. The results of the treatment have not been promising, and the annual costs for the therapy can be estimated to about 200,000 dollars. It is my opinion that enzyme substitution therapy has failed in inherited storage diseases.

SESSION III

BRAIN–HORMONE INTERACTIONS

Neurosecretion — Comparative and Evolutionary Aspects*

BERTA SCHARRER

*Department of Anatomy, Albert Einstein College of Medicine,
New York (U.S.A.)*

INTRODUCTION

The formulation of the neuron doctrine has established the identity of highly differentiated cellular units whose structural and functional specializations set them clearly apart from other cell types. Neurons, with their extended processes that make contact with other cells, mostly with other neurons, are designed for the reception of stimuli, the conduction of impulses, and the transmission of signals.

This orderly and generally accepted picture was disturbed by the discovery of a class of neurons whose primary activity consists in the manufacture of a specific glandular product, and whose axons terminate without establishing synaptic contact. At the time, most neurobiologists could not conceive of neurons engaged in secretory activity which is so much more pronounced than that involved in the synthesis of conventional neurotransmitters. Now, after nearly 50 years of concentrated efforts, the enigma no longer exists. Specific hormonal functions can be ascribed to these "neurosecretory neurons", and other non-conventional modes of neurochemical communication are under active investigation. But what is the rationale for the existence of these phenomena? Why, for example, should certain neurons deviate so profoundly from the norm so as to send a blood-borne messenger to the mammalian kidney resulting in water conservation? As the following account will demonstrate, part of the answer must be sought in broad evolutionary terms.

PHYLOGENY OF NEURAL SYSTEMS OF COMMUNICATION

Starting with the simplest forms of multicellular organisms, we find among the sponges what Pavans de Ceccatty (1974) interprets as a reticular neuroid tissue complex. Cells classifiable as primitive neurons and elementary synaptic contacts appear for the first time in the lowest eumetazoans, the coelenterates. What seems important in the context of the present analysis is that some of the coelenterate neurons differ from the rest in that they display cytological signs

---

* Dedicated in friendship to Professor Wolfgang Bargmann on his 70th birthday, January 27, 1976.

of neurosecretory activity comparable to those in higher animals. Furthermore, tests with isolated neurosecretory granules of *Hydra* have demonstrated the role of their content in the regulation of growth and differentiation, especially during regeneration (Lentz, 1968). There is also some evidence suggesting that neurosecretory messengers participate in the induction of gametogenesis and sex differentiation in this coelenterate (Burnett and Diehl, 1964).

Perhaps even more remarkable is the fact that, in sponges, cell types that do not even satisfy all of the criteria of primitive neurons contain cytoplasmic inclusions resembling those in neurosecretory cells. These inclusions are located in the perikarya and in bulbous swellings of the cellular processes; they stain with alcian blue and, in electron micrographs, appear as membrane-bounded granules about 100–1700 nm in diameter (Pavans de Ceccatty, 1966; Lentz, 1968). However, nothing is known about a possible role of these cellular products in the propagation of rudimentary signals.

Neurosecretory granules are plentiful in the nervous system of planarians where their active principle controls growth during development and regeneration (Lentz, 1968), as well as reproductive events (Grasso and Quaglia, 1971; Grasso and Benazzi, 1973). In annelids, an impressively large proportion (over 50%) of the neurons making up well circumscribed ganglia are of the neurosecretory type. Their products are released into the circulation to carry out several hormonal messenger functions. Among these functions are control over regeneration, reproduction and, in dimorphic species, over somatic transformations (Durchon, 1967; Hauenschild, 1974).

These few examples should suffice to support the following conclusions. Hormonal mechanisms occur in primitive metazoans where they govern a number of vital processes. Since, at this level of differentiation, "regular" glands of internal secretion are still missing, the nervous system is the only agency available for carrying out all of the existing endocrine functions. Thus, neurohormones hold the rank of the phylogenetically oldest blood-borne messengers, and the hormonal type of coordination accounts for a relatively large sector of neuronal activities in lower invertebrates. It follows that the conceptual model of the ancestral neuron is that of a functionally versatile entity endowed with the means for long distance as well as more or less localized chemical signalling.

In the course of evolution the scene shifts in more than one direction. Not only is there a staggering increase in the number of neurons, as primitive nervous systems give way to more and more elaborate structures but also a change in their functional properties. The evolution of higher integrative centers with their complex circuitries pari passu leads to neuronal specialization whereby graded responses become all-or-nothing and signals need to be rapid, precisely localized, and polarized. In other words, in the most advanced forms, the vast majority of nerve cells engage in interneuronal synaptic transmission and, in the form of neurotransmitters, make only a restricted use of chemical mediators.

This shift in functional priority, and the resulting preeminence of the "conventional neuron", seems responsible for at least some of the past conceptual difficulties in the ranks of neurobiologists primarily concerned with mammalian systems vis-à-vis the phenomenon of neurosecretion.

Another evolutionary change in design, seemingly arguing against the need for blood-borne neurochemical mediators in higher animals, is the evolvement of extraneuronal hormone sources. In arthropods, and even more so in vertebrates, the availability of a second integrative system, the endocrine apparatus proper, does permit a division of labor, and so should relieve neurons from doing double-duty.

NEUROENDOCRINE INTERACTIONS

In reality, neurohormonal activities do not disappear following the acquisition of regular endocrine glands. The manner in which they continue to function is in fact two-fold.

(1) First order neurosecretory systems, i.e., one-step control over "terminal" effector cells, remain in operation, even in mammals, as exemplified by the effects of vasopressin on kidney tubule cells and of oxytocin on the myoepithelial cells of the mammary gland. However, there is no compelling reason why higher organisms should not get along without such systems, and their existence makes little sense except in an evolutionary perspective. It is conceptually sound to interpret them as carry-overs, comparable to systems used by necessity in phylogenetically less advanced forms.

(2) In creating a new order of command, the takeover of most of the conventional hormonal functions by the endocrine apparatus has given rise to a novel use for the neurosecretory neuron. It is a highly specialized role that could not be dispensed with, and one that makes very good sense. Directives intended for hormone-producing cells must be integrated in the brain, and passed on to the first way station of the endocrine apparatus, i.e., to the adenohypophysis, or analogous invertebrate organs. As has been pointed out repeatedly in the past (Scharrer, 1970, 1972, 1974), the neurosecretory neuron with its dual capacity is ideally suited to transmit this very kind of information. Therefore, instead of having become obsolete, neurohormones have now come into their own by serving as special messengers between the two systems of integration.

So vital is this new function, that its success is assured by the availability of several mechanisms for communication, each of them with distinct adaptive features. The most prominent pathway is the special portal circulation which provides simultaneous access to various adenohypophyseal effector cells without unnecessary detour. Alternate routes for neurosecretory signals that are even more "private" will be discussed next.

NON-HORMONAL ACTIVITIES OF NEUROSECRETORY NEURONS

A rather unexpected result of the search for variants in the mode of operation of the neuroendocrine axis was that not all of the neurosecretory neurons release their products into the circulation. In vertebrates, including mammals, there is ample ultrastructural evidence that axons laden with such active materials may circumvent the vascular route and penetrate the glandular

128

parenchyma to terminate close to, or even in contiguity with, their cells of destination, for example, in the pars intermedia. The same spatial relationships have been found in the endocrine organs of insects which are avascular.

Another interesting outcome of studies stimulated by these results is that comparable "synaptoid" release sites of neurosecretory materials, suggesting close range control, are not restricted to endocrine effector cells. They also occur on somatic elements such as exocrine gland cells and muscle fibers. Furthermore, and perhaps most unexpectedly, neurosecretory neurons have been shown, in vertebrates as well as invertebrates, to establish synapse-like relationships (Fig. 1) with other neurons, some of which may themselves be of the non-conventional type.

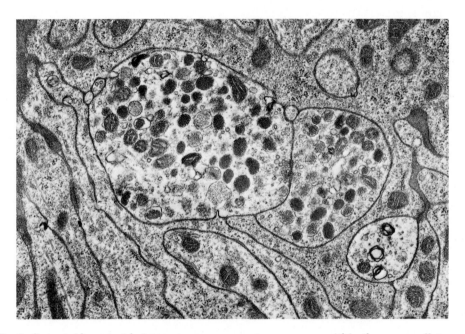

Fig. 1. Synaptoid contact between two neurosecretory neurons within the corpus allatum of an insect, *Arphia pseudonietana*. Note clustered electronlucent vesicles and "intersynaptic" space, characteristic of site of release of neurochemical mediator. (Specimen courtesy of Dr. S.N. Visscher.) × 21,000.

The realization that, at least in certain special situations, peptidergic neurosecretory mediators may operate in a manner comparable to that of neurotransmitters has added a new and important facet to the "gestalt" of the classical neurosecretory neuron.

NON-CONVENTIONAL INTERNEURONAL COMMUNICATION

Let us now briefly focus on some of these non-conventional forms of chemical neuron-to-neuron signalling, since indications for their existence are not based on ultrastructural criteria alone (Dyer and Dyball, 1974). Physiological experiments in arthropods as well as mammals have shown that neurosecretory messengers, delivered either at close range or via circulatory channels, elicit a number of specific responses from certain kinds of neurons.

Neurohormonal stimulation is responsible for elaborately patterned behavioral sequences characteristic of postembryonic development and reproductive events in crustaceans and insects. To cite only one example, in the moth *Cecropia*, a neurosecretory factor, called "eclosion hormone", triggers a series of stereotyped movements, preprogrammed in the abdominal ganglia, that bring about the terminal molt, and then turns off the responsible motor neurons that are no longer needed (Truman and Riddiford, 1974).

Similarly, some conventional vertebrate neurons are capable of responding to neurosecretory stimuli. Among them are dopaminergic cells in the mammalian central nervous system that are attuned to hypothalamic messengers such as TRF (thyrotropin releasing factor), the effect being comparable to that elicited by L-DOPA (Plotnikoff et al., 1972). There is also direct neurochemical evidence suggesting that such a peptidergic hypothalamic factor affects the synthesis of the neurotransmitter dopamine (see Friedman et al., 1973) and activates noradrenergic neurons (Constantinidis et al., 1974).

Reports on behavioral alterations attributable to non-conventional neuroregulators originating in the hypothalamus include antidepressant effects in humans (Ehrensing and Kastin, 1974; Horst and Spirt, 1974) and facilitation of lordosis behavior in estrogen-primed, hypophysectomized, ovariectomized rats (Pfaff, 1973).

These, and an increasing number of related data, suggest that TRF has a modulating effect on synaptic, especially monoaminergic, transmission. Apparently, this role evolved before that of controlling thyrotropin release, and it seems to be of a more general importance (Grimm-Jørgensen et al., 1975; McCann and Moss, 1975).

Of equal interest are recent experimental data suggesting a broader role for the posterior lobe hormones. In addition to their well known first order neurohormonal activity, neurohypophyseal hormones are responsible for antidromic excitatory stimuli. They seem to participate in the processing of certain neural signals resulting in motor responses, learning, glucose uptake, etc. (Sterba, 1974 and de Wied et al., Chapter 11, pp. 181–194 in this volume). Moreover, effects that differ from the conductance changes evoked by conventional neurotransmitters, and that may represent a new form of information transfer, can be elicited in certain neurosecretory neurons of molluscs by the application of vasopressin and related peptides (Barker and Gainer, 1974). The role of oxytocin as a prohormone, second order, is referred to below.

In a number of cases, the extracellular route to the neuronal receptor cells is still under investigation, but since some of the effects persist in the absence of the pituitary, the pathway can be said to differ from that used by the same neurochemical mediators in their hypophyseotropic role. Incomplete though they are, the existing data on psychotropic and other non-conventional effects of neurosecretory mediators have opened a new and promising chapter in biomedical research.

CHEMICAL EVOLUTION OF NEUROSECRETORY MEDIATORS

The biosynthetic activity of classical neurosecretory neurons differs from that of conventional nerve cells not only in quantity but also in quality. Even though much of our present knowledge of the chemical identities of neuromediators relates to mammalian systems, certain evolutionary trends are beginning to emerge.

In contradistinction to regular neurotransmitters, neurosecretory products of invertebrates as well as vertebrates are predominantly proteinaceous. Another distinguishing feature is that biologically active polypeptides, e.g., vasopressin, are bound by non-covalent forces to special carrier proteins (neurophysins; see Walter, 1975; Watkins, 1975). Both components make a strikingly parallel and sudden appearance early during fetal development (Pearson et al., 1975), and the possibility exists that neurophysins may actually play a more active role than that originally conceived (Pilgrim, 1974).

Much information is being amassed on the occurrence and precise localization of such peptides and their affiliated neurophysins within the neurosecretory systems of various animals by the use of immunochemical, including immunoelectron microscopic, methods (see Zimmerman, 1976). Moreover, the availability of synthetically produced neurohormones and their analogues represents a valuable tool for the differential determination of their functional roles.

A great deal has been learned from comparative biochemical studies, encompassing the entire vertebrate series, on the phylogenetic distribution of several molecular species of neurohypophyseal hormones. By comparison, data on the chemical identities of hypophyseotropins in non-mammalian species are much more scanty (Dubois et al., 1974). What can be said about either of these two groups of neurohormones is that, in spite of certain variations in amino acid composition — presumably resulting from successive gene duplications — there is on the whole an impressive similarity in their activity spectrum and chemical structure (see Acher, 1974a; Heller, 1974; Wallis, 1975). Furthermore, there is increasing evidence suggesting a common evolutionary origin for representatives of both families of hypothalamic hormones (Carraway and Leeman, 1975).

By the same token, the neurophysins appear as a phylogenetically old and strikingly homologous class of neuronal products (Capra and Walter, 1975). Such special proteins have been identified by their cross-reaction with antihuman antisera not only in neurosecretory neurons of mammals and birds, but also of teleosts and cyclostomes (see Zimmerman, 1976).

Comparable data in invertebrates are still sporadic, but histochemical and biochemical parallelisms strongly suggest the existence of analogous proteinaceous compounds in lower forms (see Scharrer and Weitzman, 1970). To cite one specific case, a crustacean chromatophorotropin has been identified as a small peptide with N- and C-terminal regions corresponding to those of some of the vertebrate hypophyseotropins (Fernlund and Josefsson, 1972). Furthermore, a chemically synthesized octapeptide has been shown to concentrate the pigments of two types of crustacean effector cells both in vitro and in vivo (Josefsson, 1975).

Another case in point is the recent demonstration of immunoreactive TRF among invertebrates, i.e., in the circumesophageal ganglia of various gastropods, in amounts comparable to those in cerebral cortical tissue of some vertebrates (Grimm-Jørgensen et al., 1975).

The postulation of this chemical parallelism is indirectly supported also by striking cytophysiological similarities. Throughout the metazoan series, the ultrastructural parameters of the dynamics of production, storage, and discharge of neurosecretory materials are the same. Active peptides and carrier proteins, when present, are packaged within the cells' typical secretory granules from which they are released together, as suggested by electron microscopic signs of exocytosis (Douglas, 1974).

What can be inferred from these observations, incomplete though they are, about the phylogenetic origin and mutual relationships of the components of neurosecretory materials? Did the original blueprint call for the concomitant·de novo synthesis of active peptides on one hand, and of hormonally "silent" carrier proteins on the other? Or, was there initially one ancestral protein molecule which gradually gave rise to classes of compounds with different functions? On conceptual grounds, the latter possibility would seem to be the more likely (cf. Acher, 1974a, b). It is also in line with certain views based on isotope studies pertaining to the origin of the materials within presently existing neurosecretory systems.

As proposed by Sachs et al. (1969), active polypeptides may be derived from a high molecular weight precursor molecule synthesized in the perikarya of magnocellular hypothalamic neurons. During the maturation of the neurosecretory granules, a similar enzymatic breakdown mechanism could well give rise to the neurophysins, following a common ancestral pattern of protein biosynthesis (see also Pilgrim, 1974). Neurohormone and carrier might even share one and the same macromolecular precursor.

In turn, an active peptide, e.g., oxytocin, can act as precursor for other hormonal factors, such as the hypophyseotropin MIF (MSH-release inhibiting factor), a tripeptide fragment released by further enzymatic action.

The large protein precursor, being presumably inactive itself, qualifies as a prohormone, first order, comparable to proinsulin. Conversely, the polypeptide hormone, in its capacity as precursor for a smaller peptide with an endocrine activity entirely different from that of the parent principle, can be classified as a prohormone, second order (see Walter, 1974; Schwartz and Walter, 1974).

In short, we are dealing with a special principle of hormone economy. The classical neurosecretory products of the present are distinctive but closely related proteinaceous entities which, in the course of a long evolutionary history, have undergone molecular modulations and have acquired the capacity for multiple and varied uses. Some signs of this progression are reflected in neuroendocrine patterns of lower forms today, and perhaps also in the molecular events during ontogenetic development (Pearson et al., 1975).

We might add that, to some degree, this principle of diversification also applies to aminergic neurons. For the most part their neurochemical messengers function at close range, dispatching regular synaptic signals to other neurons or endocrine effector cells (Fuxe et al., 1974; Terlou, 1974), yet in special instances the same messengers may act as non-classical (B-type) neurohormones (see, for example, Hinks, 1967).

THE PLACE OF NEUROSECRETION IN NEUROCHEMICAL MEDIATION

As has become apparent, the degree of flexibility with which neurosecretory neurons seem to operate in transmitting neurally derived information to various receptors is certainly impressive. Nevertheless, within the total framework of neurobiology, the activities of these extraordinary cells constitute a very small proportion, designed to meet a number of special requirements.

Therefore, in past efforts to determine the origin of neurosecretory neurons, it could be argued that the capacity for glandular activity above and beyond that of conventional neurons is a secondary phenomenon, the result of progressive specialization which appeared relatively late in phylogeny (e.g. Hanström, 1954; Gabe, 1966). According to a converse proposition, neurosecretory neurons are derived from glandular elements originally located in the epidermis and subsequently incorporated into nervous centers where they secondarily acquired neuronal properties (Clark, 1956). Both of these views lack sufficient support.

CONCLUSIONS

On the basis of the current information referred to above, the most reasonable scheme for the phylogenetic derivation of neurosecretory neurons seems to lie between these two extremes. It is based on the simple premise that neurons originate from undifferentiated epithelial cells whose basic endowments include excitability and conductivity, as well as the capacity for elaboration of physiologically active substances. Having been passed on to the primitive neuron, these inherent properties are not discarded in the course of further differentiation.

It is the degree to which they become either reduced or further developed that eventually leads to the evolutionary separation into various classes of neurons, and that determines their rank within a series arranged according to the different modes of neurochemical communication in operation.

At one end of the line is the synaptic type of chemical transmission characteristic of the great majority of conventional neurons. In this kind of cell the demands for secretory activity, though still in operation, have become very much reduced, while its bioelectric activity has gained predominance. At the opposite end of the spectrum is the type of communication carried out by classical neurosecretory neurons that dispatch their messengers via the general circulation and in which impulse conduction serves the release of neurohormones (Cross, 1974). Since these substances, in order to be effective, must be available in substantial amounts, comparable in fact to those of regular hormones, biosynthetic activity has top priority in such neurons. Between these two endpoints, various gradations of secretory activity encompass mechanisms in which the neurochemical messenger may reach its destination via semiprivate circulatory channels or via alternate non-vascular routes. Quite obviously, the shorter the extracellular pathway, the smaller are the demands on the synthetic machinery for producing appropriate amounts of the respective messenger substances.

The recognition of these intermediate types of neurochemical activity has removed the sharp dividing line between classical neurosecretory and conventional neurons, and the phenomenon of neurosecretion, once so difficult to assimilate, now blends into a continuum. What used to be considered a dichotomy between two classes of neural elements, has turned out to constitute a spectrum of neurochemical activities. What has also become clear is that the pluripotential neurosecretory neuron, in its various forms, has remained closer to the nerve cell precursor than has the conventional neuron. The inherited capacity for secretory activity has been put to use in various ways at every level of the evolutionary scale, and hormones derived from neural elements have remained indispensible even after the appearance of the endocrine system proper.

SUMMARY

The rationale for the existence of neurosecretory phenomena, and their place within the range of neurochemical mediation, is inherent in their evolutionary history. Signs of neurosecretory activity, i.e., the specialization of certain neurons for the production of neurohormones, are found in all metazoans. These hormones are thus phylogenetically the oldest, and also the only blood-borne messengers operating in the more primitive invertebrates which lack "regular" glands of internal secretion.

The recognition of neuronal types capable of several intermediate modes of neurochemical communication has removed the sharp dividing line between classical neurosecretory cells and conventional neurons, and the phenomenon of neurosecretion, once so difficult to assimilate, now blends into a spectrum of neurochemical activities.

The conceptual model of the ancestral neuron, considered to be the phylogenetic derivative of an undifferentiated and pluripotential epithelial cell, is that of a functionally versatile structure, equally endowed for the dispatch of long distance and localized chemical signals. The neurosecretory neuron has remained closer to the nerve cell precursor than has the conventional neuron with its specialization for synaptic transmission. Furthermore, the inherited capacity for secretory activity has been put to good use by neurosecretory neurons in various ways at every level of the evolutionary scale.

ACKNOWLEDGEMENT

Parts of the studies referred to in this chapter have been supported by Research Grants NB-05219, NB-00840, and 5 PO 1 NS-07512 from the U.S.P.H.S.

134

REFERENCES

Acher, R. (1974a) Chemistry of the neurohypophysial hormones: an example of molecular evolution. In *Handbook of Physiology, Sect. 7, Endocrinology, Vol. 4, Pt. 1*, R.O. Greep and E.B. Astwood, (Eds.), American Physiol. Soc., Washington, D.C., pp. 119–130.

Acher, R. (1974b) Recent discoveries in the evolution of proteins. *Angew. Chemie*, (Int. Ed.), 13: 186–197.

Barker, J.L. and Gainer, H. (1974) Peptide regulation of bursting pacemaker activity in a molluscan neurosecretory cell. *Science*, 184: 1371–1373.

Burnett, A.L. and Diehl, N.A. (1964) The nervous system of *Hydra*. III. The initiation of sexuality with special reference to the nervous system. *J. exp. Zool.*, 157: 237–249.

Capra, J.D. and Walter, R. (1975) Primary structure and evolution of neurophysins. *Ann. N.Y. Acad. Sci.*, 248: 397–407.

Carraway, R. and Leeman, S.E. (1975) The amino acid sequence of a hypothalamic peptide, neurotensin. *J. biol. Chem.*, 250: 1907–1911.

Clark, R.B. (1956) On the origin of neurosecretory cells. *Ann. Sci. nat. Zool.*, 18: 199–207.

Constantinidis, J., Greissbühler, F., Gaillard, J.M., Hovaguinian, T. and Tissot, R. (1974) Enhancement of cerebral noradrenaline turnover by thyrotropin-releasing hormone: evidence by fluorescence histochemistry. *Experientia (Basel)*, 30: 1182–1183.

Cross, B.A. (1974) The neurosecretory impulse. In *Neurosecretion — the Final Neuroendocrine Pathway*, F. Knowles and L. Vollrath, (Eds.), Springer-Verlag, Berlin, pp. 115–128.

Douglas, W.W. (1974) Involvement of calcium in exocytosis and the exocytosis-vesiculation sequence. *Biochem. Soc. Symp.*, 39: 1–28.

Dubois, M.P., Barry, J. et Leonardelli, J. (1974) Mise en évidence par immunofluorescence et répartition de la somatostatine (SRIF) dans l'éminence médiane des Vertébrés (Mammifères, Oiseaux, Amphibiens, Poissons). *C.R. Acad. Sci. (Paris), sér., D*, 279: 1899–1902.

Durchon, M. (1967) L'endocrinologie des vers et des mollusques. Coll. *Les Grands Problèmes de la Biologie*. Masson, Paris, 241 pp.

Dyer, R.G. and Dyball, R.E.J. (1974) Evidence for a direct effect of LRF and TRF on single unit activity in the rostral hypothalamus. *Nature (Lond.)*, 252: 486–488.

Ehrensing, R.H. and Kastin, A.J. (1974) Melanocyte-stimulating hormone-release inhibiting hormone as an antidepressant. A pilot study. *Arch. gen. Psychiat.*, 30: 63–65.

Fernlund, P. and Josefsson, L. (1972) Crustacean color-change hormone: amino acid sequence and chemical synthesis. *Science*, 177: 173–175.

Friedman, E., Friedman, J. and Gershon, S. (1973) Dopamine synthesis: stimulation by a hypothalamic factor. *Science*, 182: 831–832.

Fuxe, K., Hökfelt, T., Jonsson, G. and Löfström, A. (1974) Aminergic mechanisms in neuroendocrine control. In *Neurosecretion — the Final Neuroendocrine Pathway*, F. Knowles and L. Vollrath (Eds.), Springer-Verlag, Berlin, pp. 269–275.

Gabe, M. (1966) *Neurosecretion, Int. Ser. Monogr. Biol. Vol. 28*, Pergamon Press, Oxford, 872 pp.

Grasso, M. and Benazzi, M. (1973) Genetic and physiologic control of fissioning and sexuality in planarians, *J. Embryol. exp. Morph.*, 30: 317–328.

Grasso, M. and Quaglia, A. (1971) Studies on neurosecretion in planarians III. Neurosecretory fibres near the testes and ovaries of *Polycelis nigra*. *J. submicr. Cytol.*, 3: 171–180.

Grimm-Jørgensen, Y., McKelvy, J.F. and Jackson, I.M.D. (1975) Immunoreactive thyrotrophin releasing factor in gastropod circumoesophageal ganglia. *Nature (Lond.)*, 254: 420.

Hanström, B. (1954) On the transformation of ordinary nerve cells into neurosecretory cells. *Kgl. Fysiogr. Sällsk. Lund. Förh.*, 24: 75–82.

Hauenschild, C. (1974) Endokrine Beeinflussung der geschlechtlichen Entwicklung einiger Polychaeten. *Fortschr. Zool.*, 22: 75–92.

Heller, H. (1974) Molecular aspects in comparative endocrinology. *Gen. comp. Endocr.*, 22: 315–332.

Hinks, C.F. (1967) Relationship between serotonin and the circadian rhythm in some nocturnal moths. *Nature (Lond.)*, 214: 386–387.

Horst, W.D. and Spirt, N. (1974) A possible mechanism for the anti-depressant activity of thyrotropin releasing hormone. *Life Sci.*, 15: 1073–1082.

Josefsson, L. (1975) Structure and function of crustacean chromatophorotropins. *Gen. comp. Endocr.*, 25: 199–202.

Lentz, T.L. (1968) *Primitive Nervous Systems*. Yale Univ. Press, New Haven, Conn.

McCann, S.M. and Moss, R.L. (1975) Putative neurotransmitters involved in discharging gonadotropin-releasing neurohormones and the action of LH-releasing hormone on the CNS. *Life Sci.*, 16: 833–852.

Pavans de Ceccatty, M. (1966) Ultrastructures et rapports des cellules mésenchymateuses de type nerveux de l'Éponge *Tethya lyncurium Lmk. Ann. Sci. nat. Zool.*, 8: 577–614.

Pavans de Ceccatty, M. (1974) The origin of the integrative systems: a change in view derived from research on coelenterates and sponges. *Perspect. Biol. Med.*, 17: 379–390.

Pearson, D.B., Goodman, R. and Sachs, H. (1975) Stimulated vasopressin synthesis by a fetal hypothalamic factor. *Science*, 187: 1081–1082.

Pfaff, D.W. (1973) Luteinizing hormone-releasing factor potentiates lordosis behavior in hypophysectomized ovariectomized female rats. *Science*, 182: 1148–1149.

Pilgrim, C. (1974) Histochemical differentiation of hypothalamic areas. In *Integrative Hypothalamic Activity, Progress in Brain Research*, Vol. 41, D.F. Swaab and J.P. Schadé (Eds.), Elsevier, Amsterdam, pp. 97–110.

Plotnikoff, N.P., Kastin, A.J., Anderson, M.S. and Schally, A.V. (1972) Oxotremorine antagonism by a hypothalamic hormone, melanocyte-stimulating hormone release-inhibiting factor (MIF). *Proc. Soc. exp. Biol. (N.Y.)*, 140: 811–814.

Sachs, H., Fawcett, P., Takabatake, Y. and Portanova, R. (1969) Biosynthesis and release of vasopressin and neurophysin. *Recent Progr. Hormone Res.*, 25: 447–491.

Scharrer, B. (1970) General principles of neuroendocrine communication. In *The Neurosciences: Second Study Program*, F.O. Schmitt (Ed.), The Rockfeller University Press, New York, pp. 519–529.

Scharrer, B. (1972) Neuroendocrine communication (neurohormonal, neurohumoral, and intermediate). In *Topics in Neuroendocrinology, Progress in Brain Research*, Vol. 38, J. Ariëns Kappers and J.P. Schadé (Eds.), Elsevier, Amsterdam, pp. 7–18.

Scharrer, B. (1974) The spectrum of neuroendocrine communication. In *Recent Studies of Hypothalamic Function, Int. Symp. Calgary 1973*, Karger, Basel, pp. 8–16.

Scharrer, B. and Weitzman, M. (1970) Current problems in invertebrate neurosecretion. In *Aspects of Neuroendocrinology*, W. Bargmann and B. Scharrer (Eds.), Springer-Verlag, Berlin, pp. 1–23.

Schwartz, I.L. and Walter, R. (1974) Neurohypophyseal hormones as precursors of hypophysiotropic hormones. *Israel J. med. Sci.*, 10: 1288–1293.

Sterba, G. (1974) Ascending neurosecretory pathways of the peptidergic type. In *Neurosecretion — the Final Neuroendocrine Pathway*, F. Knowles and L. Vollrath (Eds.), Springer-Verlag, Berlin, pp. 38–47.

Terlou, M., Goos, H.J.T. and van Oordt, P.G.W.J. (1974) Hypothalamic regulation of pars intermedia activity in amphibians. *Fortschr. Zool.*, 22: 117–133.

Truman, J.W. and Riddiford, L.M. (1974) Hormonal mechanisms underlying behavior. In *Advances in Insect Physiology*, Vol. 10, J.E. Treherne, M.J. Berridge and V.B. Wigglesworth (Eds.), Academic Press, London, pp. 297–352.

Wallis, M. (1975) The molecular evolution of pituitary hormones. *Biol. Rev.*, 50: 35–98.

Walter, R. (1974) Oxytocin and other peptide hormones as prohormones. In *Psychoneuroendocrinology*, N. Hatotani (Ed.), Karger, Basel, pp. 285–294.

Walter, R. (1975) Neurophysins: carriers of peptide hormones. *Ann. N.Y. Acad. Sci.*, 248: 512 pp.

Watkins, W.B. (1975) Immunohistochemical demonstration of neurophysin in the hypothalamoneurohypophysial system. *Int. Rev. Cytol.*, 41: 241–284.

de Wied, D., van Wimersma Greidanus, T.B., Bohus, B., Urban, I. and Gispen, W.H. (1976) Vasopressin and memory consolidation. In *Perspectives in Brain Research, Progress in Brain Research, Vol. 45*, M. Corner and D.F. Swaab (Eds.), Elsevier, Amsterdam, pp. 181–194.

Zimmerman, E.A. (1976) Localization of hypothalamic hormones by immunocytochemical techniques. In *Frontiers in Neuroendocrinology, Vol. 4*, L. Martini and W.F. Ganong (Eds.), Raven Press, New York, pp. 25–62.

DISCUSSION

R. LEVI-MONTALCINI: Could you say something about the nature and the function of the electrical activity of neurosecretory cells? We studied some of these cells in vitro, and found that they closely resembled the conventional neuron.

B. SCHARRER: Various investigators (e.g., Cross, 1974) have shown that neurosecretory cells exhibit more or less typical action potentials whose discharge frequency can be influenced by certain physiological stimuli. The resulting depolarization is probably responsible for the discharge of the neurosecretory material.

R. STOECKART: From your presentation it is clear that you are against the idea of dividing neurons into secretory neurons and non-secretory neurons. There seems to be a continuous transition between these two cell types. Pearse's idea, on the contrary, is that the neuroendocrine system is derived from the neural crest, just as the rest of the proteinaceous hormone-producing endocrine system.

B. SCHARRER: I would certainly not go as far as that. I would classify the neurosecretory cells as neurons, and not just as endocrine cells. You brought up a very interesting point, though. In the early days of neuroendocrinology, there appeared to be a clear-cut dichotomy between an "endocrine neuron" and a classical, conventional neuron. We have since come to recognize a number of intermediate stages, which bring us to the conclusion that we are dealing with an entire spectrum of possible modes of neurochemical communication. You will have no trouble in establishing the endpoints, i.e., conventional synaptic versus neurohormonal signals. But in the intermediate area of this spectrum you find non-conventional types in which the neurochemical mediator cannot be classified as either hormonal or neurohumoral. Furthermore, there are, aside from peptidergic neurosecretory cells, aminergic neurons whose product seems to be released into the circulation and thus qualifies as a neurohormone.

J. OLDS: I have heard reports of endings that contain both apparently catecholamine-containing vesicles and possibly peptide-containing vesicles, and I wonder what you think about the possibility that a neuron might ignore Dale's principle, and transport both a protein and a more transmitter-like message.

B. SCHARRER: The answer is quite simple: I am prepared to abandon Dale's principle as soon as we have compelling reasons to do so. I do not know of any conclusive evidence for such dual function in a conventional neuron. The presence of more than one putative neurochemical mediator in several types of giant neurons of the gastropod *Aplysia* may be explained by the possible fusion of genetically heterogeneous nerve cells in the course of development (Brownstein et al., 1974).

M. KARASEK: I would like to ask you about the substances which are stained by a mixture of zinc iodide and osmium tetroxide according to Champy-Maillet. Of course, I know that it is not a specific method for the staining of microvesicles and synaptic vesicles, but I should like to mention that in our studies in Poland, using rats (Pawliokowski et al., 1973) we found that in stimulated neurosecretory endings the microvesicles are completely clear, but in non-stimulated neurosecretory tissues these microvesicles are heavily stained with this mixture. What can be the nature of the substance stained by this method?

B. SCHARRER: I have used this method in insect neuroendocrine organs that are comparable to the posterior pituitary. I have not found differences in the ratios of filled to empty vesicles in the stimulated versus non-stimulated conditions. Although this was the original assumption, we do not think anymore that we are demonstrating either cholinergic or adrenergic terminals by this method. I think your observation is interesting, and the fact that we could not see such differences does not contradict it; but I cannot make any comment on the actual nature of the substance involved.

A. TIXIER-VIDAL: Is there any evidence from ontogenetic studies that the neurosecretory neuron is the most primitive type of neuron?

B. SCHARRER: Only to the extent that, in ontogenetically very early stages, mammalian neurosecretory neurons (for example, those in the neural lobes of fetal sheep and seals) contain vasotocin rather than either vasopressin or oxytocin (Vizsolyi and Perks, 1969). Vasotocin is often considered to be an ancestral molecule: its presence in submammalian vertebrates speaks for that. The fact that in the fetus this more "primitive" molecule takes the place of the neurohypophyseal hormone subspecies that are characteristic of mammals at later stages of development might be interpreted as an indication that the neurosecretory neuron is more pluripotential, i.e., less fully differentiated, than the conventional neuron.

REFERENCES

Brownstein, M.J., Saavedra, J.M., Axelrod, J., Zeman, G.H. and Carpenter, D.O. (1974) Coexistence of several putative neurotransmitters in single identified neurons of *Aplysia. Proc. nat. Acad. Sci. (Wash.)*, 71: 4662–4665.

Cross, B.A. (1974) The neurosecretory impulse. In *Neurosecretion — The Final Neuroendocrine Pathway*, F. Knowles and L. Vollrath (Eds.), Springer-Verlag, Berlin, pp. 115–128.

Pawliokowski, M., Karasek, M. and Kepczynska, M. (1973) Ultrastructure of neurosecretory endings in rat neurohypophysis in different functional states, investigated according to Champy-Maillet method. *Folia histochem. cytochem.*, 11: 349–350.

Vizsolyi, E. and Perks, A.M. (1969) New neurohypophyseal principle in foetal mammals. *Nature (Lond.)*, 223: 1169–1170.

Hormones and Brain Development

R. BALÁZS

MRC Developmental Neurobiology Unit, Carshalton (Great Britain)

INTRODUCTION

In this paper I will consider the influence of metabolic factors — especially hormones and, to some extent, nutrition — on the structural and biochemical development of the rat brain, in an attempt to reach certain generalizations as to mechanisms that may be involved in impairments of brain functions frequently manifested after exposure to metabolic insults during early life. I will rely heavily in this presentation on results obtained by our own group, and I am indebted to the important contribution to these studies of my colleagues in the Unit and of visiting scientists (see Acknowledgements).

ASSEMBLY OF CELLS

Interference with cell formation

The cerebellum serves as a good model to study cell formation and the consequences of interference with the proliferation and assembly of cells in the brain (Balázs, 1973b). In the rat cerebellum 97% of the final cell number, including the majority of the nerve cells, is acquired during the first 3 weeks after birth (Patel et al., 1973), thus permitting relative ease in experimentation. Cell replication in the brain takes place predominantly at circumscribed sites, such as the subependymal layer (SEL) of the forebrain ventricles (Altman, 1969). The germinal site in the cerebellum, the external granular layer (EGL), constitutes a continuous layer adjacent to the surface during the period of active cell proliferation, thus facilitating an appraisal of the replicating capacity of the whole structure. Finally, there is a chronological order in the formation of the different nerve cell types (Altman, 1969), the role of which is relatively well-known in the cerebellar circuits (Eccles et al., 1967).

The experimental evidence is now quite extensive, indicating that metabolic imbalance during the early postnatal period can influence cell proliferation in the brain. These results have recently been reviewed (Balázs, 1973a, 1976), so that it will suffice here to mention that, in the hyperthyroid state, the rate of cell acquisition in the cerebellum is apparently accelerated during the first few days after birth (Gourdon et al., 1973; Weichsel, 1974), while active cell proliferation comes to a premature end in the second week (Balázs et al., 1971). In comparison with controls, in the cerebellum of thyroid-deficient rats cell numbers are reduced in the second week, but they become similar by the fifth week (Balázs et al., 1968; Gourdon et al., 1973). These changes seem to occur preferentially in the cerebellum (Patel et al., 1976). Recent studies have shown that one of the factors involved in the transient decrease of cell numbers is a reduction of replicating cells in the EGL during the second week (Nicholson and Altman, 1972a; Lewis et al., 1976), whereas the "catch-up" in cell numbers is related to the persistence of the EGL for a longer time than in controls (Legrand, 1967; Hamburgh, 1968; Nicholson and Altman, 1972a, Patel et al., 1976; Lewis et al., 1976).

Corticosteroids in high doses resulted in a severe inhibition of mitotic activity in the brain which, however, was restored soon after cessation of the treatment (Howard, 1965; Cotterrell et al., 1972). Nevertheless, cell numbers in the brain were permanently reduced after corticosteroid treatment in infancy. It has been claimed that administration of growth hormone during gestation leads to an increase in cell acquisition in the brain (Zamenhof et al., 1966; Sara et al., 1974), but we were unable to reproduce these results (Cotterrell, 1971). Zamenhof et al. (1971) have recently obtained results similar to our negative findings, but they now claim that treatment with growth hormone prevents the depression of cell aquisition caused by nutritional deprivation in pregnant rats.

Undernutrition frequently accompanies experimentally induced abnormal hormonal state, and thus we also investigated its influence on cell proliferation in the brain (Patel et al., 1973; Lewis et al., 1975). Previous results were confirmed concerning the depression of cell aquisition caused by under-nutrition during the suckling period (for reviews see Winick, 1969; Dobbing and Smart, 1974). However, in a series of extensive studies, in which the contribution of Drs. Paul Lewis and Ambrish Patel are of major importance, we established that the mechanisms underlying this effect differ conspicuously from those in an abnormal hormonal state, such as thyroid deficiency (for review see Balázs et al., 1975a). The most prominent difference between these conditions relates to their effect on the generation cycle of the dividing cells. Undernutrition results in a selective and marked prolongation of the S phase, while the G_1 phase is severely curtailed (Lewis et al., 1975). In contrast, cell cycle parameters appear to be normal in the germinal cells in thyroid deficiency (Lewis et al., 1976).

Permanent changes in brain function are frequently associated with metabolic imbalance occurring during the period of active brain development (Eayrs 1971; Dobbing and Smart, 1974; Tizard, 1974). It has been proposed earlier that the functional effects of insults may depend, in part, on the time of interference with cell formation, which in turn determines the cell types affected (Balázs 1972; Barnes and Altman, 1973). The salient points of this hypothesis can be demonstrated by considering the cerebellum as a model, because of the advantages already discussed in the introduction to this section. The functional plan of the cerebellar cortex is based on a population of large neurons, the Purkinje cells: these are the only efferent cells in the cortex and they are formed prenatally. The Purkinje cells receive inputs from outside through 3 afferent systems: two excitatory afferents — the climbing fibers and the mossy fibers — and one inhibitory afferent originating in the locus coeruleus. The functioning of both the input and the output systems is modulated by internal circuits in which the cerebellar cortical interneurons play an important role. The "birthdays" of the various types of interneurons have recently been established (Altman, 1969). In the rat, the generation of the inhibitory interneurons is finished by the end of the second postnatal week; the Golgi cells are formed in the perinatal period, the basket and the stellate cells at about the end of the first and second weeks, respectively. The only excitatory nerve cell, the granule cell, is by far the most numerous cell type in the cerebellar cortex, constituting approximately half the total cell number, and about 50% of these cells are formed in the third week after birth. Assuming that the chronological order in the generation of cell-types holds stringently even under pathological conditions, the balance of excitatory and inhibitory intracerebellar influences on the Purkinje cells will be differently affected, depending on whether the interference with cell formation occurs during the first two postnatal weeks, thus affecting the inhibitory interneurons, or in the third week, when the excitatory granule cells would be influenced exclusively. Furthermore, the localization of synapses on the postsynaptic cell affects the efficiency of polarization of the cell by postsynaptic stimulation (Rall, 1970). The terminals of the basket cells are strategically localized around the initial axon segments of the Purkinje cells, while those of the stellate cells are on the dendrites of the Purkinje cells. Thus, it is expected that an insult in the first postnatal week, when the basket cells are formed, would lead to more drastic consequences than one in the second week, when the stellate cells are formed.

Cell death

This process usually accompanies cell formation. Table I shows that the proportion of degenerating cells in the cerebellar germinal site, the EGL, is relatively low during the period of active postnatal cell proliferation. However, abnormally high cell loss may occur under certain conditions. For example, Lewis (1975) has observed that the pyknotic index in the EGL of 12-day-old undernourished rats is 1·3%. On the other hand, in thyroid deficiency the loss of germinal cells is not statistically significantly different from controls, but the death of differentiated cells is dramatically elevated during the second week of life (Table I). It has been estimated that the mean survival time for pyknotic nuclei in neural tissue is 9–13 hr (Lewis, 1975), and thus a pyknotic index of 1·2% in the internal granular layer of the thyroid deficient cerebellum at day 12 signifies a loss of approximately 1% of the total cerebellar cell number in 24 hr (Lewis et al., 1976).

The observations indicated that, while the replicating and the migrating cells are relatively unaffected, certain conditions in thyroid deficiency are unfavorable for the survival of a fraction of differentiated cells. The effects of thyroid deficiency on the structural development of the cerebellar cortex provide an important lead in identifying such adverse conditions.

One of the most remarkable of these effects is a severe retardation of the dendritic arborization of the Purkinje cells (Legrand, 1967). The granule cells,

TABLE I

EFFECT OF THYROID DEFICIENCY AND UNDERNUTRITION ON CELL DEGENERATION (PYKNOTIC INDICES, %) IN THE CEREBELLUM

One thousand nuclei were counted in the external granular layer and in the internal granular layer (IGL) (the latter results refer to the nodule, but they were similar to those obtained in the paramedian lobule): the pyknotic index was calculated as the percentage of degenerating nuclei. The results, which are usually the means of 10 animals in each group, were analyzed after transformation taking squaring roots (Lewis et al., 1976) by analysis of variance, using a 3-way classification. Thyroid deficiency was induced by giving to mother rats 50 mg propylthiouracil daily from the 18th day of gestation onwards. Undernutrition was effected by halving the normal diet of mother rats from the 6th day of pregnancy throughout the experimental period. The results for the hypothyroid and undernourished groups, respectively, are taken from Lewis et al. (1976) and Lewis (1975); the pyknotic indices in the undernourished IGL are unpublished observations of Dr. P.D. Lewis.

Age (days)	External granular layer			Internal granular layer		
	Control	Hypothyroid	Undernourished	Control	Hypothyroid	Undernourished
6	0·39	0·20	0·25	0·16	0·16	0·17
12	0·58	0·90	1·30*	0·06	1·20*	0·24
21	0·36	0·97	0·38	0·10	0·21	0·14

* Difference between experimental and control groups significant ($P < 0.01$).

generated in the EGL, migrate through the molecular layer to their final position below the Purkinje cells, and they establish abundant synaptic contact through their axons, the parallel fibers, with the spiny branchlets of the Purkinje cell dendrites (Eccles et al., 1967; Palay and Chan-Palay, 1974). In thyroid deficiency, the availability of synaptic sites for the parallel fibers is drastically reduced because of the hypoplasia of the dendritic tree of the Purkinje cells, and this is further aggravated by a substantial decrease in the number of basket cells (Nicholson and Altman, 1972a; Clos and Legrand, 1973). It is proposed, therefore, that in accordance with the redundancy hypothesis of Hamburger and Levi-Montalcini (1949), death of a number of the granule cells is consequent upon a severe deficit in available postsynaptic sites for the termination of their axons. The relationship in the lack of synapse formation between parallel fibers and Purkinje cell dendrites, and granule cell death, has also been observed recently in a "cerebellar" mutant mouse, the "staggerer" (Sotelo and Changeux, 1974).

Compensatory mechanisms

In the course of our studies on the effect of metabolic imbalance on cell acquisition we also observed powerful compensatory mechanisms in the developing brain. In thyroid deficiency the two major factors contributing to the reduction in cerebellar cell numbers during the second week are a decrease in the number of germinal cells and an increase in the death of granule cells. In this condition, cell numbers are restored to normal mainly as a result of a prolongation of the period of active cell proliferation in the cerebellar cortex. This was shown by the observation that the rate of in vivo DNA synthesis, used as an index of mitotic activity, is even higher at day 21 than at day 12, when it peaks in the control, and is 3–4 times the normal value by the end of the third week (Patel et al., 1976). These results are consistent with morphological observations demonstrating that the EGL, which disappears in controls by about 24 days after birth, persists for about 10 days longer as a multicellular layer containing labeled cells after [^{3}H] thymidine administration (Legrand, 1967; Hamburgh, 1968; Nicholson and Altman, 1972a; Lewis et al., 1976). Furthermore, the dendritic tree of the Purkinje cells develops considerably, even in thyroid-deficient animals, after the second week of life; thus, although it remains hypoplastic in comparison with controls, new synaptic contact sites do become available for the axons of the granule cells. It must be emphasized, however, that restoration of normal cell number does not necessarily mean normal cellular composition. Indeed, it has been observed that in thyroid deficiency the number of basket cells is permanently reduced, and that of glia increased (Nicholson and Altman, 1972a; Clos and Legrand, 1973).

The DNA synthesis phase of the cell cycle is markedly prolonged in the brain of animals undernourished during early life. In other proliferating tissues the lengthening of the S phase is accompanied by a similar prolongation of the cell cycle time (for references see Balázs and Patel, 1973). In the brain, however, a selective regulatory process comes into operation, and the prolongation of the generation time is much less than that of the S phase because of a virtual elimination of the G_1 phase (Lewis et al., 1975). However, it is not yet known whether or not such a drastic effect on the cell cycle, in cells which are near to their terminal division, will have any adverse consequences on differentiated functions. In this context, the recent findings of Vonderhaar and Topper (1974) may be of great importance: these authors have observed that some processes occurring during a limited period in the G_1 phase are critical in terms of the final differentiation of certain cells.

There are also powerful safety factors built into the structural design of the CNS as a consequence of convergence and divergence of neuronal inter-connections, and the abundant reiteration of neuronal circuits with the same function.

INTERFERENCE WITH MATURATION

An effect on the assembly of cells is evidently only one of the factors contributing to behavioral anomalies which may develop after insults of various kinds in early life. Interference with neuronal differentiation and the development of neuronal circuits is also of great importance, and there are clear indications that certain hormones and nutrition can influence these processes (for review, see Baláżs, 1974; Dobbing and Smart, 1974).

Brain maturation can be followed in terms of morphological and biochemical estimates, such as dendritic arborization, synaptogenesis, myelination and changes with age in cerebral chemical constituents including enzyme activities. However, the differentiation of cells is manifested not only in quantitative changes but also in qualitative alterations. Two biochemical markers of this kind have been used in our laboratory: these are (1) the conversion of glucose carbon into amino acids, as an indicator of the fate of labeled glucose, and (2) the glutamine/glutamate specific radioactivity ratio after the administration of labeled amino acids or fatty acids, as an index of the appearance of the signs of metabolic compartmentation of glutamate. Both markers are related to changes in the metabolic pattern of brain tissue, and have been found to be sensitive indicators of brain development as affected by various experimental conditions (for review see Patel and Baláżs, 1975). Using these indices, it has been observed that brain maturation is significantly retarded in thyroid deficiency and undernutrition, whereas it is advanced after neonatal treatment with thyroid hormone (Table II). The information is less complete on the effects of corticosteroid treatment, but it would appear that the biochemical development of the brain is not much influenced (Cotterrell, 1971), although Schapiro et al. (1970) have observed that the appearance of certain innate behavioral patterns is retarded under their experimental regimen.

The requirement for thyroid hormone in neuronal maturation deserves special attention. This is generally accepted since the pioneering studies of Eayrs (1955) demonstrating that in thyroid deficiency the growth of the nerve fibers and the dendritic arborization of neurons were severely retarded (for other estimates see Table II). However, it would appear that, besides a reduction in neuronal process formation, thyroid deficiency also results in qualitative changes in the development of neuronal circuits. Again the cerebellar cortex offers certain advantages in this type of study, since it is

TABLE II

EFFECT OF THYROID HORMONE AND UNDERNUTRITION ON BRAIN MATURATION

The results are expressed as a percentage of the control values at the ages indicated. During normal development all estimates showed substantial increases, and at day 10, as a percentage of the values in adults, they were 25–30% in (1) and (2), about 2% in (3) and about 25% in (4). (1) and (2) refer to the forebrain, and (3) and (4) to the cerebellar cortex. Cragg (1970 and 1972) has estimated the number of nerve terminals per neuron in the cerebral cortex at 3–5 weeks after birth: as a percentage of control values, the estimates were about 60% in undernutrition and 78% in thyroid deficiency.

Age (days)	Thyroid deficiency					Hyperthyroidism					Undernutrition			
	10	14	18	24	35	10	12	15	21	30	9	14	21	35
(1) Fate of glucose[a,b]	75	76	53* (19)			120	164	117* (14)	104 (18)		44	46 (15)	49	
(2) Compartmentation of glutamate[c,d]	88* (12)		81	53* (25)		131 (9)	109	110	110		60	66 (15)	50	
(3) Axon terminal density[e,f]	50			78	73* (30)	300		176	104	61		83		93
(4) Dendritic arborization of Purkinje cells[g,h]	25	39	53	62	40	161 (9)	147					58	57 (18)	

* The ages when these estimates were obtained are given in brackets.
[a] Cocks et al. (1970); [b] Balázs and Patel (1973); [c] Patel and Balázs (1971); [d] Patel et al. (1975); [e] Nicholson and Altman (1972b); [f] Rebière (1973); [g] Legrand (1967); [h] Rebière and Legrand (1972).

possible to follow with electron microscopic investigation the development of the two major cerebellar circuits (Hajós et al., 1973).

In the immature animal the *climbing fiber-Purkinje cell circuit* is characterized by powerful synapses involving large spines which emerge from the bodies of the Purkinje cells (Larramendi, 1969). Since, during the first few postnatal weeks, the other main circuit is still in the process of being formed, it is evident that in the immature animal the climbing fiber-Purkinje cell circuit is dominant. With maturation, however, the climbing fiber contacts move up completely to the dendrites of the Purkinje cells, and consequently the developmental state of this circuit can be judged by surveying the Purkinje cells for somatic hooks.

In the *mossy fiber-granule cell-Purkinje cell circuit* the afferent input is transmitted to the Purkinje cells through the granule cells in the cerebellar glomeruli in the internal granular layer. During development this circuit gains progressively in importance, becoming the most abundant synaptic type (parallel fiber-Purkinje cell synapses) in the adult cerebellar cortex. The ultrastructural appearance of the glomerulus is a good indicator of the maturational state of this circuit. In the immature animal, the mossy fiber terminals are relatively small but, even more significantly, the electron-dense dendritic trunks of the granule cells are already engaged in multiple synaptic contact with the terminal. With maturation the mossy fiber terminal becomes one of the largest presynaptic structures in the CNS (longitudinal diameter about 20 μm), and the granule cell dendrites, which are rendered electron translucent, are now digitated; each digit is involved in a synaptic contact with the terminal.

Hajós et al. (1973) observed that in thyroid deficiency the reorganization of the climbing fiber-Purkinje cell circuit was significantly delayed, although the somatic hooks did ultimately disappear from the Purkinje cells. The development of the cerebellar glomeruli was severely retarded: the mossy fiber rosettes were relatively small and the granule cell dendrites maintained an immature ultrastructural appearance. It seems, therefore, that in thyroid deficiency an immature "wiring pattern" persists for a longer time, and the balance between the two major circuits is shifted in favor of the climbing fiber-Purkinje cell circuit. These conclusions are supported by electro-physiological observations (Crepel, 1974, 1975), which are consistent with a marked retardation of the maturation of the mossy fiber-granule cell-Purkinje cell circuit, while the effects are less severe on the climbing fiber response of the Purkinje cells.

The motor coordination of hypothyroid animals seems to be impaired (Eayrs and Lishman, 1955), and the observed changes in the "wiring pattern" in the cerebellum may be instrumental in this functional deficit. Similar changes in synaptic organization may be involved in the impaired performance of hypothyroid animals in tests of adaptive behavior, and may underly mental retardation frequently seen in human cretins (Eayrs, 1968). However, our understanding of the meaningful correlations between the physical and behavioral changes is still very limited. For example, the behavioral effects of neonatal thyroid deficiency can only be corrected by remedial treatment initiated during the first fortnight after birth. In contrast, it appears that, as far as it is possible to determine by current cytological techniques, the structural alterations in the CNS can be reversed to a great extent by remedial treatment started even at a later age (Eayrs, 1971). Similarly, the electrophysiological responses of the Purkinje cells are also restored nearly to normal by making thyroid-deficient rats euthyroid after the first month of life (Crepel, 1975).

PERSPECTIVES FOR FUTURE RESEARCH

"Organizing" effect of hormones in the CNS: development of neuroendocrine circuits

It appears that hormonal imbalance in early life can also influence, relatively selectively, the differentiation of certain types of nerve cells. For example, it has been reported that treatment with corticosteroids at birth leads to a marked reduction in adulthood in the amount of growth hormone releasing factor, which is probably produced by specific neurosecretory nerve cells in the hypothalamus (Sawano et al., 1969). A similar mechanism may be involved in both the degranulation in thyroid deficiency of pituitary acidophil cells, which synthesize growth hormone, and in the chronic impairment of the functioning of the hypothalamic-pituitary-thyroid system, which has been reported to develop after neonatal treatment with thyroid hormone (Eayrs and Holmes, 1964; however, see Schreiber and Kmentová, 1965–1966). However, the best-known example of hormonal influence on the differentiation of circumscribed parts of the CNS is the effect of gonadal hormones in early life on the sexual differentiation of the brain. I will consider, rather than hard facts, only certain aspects of this experimental paradigm, indicating my own prejudice concerning perspectives for future research.

During a limited period, until approximately the 10th postnatal day, gonadal hormones have a lasting influence on reproductive activity and sexual behavior in rats. In the adult female, treated with gonadal hormones during the critical period, the pattern of gonadotrophin secretion is non-cyclic, i.e. of the male type, and these animals are in persistent estrus. It has been established that "masculinization" is the result of alterations in central components of the neuroendocrine circuit regulating reproductive activity (for reviews see Flerkó, 1971; Gorski, 1971; McEwen et al., 1972; Balázs, 1973b). The neuroendocrine circuit concerned with gonadotrophin secretion shows organizational features characteristic of neuronal networks in general. In an utterly simplified manner, the functioning of the network depends on the nature of the transmitter liberated at the synaptic junction, on the presence of receptors for transmitters and hormones, and on the localization of terminals on the postsynaptic cell.

It is proposed that the organization of the neuroendocrine circuit may be altered by changing the characteristics of certain units at the time of assembly. This hypothesis relies heavily on the observation that "masculinization" can only be effected during a limited period, when it seems that relevant nerve cells are not yet fully committed. This view is supported by the following observations. During the critical period, the activities of the known transmitter enzymes (for references see Balázs, 1973b) and specific hormone receptor activities (Vértes et al., 1973) are low in comparison with the adult values.

Furthermore, the rapid phase of formation of neuronal processes also starts after the critical period (see Balázs, 1973b). There is limited evidence indicating that some of the above properties are sexually dimorphic and that they may be influenced during development by hormonal and neuronal factors (see Balázs, 1974). It must be emphasized that much of the evidence has been obtained on non-CNS tissues including model systems, such as cultured cells of nervous tissue origin. It has been observed that the biosynthesis of certain enzymes critical in transmitter production is controlled by hormones. For example, corticosteroids are involved in the regulation of tryptophan hydroxylase (Azmitia and McEwen, 1974), phenethylamine N-methyltransferase (Axelrod, 1973; for CNS see Moore and Phillipson, 1975), and recent observations suggest that they act as modulatory agents in the transsynaptic induction of tyrosine hydroxylase (Goodman et al., 1975). ACTH seems to be needed for the maintenance of the basal level of tyrosine hydroxylase and dopamine β-hydroxylase in the peripheral nervous system (Axelrod, 1973). It is especially important that cyclic-AMP can induce the synthesis of certain transmitter enzymes in some neuronal systems, and that in certain model systems the inducing effect of noradrenaline seems to be mediated through cyclic-AMP (Werner et al., 1971; Waymire et al., 1972; Keen and McLean, 1972; Mackay and Iversen, 1974). There is good evidence indicating that cyclic nucleotides are involved in the regulation of multiplication and differentiation of cells, including cells of nervous tissue origins (for review see Rutter et al., 1973). Besides these hormonal mechanisms, there is evidence that the biosynthesis of transmitter enzymes is also controlled by neuronal influences. A transsynaptic induction of the hydroxylating enzymes of catecholamine synthesis has been demonstrated (Axelrod, 1973), also affecting the CNS (Thoenen, 1970).

There is some evidence, although still controversial, that treatment with androgens in early life can influence the estrogen receptor activity in the critical parts of the hypothalamus (for review see Vértes et al., 1973; however, see Maurer and Wooley, 1974). Finally, Raisman and Field (1973) have demonstrated that in the preoptic nucleus the localization of certain synapses on postsynaptic cells is sexually dimorphic, and is also influenced by androgenization.

On the basis of these considerations, I should like to propose that an important area for future research should be concerned with testing the hypothesis that hormones may modify neuroendocrine circuits by influencing, at a critical stage, the differentiation of nerve cells in terms of transmitter production mechanisms, and the endowment of cells with specific hormonal and transmitter receptors.

Isolation of morphological structures of the brain:
prelude to the study of the effects of hormones
at the molecular level

Finally, I should like to consider briefly certain new technical developments in which our group has been deeply involved. We believe that these new techniques may significantly contribute to the elucidation at the molecular level of the effects of metabolic imbalance on the developing brain. It must be

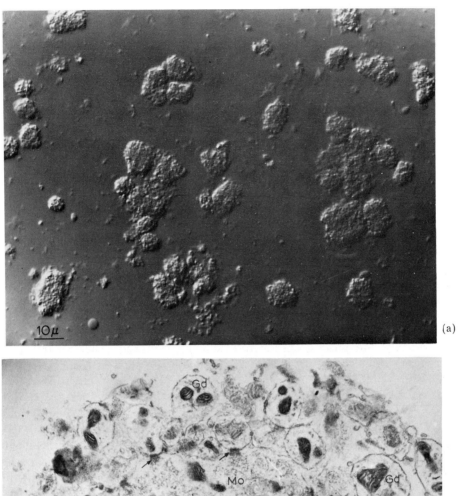

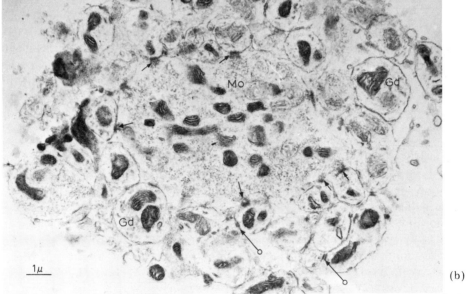

Fig. 1. Preparations of glomerulus particles from rat cerebellum. a: appearance of the preparation in Nomarski interference contrast microscope. b: electron microscopic view of one glomerulus particle; the center of the particle is occupied by the mossy fiber terminal (Mo), which is surrounded by the dendritic digits of the granule cells (Gd). Synaptic specializations (arrows) and interdendritic puncta adhaerentia (ringed arrows) are indicated.
(Reproduced from Hajós et al., 1975, by permission of J. Neurochem.)

remembered that interpretation of the biochemical results on the whole tissue is very difficult because of the extreme heterogeneity of the brain. Thus, as a preliminary to prying deeper, for example, into the mechanisms of hormonal effects in the CNS during development, preparations containing well-defined morphological structures in high purity and sufficient yield must become available.

Isolation of large pieces of the cerebellar glomeruli (glomerulus particles) in a pure form

I have described above, as one of the characteristic structural changes seen in thyroid deficiency, the retarded maturation of the cerebellar glomeruli. It is evident that in order to understand the biochemical changes associated with the development of this complex synapse, under both normal and abnormal conditions, we need to obtain this structure in an isolated form. In collaboration with Drs. F. Hajós, G. Wilkin, R. Tapia (National University of Mexico) and G.L.A. Reynièrse (St. Elisabeth Hospital, Leiderdorp, The Netherlands), we have succeeded in this aim (Hajós et al., 1974; Tapia et al., 1974; Balázs et al., 1975c); over 90% of the final preparation is composed of glomerulus particles with well-preserved structural integrity (Fig. 1). With the help of Prof. J.E. Wilson (University of Michigan, East Lansing, U.S.A.) we have also started to characterize the glomerulus particles in terms of enzyme composition and more complex biochemical properties, such as transport of amino acids (Wilson et al., 1975). To indicate the type of enquiry which the availability of this preparation made possible, I want to mention only one example. It is currently often assumed that nerve cells are specific not only in terms of the transmitter they release, but also in terms of the transmitter which they accumulate via a high affinity transport system (e.g., Iversen, 1971; Kuhar, 1973). Since suitable preparations have not been hitherto available, it was not possible to confirm this hypothesis which, however, could be tested with the help of the glomerulus particles. This preparation is composed almost exclusively of neuronal processes, the excitatory mossy fiber terminal, the amputated dendritic digits of the granule cells and the inhibitory terminals of the Golgi cells; these different structures can be clearly identified by electron microscopy. Furthermore, we established that the glomerulus particles exhibit high affinity uptake of $[^3H]$GABA (Wilkin et al., 1974), which is considered the inhibitory transmitter of the Golgi cells (Bisti et al., 1971; Curtis, 1975). We observed, in collaboration with Drs. F. Schon and J.S. Kelly (MRC Neurochemical Pharmacology Unit, Cambridge) that $[^3H]$GABA was taken up almost exclusively into the inhibitory Golgi terminals (Fig. 2) (Wilkin et al., 1974) where, according to McLaughlin et al. (1974), glutamate decarboxylase is also concentrated. These investigations supported the hypothesis that high affinity uptake processes for a particular transmitter substance, GABA, are present exclusively in those nerve terminals which are known from neurophysiological studies to release that substance. Further studies are currently in progress to test the limits of this specificity.

We have also learnt a very important lesson from the work in which biochemical and electron microscopic techniques were used in conjunction to isolate the glomerulus particles: it seems that, granted a characteristic

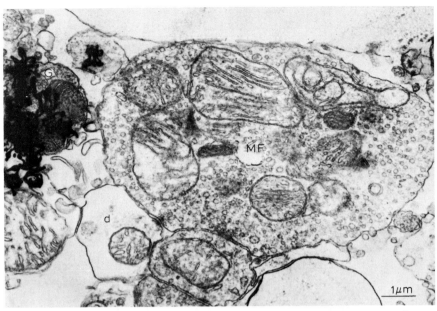

Fig. 2. The inhibitory Golgi axon terminals are the selective sites of high affinity [³H]GABA uptake in the glomerulus particles. After the preparations had been incubated in the presence of 2·5 μM [³H]GABA at 37°C for 6 min in buffered saline, they were processed for electron microscopic autoradiography. One glomerulus particle is shown: the mossy fiber terminal (MF) and the granule cell dendrites (d) are devoid of silver grains which, however, are concentrated over a small terminal identifiable by several criteria as a Golgi axon terminal (G). Quantitative studies on silver grain distribution showed that the inhibitory terminals concentrated [³H]GABA over 100 times more than the excitatory mossy fiber terminals. (Reproduced from Wilkin et al., 1974, by permission of Nature.)

ultrastructural appearance, conditions can be found which permit the rupture of cells and, at the same time, the preservation of structures which are larger and maintain a more complex level of organization than the usual subcellular organelles hitherto prepared from brain tissue.

Preparation of cell bodies from the developing cerebellum with preservation of a high degree of morphological integrity

Our descriptive knowledge about the effects of thyroid hormone or undernutrition on brain development is quite respectable, but we know very little about the mechanisms which underly, for example, the thyroid hormone requirement of the Purkinje cells for dendritic arborization or the changes in cell cycle parameters in undernutrition. To approach these and similar basic questions preparations of specific cell types are badly needed. Some progress has already been made in this direction (e.g., for cerebellum, Bocci, 1966; Cohen et al., 1973; Barkley et al., 1973; Yanagihara and Hamberger, 1973), but the parallel preservation of both ultrastructure and metabolic activity of the isolated cells presented a major obstacle which has not been satisfactorily resolved (Johnston and Roots, 1970). In collaboration with Dr. J. Cohen, Dr. G.R. Dutton and Mr. N. Currie (Open University, Milton Keynes) we have

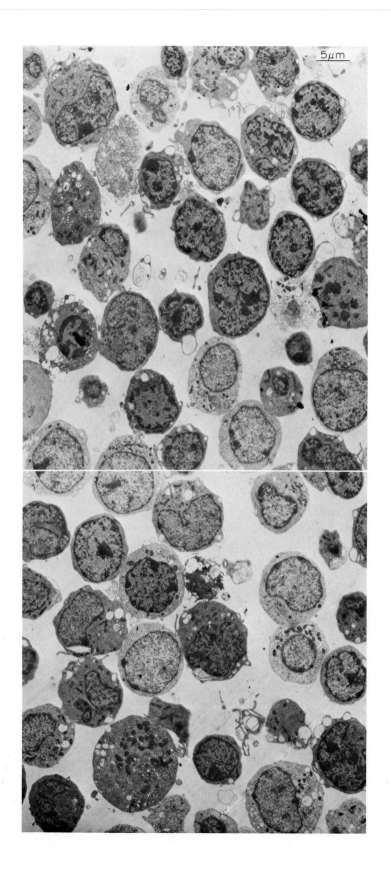

made certain advances to meet these criteria (Cohen et al., 1974; Balázs et al., 1975b).

Fig. 3 shows the morphological preservation of the "cells" obtained from dissociated cerebellar tissue; it is especially important that the plasma membranes are continuous and the mitochondria are well-preserved. The biochemical integrity of the preparations was indicated by observations showing that the "cells" exhibited good respiratory control, they accumulated K^+ ions against a concentration gradient and synthesized proteins at a linear rate for hours.

In current studies we have succeeded in obtaining fractions which are relatively enriched in the perikarya of Purkinje cells and proliferating cells respectively. Furthermore, the viability of the cell suspension was also demonstrated by tissue culture studies. We hope, therefore, that these preparations will facilitate the study of the contribution of various cell types to the overall biochemistry and the development of the cerebellum, and they will also promote our understanding of hormonal influences in the CNS.

ACKNOWLEDGEMENTS

I want to acknowledge in particular the collaboration in developmental studies of Prof. J.T. Eayrs (Dept. Anatomy, University of Birmingham) who introduced me to this field of research, Drs. Mary Cotterrell (from our Unit), F. Hajós (1st Dept. Anatomy, Semmelweis Medical School, Budapest), A.L. Johnson (MRC Statistical Research and Services Unit, London), S. Kovács (Dept. Physiology, University of Pécs), P.D. Lewis (Royal Postgraduate Medical School, Hammersmith Hospital), A.J. Patel (from our Unit), and A. Rabié (Laboratoire de Physiologie Comparée, Montpellier) for their important contributions to these studies. I am grateful to my former Director, Dr. D. Richter, whose deep interest was a strong stimulating influence in my work.

REFERENCES

Altman, J. (1969) DNA metabolism and cell proliferation. In *Handbook of Neurochemistry*, Vol. 2, A. Lajtha (Ed.), Plenum Press, New York, pp. 137–182.

Axelrod, J. (1973) The fate of noradrenaline in the sympathetic neurone. *Harvey Lect.*, 67: 175–197.

Azmitia, E.C., Jr. and McEwen, B.S. (1974) Adrenalcortical influence on rat brain tryptophan hydroxylase activity. *Brain Res.*, 78: 291–302.

Fig. 3. Montage of low-power electron micrographs of cell body suspension derived from dissociated cerebellar tissue of 14-day-old rats. There is little debris in the preparation, and, although some perikarya show signs of damage (cytoplasmic vacuoles and blebbing), the majority is well-preserved. On the basis of the ultrastructure various "cell"-types could be distinguished: the cytoplasm of the different perikarya varies substantially in terms of electron density, relative amounts of Golgi apparatus, endoplasmic reticulum, ribosomes and mitochondria. Notable differences among the nuclei include size, shape and electron density (condensed vs. dispersed chromatin). (From Wilkin et al., 1976.)

Balázs, R. (1972) Hormonal aspects of brain development. In *The Brain in Unclassified Mental Retardation, I.R.M.R. Study Group No. 3*, J.B. Cavanagh (Ed.), Churchill-Livingstone, London, pp. 61–72.

Balázs, R. (1973a) Effects of disturbing metabolic balance, in the early postnatal period, on brain development. In *Inborn Errors of Metabolism*, F.A. Hommes and C.J. Van Den Berg (Eds.), Academic Press, New York, pp. 33–53.

Balázs, R. (1973b) Hormonal influences on brain development. In *Biochemistry and Mental Illness, Biochem. Soc. Special Publ. No. 1*, L.L. Iversen and S.P.R. Rose (Eds.), The Biochemical Society, London, pp. 39–57.

Balázs, R. (1974) Influence of metabolic factors on brain development. *Brit. med. Bull.*, 30: 126–134.

Balázs, R. (1976) Effect of thyroid hormone and undernutrition on cell acquisition in the rat brain. In *Thyroxine and Brain Development*, G.D. Grave (Ed.), in press.

Balázs, R. and Patel, A.J. (1973) Factors affecting the biochemical maturation of the brain. Effect of undernutrition during early life. In *Neurobiological Aspects of Maturation and Aging, Progress in Brain Research, Vol. 40*, D.H. Ford (Ed.), Elsevier, Amsterdam, pp. 115–128.

Balázs, R., Kovács, S., Teichgräber, P., Cocks, W.A. and Eayrs, J.T. (1968) Biochemical effects of thyroid deficiency on the developing brain. *J. Neurochem.*, 15: 1335–1349.

Balázs, R., Kovács, S., Cocks, W.A., Johnson, A.L. and Eayrs, J.T. (1971) Effect of thyroid hormone on the biochemical maturation of rat brain: postnatal cell formation. *Brain Res.*, 25: 555–570.

Balázs, R., Lewis, P.D. and Patel, A.J. (1975a) Effects of metabolic factors on brain development. In *Growth and Development of the Brain*, M.A.B. Brazier (Ed.), Raven Press, New York, pp. 83–115.

Balázs, R., Wilkin, G.P., Wilson, J.E., Cohen, J. and Dutton, G.R. (1975b) Biochemical dissection of the cerebellum — isolation of perikarya from the cerebellum with well-preserved ultrastructure. In *Metabolic Compartmentation and Neurotransmission*, S. Berl and D. Schneider (Eds.), Plenum Press, New York, pp. 363–383.

Balázs, R., Hajós, F., Johnson, A.L., Reynièrse, G.L.A., Tapia, R. and Wilkin, G.P. (1975c) Subcellular fractionation of rat cerebellum: an electron microscopic and biochemical investigation. III. Isolation of large fragments of the cerebellar glomeruli. *Brain Res.*, 86: 17–30.

Barkley, D.S., Rakic, L.L., Chaffee, J.K. and Wong, D.L. (1973) Cell separation by velocity sedimentation of postnatal mouse cerebellum. *J. Cell Physiol.*, 81: 271–280.

Barnes, D. and Altman, J. (1973) Effects of different schedules of early undernutrition on the preweaning growth of the rat cerebellum. *Exp. Neurol.*, 38: 406–419.

Bisti, S., Iosif, G. and Strata, P. (1971) Suppression of inhibition in the cerebellar cortex by picrotoxin and bicuculline. *Brain Res.*, 28: 591–593.

Bocci, V. (1966) Enzyme and metabolic properties of isolated neurones. *Nature (Lond.)*, 212: 826–827.

Clos, J. and Legrand, J. (1973) Effects of thyroid deficiency on the different cell populations of the cerebellum in the young rat. *Brain Res.*, 63: 450–455.

Cocks, J.A., Balázs, R., Johnson, A.L. and Eayrs, J.T. (1970) Effect of thyroid hormone on the biochemical maturation of rat brain: conversion of glucose-carbon into amino acids. *J. Neurochem.*, 17: 1275–1285.

Cohen, J., Mareš, V. and Lodin, Z. (1973) DNA content of purified preparations of mouse Purkinje neurons isolated by a velocity sedimentation technique. *J. Neurochem.*, 20: 651–657.

Cohen, J., Dutton, G.R., Wilkin, G.P., Wilson, J.E. and Balázs, R. (1974) A preparation of viable cell perikarya from developing rat cerebellum with preservation of a high degree of morphological integrity. *J. Neurochem.*, 23: 899–901.

Cotterrell, M. (1971) *The Effects of Growth Hormone and Corticosteroid Treatment on the Biochemical Maturation of Rat Brain*. M.Sc. Thesis, Council for National Academic Awards, U.K.

Cotterrell, M., Balázs, R. and Johnson, A.L. (1972) Effects of corticosteroids on the biochemical maturation of rat brain: postnatal cell formation. *J. Neurochem.*, 19: 2151–2167.

Cragg, B.G. (1970) Synapses and membraneous bodies in experimental hypothyroidism. *Brain Res.*, 18: 297–307.

Cragg, B.G. (1972) The development of cortical synapses during starvation in the rat. *Brain*, 95: 143–150.

Crepel, F. (1974) Excitatory and inhibitory processes acting upon cerebellar Purkinje cells during maturation in the rat: influence of hypothyroidism. *Exp. Brain Res.*, 20: 403–420.

Crepel, F. (1975) Consequences of hypothyroidism during infancy on the function of the cerebellar neurons in the adult rat. *Brain Res.*, 85: 157–160.

Curtis, D.R. (1975) Gamma-aminobutyric and glutamic acids as mammalian central transmitters. In *Metabolic Compartmentation and Neurotransmission*, S. Berl and D. Schneider (Eds.), Plenum Press, New York, pp. 11–36.

Dobbing, J. and Smart, J.L. (1974) Vulnerability of developing brain and behaviour. *Brit. med. Bull.*, 30: 164–168.

Eayrs, J.T. (1955) The cerebral cortex of normal and hypothyroid rats. *Acta Anat. (Basel)*, 25: 160–183.

Eayrs, J.T. (1968) Developmental relationships between brain and thyroid. In *Endocrinology and Human Behaviour*, R.P. Michael (Ed.), Oxford University Press, London, pp. 239–255.

Eayrs, J.T. (1971) Thyroid and the developing brain: anatomical and behavioural effects. In *Hormones in Development*, M. Hamburgh and E.J.W. Barrington (Eds.), Appleton-Century-Crofts, New York, pp. 345–355.

Eayrs, J.T. and Holmes, R.L. (1964) Effect of neonatal hyperthyroidism on pituitary structure and function in the rat. *J. Endocr.*, 29: 71–81.

Eayrs, J.T. and Lishman, W.A. (1955) The maturation of behavior in hypothyroidism and starvation. *Brit. J. Anim. Behav.*, 3: 17–24.

Eccles, J.C., Ito, M. and Szentágothai, J. (1967) *The Cerebellum as a Neuronal Machine*, Springer, Berlin.

Flerkó, B. (1971) Steroid hormones and the differentiation of the CNS. In *Current Topics in Experimental Endocrinology, Vol. 1*, L. Martini and V.H.T. James (Eds.), Academic Press, New York, pp. 41–80.

Goodman, R., Otten, U. and Thoenen, H. (1975) Organ culture of the rat adrenal medulla: a model system for the study of trans-synaptic enzyme induction. *J. Neurochem.*, 25: 423–427.

Gorski, R.A. (1971) Gonadal hormones and the perinatal development of neuroendocrine function. In *Frontiers of Neuroendocrinology*, L. Martini and W.F. Ganong (Eds.), Oxford University Press, London, pp. 237–290.

Gourdon, J., Clos, J., Coste, C., Dainat, J. and Legrand, J. (1973) Comparative effects of hypothyroidism, hyperthyroidism and undernutrition on the protein and nucleic acid contents of the cerebellum in the young rat. *J. Neurochem.*, 21: 861–871.

Hajós, F., Patel, A.J. and Balázs, R. (1973) Effect of thyroid deficiency on the synaptic organization of the rat cerebellar cortex. *Brain Res.*, 50: 387–401.

Hajós, F., Tapia, R., Wilkin, G.P., Johnson, A.L. and Balázs, R. (1974) Subcellular fractionation of rat cerebellum: an electronmicroscopic and biochemical investigation. I. Preservation of large fragments of the cerebellar glomeruli. *Brain Res.*, 70: 261–279.

Hajós, F., Wilkin, G., Wilson, J.E. and Balázs, R. (1975) A rapid procedure for obtaining a preparation of large fragments of the cerebellar glomeruli in high purity. *J. Neurochem.*, 24: 1277–1278.

Hamburger, V. and Levi-Montalcini, R. (1949) Proliferation, differentiation and degeneration in the spinal ganglia of the chick embryo under normal and experimental conditions. *J. exp. Zool.*, 111: 457–500.

Hamburgh, M. (1968) An analysis of the action of thyroid hormone on development based on in vivo and in vitro studies. *Gen. comp. Endocr.*, 10: 198–213.

Howard, E. (1965) Effects of corticosterone and food restriction on growth and on DNA, RNA and cholesterol contents of the brain and liver in infant mice. *J. Neurochem.*, 12: 181–191.

Iversen, L.L. (1971) Role of transmitter uptake mechanisms in synaptic neurotransmission. *Brit. J. Pharmacol.*, 41: 571–591.

156

Johnston, P.V. and Roots, B.I. (1970) Neuronal and glial perikarya preparations: an appraisal of present methods. *Int. Rev. Cytol.*, 29: 265–280.

Keen, P. and McLean. W.G. (1972) Effect of dibutyryl cyclic-AMP on levels of dopamine β-hydroxylase in isolated superior cervical ganglia. *Arch. Pharmacol.*, 275: 465–469.

Kuhar, M.J. (1973) Neurotransmitter uptake: a tool in identifying neurotransmitter-specific pathways. *Life Sci.*, 13: 1623–1634.

Larramendi, L.M.H. (1969) Analysis of synaptogenesis in the cerebellum of the mouse. In *Neurobiology of Cerebellar Evolution and Development*, R. Llinás (Ed.), AMA Educ. and Res. Found., Chicago, Ill., pp. 803–843.

Legrand, J. (1967) Analyse de l'action morphogénétique des hormones thyroidiennes sur le cervelet du jeune rat. *Arch. Anat. micr. Morph. exp.*, 56: 205–244.

Lewis, P.D. (1975) Cell death in the germinal layers of the postnatal rat brain. *Neuropath. appl. Neurobiol.*, 1: 21–29.

Lewis, P.D., Balázs, R., Patel, A.J. and Johnson, A.L. (1975) The effect of undernutrition in early life on cell generation in the rat brain. *Brain Res.*, 83: 235–247.

Lewis, P.D., Patel, A.J., Johnson, A.L. and Balázs, R. (1976) Effect of thyroid deficiency on cell aquisition in the postnatal rat brain: a quantitative histological study. *Brain Res.*, 104: 49–62.

Mackay, A.V.P. and Iversen, L.L. (1974) Regulation of tyrosine hydroxylase synthesis in organ-cultured sympathetic ganglia. *Biochem. Soc. Trans.*, 2: 669–673.

Maurer, R.A. and Woolley, D.E. (1974) ^{3}H-Estradiol distribution in normal and androgenized female rats using an improved hypothalamic dissection procedure. *Neuroendocrinology*, 14: 87–94.

McEwen, B.S., Zigmond, R.E. and Gerlach, J.L. (1972) Sites of steroid binding and action in the brain. In *The Structure and Function of Nervous Tissue, Vol. 5*, G.H. Bourne (Ed.), Academic Press, New York, pp. 205–291.

McLaughlin, B.J., Wood, J.G., Saito, K., Barber, R., Vaughn, J.E., Roberts, E. and Wu, J.-E. (1974) The fine structural localization of glutamate decarboxylase in synaptic terminals of rodent cerebellum. *Brain Res.*, 76: 377–391.

Moore, K.E. and Phillipson, O.T. (1975) Effects of dexamethasone on phenylethanolamine N-methyltransferase and adrenaline in the brains and superior cervical ganglia of adult and neonatal rats. *J. Neurochem.*, 25: 289–294.

Nicholson, J.L. and Altman, J. (1972a) The effects of early hypo- and hyperthyroidism on the development of rat cerebellar cortex. I. Cell proliferation and differentiation. *Brain Res.*, 44: 13–23.

Nicholson, J.L. and Altman, J. (1972b) Synaptogenesis in the rat cerebellum: effects of early hypo- and hyper-thyroidism. *Science*, 176: 530–532.

Palay, S.L. and Chan-Palay, V. (1974) *Cerebellar Cortex, Cytology and Organization*, Springer, Berlin.

Patel, A.J. and Balázs, R. (1971) Effect of thyroid hormone on metabolic compartmentation in the developing rat brain. *Biochem. J.*, 121: 469–481.

Patel, A.J. and Balázs, R. (1975) Factors affecting the development of metabolic compartmentation in the brain. In *Metabolic Compartmentation and Neurotransmission*, S. Berl and D. Schneider (Eds.), Plenum Press, New York, pp. 385–395.

Patel, A.J., Balázs, R. and Johnson, A.L. (1973) Effect of undernutrition on cell formation in the rat brain. *J. Neurochem.*, 20: 1151–1165.

Patel, A.J., Atkinson, D.J. and Balázs, R. (1975) Effect of undernutrition on metabolic compartmentation of glutamate and on incorporation of [14C]leucine into protein in the developing rat brain. *Develop. Psychobiol.*, 8: 453–464.

Patel, A.J., Rabié, A., Lewis, P.D. and Balázs, R. (1976) Effect of thyroid deficiency on postnatal cell formation in the rat brain: a biochemical investigation. *Brain Res.*, 104: 33–48.

Raisman, G. and Field, P.M. (1973) Sexual dimorphism in the neuropil of the preoptic area of the rat and its dependence on neonatal androgen. *Brain Res.*, 54: 1–29.

Rall, W. (1970) Cable properties of dendrites and effects of synaptic location. In *Excitatory Synaptic Mechanisms*, P. Andersen and J.K.S. Jansen (Eds.), Universitetsforlaget, Oslo, pp. 175–187.

157

Rebière, A. (1973) Aspects quantitatifs de la synaptogenèse dans le cervelet du rat sous-alimenté dès la naissance. Comparaison avec l'animal rendu hypothyroïdien. *C.R. Acad. Sci. (Paris)*, 276: 2317-2320.

Rebière, A. et Legrand, J. (1972) Effects comparés de la sous-alimentation de l'hypothyroïdisme et de l'hyperthyroïdisme sur la maturation histologique de la zone moléculaire du cortex cérébelleux chez le jeune rat. *Arch. Anat. micr. Morph. exp.*, 61: 105-126.

Rutter, W.J., Pictet, R.L. and Morris, P.W. (1973) Toward molecular mechanisms of developmental processes. *Ann. Rev. Biochem.*, 42: 601-646.

Sara, V.R., Lazarus, L., Stuart, M. and King, T. (1974) Fetal brain growth: selective action by growth hormone. *Science*, 186: 446-447.

Sawano, S., Arimura, A., Schally, A.V., Redding, T.W. and Schapiro, S. (1969) Neonatal corticoid administration: effects upon adult pituitary growth hormone and hypothalamic growth hormone-releasing hormone activity. *Acta. endocr. (Kbh.)*, 61: 57-67.

Schapiro, S., Salas, M. and Vukovich, K. (1970) Hormonal effects on ontogeny of swimming ability in the rat: assessment of central nervous system development. *Science*, 168: 147-151.

Schreiber, V. and Kmentová, V. (1965-1966) Thyroxine in the early postnatal period: minimal changes in thyroid function. *Neuroendocrinology*, 1: 121-128.

Sotelo, C. and Changeux, J.-P. (1974) Transsynaptic degeneration 'en cascade' in the cerebellar cortex of staggerer mutant mice. *Brain Res.*, 67: 519-526.

Tapia, R., Hajós, F., Wilkin, G., Johnson, A.L. and Balázs, R. (1974) Subcellular fractionation of rat cerebellum: an electron microscopic and biochemical investigation. II. Resolution of morphologically characterized fractions. *Brain Res.*, 70: 285-299.

Thoenen, H. (1970) Induction of tyrosine hydroxylase in peripheral and central adrenergic neurones by cold-exposure of rats. *Nature (Lond.)*, 228: 861-862.

Tizard, J. (1974) Early malnutrition, growth and mental development in man. *Brit. med. Bull.*, 30: 169-174.

Vértes, M., Barnea, A., Lindner, H.R. and King, R.J.B. (1973) Studies in androgen and estrogen uptake by rat hypothalamus. In *Receptors for Reproductive Hormones*, B.W. O'Malley and A.R. Mears (Eds.), Plenum Press, New York, pp. 137-173.

Vonderhaar, B.K. and Topper, Y.J. (1974) A role of the cell cycle in hormone-dependent differentiation. *J. Cell Biol.*, 63: 707-712.

Waymire, J.C., Weiner, N. and Prasad, K.N. (1972) Regulation of tyrosine hydroxylase activity in cultured mouse neuroblastoma cells: elevation induced by analogs of adenosine $3':5'$-cyclic monophosphate. *Proc. nat. Acad. Sci. (Wash.)*, 69: 2241-2245.

Weichsel, M.E., Jr. (1974) Effect of thyroxine on DNA synthesis and thymidine kinase activity during cerebellar development. *Brain Res.*, 78: 455-465.

Werner, I., Peterson, G.R. and Shuster, L. (1971) Choline acetyltransferase and acetylcholinesterase in cultured brain cells from chick embryos. *J. Neurochem*, 18: 141-151.

Wilkin, G., Wilson, J.E., Balázs, R., Schon, F. and Kelly, J.S. (1974) How selective is high affinity uptake of GABA into inhibitory nerve terminals? *Nature (Lond.)*, 252: 397--399.

Wilkin, G.P., Balázs, R., Wilson, J.E., Cohen, J. and Dutton, G.R. (1976) Preparation of cell bodies from the developing cerebellum: structural and metabolic integrity of the isolated "cells". *Brain Res.*, in press.

Wilson, J.E., Wilkin, G.P. and Balázs, R. (1975) Metabolic properties of a purified preparation of large fragments of the cerebellar glomeruli: glucose metabolism and amino acid uptake. *J. Neurochem.*, 26: 957-965.

Winick, M. (1969) Malnutrition and brain development. *J. Pediat.*, 74: 667-679.

Yanagihara, T. and Hamberger, A. (1973) A method for separation of Purkinje cell and granular cell-enriched fractions from rabbit cerebellum. *Brain Res.*, 59: 445-448.

Zamenhof, S., Mosley, J. and Schuller, E. (1966) Stimulation of the proliferation of cortical neurons by prenatal treatment with growth hormone. *Science*, 152: 1396-1397.

Zamenhof, S., Van Marthens, E. and Grauel, L. (1971) Prenatal cerebral development: effect of restricted diet reversal by growth hormone. *Science*, 174: 954-955.

DISCUSSION

P.B. BRADLEY: Many years ago we did some studies on electrophysiological concomitants of hypothyroidism, together with John Eayrs. We thought that we were able to distinguish between the morphological changes which this neonatally induced hypothyroidism produced, and the metabolic effects, particularly in terms of electrophysiological responses. The main morphological change was seen in the cerebellar cortex. This was a change in connectivity rather than in cell numbers. My question is whether you have been able to distinguish between metabolic and anatomical effects in your particular studies.

R. BALÁZS: First of all I should like to say that I owe a lot to Prof. Eayrs, who introduced me into this field of research. At the beginning of our work we received experimental animals from him, so I suppose that thyroid deficiency was induced in the same way as in your studies. However, it seems that the consequences, in terms of the morphology and biochemistry of the CNS, as well as behavior, are very similar whether thyroid deficiency is induced by giving ^{131}I or by using drugs. I think what you really have in mind is the question of reversibility. One has to consider here that it is an extremely difficult task to find the proper correlations between physical and behavioral changes. Since, during the period that we are studying, almost everything is subject to developmental changes, it is very easy to fall into the pitfall of believing that certain estimates are correlated. In this context recent results of Eayrs (1971) are of great importance: by implementing replacement treatment at different times after birth he has found that the structural changes after neonatal thyroidectomy are relatively reversible, whereas the behavioral alterations are not. Functionally relevant processes must therefore occur during a limited period of structural development.

A. TIXIER-VIDAL: Your finding that in undernutrition the rate of the G_1 phase is modified is very fascinating. The hypothesis that you put forward is interesting with regard to the possibility of induction of differentiation during the G_1 phase, during the last division in the cerebellum. But in the hypothalamus the situation is very different. According to recent findings, the last division in the fetal lamb hypothalamus occurs between 12 and about 15 weeks of fetal life, but the maturation of the hypothalamic cells takes a very long time after the last division. Could you comment on this?

R. BALÁZS: I think that interference with cell formation is only one of the factors which may lead to functional defects. Interference with the maturation of cells is also of great importance. In fact, depending on species and developmental stage the latter may often provide even more insight into mechanisms underlying impaired functional performance.

E. MEISAMI: I was wondering whether in any other species there is evidence that cell proliferation during earlier stages of nervous system development is also regulated by thyroid hormones.

R. BALÁZS: The rat is an extremely good species for experimental purposes, but it is not the best model of human cretinism. In man, the thyroid gland starts to function at the end of the first trimester, that means *before* the major proportion of the nerve cells is formed (Dobbing and Sands, 1970). In the rat it starts to function at the 18th day of gestation, *after* the completion of the formation of the major fraction of the nerve cells in the forebrain: two completely different situations! In part because of expedience we try to simplify complex situations. It is much easier to influence experimentally the development of the CNS in the baby rat, in which the relevant processes proceed actively after birth (at least in certain parts of the brain) than in other species in which they occur predominantly during gestation, when the powerful compensatory mechanisms of the mother must first be overcome. Nevertheless, we must be aware of the limitations of our models.

E. MEISAMI: Is there any electrophysiological study of the cerebellum in hypothyroid animals?

R. BALÁZS: Crepel (1974, 1975), from Paris, has done detailed electrophysiological work on the cerebellum of thyroid-deficient rats. His results are consistent with a slight delay in the appearance of the adult pattern of the Purkinje cell response to climbing fiber stimulation, and with a severe (although not persistent) retardation of the development of the granule cell-Purkinje cell circuit.

REFERENCES

Crepel, F. (1974) Excitatory and inhibitory processes acting upon cerebellar Purkinje cells during maturation in the rat: influence of hypothyroidism. *Exp. Brain Res.*, 20: 403–420.
Crepel, F. (1975) Consequences of hypothyroidism during infancy on the functions of cerebellar neurons in the adult rat. *Brain Res.*, 85: 157–160.
Dobbing, J. and Sands, J. (1970) Timing of neuroblast multiplication in developing human brain. *Nature (Lond.)*, 226: 639–640.
Eayrs, J.T. (1971) Thyroid and the developing brain: anatomical and behavioural effects. In *Hormones in Development*, M. Hamburgh and E.J.W. Barrington (Eds.), Appleton-Century-Crofts, New York, pp. 345–355.

The Molecules of Neurosecretion: Their Formation, Transport and Release

B.T. PICKERING

*Department of Anatomy, University of Bristol,
Bristol (Great Britain)*

INTRODUCTION

The concept of neurosecretion was received with great scepticism when first propounded by Ernst Scharrer (1928), since the idea that a nerve cell could indulge in secretory activity akin to an endocrine cell was completely alien to the accepted properties of neurons. However, neurosecretion is now a well documented and completely accepted phenomenon (see Scharrer, p. 125, in this volume). Not only is it, by now, well known that neurons are capable of secretion (Smith, 1971a), but I shall attempt to show that they are ideal models for studying the properties of secretory cells in general.

One may consider 3 phases in the secretion of substances from cells:

(1) synthesis of the molecules to be secreted;

(2) transport of the molecules from the synthesis site to the release site, and

(3) release, i.e., transfer of molecules from inside to outside the cell.

The great advantage that the neurosecretory neuron offers for the study of these individual components of secretion is that, unlike most other secretory cells, it has discrete anatomical compartments in which each process occurs. Thus, in general, synthesis takes place in the perikaryon, intracellular transport can be readily studied in the axon, and release occurs predominantly from the nerve terminal. These are sweeping generalizations and, as such, are not strictly true but I shall review what is known about the processes in the hypothalamo-neurohypophyseal neuron, and attempt to point out some similarities and differences with other endocrine neurons, with "ordinary" neurons and with non-neuronal secretory cells.

FORMATION

The hypothalamo-neurohypophyseal system

There are two main groups of hypothalamo-neurohypophyseal neurosecretory neurons terminating in the neural lobe of the pituitary gland: those with perikarya in the supraoptic nucleus of the hypothalamus and those which stem from the paraventricular nucleus. Biochemically also, these neurosecretory neurons can be divided into two groups: those which produce oxytocin and those which synthesize vasopressin; but, contrary to early suggestions, these two subdivisions are not equivalent, since both hypothalamic nuclei contain both oxytocin-neurons and vasopressin-neurons (Sokol, 1970; Burford et al., 1972, 1974; Zimmerman et al., 1974, 1975; Vandesande et al., 1975). Along with the neurohypophyseal hormones, these neurons synthesize and secrete a family of sulfur-rich proteins, the neurophysins, which are present in the same secretory granules as the hormones (Ginsburg and Ireland, 1963, 1966; Dean and Hope, 1966, 1967). The neurophysins specifically bind the hormones (van Dyke et al., 1942; Archer et al., 1955) and have been thought of in the past as "carrier molecules" necessary to keep the hormones within the secretory granules during their passage from the hypothalamus to the neurohypophysis (Sawyer, 1961; Ginsburg, 1968). However, the inter-dependence of hormone and neurophysin syntheses and the increasing evidence that vasopressin and oxytocin are each stored in the gland in association with a specific neurophysin (Dean et al., 1968; Burford et al., 1971; Robinson et al., 1971; Pickup et al., 1973; Legros and Louis, 1974; Legros et al., 1974) have given rise to the hypothesis that each hormone and its specific neurophysin may originate from a common biosynthetic precursor protein (Sachs et al., 1969; Pickering et al., 1971). The existence of such a precursor in the biosynthetic pathway to vasopressin was demonstrated in Sachs' laboratory some ten years ago (Sachs and Takabatake, 1964; Takabatake and Sachs, 1964). The nature of this precursor is still unknown but the simplest hypothesis would be that it represents the hormone and its specific neurophysin in covalent linkage. At first sight one might suggest that such a linkage would be likely to involve the free NH_2-terminal group of the hormone since the carboxyl group is blocked (Hope and Pickup, 1974), but it may be that the very fact that the carboxyl is amidated is evidence that this group has been part of a peptide link. On the basis of immunohistochemical studies of the pars intermedia of several species, and the presence of a peptide having the sequence of the 22 carboxyterminal residues of ACTH, Scott et al. (1974a, b) have proposed that the tridecapeptide amide α-MSH arises from ACTH by a series of proteolylic steps. Bradbury et al. (1975) have evidence to suggest that α-MSH is formed by transamidation of a Val-Gly bond to give the terminal -Val(NH_2) of the hormone, and that this Val-Gly bond is present in a protein which may be a precursor for both ACTH and MSH. Such a conclusion prompted D.G. Smyth (personal communication) to suggest that the neurohypophyseal hormones might also arise from their prohormones by transamidation, in this case transamidation of a glycyl bond would give the terminal glycinamide of the hormones. If we believe that the precursor is hormone covalently linked to neurophysin, its structure would be similar to that shown in Fig. 1 and the sensitive bond would be the glycylalanine one. It is interesting, in this respect, that all of the neurophysins studied to date have an NH_2-terminal alanine (Pickering and Jones, 1976) and that the -Gly-Ala-bond is particularly susceptible to transamidation (D.G. Smyth, personal communication).

Comparison of the ratio of oxytocin to vasopressin in the hypothalamus with that in the neurohypophysis has led to the suggestion that the final maturation of the precursor probably takes place after its sequestration in the secretory granule, and during intra-axonal transport to the neurohypophysis (see Pickering et al., 1971). Such a situation requires the presence of an enzyme ("maturase") within the granule. From a study of the turnover of the individual neurophysins in the rat hypothalamo-neurohypophyseal neuron, we (Burford and Pickering, 1973; Pickering et al., 1974) have concluded that in the rat the minor (third) neurophysin component arises in the granule from the proteolysis of oxytocin-neurophysin after the granules have arrived in the gland, and that this too requires the presence of an enzyme within the granule. Thus, the current hypothesis which we favor for the biosynthesis of neurohypophyseal hormones (see Fig. 2) holds that a prohormone is

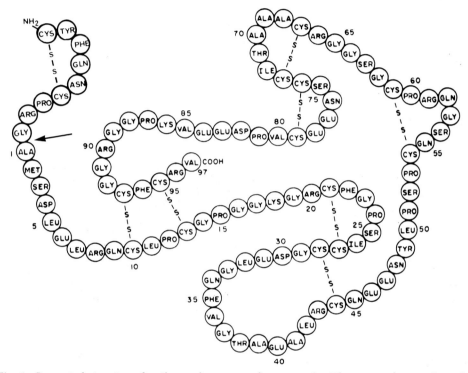

Fig. 1. Suggested structure for the prohormone of vasopressin. The arrow shows where the transamidase would act (Smyth, personal communication). The primary structure of bovine neurophysin II is from Schlesinger et al. (1972).

synthesized by the ribosomal system in the perikaryon of the neurosecretory neuron, that it is packaged into neurosecretory granules along with a "maturase" and that during transport to the nerve terminal it is cleaved to give neurophysin plus hormone. In the oxytocin-producing neurons, the specific neurophysin (oxytocin-neurophysin) is further slowly digested to give the minor neurophysin component (Pickering et al., 1975).

Such a situation also occurs in a bona fide secretory cell, e.g., the β-cell of the pancreatic islets (Fig. 2). Here proinsulin is packaged into secretory granules in the Golgi apparatus, and during transport towards the cell periphery is cleaved to give insulin and "C" peptide (see Steiner et al., 1973).

164

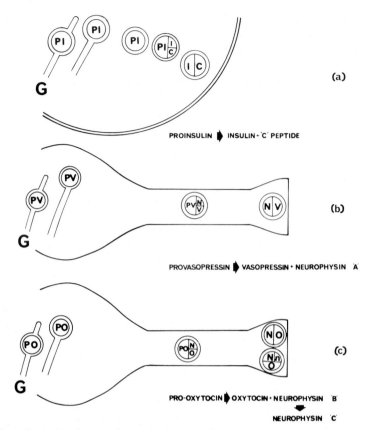

Fig. 2. Hypothetical scheme comparing biosynthesis in the neurosecretory cells of the hypothalamo-neurohypophyseal tract with those in the β-cells of the Islets of Langerhans. Abbreviations: a: G, Golgi apparatus; PI, proinsulin; I, insulin; C, "c" peptide. b: PV, provasopressin; V, vasopressin; N, neurophysin "A". c: PO, pro-oxytocin; O, oxytocin; N, neurophysin "B"; n, neurophysin "C".

"Ordinary" neurons

In the adrenergic neuron, noradrenaline is synthesized from tyrosine by the following scheme:

$$\text{tyrosine} \rightarrow \text{dihydroxphenylalanine (DOPA)} \rightarrow \text{dihydroxyphenylethylamine (dopamine)}$$
$$\downarrow$$
$$\text{dopamine-}\beta\text{-hydroxylase}$$
$$\downarrow$$
$$\text{noradrenaline}$$

The enzyme dopamine-β-hydroxylase (DBH) is located within the dense-cored secretory granules which are characteristic of aminergic neurons and which also contain a large proportion of the noradrenaline stored within the axon terminals of such neurons (De Potter, 1971). Thus, to the extent that the final step in the synthesis of their secretory product occurs within the secretory granules, the noradrenergic and the hypothalamo-neurohypophyseal neurons have analogous biosynthetic mechanisms. Furthermore, although the relative amount of DBH in the granules (DBH/mg protein) is constant throughout the length of the splenic nerve, the intragranular ratio, noradrenaline:DBH, increases in granule preparations made from portions of the neuron further and further from the perikaryon (Klein, 1974; Lagercrantz et al., 1974). Thus, again, the production of active substance continues during transport of the secretory granule from the site of its formation to its release site. However, in the case of the adrenergic neuron this increased production represents de novo synthesis rather than maturation of an existing precursor. Whereas in the hypothalamo-neurohypophyseal neuron and in the β-cell of the pancreas the granule contains both an enzyme and its substrate, in the adrenergic neuron

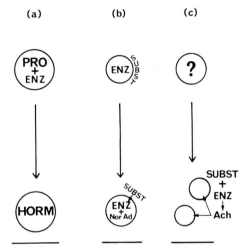

Fig. 3. The intragranular events in (a) neurosecretory cells (and other polypeptide secretory cells), (b) adrenergic neurons and (c) cholinergic neurons. a: both the enzyme (ENZ) and its substrate (prohormone, PRO) are transported from the Golgi apparatus to the release site. b: only the enzyme (DBH) is carried in the granule while the substrate (dopamine) is picked up en route. c: both the enzyme (ChAc) and the substrates (acetyl coenzyme A + choline) are cytoplasmic and vesicle transport seems to be necessary only to replenish the storage organelles themselves, although the ? is meant to denote the uncertainty in this system.

only the enzyme is packaged by the Golgi apparatus and the substrate (dopamine) is presumably picked up while the granule is in transit.

In cholinergic neurons the situation is still far from clear (for review see Dahlström et al., 1974). The active secretory product, acetylcholine, is made in the cytoplasmic compartment by the transfer of an acetyl group from acetyl coenzyme A to choline under the influence of the enzyme choline acetyltransferase (ChAc). This reaction occurs throughout the neuron and especially at the axon terminus, where the acetylcholine so formed is taken up into the synaptic vesicles (Whittaker, 1969). The uncertainty at present seems to be the nature of the subcellular components into which the acetylcholine, formed in the proximal part of the neuron, is gathered, and whether some of the ChAc may be packaged in the same or similar vesicles for transport down the axon (Dahlström et al., 1974). An attempt to summarize the intragranular events in all of these cell types is shown in Fig. 3, although no suggestion has been made to account for the presence of the chromogranins (apart from DBH), the soluble proteins present in adrenergic neurons (Banks and Helle, 1971), since I know of no evidence on which to base such a suggestion.

Hypothalamic releasing hormones

The hypothalamic hormones which influence the release of anterior pituitary hormones are all small polypeptides, and those isolated until now range from 3 to 14 residues (Bøler et al., 1969; Burgus et al., 1969; Matsuo et al., 1971; Brazeau et al., 1973). Like the neurohypophyseal hormones they are synthesized in hypothalamic neurons which, in this case, terminate in the median eminence in association with the primary capillary plexus of the hypophyseal portal system. Also like the neurohypophyseal hormones, many of the hypothalamic hormones have been localized in dense-cored secretory granules (Pelletier et al., 1974a, b), some of which have been harvested by differential centrifugation (Ishii, 1970; Mulder, 1970; Fink et al., 1972a, b; Taber and Karavolas, 1975). In view of these similarities it seemed reasonable to suggest that the biosynthesis of these two groups of peptides would also follow a similar pattern, namely, that the hypothalamic hormone would be formed by the cleavage in granulo of a protein precursor (Cross et al., 1975). Indeed, two of the peptides purified to date have carboxyterminal amides and the other has an amino terminal alanine, so that they could indeed all arise from such prohormones by the transamidation reaction proposed by Smyth and his colleagues.

There is, however, a large body of evidence from Reichlin's laboratory (Reichlin, 1973) that, far from being formed from prohormones, the hypothalamic releasing hormones are synthesized by direct condensation of amino acids under the influence of soluble synthetase enzymes. Thus, radioactive thyrotropin-releasing hormone (TRH) could be formed from labeled proline by a ribosome-free cell sap fraction, and this synthesis did not require RNA (Mitnick and Reichlin, 1971, 1972). Similar conclusions have been made for the synthesis of growth hormone-releasing hormone (GH-RH) and prolactin-releasing hormone (PRH) (Reichlin and Mitnick, 1973; Mitnick et al., 1973). In the newt (*Triturus viridescens*), too, Grimm-Jørgensen and McKelvy (1974) showed that TRH synthesis occurred in the presence of inhibitors of conventional ribosomal protein synthesis (chloramphenicol, cycloheximide and diphtheria toxin) but ribonuclease completely abolished synthesis so that in this amphibian system intact RNA is required.

In the absence of confirmatory evidence from other laboratories, the mechanism of biosynthesis of releasing factors must remain an open question. On the one hand, analogy with the other peptidergic neurosecretory system makes the prohormone hypothesis attractive, and this is supported both by the presence of similar electron-dense secretory granules and by the occurrence of appropriate terminal amino acids in each peptide. On the other hand, the work of the Reichlin and McKelvy groups suggests a cytoplasmic ribosome-free synthesis, with the active products then being taken up by the secretory granule much the same as in the cholinergic neuron. Between these extremes lies the possibility that the releasing-hormone cells synthesize their products in the same way as do adrenergic neurons, and that in vivo the Reichlin "synthetase" is sequestered in the granules. Moreover, it is possible that each of the 3 mechanisms may be used for one or other of the releasing hormones, since there is no reason to assume that they will all be treated alike.

TRANSPORT

Radioactive neurohypophyseal hormones and associated neurophysins begin to arrive in the neural lobe of the pituitary gland between 1 and 2 hr after the presentation of a labeled amino acid to the hypothalamus (Jones and Pickering, 1970, 1972; Norström and Sjöstrand, 1971; Burford and Pickering, 1973). When neurosecretory granule membranes were labeled, by giving · rats intracisternal injections of $[^3H]$ choline, they showed a similar time course of arrival in the gland as their contents (Pickering et al., 1975; Swann and Pickering, 1976). Thus the neurosecretory granules are transported along the hypothalamo-neurohypophyseal tract at velocities in excess of 3 mm/hr. By crushing neurons of the sympathetic nervous system and measuring the rate of increase of noradrenaline proximal to the crush, Dahlström and her colleagues (e.g., Dahlström and Häggendal, 1966, 1967) have estimated that adrenergic granules are transported at 2–10 mm/hr. There also appear to be present in cholinergic neurons some vesicles which transport ACh at velocities of the order of 5 mm/hr (Dahlström et al., 1974). It would appear that all of these rapid transport processes involve, in some way, the microtubule system, since colchicine and vinblastine inhibit such processes in all these neuronal systems (Dahlström, 1968; Norström et al., 1971; Flament-Durand and Dustin, 1972; Dahlström et al., 1974), and these compounds appear to work by disaggregating microtubules (Malawista, 1965; Schmitt, 1968). It is probable that a similar mechanism is concerned in the intracellular movement of granules in other secretory cells although their morphology makes them less amenable to study than neurons. Certainly colchicine will inhibit hormone release under appropriate conditions (Lacy et al., 1968; Sheterline et al., 1975) although under others it may have the reverse effect (Sundberg et al., 1973). It has been proposed (Schmitt, 1969) that rapid transport in nerves (and thus perhaps in all cells) is brought about by an interaction of storage vesicle and microtubule which is akin to the sliding-filament mechanism for muscle contraction. Thus it may be suggested that one of the functions of secretory granules is to facilitate the rapid transport of secretory products from the site of synthesis to the release site.

RELEASE

Turning now to the release of the molecules of neurosecretion, I propose to focus on two aspects of the process. Firstly the availability of molecules for release, and secondly the fate of the storage vesicle once it has released its contents. Sachs (1971) found that the radioactive vasopressin released by dog pituitary glands 10 days after labeling had a higher specific radioactivity than did the hormone remaining in the gland. Thus there is a preferential release of newly synthesized hormone. In an extension of these findings (Fig. 4) we have found that rat neural lobes taken at increasing times after an intracisternal injection of [^{35}S]cysteine release a progressively decreasing proportion of their stored radioactive protein (neurophysin) when stimulated in vitro (Wong and Pickering, 1976). Thus the neurosecretory product becomes less and less available for release as the time after it entered the gland increases. Electron microscope autoradiography provided the explanation for these findings (Heap

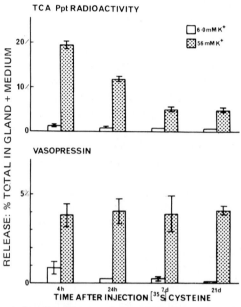

Fig. 4. The proportion of radioactive protein released by rat neurohypophysis in vitro at various times after labeling. Rats were given intracisternal injections of [^{35}S]cysteine and at various times after injection their neural lobes were removed and incubated in vitro. Release was stimulated by increasing the [K^+] in the medium and the radioactivity of the TCA-precipitable protein thus released was expressed as a percentage of the total TCA-precipitable protein present in the gland at the commencement of the incubation. Note that the radioactive protein is less and less available for release as time goes on, although the proportion of vasopressin released remains the same. (Drawn from the results of Wong and Pickering, 1976.)

et al., 1975) since it could be shown that after intracisternal injection of [^{35}S]cysteine into rats, radioactive granules could first be seen in terminal dilatations of the axons ("nerve endings") which abut on basement membrane (Morris, 1976) and then, as the time after injection increased, appeared in greater proportion deeper and deeper inside the non-terminal dilatations ("nerve-swellings"). Thus it appears that in the neurohypophyseal system the hormone granules follow a prescribed route (Fig. 5) through the neuron, being taken first to the release site and then carried into the storage sites (Cross et al., 1975; Heap et al., 1975). Also in the β-cell of the pancreas there is evidence for preferential release of newly synthesized insulin and this, together with the effects of colchicine, has been taken as evidence for a microtubule-mediated transport from the Golgi apparatus to the release site before equilibration with the storage pool of hormone (Howell and Lacy, 1971). Although there is similar evidence in both adrenergic and cholinergic neurons for the preferential release of newly synthesized transmitter (Kopin et al., 1968; Collier, 1969), it is much more difficult to equate this with granules being transported initially to release sites because, in these systems, the situation is complicated by local synthesis and re-uptake into the storage vesicles.

It now seems generally accepted that most, if not all, secretory cells which store their product in membrane-bound vesicles release it by the process of

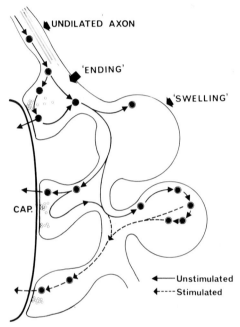

Fig. 5. Scheme for the movement of neurosecretory granules through the compartments of the hypothalamo-neurohypophyseal neuron within the neural lobe of the pituitary gland. (From Heap et al., 1975.)

exocytosis (emiocytosis), first described for the exocrine pancreas and the anterior pituitary (Palade, 1959; Farquhar, 1961). The hypothalamo-neurohypophyseal neuron is no exception to this generalization (for review see Douglas, 1973; Dreifuss, 1975) and argument has centered around the mechanism for retrieval of the granular membrane after the granule has fused with the plasmalemma and discharged its contents. In addition to the large (about 150 nm) electron-dense neurosecretory granules, the hypothalamo-neurohypophyseal neurons contain so-called "small vesicles" of the order of 40 nm in diameter (Palay, 1957). These "small vesicles" have been suggested to represent a phase in the membrane recapture process (Douglas et al., 1971; Douglas, 1973) since they appear to increase in number as a result of stimulation of the gland and to become labeled with extracellular marker

(Douglas et al., 1971; Santolaya et al., 1972). When the profiles of the axon dilatations seen in electron micrographs are classified according to whether they contain "small vesicles" ("endings") or not ("swellings") it becomes apparent that a much greater proportion of "endings" than "swellings" are associated with basement membrane (Morris, 1976). In addition, after an intracisternal injection of [^{35}S] cysteine radioactive granules appear in endings

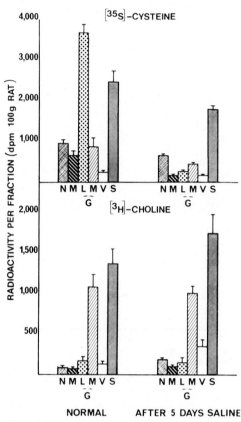

Fig. 6. Subcellular distribution of radioactivity after the intracisternal injection of either [^{35}S]cysteine or [^{3}H]choline. Animals were killed either after 5 days with access to normal drinking water or after 5 days during which the rats had 2% NaCl to drink. Note that saline treatment depleted the gland of ^{35}S radioactivity but that ^{3}H was unaffected both with regard to total amount and to distribution. Abbreviations: N, nuclear fraction; M, mitochondrial fraction; GL, granule contents; GM, granule membranes; V, microsomal (small vesicle) fraction; S, final supernatant. (From Pickering et al., 1975.)

first and then move into swellings, and the profiles of radioactive "endings" are in the main restricted to the low end of the distribution of diameters of axonal dilatations (Heap et al., 1975). All of these observations are compatible with "small vesicles" being associated with the process of hormone release. When, however, we labeled the membrane of the neurosecretory granules with [^{3}H]choline and took glands from rats at periods of 4 hr to 4 weeks after labeling, we could find no evidence of a movement of radioactivity from the subcellular fraction containing the granule membranes to that containing the "small vesicles" (Swann and Pickering, 1976). Since, in unstressed rats, this could have resulted from a rapid rate of metabolism of the "small vesicles", arising from a slow rate of release, we stimulated hormone release in labeled animals by giving them 2% NaCl to drink for 5 days prior to removal of the glands (Jones and Pickering, 1969). This treatment led to the expected loss of ^{35}S-labeled granular contents. However, the ^{3}H-label in the granular membrane did not move into the "small vesicle" fraction in equivalent amounts but largely remained in the granular fraction (Fig. 6). Accepting that hormone release has occurred by exocytosis, since the neurophysin proteins have also been discharged, these results suggest that the granular membrane has been recaptured not as small vesicles but as a vesicle whose dimensions afford it the centrifugal properties of the intact granule. Interestingly, by measuring the amount of extracellular marker taken up by neurohypophysis stimulated in vitro, Nordmann et al. (1974) have come to similar conclusions, and Castel (1974) showed that osmotic stress caused mice to take up extracellular markers into the neurohypophysis enclosed in what she called macropinocytotic vesicles.

Similarly, in the sympathetic neuron, side by side release of the protein and noradrenaline contained in the secretory granules is compatible with release by exocytosis (for review see Smith, 1971b). Noradrenergic granules comprise two main populations: large (about 69 nm), which are found throughout the neuron, and smaller (about 44 nm), which are restricted to the axon termini (Fillenz, 1971). The smaller vesicles in the splenic nerve, although containing noradrenaline, contain little DBH (De Potter, 1971) and that which they do contain is membrane bound (Potter, 1967). This may not, however, apply to all sympathetic neurons, since Bisby et al. (1973) found a considerable proportion of the DBH of the vas deferens in small vesicles, although even here it is much less than the proportion of noradrenaline in such vesicles, and they did not determine if it was soluble or membrane bound. De Potter (1974) has shown that stimulation of the splenic nerve can lead to a transformation of large vesicles into smaller vesicles and it may be that the latter are formed as a result of granule membrane recapture after exocytosis. These smaller vesicles can take up noradrenaline and, by virtue of their membrane-bound DBH, probably synthesize it (De Potter, 1974) and so maintain terminal stores. It is interesting to note that the neurohypophyseal granule contains some membrane-bound neurophysin and that this too is retained when the non-bound granular contents are released in response to saline stimulation (Fig. 6).

In cholinergic neurons acetylcholine is stored in the synaptic vesicles (Whittaker, 1959) whose fusion with the membrane allows the release of "quanta" of transmitter (Katz, 1969). In an elegant series of experiments with a frog neuromuscular preparation, Heuser and Reese (1973) have obtained evidence for recycling of synaptic vesicles. Preparations stimulated in the presence of horseradish peroxidase (HRP) took up the enzyme and it was later found in the synaptic vesicles. By stimulating such an HRP-labeled preparation they could demonstrate release of the protein, thus completing the cycle. The primary origin of the synaptic vesicles of cholinergic neurons is still not clear: they are rarely seen in axons but recent evidence (see Dahlström et al., 1974) suggests that these neurons may contain larger electron-dense vesicles which

172

may be the primary secretory granules bringing the membrane destined for the synaptic vesicles, together with some of the choline acetylase and acetylcholine, from the perikaryon to the nerve terminal.

A summary of the membrane recapture processes is shown in Fig. 7 (modified from Douglas, 1973). It may be suggested that the prime function of secretory vesicles is for the storage and quantal release of secretory product. The neuroendocrine cell, with its low turnover, can supply its needs both for new "transmitter" and vesicle membrane by synthesis in the perikaryon, so that its granule can be used for the maturation of prohormone and intra-axonal transport of "transmitter" just as in a non-neuronal secretory cell, where the

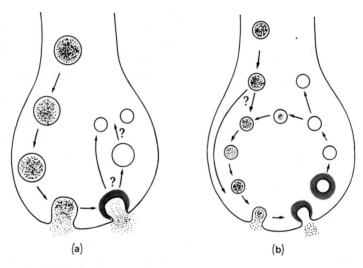

(a)   (b)

Fig. 7. Comparison of the mechanisms for membrane recapture in (a) neurosecretory and (b) adrenergic and cholinergic neurons. a: membrane recapture is shown to occur either in the form of small vesicles or via the so-called large vesicles discussed in the text. The possibility (?) that small vesicles arise from the large vesicles is indicated, but the possibility that they are derived from recapture of indifferent parts of the plasmalemma is not depicted. b: the recycling of storage vesicles is shown; the possibility that the smaller organelles are derived initially from the transport of larger vesicles from the perikaryon is indicated. (After Douglas, 1973.)

distance (and hence the time required for transport) between synthesis site and release site is much less than in a neuron. By transporting an enzyme without its substrate the noradrenergic neuron, on the other hand, is able to keep up transmitter stores by local synthesis at the release site — especially if the recaptured membrane retains some of the enzyme — and hence maintain turnover at a greater rate than in a neurosecretory neuron. This increased turnover can be further enhanced by the re-uptake of unused transmitter into the recycled vesicles. In cholinergic neurons little, if any, transmitter is taken back into the axon and the maintenance of terminal stores is largely by local synthesis. It is thus advantageous that in this system the enzyme (ChAc) is cytoplasmic and not lost during exocytosis of the transmitter, and it may well be that the increasing reliance on cytoplasmic synthesis from neurosecretory through adrenergic to cholinergic neurons (Fig. 3), is related to an increasing need for the rapid restitution of transmitter levels at the nerve terminal.

CONCLUSIONS AND SUMMARY

In this brief essay I have attempted to show that the neurosecretory neuron, far from being an oddity, shows a great deal of functional similarity both to secretory cells and to "ordinary" neurons. In each type of cell the secretory product is synthesized and transported to its release site where it is stored in vesicles prior to expulsion from the cell by exocytosis. The storage vesicle, besides playing an integral part in the release process, is also important for transport from synthesis site to release site as well as for the provision of the environment for the final stages of the synthetic process.

Perhaps my major hope, however, is that I have persuaded some readers to share my belief that the neuron, and particularly the neurosecretory neuron, is an ideal cell for the study of secretion generally. By studying the perikaryon, axon and nerve terminal separately it is possible to biochemically dissect the secretory process, and the recent success of Sachs and his colleagues to maintain neurosecretory neurons in vitro (Pearson et al., 1975) adds a new dimension to this possibility.

ACKNOWLEDGEMENTS

While I must take full responsibility for all errors and omissions, I should like to record my appreciation of the discussions with my colleagues, Drs. J.F. Morris and P. Keen, which encouraged me to attempt to draw analogies between the various neuronal systems. It is also a pleasure to acknowledge the collaboration of Drs. G.D. Burford, C.W. Jones, M.A. McPherson, R.W. Swann and T.M. Wong in the experimental work referred to, which was supported by grants from the Medical Research Council and the Royal Society.

REFERENCES

Acher, R., Manoussos, G. et Olivry, G. (1955) Sur les relations entre l'ocytocine et la vasopressine d'une part et la protéine de van Dyke d'autre part. *Biochim. biophys. Acta (Amst.)*, 16: 155–156.

Banks, P. and Helle, K.B. (1971) Chromogranins in sympathetic nerves. *Phil Trans. B*, 261: 305–310.

Bisby, M.A., Fillenz, M. and Smith, A.D. (1973) Evidence for the presence of dopamine-β-hydroxylase in both populations of noradrenaline storage vesicles in sympathetic nerve terminals of the rat vas deferens. *J. Neurochem.*, 20: 245–248.

Bøler, J., Enzmann, F., Folkers, K., Bowers, C.Y. and Schally, A.V. (1969) The identity of chemical and hormonal properties of the thyrotropin releasing hormone and pyroglutamyl-histidyl-proline amide. *Biochem. biophys. Res. Commun.*, 37: 705–710.

Bradbury, A.F., Snell, C.R. and Smyth, D.G. (1975) Biosynthesis of melanocyte and adrenocorticotrophic hormones. In *Proc. IV Amer. Peptide Symp.*, in press.

Brazeau, P., Vale, W., Burgus, R., Ling, N., Butcher, M., Rivier, J. and Guillemin, R. (1973) Hypothalamic polypeptide that inhibits the secretion of immunoreactive pituitary growth hormone. *Science*, 179: 77–79.

174

Burford, G.D. and Pickering, B.T. (1973) Intra-axonal transport and turnover of neurophysins in the rat. A proposal for a possible origin of the minor neurophysin component. *Biochem. J.*, 136: 1047–1052.

Burford, G.D., Jones, C.W. and Pickering, B.T. (1971) Tentative identification of a vasopressin-neurophysin and an oxytocin-neurophysin in the rat. *Biochem. J.*, 124: 809–813.

Burford, G.D., Dyball, R.E.J., Moss, R.L. and Pickering, B.T. (1972) Preferential labelling of "oxytocin-neurophysin" by injection of [^{35}S]cysteine into the paraventricular nucleus of the rat. *J. Physiol. (Lond.)*, 222: 156–157P.

Burford, G.D., Dyball, R.E.J., Moss, R.L. and Pickering, B.T. (1974) Synthesis of both neurohypophysial hormones in both the paraventricular and supraoptic nuclei of the rat. *J. Anat. (Lond.)*, 117: 261–269.

Burgus, R., Dunn, T.F., Desiderio, D. et Guillemin, R. (1969). Structure moléculaire du facteur hypothalamique hypophysiotrope TRF d'origine ovine: mise en évidence par spectrométrie de masse de la séquence PGA-His-Pro-NH$_2$. *C.R. Acad. Sci. (Paris)*, 269: 1870–1873.

Castel, M. (1974) In vitro uptake of tracers by neurosecretory axon terminals in normal and dehydrated mice. *Gen. comp. Endocr.*, 22: 336–337.

Collier, B. (1969) The preferential release of newly synthesized transmitter by a sympathetic ganglion. *J. Physiol. (Lond.)*, 205: 341–352.

Cross, B.A., Dyball, R.E.J., Dyer, R.G., Jones, C.W., Lincoln, D.W., Morris, J.F. and Pickering, B.T. (1975) Endocrine neurones. *Recent Progr. Hormone Res.*, 31: 243–294.

Dahlström, A. (1968) Effect of colchicine on transport of amine storage granules in sympathetic nerves of rat. *Europ. J. Pharmacol.*, 5: 111–113.

Dahlström, A. and Häggendal, J. (1966) Studies on the transport and life span of amine storage granules in a peripheral adrenergic neurone system. *Acta physiol. scand.*, 67: 278–288.

Dahlström, A. and Häggendal, J. (1967) Studies on the transport and life span of amine storage granules in the adrenergic neurone system of the rabbit sciatic nerve. *Acta physiol. scand.*, 69: 153–157.

Dahlström, A., Häggendal, J., Heilbronn, E., Heiwall, P-O. and Saunders, N.R. (1974) Proximodistal transport of acetylcholine in peripheral cholinergic neurons. In *Dynamics of Degeneration and Growth in Neurons*, K. Fuxe, L. Olson and Y. Zotterman (Eds.), Oxford, Pergamon Press, pp. 275–289.

De Potter, W.P. (1971) Noradrenaline storage particles in splenic nerve. *Phil. Trans. B*, 261: 313–317.

De Potter, W.P. (1974) Release of amines from sympathetic nerves. *Biochem. Pharmacol.*, Suppl. Part 1: 372–376.

Dean, C.R. and Hope, D.B. (1966) Protein constituents of neurosecretory granules isolated from the posterior lobes of bovine pituitary glands. *Biochem. J.*, 101: 17–18P.

Dean, C.R. and Hope, D.B. (1967) The isolation of purified neurosecretory granules from bovine pituitary posterior lobes. Comparison of granule protein constituents with those of neurophysin. *Biochem. J.*, 104: 1082–1088.

Dean, C.R., Hope, D.B. and Kažić, T. (1968) Evidence for the storage of oxytocin with neurophysin-I and of vasopressin with neurophysin-II in separate neurosecretory granules. *Brit. J. Pharmacol.*, 34: 192P.

Douglas, W.W. (1973) How do neurons secrete peptides? Exocytosis and its consequences, including "sympathetic vesicle" formation, in the hypothalamo-neurohypophysial system. In *Drug Effects on Neuroendocrine Regulation, Progress in Brain Research*, *Vol. 39*, E. Zimmermann, W.H. Gispen, B.H. Marks and D. de Wied (Eds.), Elsevier, Amsterdam, pp. 21–39.

Douglas, W.W., Nagasawa, J. and Schulz, R. (1971) Electron microscopic studies on the mechanism of secretion of posterior pituitary hormones and significance of microvesicles (synaptic vesicles): evidence of secretion by exocytosis and formation of microvesicles as a by-product of this process. *Mem. Soc. Endocr.*, 19: 353–378.

Dreifuss, J.J. (1975) A review on neurosecretory granules: their contents and mechanisms of release. *Ann N.Y. Acad. Sci.*, 248: 184–201.

Farquhar, M.G. (1961) Origin and fate of secretory granules in cells of the anterior pituitary gland. *Trans. N.Y. Acad. Sci.*, 23: 346–351.

Fillenz, M. (1971) Fine structure of noradrenaline storage vesicles in nerve terminals of the rat vas deferens. *Phil. Trans. B*, 261: 319–323.

Fink, G., Lee, V.W.K., Smith, G.C. and Tibbals, S. (1972a) Subcellular localization of corticotrophin and luteinizing hormone releasing activity in bovine median eminence. *J. Anat. (Lond.)*, 111: 494–495.

Fink, G. Smith, G.C., Tibbals, J. and Lee, V.W.K. (1972b) LRF and CRF release in subcellular fractions of bovine median eminence. *Nature New Biol.*, 239: 57–59.

Flament-Durand, J. and Dustin, P. (1972) Studies on the transport of secretory granules in the magnocellular hypothalamic neurons. I. Action of colchicine on axonal flow and neurotubules in the paraventricular nuclei. *Z. Zellforsch.*, 130: 440–454.

Ginsburg, M. (1968) Production, release, transportation and elimination of the neurohypophysial hormones. In *Handbook Exp. Pharmacol.*, Vol. 23, pp. 286–371.

Ginsburg, M. and Ireland, M. (1963) Isolation, hormone-binding capacity and sub-cellular distribution of neurophysin. *J. Physiol. (Lond.)*, 169: 114–115P.

Ginsburg, M. and Ireland, M. (1966) The role of neurophysin in the transport and release of neurohypophysial hormones. *J. Endocr.*, 35: 289–298.

Grimm-Jørgensen, Y. and McKelvy, J.F. (1974) Control of the in vitro biosynthesis of thyrotropin releasing factor (TRF) in the red spotted newt (*Triturus viridescens*). *Abstr. 56th Meeting of The Endocrine Society*, Abstr. 20.

Heap, P.F., Jones, C.W., Morris, J.F. and Pickering, B.T. (1975) Movement of neurosecretory product through the anatomical compartments of the neural lobe of the pituitary gland. An electron microscopic autoradiographic study. *Cell. Tissue Res.*, 156: 483–497.

Heuser, J.E. and Reese, T.S. (1973) Evidence for recycling of synaptic membrane during transmitter release at the frog neuromuscular junction. *J. Cell Biol.*, 57: 315–344.

Hope, D.B. and Pickup, J.C. (1974) Neurophysins. In *Handbook of Physiology, Section 7 (Endocrinology)*, Vol. IV, Pt. 1, pp. 173–189.

Howell, S.L. and Lacy, P.E. (1971) Biochemical and ultrastructural studies of insulin storage granules and their secretion. *Mem. Soc. Endocr.*, 19: 469–480.

Ishii, S. (1970) Association of luteinizing hormone-releasing factor with granules separated from equine hypophysial stalk. *Endocrinology*, 86: 207–216.

Jones, C.W. and Pickering, B.T. (1969) Comparison of the effects of water deprivation and sodium chloride imbibition on the hormone content of the neurohypophysis of the rat. *J. Physiol. (Lond.)*, 203: 449–458.

Jones, C.W. and Pickering, B.T. (1970) Rapid transport of neurohypophysial hormones in the hypothalamoneurohypophysial tract. *J. Physiol. (Lond.)*, 208: 73–74P.

Jones, C.W. and Pickering, B.T. (1972) Intra-axonal transport and turnover of neurohypophysial hormones in the rat. *J. Physiol. (Lond.)*, 227: 553–564.

Katz, B. (1969) *The Release of Neural Transmitter Substances*. Liverpool University Press, Liverpool.

Klein, R.L. (1974) A large second pool of norepinephrine in the highly purified vesicle fraction from bovine splenic nerve. *Biochem. Pharmacol.*, Suppl., Pt. 1: 330–332.

Kopin, I.J., Breese, G.R., Krauss, K.R. and Weise, V.K. (1968) Selective release of newly synthesized norepinephrine from the cat spleen during sympathetic nerve stimulation. *J. Pharmacol. exp. Ther.*, 161: 271–278.

Lacy, P.E., Howell, S.L., Young, D.A. and Fink, C.J. (1968) New hypothesis for insulin secretion. *Nature (Lond.)*, 219: 1177–1178.

Lagercrantz, H., Kirksey, D.F. and Klein, R.L. (1974) On the development of sympathetic nerve vesicles during axonal transport: density gradient analysis of dopamine β-hydroxylase in bovine splenic nerve; *J. Neurochem.*, 23: 769–773.

Legros, J.J. and Louis, F. (1974) Identification of a vasopressin-neurophysin and of an oxytocin-neurophysin in man. *Neuroendocrinology*, 13: 371–375.

Legros, J.J., Reynaert, R. and Peeters, G. (1974) Specific release of bovine neurophysin I during milking and suckling in the cow. *J. Endocr.*, 60: 327–332.

Malawista, S.E. (1965) On the action of colchicine. The melanocyte model. *J. exp. Med.*, 122: 361–384.

Matsuo, H., Baba, Y., Nair, R.M.G., Arimura, A. and Schally, A.V. (1971) Structure of LH- and FSH-releasing hormone. I. The proposed amino acid sequence. *Biochem. biophys. Res. Commun.*, 43: 1334–1339.

Mitnick, M. and Reichlin, S. (1971) Thyrotropin-releasing hormone: biosynthesis by rat hypothalamic fragments in vitro. *Science*, 172: 1241–1243.

Mitnick, M. and Reichlin, S. (1972) Enzymatic synthesis of thyrotropin-releasing hormone (TRH) by hypothalamic "TRH synthetase". *Endocrinology*, 91: 1145–1153.

Mitnick, M., Valverde, R.C. and Reichlin, S. (1973) Enzymatic synthesis of prolactin-releasing factor (PRF) by rat hypothalamic incubates and by extracts of rat hypothalamic tissue: evidence for "PRF synthetase". *Proc. Soc. exp. Biol. (N.Y.)*, 143: 418–421.

Morris, J.F. (1976) Distribution of neurosecretory granules among the anatomical compartments of the neurosecretory processes. A quantitative ultrastructural approach to hormone storage in the neural lobe. *J. Endocr.*, 68: 225–234.

Mulder, A.H. (1970) On the subcellular localization of corticotropin releasing factor (CRF) in the rat median eminence. In *Pituitary, Adrenal and the Brain, Progress in Brain Research, Vol. 32*, D. de Weid and J.A.W.M. Weijnen (Eds.), Elsevier, Amsterdam, pp. 33–41.

Nordmann, J.J., Dreifuss, J.J., Baker, P.F., Ravazzola, M., Malaisse-Legae, F. and Orci, L. (1974) Secretion-dependent uptake of extracellular fluid by the rat neurohypophysis. *Nature (Lond.)*, 250: 155–157.

Norström, A. and Sjöstrand, J. (1971) Transport and turnover of neurohypophysial proteins of the rat. *J. Neurochem.*, 18: 2007–2016.

Norström, A., Hansson, H.-A. and Sjöstrand, J. (1971) Effects of colchicine on axonal transport and ultrastructure of the hypothalamo-neurohypophysial system of the rat. *Z. Zellforsch.*, 113: 271–293.

Palade, G.E. (1959) Functional changes in the structure of cell components. In *Subcellular Particles*, T. Hayashi (Ed.), Ronald Press, New York, pp. 64–83.

Palay, S.L. (1957) The fine structure of the neurohypophysis. In *Ultrastructure and Cellular Chemistry of Neural Tissue*, H. Waelsch (Ed.), Hueber, New York, pp. 31–49.

Pearson, D., Shainberg, A., Osinchak, J. and Sachs, H. (1975) The hypothalamo-neurohypophysial complex in organ culture: morphologic and biochemical characteristics. *Endocrinology*, 96: 982–993.

Pelletier, G., Labrie, F., Arimura, A. and Schally, A.V. (1974a) Electron microscopic immunohistochemical localization of growth hormone-release inhibiting hormone (somatostatin) in the rat median eminence. *Amer. J. Anat.*, 140: 445–450.

Pelletier, G., Labrie, F., Puviani, R., Arimura, A. and Schally, A.V. (1974b) Immunohisto-chemical localization of luteinizing hormone-releasing hormone in the rat median eminence. *Endocrinology*, 95: 314–317.

Pickering, B.T. and Jones, C.W. (1976) The Neurophysins. In *Hormonal Proteins and Peptides*, C.H. Li (Ed.), Academic Press, New York, in press.

Pickering, B.T., Jones, C.W. and Burford, G.D. (1971) Biosynthesis and intra-neuronal transport of neurosecretory products in the hypothalamo-neurohypophysial system. In *Neurohypophysial Hormones. CIBA Fndn Study Grp No. 39*, G.E.W. Wolstenholme and J. Birch (Eds.), Churchill-Livingstone, London, pp. 58–74.

Pickering, B.T., Jones, C.W. and Burford, G.D. (1974) Biochemical aspects of the hypothalamo-neurohypophysial neurone. In *Neurosecretion — The Final Neuroendocrine Pathway*, F.G.W. Knowles and L. Vollrath (Eds.), Springer-Verlag, Berlin, pp. 72–85.

Pickering, B.T., Jones, C.W., Burford, G.D., McPherson, M.A., Swann, R.W., Heap, P.F. and Morris, J.F. (1975) The role of neurophysin proteins: suggestions from the study of their transport and turnover. *Ann. N.Y. Acad. Sci.*, 248: 15–35.

Pickup, J.C., Johnston, C.I., Nakamura, S., Uttenthal, L.O. and Hope, D.B. (1973) Subcellular organization of neurophysins, oxytocin, [8-lysine]-vasopressin and adenosine triphosphatase in porcine posterior pituitary lobes. *Biochem. J.*, 132: 361–371.

Potter, L.T. (1967) Role of intraneuronal vesicles in the synthesis, storage and release of noradrenaline. *Circulat. Res.*, 21, Suppl. 3: 13–24.

Reichlin, S. (1973) Hypothalamic-pituitary function. In *Endocrinology*, R.O. Scow, F.J.G. Ebling and I.W. Henderson (Eds.), American Elsevier, New York, pp. 1–16.

Reichlin, S. and Mitnick, M. (1973) Enzymatic synthesis of growth hormone releasing factor (GH-RF) by rat incubates and by extracts of rat and porcine hypothalamic tissue. *Proc. Soc. exp. Biol. (N.Y.)*, 142: 497–501.

Robinson, A.G., Zimmerman, E.A. and Frantz, A.G. (1971) Physiologic investigation of posterior pituitary binding proteins neurophysin I and neurophysin II. *Metabolism*, 20: 1148–1155.

Sachs, H. (1971) Secretion of neurohypophysial hormones. *Mem. Soc. Endocr.*, 19: 965–973.

Sachs, H. and Takabatake, Y. (1964) Evidence for a precursor in vasopressin biosynthesis. *Endocrinology*, 75: 943–948.

Sachs, H., Fawcett, C.P., Takabatake, Y. and Portanova, R. (1969) Biosynthesis and release of vasopressin and neurophysin. *Recent Progr. Hormone Res.*, 25: 447–491.

Santolaya, R.C., Bridges, T.E. and Lederis, K. (1972) Elementary granules, small vesicles and exocytosis in the neurohypophysis after acute haemorrhage. *Z. Zellforsch.*, 125: 277–288.

Sawyer, W.H. (1961). Neurohypophyseal hormones. *Pharmacol. Rev.*, 13: 225–277.

Scharrer, E. (1928) Die Lichtempfindlichkeit blindes Eltritzen (Untersuchungen über das Zwischenhirn der Fische. I. *Z. vergl. Physiol.*, 7: 1–38.

Schlesinger, D.H., Frangione, B. and Walter, R. (1972) Structure of bovine neurophysin II. *Proc. nat. Acad. Sci. (Wash.)*, 69: 3350–3354.

Schmitt, F.O. (1968) Fibrous proteins — neuronal organelles. *Proc. nat. Acad. Sci. (Wash.)*, 60: 1092–1101.

Schmitt, F.O. (1969) Fibrous proteins and neuronal dynamics. In *Cellular Dynamics of the Neuron*, S.H. Barondes (Ed.), Academic Press, New York, pp. 95–111.

Scott, A.P., Lowry, P.J., Ratcliffe, J.G., Rees, L.H. and Landon, J. (1974a) Corticotrophin-like peptides in the rat pituitary. *J. Endocr.*, 61: 355–367.

Scott, A.P., Lowry, P.J., Bennett, H.P.J., McMartin, C. and Ratcliffe, J.G. (1974b) Purification and characterization of porcine corticotrophin-like intermediate lobe peptide. *J. Endocr.*, 61: 369–380.

Sheterline, P., Schofield, J.G. and Mira, F. (1975) Colchicine binding to bovine anterior pituitary slices and inhibition of growth hormone release. *Biochem. J.*, 148: 435–459.

Sokol, H.W. (1970) Evidence for oxytocin synthesis after electrolytic destruction of the paraventricular nucleus in rats with hereditary diabetes insipidus. *Neuroendocrinology*, 6: 90–97.

Smith, A.D. (1971a) Summing up: some implications of the neuron as a secreting cell. *Phil. Trans. B*, 261: 423–437.

Smith, A.D. (1971b) Secretion of proteins (chromogranin A and dopamine β-hydroxylase) from a sympathetic neuron. *Phil. Trans. B*, 261: 363–370.

Steiner, D.F., Rubenstein, A.H., Peterson, J.D., Kemmler, W. and Tager, H.S. (1973) Proinsulin and polypeptide hormone biosynthesis. In *Endocrinology*, R.O. Scow, F.J.G. Ebling and I.W. Henderson (Eds.), American Elsevier, New York, pp. 561–566.

Sundberg, D.K., Krulich, L. Fawcett, C.P., Illner, P. and McCann, S.M. (1973) The effect of colchicine on the release of rat interior pituitary hormone in vitro. *Proc. Soc. exp. Biol. (N.Y.)*, 142: 1097–1100.

Swann, R.W. and Pickering, B.T. (1976) Incorporation of radioactive precursors into the membrane and contents of the neurosecretory granules of the rat neurohypophysis as a method of studying their fate. *J. Endocr.*, 68: 95–108.

Taber, C.A. and Karavolas, H.J. (1975) Subcellular localization of LH releasing activity in the rat hypothalamus. *Endocrinology*, 96: 446–452.

Takabatake, Y. and Sachs, H. (1964) Vasopressin biosynthesis. III. In vitro studies. *Endocrinology*, 75: 934–942.

Vandesande, F., Dierickx, K. and De May, J. (1975) Identification of the vasopressin-neurophysin II and the oxytocin-neurophysin I producing neurons in the bovine hypothalamus. *Cell Tissue Res.*, 156: 189–200.

Van Dyke, H.B., Chow, B.F., Greep, R.O. and Rothen, A. (1942) The isolation of a protein from the pars neuralis of the ox pituitary with constant oxytocic, pressor and diuresis-inhibiting activities. *J. Pharmacol.*, 74: 190–209.

Whittaker, V.P. (1959) The isolation and characterization of acetylcholine-containing particles from brain. *Biochem. J.*, 72: 694–706.

Whittaker, V.P. (1969). The nature of the acetylcholine pools in brain tissue. In *Mechanisms of Synaptic Transmission, Progress in Brain Research, Vol. 31*, K. Akert and P.G. Waser (Eds.), Elsevier, Amsterdam, pp. 211–222.

Wong, T.M. and Pickering, B.T. (1976) Last in, first out in the rat neurohypophysis. *Gen. comp. Endocr.*, in press.

Zimmerman, E.A., Robinson, A.G., Husain, M.K., Acosta, M., Franz, A.G. and Sawyer, W.H. (1974) Neurohypophysial peptides in the bovine hypothalamus: the relationship of neurophysin I to oxytocin and neurophysin II to vasopressin in supraoptic and paraventricular regions. *Endocrinology*, 95: 931–936.

Zimmerman, E.A., Defendini, R., Sokol, H.W. and Robinson, A.G. (1975) The distribution of neurophysin-secreting pathways in the mammalian brain: light microscopic studies using the immunoperoxidase technique. *Ann. N.Y. Acad. Sci.*, 248: 92–111.

DISCUSSION

S.P.R. ROSE: If the transport down the axon of the neurosecretory particles is blocked, would it then be possible to isolate the hormones bound to the neurophysins?

B.T. PICKERING: Since the enzyme is situated inside the granule, the cleavage is not dependent on the location of the granules but only on the time elapsed after their formation.

B. SCHARRER: I should like to make a brief comment: when you propose this neurosecretory system as a model for the study of secretory cells you should limit the analogy to proteinaceous systems.

B.T. PICKERING: I agree with you. I tried to get around this by talking about secretory cells containing granules. However, I intended to restrict the discussion to cells releasing proteinaceous material because I cannot explain steroid secretion in this way.

D.F. SWAAB: I was very impressed by your data obtained by autoradiography in which you showed the movement of vesicles from the terminals into the swellings. Do you have any evidence that the radioactivity is appearing afterwards over the pituicytes?

B.T. PICKERING: The proportion of radioactivity over the pituicytes was the same at every time period studied. I am not sure how to interpret these pituicyte results. I certainly cannot say, at present, whether there is indeed a movement from the ending into the swelling, and then to the pituicyte.

A. TIXIER-VIDAL: I have two questions about your experiments on the rate of accumulation of radioactivity after intracisternal injection of [^{35}S]cysteine. My first question is: would it be possible to follow at the same time the data of neurophysin, of vasopressin and oxytocin by immunoprecipitation? And my second question is: did you try to measure the same data at the level of the cell body in the supraoptic and paraventricular nuclei?

B.T. PICKERING: To answer your first question: in fact when C.W. Jones and I began this work we looked at the incorporation of radioactivity into the hormones oxytocin and vasopressin, not by immunoprecipitation but by actual isolation of the neurohormones. When, with G.D. Burford, we went on to study the neurophysins, we found that the turnover of these proteins (as judged by the decay constants for the decline in radioactivity after it had reached its peak) was not significantly different from that of the hormone. However, since the neurophysin measurements were not made in parellel with those of the hormones in the same animals, we have not done exactly what you propose. As to your second question, we are currently attempting this very thing. The problem is one of purification: in the neural lobe studies, the animal itself does the first purification step, since we give radiocysteine to the hypothalamus and then look at the gland, in which almost all of the radioactivity found has been transported along the axons. In studying the hypothalamus, we are looking for a small amount of radioactive precursor, neurophysin and hormone, in the face of a large background of radioactivity. I hope that immuno-affinity chromatography might help us to achieve a rapid separation of neurophysin-like proteins from the hypothalamus of a single rat, and preliminary results look promising. (McPherson and Pickering, 1975.)

REFERENCE

McPherson, M.A. and Pickering, B.T. (1975) *J. Endocr.*, 67: 43P.

Vasopressin and Memory Consolidation

D. de WIED, Tj.B. van WIMERSMA GREIDANUS, B. BOHUS, I. URBAN
and W.H. GISPEN

*Rudolf Magnus Institute for Pharmacology, Medical Faculty, University of Utrecht,
Utrecht (The Netherlands)*

INTRODUCTION

Vasopressin is one of the hormones which is stored and released by the posterior lobe of the pituitary. The name vasopressin is based on the pressor action of the hormone which is caused by contraction of peripheral blood vessels. However, in much lower concentrations it acts to conserve body water by concentrating the urine, thus reducing the amount of water required to excrete waste solutes. The term antidiuretic hormone (ADH) may therefore be more adequate for this substance.

ADH is a nonapeptide which is synthesized in cell bodies of neurosecretory neurons, situated in the anterior hypothalamus, in particular in the supraoptic and paraventricular nuclei (Sachs et al., 1969; Scharrer, pp. 125–137 in this volume). It is bound to a specific protein, neurohypophysin II, which is found throughout the entire neurosecretory neuron. The hormone protein complex is packed in granules from which it is released by exocytosis, which involves fusion of the granule with the plasma membrane and subsequent diffusion of its contents into the bloodstream (Douglas, 1973; Pickering, pp. 161–179 in this volume). High quantities of vasopressin-neurophysin have also been found in the hypophyseal portal vessel system (Zimmermann et al., 1973). In addition, morphological evidence points to connections between neurosecretory cells and the infundibular recess of the third ventricle (Wittkowski, 1968). These findings indicate that vasopressin may be secreted into portal blood and cerebrospinal fluid (CSF) from neuron terminals (Goldsmith and Zimmermann, 1975). Thus, the hypothalamic-neurohypophyseal system not only uses the general circulation for peripheral effects of posterior pituitary principles, but also the portal vessel system for regulation of anterior pituitary function, and the CSF for action on the central nervous system.

The latter function has been disclosed only recently, and is involved in memory processes. Memory is defined here as the retention of acquired behavior. According to current points of view memory storage in general comprises at least two stages. The first stage represents a very short period immediately after the learning experience, and involves electrical events with metabolic processes which accompany these events. This stage can be erased easily. It is transformed into a stage of a more permanent character, the so-called "long-term" memory. This consolidation process is accompanied by growth of axon collaterals, inducing changes in connectivity within the neural network, and also involves metabolic changes (Entingh et al., 1975; Matthies, 1974; Perumal et al., 1975).

EFFECT OF VASOPRESSIN ANALOGUES ON ACQUISITION AND MAINTENANCE OF ACTIVE AND PASSIVE AVOIDANCE BEHAVIOR

It is probably the consolidating phase of the memory process which is affected by vasopressin and its analogues. This notion arose from our observations in the early sixties when it was found that removal of the posterior lobe of the pituitary interfered with the maintenance of a conditioned avoidance response (de Wied, 1965). Shuttle-box avoidance behavior of posterior lobectomized rats markedly differs from that of sham-operated control animals. Although acquisition of the avoidance response is normal in the posterior lobectomized rat, the rate of extinction is much faster. Pitressin, a relatively crude extract of posterior pituitary origin, in amounts which normalize the water intake of the mildly diabetic posterior lobectomized rat, at the same time restores the ability to maintain non-reinforced avoidance behavior. Pitressin was subsequently found to increase resistance to extinction of shuttle-box avoidance behavior in intact rats (de Wied and Bohus, 1966). The same was found for purified lysine-vasopressin (LVP) on extinction of a pole-jumping one-way avoidance procedure (de Wied, 1971; van Wimersma Greidanus et al., 1973). A single subcutaneous injection of a moderate amount of this peptide increased resistance to extinction of the avoidance response which lasted several days, depending on the dose administered. Since the effect extended beyond the demonstrable presence of the peptide in the body, these studies indicated that vasopressin triggers a long-term effect on the maintenance of avoidance behavior probably by facilitating consolidation.

The inhibitory effect of vasopressin on extinction of active avoidance behavior might be explained by an increase in the general level of activity. However, administration of this peptide does not affect rearing, grooming or ambulation in a so-called "open-field" situation. In addition, vasopressin also affects passive avoidance behavior, as studied in a simple step-through one-trial passive avoidance situation (Ader and de Wied, 1972). In this situation, it facilitates retention of passive avoidance behavior, and the effect once again is of a long-term nature. Subsequent experiments indicated that the behavioral effect of vasopressin is independent of its vasopressor and antidiuretic activities. Desglycinamide-lysine-vasopressin (DG-LVP), which was isolated from hog pituitary material (Lande et al., 1971), is practically devoid of classical endocrine activities (de Wied et al., 1972). It effectively normalizes the lower rate of acquisition of shuttle-box avoidance behavior of hypophysectomized rats and, like vasopressin, it induces a long-term resistance to extinction of active and passive avoidance behavior.

VASOPRESSIN ANALOGUES ON APPROACH BEHAVIOR AND
RETROGRADE AMNESIA

Vasopressin analogues do not seem to affect extinction of a food running response in rats. Garrud et al. (1974) failed to observe an effect of LVP or DG-LVP on extinction of a straight runway approach response for food in food-deprived rats. Although DG-LVP is practically devoid of antidiuretic activity, an interaction between the peptide, hunger drive and water metabolism cannot be excluded. However, the behavior of food-deprived rats in a continual punishment situation, which were trained to hold a lever down for 8 sec in order to obtain a food reward, can be affected by vasopressin. When electric shock was introduced after training to a stable level contingent upon the completion of an 8 sec lever hold at the same time as the food, administration of lysine-vasopressin prolonged the time needed to make the next response after each shock, and increased the efficiency with which the animals performed. The latter effect may have been due to the vasopressin-induced increased tendency to freezing (Garrud, 1975). However, vasopressin is also active in approach behavior. It was found to increase resistance to extinction of sexually rewarded learning behavior. Male rats trained in a T-maze to run for a receptive female chose the correct arm of the maze at a significantly higher percentage following DG-LVP treatment after each acquisition session. The effect again is of a long-term nature. Copulation reward appeared to be essential for this effect since non-rewarded rats do not make more correct choices than do placebo-treated animals after cessation of the treatment (Bohus, in preparation). DG-LVP also delays the disappearance of intromission and ejaculatory behavior of male rats following castration. Thus, vasopressin analogues not only affect the maintenance of aversively motivated behavior but also extinction of a hormone determined behavioral pattern. Evidence for an effect on memory processes was further obtained when it appeared that vasopressin analogues could reverse amnesia. Lande et al. (1972) found that DG-LVP protects against puromycin-induced memory loss in mice. Rigter et al. (1974) demonstrated that amnesia for a one trial passive avoidance response in rats, as induced by CO_2 or by electroconvulsive shock, is reversed by treatment with DG-LVP immediately after the learning trial. These authors suggested that the peptide promotes memory consolidation either by facilitating the consolidating process or by protecting memory consolidation from the adverse effects of the amnesic treatment. The possibility that vasopressin influences retrieval was considered as well since DG-LVP exhibited antiamnesic effects also if injected 1 hr prior to the retention test.

BEHAVIORAL AND ASSOCIATED ENDOCRINE DEFECTS IN
HEREDITARY DIABETES INSIPIDUS RATS

The availability of rats with hereditary diabetes insipidus (DI) provided a model to study memory function in the absence of vasopressin. Homozygous hereditary DI rats of the Brattleboro strain (HO-DI) lack the ability to synthetize vasopressin while their heterozygous litter mates (HE-DI) have a relatively normal water metabolism (Valtin, 1967; Valtin et al., 1965; Valtin and Schroeder, 1964). HO-DI rats are inferior in acquiring and maintaining active and passive avoidance behavior (Bohus et al., 1975). The behavioral deficits are most obvious in a step-through one-trial passive avoidance paradigm. The rate of acquisition of a shuttle-box avoidance response is slower in HO-DI rats as compared to that of heterozygous litter mates or homozygous normal rats of the Brattleboro strain. These are identical to Wistar strain rats in shuttle-box avoidance and passive avoidance behavior.

Extinction of the behavior is very rapid in HO-DI and somewhat less rapid in HE-DI as compared to that of Wistar rats. The rate of acquisition of the pole-jumping response appeared to be the same in HO-DI and HE-DI rats but Wistar rats acquire the response much faster. Extinction is very rapid in HO-DI rats, somewhat slower in HE-DI animals and least rapid in the Wistar rats. Memory function of HO-DI rats is completely impaired in a one-trial passive avoidance situation when retention is tested 24 hr or later following shock exposure. Arginine-vasopressin (AVP) and DG-LVP given immediately after the learning trial readily restore passive avoidance behavior in HO-DI rats (de Wied et al., 1975). This favors the hypothesis that memory rather than learning processes are disturbed in the absence of vasopressin. Indeed, HO-DI rats are able to acquire "fear" motivated responses in the shuttle-box or in the pole-jumping test. Furthermore, full retention of passive avoidance behavior is obtained in HO-DI rats when retention is tested shortly after the learning trial. The main disturbance is in the ability to maintain the behavior. The passive avoidance response is only partially absent 3 hr after, and completely gone 24 hr after the learning trial (de Wied et al., 1975; van Wimersma Greidanus et al., 1975). These observations suggest that consolidation of memory is selectively impaired in the absence of vasopressin.

Vasopressin levels in eye plexus blood are augmented during passive avoidance response and the rate of increase is related to avoidance latency, which in turn is related to shock intensity (Thompson and de Wied, 1973). It might be, therefore, that an association between endogenous release of vasopressin and specific environmental cues is of physiological significance in the maintenance of new behavior patterns (Bohus et al., 1972). The pituitary-adrenal response also shows a marked relationship with passive avoidance behavior in DI rats (Fig. 1). At the immediate retention test, when full passive avoidance behavior is displayed by HO-DI rats, an elevation of plasma corticosterone is found which is of the same magnitude as that of HE-DI rats. At the 3 hr retention test a partial avoidance behavior is associated with a reduced corticosterone response, while retention impairment is coupled with the absence of a significant increase in plasma corticosterone (Bohus et al., 1975) These observations, therefore, indicate that the absence of vasopressin in HO-DI rats, which results in an impairment of a psychological mechanism, also results in an impairment of the accompanying endocrine response in an otherwise "fear" provoking environment. This would suggest that the behavioral effect of vasopressin is mediated by ACTH or other pituitary hormones but vasopressin effectively restores avoidance behavior in hypophysectomized rats (Bohus et al., 1973; Lande et al., 1971).

PITUITARY ADRENAL RESPONSE

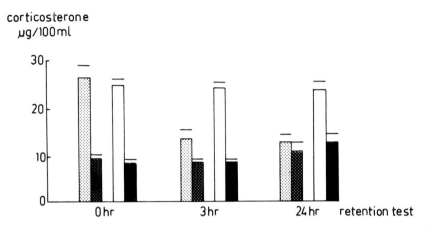

PASSIVE AVOIDANCE BEHAVIOUR

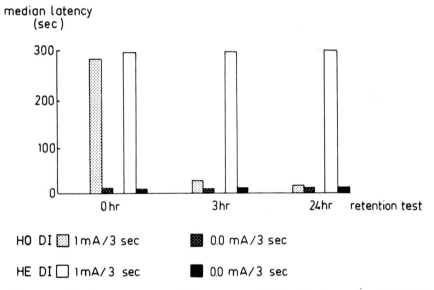

Fig. 1. Plasma corticosterone response in homozygous (HO) and heterozygous (HE) diabetes insipidus (DI) rats during passive avoidance retention. Rats (6–10 per group) were exposed to electric shocks (1 mA) or sham shock for 3 sec in the dark box and tested for retention at various intervals after the learning trial. Plasma corticosterone was determined in trunk blood from rats decapitated 15 min after the onset of the retention test.

STRUCTURE-ACTIVITY STUDIES

In an attempt to determine the active core of the vasopressin molecule in memory consolidation, the potency of a number of vasopressin analogues was assayed on extinction of the avoidance response in the pole-jumping test (de Wied et al., 1975). AVP appeared to be the most potent peptide followed by LVP. Removal of the glycinamide (DG-LVP and DG-AVP) decreases the potency to approximately 50%. Oxytocin and vasotocin are equally effective and possess about 20% of the activity of AVP. Pressinamide (PA) has retained only 10% of the behavioral potency.

$$\frac{AVP}{LVP} \quad H-Cys-Tyr-Phe-Glu-Asn-Cys-Pro-\frac{Arg}{Lys}-Gly-NH_2$$

$$PA \quad H-Cys-Tyr-Phe-Glu-Asn-Cys-NH_2$$

Thus, removal of the C-terminal part leads to a drastic decrease in potency. It may be that this portion of the molecule protects the active moiety against metabolic degradation en route to the central nervous system (CNS). Indeed, if PA is administered via one of the lateral ventricles only twice as much as AVP is needed for an equipotent effect on extinction of the pole-jumping avoidance response. In addition, AVP is 200 and PA 1000 times more active when given through this route. This suggests that the receptor in the brain interacts with only a part of the molecule, presumably located in the ring structure. The isolation of these receptors may eventually reveal the essential requirements for the memory consolidating effect of vasopressin analogues.

CSF AS A TRANSPORT MEDIUM FOR THE BEHAVIORAL EFFECT OF VASOPRESSIN

The potency of intraventricularly administered vasopressin suggests that its memory effect results from release from its production sites in the anterior hypothalamus into the CSF. Indeed, intracerebroventricular administration of vasopressin antiserum immediately after the learning trial induces an almost complete deficit in retention of passive avoidance behavior when tested at various intervals after the learning trial (van Wimersma Greidanus et al., 1975a). In contrast, avoidance latencies of control animals treated with rabbit serum or animals treated with oxytocin- or growth hormone-antiserum continue to avoid maximally. Only if animals treated with vasopressin antiserum are tested at 2 min, 1 hr or at 2 hr after the learning trial is maximum avoidance obtained. Thus, as in HO-DI rats, long-term memory rather than learning itself is disrupted in rats in which vasopressin in the CSF has been neutralized by antibodies. Peripheral (i.v.) injection of 100 times as much vasopressin antiserum as required to neutralize the peptide in the general circulation, as indicated by a virtual absence of vasopressin in the urine and by a marked increase in urine production, still fails to affect passive avoidance behavior.

These results indicate that centrally released rather than circulating vasopressin is involved in the behavioral effect of this nonapeptide.

LOCUS OF ACTION IN THE BRAIN

Localization of the site of the behavioral effect of vasopressin was attempted by intracerebral administration of the peptide and by lesion experiments. Microinjections of small amounts (0·1 μg) of LVP into the posterior thalamic area, including the parafascicular nuclei, result in an increased resistance to extinction of the pole-jumping avoidance response. Other brain areas, including the ventromedial and anteromedial parts of the thalamus, the posterior hypothalamus, the substantia nigra, the reticular formation, the substantia grisea, the putamen and the dorsal hippocampal complex proved to be ineffective sites with this technique (van Wimersma Greidanus et al., 1973, 1976). Thus, the parafascicular area seems to be a locus of action.

However, ineffective microinjections may not necessarily represent non-sensitive structures, since a unilateral microinjection of a small amount of vasopressin into a restricted area, might not be sufficient to induce functional changes which lead to overt behavioral manifestations. Rats bearing lesions in the parafascicular area were therefore employed to confirm the significance of this region for the memory consolidating effect of LVP. Although the behavioral effect of the peptide is indeed significantly reduced, long-term resistance to extinction could still be obtained by a factor three increase of the dose of LVP. These nuclei therefore may be involved in but not essential for the memory consolidating effect of vasopressin. Marked behavioral changes have been reported in rats following ablation of the septum or following dorsal hippocampectomy. Both regions have been implicated in learning and memory processes (Altman et al., 1973; Fried, 1972; Isaacson and Kimble, 1972; Olds, 1972). Indeed, destruction of rostral septal or dorsal hippocampal areas prevents the memory consolidating effect of vasopressin (van Wimersma Greidanus et al., 1976). It is possible, therefore, that vasopressin acts on midbrain limbic circuits, including septal and hippocampal structures, in such a way as to facilitate the storage and/or retrieval of acquired behavior.

DIABETES INSIPIDUS AND PARADOXICAL SLEEP

Electrophysiological data support the hypothesis that the hippocampus is involved in the memory consolidating effect of vasopressin analogues. Rhythmic slow activity (RSA) during paradoxical sleep (PS) episodes contain substantially slower hippocampal theta frequencies in HO-DI rats as compared to HE-DI or homozygous normal rats (Urban and de Wied, 1975).

Differences are found in various spectral parameters and the peak frequency of RSA of HO-DI rats is approximately 1 Hz lower than that of controls. Thus, PS causes a difference in RSA in the absence of vasopressin. Administration of DG-AVP enhances the generation of higher frequencies and almost completely restores the spectrum of hippocampal frequencies to control values. PS deprivation leads to consolidation deficits (Fishbein, 1971; Leconte and Bloch, 1970; Stern, 1971). It might be, therefore, that the impaired memory of HO-DI rats is due to the different quality of PS found in these animals. Drugs which facilitate memory functions enhance the generation of theta frequencies in the post-learning period (Longo and Loizzo, 1973), suggesting that changes in hippocampal theta activity may be related to memory consolidation. Landfield et al. (1972) maintain that theta activity in the post-learning period may reflect a brain state which is optimal for memory storage. Hypophysectomized rats which also show learning deficits (de Wied, 1964) have shorter PS episodes and lack the normally present PS circadian rhythmicity (Valatx et al., 1975). PS is also markedly disturbed in the chronic pontine cat without hypothalamus or pituitary gland (Jouvet, 1965). These deficits can be restored by treatment with various pituitary principles (Jouvet, 1965).

VASOPRESSIN ANALOGUES AND THE DEVELOPMENT OF RESISTANCE TO THE ANALGESIC ACTION OF MORPHINE

The biochemical substrate of vasopressin analogues is as yet unknown. The protective effect of DG-LVP against puromycin-induced memory blockade in mice (Lande et al., 1972) suggests that vasopressin affects memory processes through protein synthesis. Experimental evidence for this at present is not available. Recently, Krivoy et al. (1974) reported that DG-LVP facilitates the development of resistance to the analgesic action of morphine in mice. This might suggest a physiological role of vasopressin in the development of tolerance to narcotic analgesics. Conversely, in the absence of vasopressin the development of resistance to the analgesic action of morphine as measured in rats on the hot plate, is greatly retarded (de Wied and Gispen, 1976). This disturbance can be restored by treatment with vasopressin analogues. Development of resistance to morphine analgesia may be regarded as a form of learning or memory (Cohen et al., 1965). This view is corroborated by observations showing that protein synthesis inhibitors which impair learning and memory, prevent the development of tolerance to narcotic analgesics as well (Cox and Osman, 1970). Thus, similar mechanisms as in learning and memory processes may be involved in the development of tolerance.

CONCLUSION AND SUMMARY

The hypothalamic-neurohypophyseal system possibly makes use of (a) the general circulation for peripheral effects of posterior pituitary hormones; (b) the portal vessel system for regulation of anterior pituitary function and (c) the cerebrospinal fluid for CNS activities. Evidence is presented that vasopressin and its analogues facilitate the consolidation of learned behavior patterns. Under certain conditions these peptides facilitate acquisition of active avoidance behavior and increase the resistance to extinction of active and passive avoidance behavior, and of sexually motivated approach behavior as well. Conversely, severe memory disturbances are found in the absence of vasopressin, such as occurs in hereditary diabetes insipidus rats. Intraventricular administration of minute amounts of vasopressin analogues facilitate memory consolidation. This supports the idea that the behavioral effect of these polypeptides is centrally mediated. Vasopressin antibodies, which are assumed to neutralize in situ vasopressin released into the CSF, prevent memory consolidation. Studies on paradoxical sleep in diabetes insipidus rats reveal disturbances in hippocampal theta frequencies, and strengthen the hypothesis that memory consolidation is under the influence of vasopressin analogues. The development of resistance to the analgesic action of narcotic analgesics is facilitated by administration of vasopressin analogues and markedly retarded in diabetes insipidus rats. These and other results suggest that the memory consolidating effects of vasopressin analogues are of a more general nature.

REFERENCES

Ader, R. and de Wied, D. (1972) Effects of lysine vasopressin on passive avoidance learning. *Psychon. Sci.*, 29: 46–48.

Altman, J., Brunner, R.L. and Bayer, S.A. (1973) The hippocampus and behavioral maturation. *Behav. Biol.*, 8: 557–596.

Bohus, B. Effect of DG-lysine vasopressin on sexually motivated T-maze behavior in the male rat. In preparation.

Bohus, A., Ader, R. and de Wied, D. (1972) Effects of vasopressin on active and passive avoidance behavior. *Horm. Behav.*, 3: 191–197.

Bohus, B., Gispen, W.H. and de Wied, D. (1973) Effect of lysine vasopressin and ACTH 4–10 on conditioned avoidance behavior of hypophysectomized rats. *Neuroendocrinology*, 11: 137–143.

Bohus, B., van Wimersma Greidanus, Tj.B. and de Wied, D. (1975) Behavioral and endocrine responses of rats with hereditary hypothalamic diabetes insipidus (Brattleboro strain). *Physiol. Behav.*, 14: 609–615.

Cohen, M., Keats, A.S., Krivoy, W.A. and Ungar, G. (1965) Effect of actinomycin D on morphine tolerance. *Proc. Soc. exp. Biol. (N.Y.)*, 119: 381–384.

Cox, B.M. and Osman, O.H. (1970) Inhibition of the development of tolerance to morphine in rats by drugs which inhibit ribonucleic acid or protein synthesis. *Brit. J. Pharmacol.*, 38: 157–170.

Douglas, W.W. (1973) How do neurones secrete peptides? Exocytosis and its consequences, including "synaptic vesicle" formation, in the hypothalamo-neurohypophyseal system. In *Drug Effects on Neuroendocrine Regulation, Progress in Brain Research*, Vol. 39, E. Zimmermann, W.H. Gispen, B.H. Marks and D. de Wied (Eds.), Elsevier, Amsterdam, pp. 21–39.

Entingh, D., Dunn, A., Glassman, E., Wilson, J.E., Hogan, E. and Damstra, T. (1975) Biochemical approaches to the biological basis of memory. In *Handbook of Psychology*, M.S. Gazzaniga and C. Blakemore (Eds.), Academic Press, New York, pp. 201–238.

Fishbein, W. (1971) Disruptive effects of rapid eye movement sleep deprivation on long-term memory. *Physiol. Behav.*, 6: 279–282.

Fried, P.A. (1972) The septum and behaviour: a review. *Psychol. Bull.*, 78: 292–310.

Garrud, P. (1975) Effects of lysine-8-vasopressin on punishment-induced suppression of a lever-holding response. In *Hormones, Homeostasis and the Brain, Progress in Brain Research*, Vol. 42, W.H. Gispen, Tj.B. van Wimersma Greidanus, B. Bohus and D. de Wied (Eds.), Elsevier, Amsterdam, pp. 173–186.

Garrud, P., Gray, J.A. and de Wied, D. (1974) Pituitary-adrenal hormones and extinction of rewarded behavior in the rat. *Physiol. Behav.*, 12: 109–119.

Goldsmith, P.C. and Zimmermann, E.A. (1975) Ultrastructural localization of neurophysin and vasopressin in the rat median eminence. In *Abstracts Fifty-Seventh Annual Meeting of the Endocrine Society*, p. 239.

190

Isaacson, R.L. and Kimble, D.P. (1972) Lesions of the limbic system: their effects upon hypotheses and frustration. *Behav. Biol.*, 7: 767–793.

Jouvet, M. (1965) Etude de la dualité des états de sommeil et des méchanismes de la phase paradoxale. In *Aspects Anatomo-fonctionnels de la Physiologie du Sommeil*, C.N.R.S., Paris, pp. 397–449.

Krivoy, W.A., Zimmermann, E. and Lande, S. (1974) Facilitation of development of resistance to morphine analgesia by desglycinamide[9]-lysine-vasopressin. *Proc. nat. Acad. Sci. (Wash.)*, 71: 1852–1856.

Lande, S., Witter, A. and de Wied, D. (1971) Pituitary peptides. An octapeptide that simulates conditioned avoidance acquisition in hypophysectomized rats. *J. biol. Chem.*, 246: 2058–2062.

Lande, S., Flexner, J.B. and Flexner, L.B. (1972) Effect of corticotrophin and desglycinamide[9]-lysine vasopressin on suppression of memory by puromycin. *Proc. nat. Acad. Sci. (Wash.)*, 69: 558–560.

Landfield, P.W., McGaugh, J.L. and Tusa, R.J. (1972) Theta rhythm: a temporal correlate of memory storage processes in the rat. *Science*, 175: 87–89.

Leconte, P. et Bloch, V. (1970) Déficit de la retention d'un conditionnement après privation de Sommeil Paradoxal chez le rat. *C.R. Acad. Sci. (Paris)*, Série D, 271: 226–229.

Longo, V.G. and Loizzo, A. (1973) Effects of drugs on the hippocampal theta rhythm. Possible relationships to learning and memory processes. In *Pharmacology and the Future of Man, Fifth Int. Congr. Pharmacology, Vol. 4, Brain, Nerves and Synapses*, F.E. Bloom and G.H. Acheson (Eds.), Karger, Basel, pp. 46–54.

Matthies, H. (1974) The biochemical basis of learning and memory. *Life Sci.*, 15: 2017–2031.

Olds, J. (1972) Learning and the hippocampus. *Rev. Canad. Biol.*, 31: Suppl, 215–238.

Perumal, R., Gispen, W.H., Wilson, J.E. and Glassman, E. (1975) Phosphorylation of proteins from the brains of mice subjected to short-term behavioral experiences. In *Hormones, Homeostasis and the Brain, Progress in Brain Research, Vol. 42*, W.H. Gispen, Tj.B. van Wimersma Greidanus, B. Bohus and D. de Wied (Eds.), Elsevier, Amsterdam, pp. 201–207.

Pickering, B.T. (1976) The molecules of neurosecretion: their formation, transport and release. In *Perspectives in Brain Research, Progress in Brain Research, Vol. 45*, M. Corner and D.F. Swaab (Eds.), Elsevier, Amsterdam, pp. 161–179.

Rigter, H., van Riezen, H. and de Wied, D. (1974) The effects of ACTH- and vasopressin-analogues on CO_2-induced retrograde amnesia in rats. *Physiol. Behav.*, 13: 381–388.

Sachs, H. Fawcett, P., Takabatake, Y. and Portanova, R. (1969) Biosynthesis and release of vasopressin and neurophysin. *Recent Progr. Hormone Res.*, 25: 447–491.

Scharrer, B. (1976) Neurosecretion — comparative and evolutionary aspects. In *Perspectives in Brain Research, Progress in Brain Research, Vol. 45*, M. Corner and D.F. Swaab (Eds.), Elsevier, Amsterdam, pp. 125–137.

Stern, W.C. (1971) Acquisition impairments following rapid eye movement sleep deprivation in rats. *Physiol. Behav.*, 7: 345–352.

Thompson, E.A. and de Wied, D. (1973) The relationship between the antidiuretic activity of rat eye plexus blood and passive avoidance behaviour. *Physiol. Behav.*, 11: 377–380.

Urban, I. and de Wied, D. (1975) Inferior quality of RSA during paradoxical sleep in rats with hereditary diabetes insipidus. *Brain Res.*, 97: 362–366.

Valatx, J.-L., Chouvet, G. and Jouvet, M. (1975) Sleep-waking cycle of the hypophysectomized rat. In *Hormones, Homeostasis and the Brain, Progress in Brain Research, Vol. 42*, W.H. Gispen, Tj.B. van Wimersma Greidanus, B. Bohus and D. de Wied (Eds.), Elsevier, Amsterdam, pp. 115–120.

Valtin, H. (1967) Hereditary hypothalamic diabetes insipidus in rats (Brattleboro strain). *Amer. J. Med.*, 42: 814–827.

Valtin, H. and Schroeder, H.A. (1964) Familial hypothalamic diabetes insipidus in rats (Brattleboro strain). *Amer. J. Physiol.*, 206: 425–430.

Valtin, H., Sawyer, W.H. and Sokol, H.W. (1965) Neurohypophysial principles in rats homozygous and heterozygous for hypothalamic diabetes insipidus (Brattleboro strain). *Endocrinology*, 77: 701–706.

de Wied, D. (1964) Influence of anterior pituitary on avoidance learning and escape behavior. *Amer. J. Physiol.*, 207: 255–259.

de Wied, D. (1965) The influence of the posterior and intermediate lobe of the pituitary and pituitary-peptides on the maintenance of a conditioned avoidance response in rats. *Int. J. Neuropharmacol.*, 4: 157–167.

de Wied, D. (1971) Long term effect of vasopressin on the maintenance of a conditioned avoidance response in rats. *Nature (Lond.)*, 232: 58–60.

de Wied, D. and Bohus, B. (1966) Long term and short term effects on retention of a conditioned avoidance response in rats by treatment with long acting Pitressin and α-MSH. *Nature (Lond.)*, 212: 1484–1486.

de Wied, D. and Gispen, W.H. (1976) Impaired development of tolerance to morphine analgesia in rats with hereditary diabetes insipidus. *Psychopharmacologia (Berl.)*, in press.

de Wied, D., Greven, H.M., Lande, S. and Witter, A. (1972) Dissociation of the behavioral and endocrine effects of lysine vasopressin by tryptic digestion. *Brit. J. Pharmacol.*, 45: 118–122.

de Wied, D. Bohus, B. and van Wimersma Greidanus, Tj.B. (1975) Memory deficit in rats with hereditary diabetes insipidus. *Brain Res.*, 85: 152–156.

de Wied, D., Bohus, B., Urban, I., van Wimersma Greidanus, Tj.B. and Gispen, W.H. (1975) In *Peptides: Chemistry, Structure and Biology, Proceedings of the 4th American Peptide Symposium*, R. Walter and J. Meienhofer (Eds.), Ann Arbor Sciences Publishers, pp. 635–643.

van Wimersma Greidanus, Tj.B., Bohus, B. and de Wied, D. (1973) Effects of peptide hormones on behavior. In *Progress in Endocrinology, Proc. Fourth Int. Congr. Endocrinology, Washington, D.C.*, Excerpta Medica I.C.S. No. 273, Excerpta Medica, Amsterdam, pp. 197–201.

van Wimersma Greidanus, Tj.B., Dogterom, J. and de Wied, D. (1975a) Intraventricular administration of anti-vasopressin serum inhibits memory consolidation in rats. *Life Sci.*, 16: 637–644.

van Wimersma Greidanus, Tj.B., Bohus, B. and de Wied, D. (1975b) The role of vasopressin in memory processes. In *Hormones, Homeostasis and the Brain, Progress in Brain Research, Vol. 42*, W.H. Gispen, Tj.B., van Wimersma Greidanus, B. Bohus and D. de Wied (Eds.), Elsevier, Amsterdam, pp. 135–141.

van Wimersma Greidanus, Tj.B., Bohus, B. and de Wied, D. (1976) CNS sites of action of ACTH, MSH and vasopressin, related to avoidance behavior. In *Anatomical Neuroendocrinology Proc. Conference on Neurobiology of CNS-Hormone Interactions, Chapel Hill N.C.*, W.E. Stumpf and L.D. Grant (Eds.), Karger, Basel, in press.

Wittkowski, W. (1968) Electronenmikroskopische Studien zur intraventrikulären Neurosekretion in den Recessus infundibularis der Maus. *Z. Zellforsch.*, 92: 207–216.

Zimmermann, E.A., Carmel, P.W., Husain, M.K., Ferin M., Tannenbaum, M., Frantz, A.G. and Robinson, A.G. (1973) Vasopressin and neurophysin: high concentrations in monkey hypophyseal portal blood. *Science*, 182: 925–927.

DISCUSSION

R. BALÁZS: May I ask you whether you see any change in behavior in diabetes insipidus patients?

D. DE WIED: We ourselves do not see patients, but of course we have asked this question to various clinicians. First of all there are many patients with a hereditary form of hypothalamic diabetes, and these have not been very cooperative so far. But Dr. R. Heath from New Orleans sent me a paper on a number of patients with diabetes insipidus: several of these complained about memory disturbances. In these cases however, diabetes insipidus was caused by trauma or tumors, which makes an interpretation of such findings quite impossible.

J. OLDS: First, I wish to express a view of my own and of many of my colleagues: this is potentially the most important addition to behavioral psychology that has come along in a long time. I would like to ask to what degree you think that the action of vasopressin is due to the same vasopressin that is involved in diabetes insipidus and what degree, you think, is due to some peptide that might be in the brain already?

D. DE WIED: We cannot say anything for sure, but my personal feeling is that when consolidation takes place, vasopressin affects protein synthesis in a direct way. We think that at the place where vasopressin is acting we may find growth of axon collaterals.

J. OLDS: Doesn't it seem unreasonable to you that something like this diabetes state of the animal, which would not seen to be a necessary counterpart of consolidation, should appear from your research *to be* a necessity?

D. DE WIED: This is difficult to answer. Vasopressin has many effects: it acts on the kidney, on the blood vessels, on the anterior pituitary, it has metabolic actions, etc. etc. Apparently, another of its actions is in the CNS. For this effect, the peptide is probably released from the anterior hypothalamic nuclei into the CSF. It is of course possible that it in itself causes the production of a peptide in the brain which affects memory.

H. VAN DER LOOS: How do you think vasopressin is being released into the third ventricle?

D. DE WIED: There is morphological evidence for the presence of neurosecretory material in the third ventricle.

B. SCHARRER: There are indeed branches of neurosecretory neurons that enter the third ventricle, although actual release of vasopressin has not yet been proved.

D. DE WIED: It is necessary to measure the release of vasopressin into the CSF under learning conditions.

H. VAN DER LOOS: If rats are brought to secrete vasopressin under other circumstances, will that affect memory consolidation?

D. DE WIED: I don't know, but we have found that vasopressin is released in more than normal amounts into the eye plexus blood during the retention of passive avoidance behavior.

B.T. PICKERING: I really wanted to ask a question along the same line as Dr. Old's. If we are looking at the doses of vasopressin that you have used, it seems to me likely that what you are doing is to mimic the effects of some peptide other than vasopressin. Because, even when you put your dose directly into the ventricle it is quite a large dose, in terms of vasopressin.

D. DE WIED: The lowest dose of vasopressin that we have used to affect memory consolidation (in the lateral ventricle) is 25 pg. However, the physiological role of vasopressin in this respect follows from the disturbance in memory consolidation of hereditary hypothalamic diabetes insipidus rats.

S.P.R. ROSE: The important thing in these experiments is that you have shown that endogenously produced substances can affect attention. We must, however, not forget that substances like amphetamine or strychnine have related effects on attention.

D. DE WIED: The difference with amphetamine is that it has all kind of effects on the brain.

This can be shown, for instance, in open field tests. But the peptides seem to have a more specific effect on memory consolidation.

J. OLDS: I would like to ask Dr de Wied for a comment. I imagine that you think that peptide messages are sent from some areas to other areas in the brain. Because you mentioned the cerebrospinal fluid, moreover, I suppose that you imagine that the access is better for those parts of the brain that are located closer to the cisterns and the ventricles. When a command goes out, i.e., vasopressin is secreted, it would say that it is time to pay attention. There has to be a set of neurons that sends the message, i.e., one that controls the vasopressin secretion step, but there has also to be a set of neurons that receive the message, i.e., some sort of a detection system which is waiting for the message. Am I perhaps over-exaggerating the network that you are thinking of?

D. DE WIED: No, not at all: this is in fact the line along which we are now thinking. We need, however, to have proof of the release of these peptides in the CSF. Heller et al. (1968), who were the first to find vasopressin in the CSF, tried to determine roughly where this vasopressin came from. Peripheral injections of vasopressin did not augment the vasopressin content in the CSF. This is thus one piece of evidence that the vasopressin that has been found by bioassay or radioimmunoassay in the CSF probably comes from hypothalamic sites, and not from the peripheral circulation. We felt that we could obtain more evidence by the binding of vasopressin in the CSF to specific antibodies. We assume that these antibodies will not easily leave the CSF once they are in the lateral ventricle. In this way, behavioral disturbances were obtained which were similar to those found in the diabetes insipidus animal (Bohus et al., 1975). There is quite a lot of evidence that all kinds of stressful situations release vasopressin, ACTH, prolactin, and/or growth hormone from the pituitary.

J. OLDS: Do you think that this is a different axon which is carrying the vasopressin towards the cerebrospinal fluid, from that axon that would carry vasopressin just to the vascular system of the posterior lobe?

B. SCHARRER: Well, I recall the discussion and diagrams presented by Dr. Knowles at the IVth International Symposium at Strasbourg, in 1966 (Knowles, 1967). His evidence for a bidirectional secretory capacity of certain neurosecretory neurons of lower vertebrates argues against the view that different axons carry neurosecretory material to the cerebrospinal fluid and the vascular system, respectively. The same cell whose axon terminal makes contact with a blood vessel may reach into the third ventricle with short dendritic processes. This arrangement provides two "gates" in opposite directions, but the principal destination for the secretory product seems to be the vascular system.

D. DE WIED: Is it not easier to assume that most of the stimuli cause a release in all possible directions?

B. SCHARRER: Even if it is true that release of neurosecretory material into the vascular system involves membrane depolarization comparable to that in conventional axons, discharge from the apical pole of neurosecretory neurons need not necessarily be accomplished in the same way. Moreover, if we assume that an active peptide released into the circulation has a specific function, different from that of the same substance present in the cerebrospinal fluid, obligatory simultaneous discharge in all directions would seem to be less than optimal.

J. DOGTEROM: We have just recently tried to measure vasopressin in the cerebrospinal fluid in human, dog and rat. For all three species, there appears to be a concentration of vasopressin in the cerebrospinal fluid which is about 5 or 10 times higher than in the general circulation. Simultaneous plasma determinations in dog and rat also revealed high levels, however. So we have to study whether the high concentrations in the cerebrospinal fluid are not caused by the anesthesia in these latter species, or by stress in humans. From immunofluorescence studies at the Netherlands Central Institute for Brain Research, it appears that vasopressin-containing fibers of the hypothalamo-neurohypophyseal tract are running very closely under the lining of the third ventricle. This looks as if the same fiber tract would be able to release vasopressin both into the general circulation and into the cerebrospinal fluid.

J. OLDS: I would like to ask one question about specificity. I wondered whether the Brattleboro rat might be deficient in a *variety* of vasopressin-like substances. Is there, for instance, an oxytocin deficit in the Brattleboros?

D. DE WIED: Brattleboros have about 50% of the normal oxytocin content in the pituitary, so there may be a defect also in the synthesis of this hormone. Oxytocin, moreover, has approximately 20% of the behavioral effects of vasopressin. In addition, these animals seem to have an increased vasotocin release, which could also contribute to the behavioral defects that we have seen.

J. OLDS: So you may have a whole field of peptides that can influence learning to some degree?

D. DE WIED: Yes, indeed ACTH and its analogues also have such effects. And there are now reports in the literature about such effects of releasing factors and other peptides in the brain. These peptides might give specific (but also non-specific) information to the brain.

P.B. BRADLEY: I think, in this connection, about the fact that substance P is coming back into the picture. And, of course, the morphine-like factor which has been found in the brain (Hughes et al., 1975) is also a peptide. So I think we have to consider many more of these substances.

D. DE WIED: Well, some of these peptides I have been talking about do in fact interfere with the binding of morphine (Terenius et al., 1975).

REFERENCES

Bohus, B., van Wimersma Greidanus, Tj.B. and de Wied, D. (1975) Behavioral and endocrine responses of rats with hereditary hypothalamic diabetes insipidus (Brattleboro strain). *Physiol. Behav.*, 14: 609–615.

Heller, H., Hasan, S.H. and Saifi, A.Q. (1968) Antidiuretic activity in the cerebrospinal fluid. *J. Endocr.*, 41: 273–280.

Hughes, J., Smith, T.W., Kosterlitz, H.W., Fothergill, L.A., Morgan, B.A. and Morris, H.R. (1975) Identification of two related pentapeptides from the brain with potent opiate agonist activity. *Nature (Lond.)*, 258: 557–579.

Knowles, F. (1967) Neuronal properties of neurosecretory cells. In *Neurosecretion*, F. Stutinsky (Ed.), Springer Verlag, Heidelberg, pp. 8–19.

Terenius, L., Gispen, W.H. and de Wied, D. (1975) ACTH-like peptides and opiate receptors in the rat brain: structure-activity studies. *J. Pharmacol.*, 33: 395–399.

SESSION IV

THE BRAIN AS A STRUCTURAL SYSTEM

Real Neural Networks

V. BRAITENBERG

Max-Planck-Institute for Biological Cybernetics, Tübingen (G.F.R.)

INTRODUCTION

There have been in the past years research groups and symposia on "neural networks". These were based on fleeting abstractions from electrophysiological data, quickly provided by neurologists who were eager to see their terminology become food for thought in mathematical circles. By now the mathematicians have made pure mathematics out of the original models, or "artificial intelligence", or they have given up matching their abstract developments of obsolete neurology with the intuitions of a new generation of neurologists. Yet, the "natural intelligence" of nervous tissue remains the most tantalizing subject for speculation. What fundamental facts, beliefs and warnings would we collect today from brain science in order to prompt the most realistic possible theories? And, in particular, what contributions would come from neuroanatomy?

This paper will review a few observations from comparative neuroanatomy, in order to stress a few points which are undoubtedly very relevant to future "real nerve theories", viz: (a) neuronal wiring may in some cases by very precise (fiber projections in the visual system of the fly); (b) the synaptic junctions may be functionally very diversified (lamina ganglionaris of the fly); (c) some of the wiring takes place while the nerve net is already operating (growth of dendrites in the cortex of the mouse); and (d) there are inborn constraints to this kind of plasticity (arrangement of axons in the cortex of the mouse).

THE NEURAL WIRING MAY OCCASIONALLY BE VERY PRECISE

The question of whether or not brains work like computers has sometimes been understood as being equivalent to the question of the degree to which the wiring of the nervous system is analogous to that of present day computing equipment: completely specified by the blueprint, with no loose ends, and with nothing left to chance. However, merely a look into a Golgi preparation of any

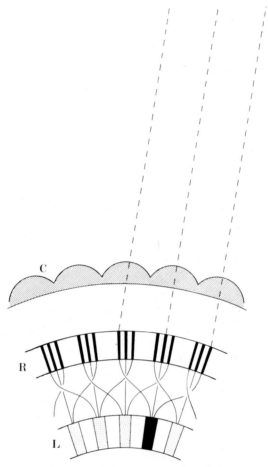

Fig. 1. Projection of the optical environment through the cornea (C) and the retina (R) onto the lamina ganglionaris (L) of the fly's compound eye. Only 3 of the 8 retinula cells are shown in each ommatidium. The fibers between R and L are so arranged that the output from all the retinula cells which look in the same direction (dotted lines) is united in the same compartment (black) of the lamina ganglionaris. (From Braitenberg, 1973).

complex neuropil does not suggest any such comparison. In addition, there are arguments concerning the limitations of genetic information capacity which indicate that the enormous number of fiber connections within the brain cannot possibly be fully specified at birth (Braitenberg, 1973). It was, on the other hand, largely a matter of taste (rather than of scientific necessity) that led some researchers to a more dynamic view of the nervous system, in which the basic neighborhood connectivities and the functional interrelations among neurons are changing all the time under the influence of experience.

In this connection it becomes interesting to stress a finding from the anatomy of the visual ganglia of insects, which shows that in certain instances the wiring is specified even down to individual nerve fibers (Fig. 1). The compound eye of the fly is composed of about 3000 nearly identical subunits, called ommatidia, each equipped with its own separate optics and containing 8 separate photosensitive elements, the rhabdomeres. Each rhabdomere is a specialized portion of one cell, the so-called retinula cell. The upper ends of 7 of these rhabdomeres in each ommatidium are arranged in a very regular pattern, localized in the focal plane (or rather focal curved surface) of the inverting optical system. This pattern is called *retinula* for a very good reason: to each rhabdomere corresponds a line of sight, and to the whole retinula 7 lines of sight, which intersect a distal plane in a pattern which is that of the retinula rotated by $180°$. The optical information discretely gathered by the elements of the retinula, and transformed by the visual pigments into depolarizations of the cell membranes, is carried down into the first-order visual ganglion — the lamina ganglionaris — through a bundle of 8 fibers emanating from the base of each ommatidium. It will come as no surprise that this nerve bundle is in fact twisted by $180°$: the miniscule portion of the visual environment seen by each ommatidium has been inverted by the lens optics, and could not fit continuously into the global picture provided by the, non-inverting, array of ommatidia (i.e. an ommatidium pointing forwards sees a portion of the environment situated in front of the animal, one pointing backward sees a posterior portion of the visual field, etc.) unless it were first re-rotated by $180°$ in the fiber bundle projecting to the ganglion.

There is even more precision to be discovered in this system: retinulae of neighboring ommatidia have their lines of sight so oriented that each is parallel, with great precision, to another line of sight in each of 6 neighboring ommatidia (Autrum and Wiedemann, 1962; Kirschfeld, 1967). This means that 7 retinula cells of 7 different ommatidia (here I simplify slightly, leaving out retinula cell number 8 which would complicate the issue, but without changing the argument) receive precisely the same visual information. The law of the retinula-to-lamina-projection is this: all the elements that look at the same point of the visual field send their axon into the same compartment of the ganglion (Braitenberg, 1967). The rigor with which this principle is carried through is especially astonishing in exceptional regions of the eye, such as near the margin (where an ommatidium has fewer neighbors than elsewhere) or near the "equator", where the arrangement of the elements in the retinula changes abruptly. Horridge and Meinertzhagen (1970) dedicated a very diligent study to the precision of this wiring and found absolutely no exceptions. It is easy to convince oneself that learning plays no part in the establishment of this type of connection, since one finds the whole arrangement ready made in the late stages of pupation, long before the compound eye has ever received visual input (except for subdued and diffuse light, which may filter through the involucre of the pupa).

To be fair, we have to point out the special situation in which this precise fiber pattern occurs: (a) it does not represent information handling *within* the nervous system, but is situated at the interface with the primary sensory organs; (b) even if in each eye 24,000 fibers follow the above rule, the genetic blueprint has to do little more than to specify the fiber projections for the 8 fibers in each ommatidium, together with the rule for how this is to be repeated (including mirror-image reflection at the equator, etc.).

THE COMPONENTS OF THE NERVOUS SYSTEM ARE NOT ALL OF ONE KIND

There are many variations in nerve net theories, all based on the supposition that neuronal networks composed of a large number of identical elements, characterized only by different thresholds and perhaps by different time constants, interconnected through synapses of only two kinds (excitatory or inhibitory), can do astonishing things if only the wiring is sophisticated enough. A recent study of synaptic junctions in the first visual ganglion of the fly, the lamina ganglionaris (Braitenberg and Burkhardt, 1976; Burkhardt and Braitenberg, 1976), has convinced us that this supposition of the homogeneity of the components may not be justified. We had undertaken a study of the visual ganglion of insects in the hope of being able eventually to relate patterns of fiber connections to the lines of flow diagrams emerging from the behavioral analysis of optomotor reactions in insects (e.g., Hassenstein and Reichardt, 1953; Reichardt, 1957; Götz, 1968). We are still very far from a complete understanding of the visual system of insects, but probably by now the lamina ganglionaris of flies is better known than any other piece of nerve structure, insofar as the typology of the elements and the pattern of their connections is concerned (Cajal, 1909; Cajal and Sanchez, 1915; Trujillo Cenóz, 1965; Braitenberg, 1967, 1970; Strausfeld, 1970, 1971; Boschek, 1971; Braitenberg and Debbage, 1974). The most interesting result of these studies has been the realization that the synaptic connections in the ganglion appear to be compatible with almost any reasonable supposition about information handling at that level. As long as we are not able to distinguish excitatory from inhibitory synapses in the histological preparations, or even to recognize threshold elements or delay lines, we will of course not be able to decide whether a system of lateral connections serves the purpose of contour enhancement, cluster analysis, movement detection or anything else.

What we did next was to contribute to the inventory of so-called synaptic specializations, by taking many electron micrographs of peculiar structures that were found in places in which signal transmission from neuron to neuron could reasonably be expected. Even if the spatial resolution of electrophysiology lags behind that of histology, so that a direct biophysical analysis of these junctions will not be available in the near future, it is still reasonable to suppose that junctions which appear different under the electron microscope are also different in their function. There are at least two kinds of presynaptic specializations in the visual ganglia of the fly, and many more kinds of postsynaptic involvement — including "synapses" which clearly look as if they were transmitting signals from neurons to glia. The most striking observations are the following (for details see Burkhardt and Braitenberg, 1976).

(1) All the synapses between retinula cell axons and second-order neurons in the lamina ganglionaris are such that one presynaptic element faces four different postsynaptic cells. The four postsynaptic elements are arranged in an array of great geometrical constancy, and the postsynaptic organelles are not the same in all elements. There is no ready explanation for the fact that one-to-many synapses should be the rule there (Fig. 2).

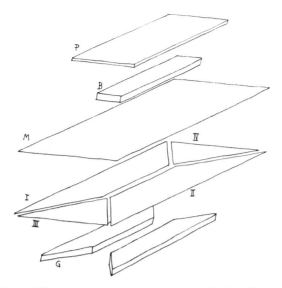

Fig. 2. Exploded view of the complex synapse between retinula cell axons and second order elements in the lamina ganglionaris of the fly, as described in Burkhardt and Braitenberg (1976). P, presynaptic plate; B, presynaptic bar; M, presynaptic membrane; I, II, III and IV, the 4 postsynaptic elements; G, the "postsynaptic bags" which are present in two of the four postsynaptic cells.

(2) Another striking observation is this: a functional connection between two neurons in the lamina ganglionaris in the fly is mediated in one instance by about 40 structures of the kind that cytologists call synapses, while in another instance by only one or two. We have no idea whether a large number of parallel contacts increases the channel capacity in some sense, i.e., either the amplitude of the signal or the reliability of the transmission.

(3) There are various kinds of neuron-to-glia contacts in the first visual ganglion of the fly. One of the most peculiar (and numerically prevalent) is the "gnarl-complex", in which what appears to be a presynaptic specialization of the neuron faces a glial lamella which, exactly the opposite of the "synapse", is invaginated adventurously into another neuron where it forms vast grape-like expansions. There are vesicles on the side of the so-called presynaptic specialization, while the glia-to-neuron membrane contact is thickened and dense, so that the whole complex may be interpreted as a synapse with a most spectacular postsynaptic specialization.

Add these structures of the fly's eye to other types of synapses in other animals, and you will realize that the wide morphological variety of junctions between neurons by itself leaves far too many degrees of freedom to the imagination of brain theorists.

NERVE NETS GROW WHILE THEY LEARN

Many neural net theories incorporate a principle by which the structure of the net changes with time as a function of the input. One of the puzzling questions in neurobiology is how macroscopical changes of nerve net operation, simulating learning in living organisms, can be obtained by imposing microscopical laws which govern changes in individual synapses as a function of the activity in pre- and/or postsynaptic neurons. The mechanisms, however, which underlie learning in natural brains, as opposed to artificial ones, are not known: evidence indicates that the actual growth of new connections may serve as a substrate of memory (e.g., Mark, 1974). Brains do in fact continue to grow while they learn, at least early in life, and in animals which are relatively mature at birth (guinea pigs) they grow less than in animals, such as rats and mice, which are born very immature (Altman, 1967). Furthermore, certain portions of the brains of animals raised in "enriched" environments tend to be larger than in animals raised under relatively deprived conditions (Rosenzweig et al., 1972). In our own laboratory, we have focussed our attention upon the growth of basal dendrites in the cerebral cortex of the mouse, which appears to be responsible for most of the cortical volume increase (about a two-fold increase in thickness) during the first two weeks of life. Since the basal dendrites are the target mainly of axon collaterals of neighboring pyramidal cells (Globus, 1971), it would seem that most of the changes in the wiring capacity of the cortex at the beginning of life represent changes in the potential connections among clusters of pyramidal cells. Whether any of these changes incorporate experience, e.g., with sensory stimuli, is of course still an open question.

The spines on dendrites of pyramidal cells have also been suspected of being embodiments of "engrams". A study by Schüz (1976) in our laboratory focussed upon the difference of the density of spines on dendrites of otherwise very similar pyramidal cells of the same region and layer. If spines are indeed indicative of memory traces, two conclusions emerged from this study. Firstly, some pyramidal cells must have been modified much more than others, which are thus, perhaps, being kept in reserve for future learning. Secondly, spine plasticity would need to be a process involving the entire dendritic tree, apical as well as basal, and not just individual segments or junctions. These findings are consistent with the idea that cortical neurons act as the detectors of correlations among the activities of different sets of afferent fibers, and then establish synapses preferentially with such sets. Apart from the advantages in terms of information theory which are given by the coding of correlated sets of neurons onto individual units, electrophysiological observations (Hubel and Wiesel, 1965; Wiesel and Hubel, 1965) on single neurons of the visual cortex indicate that such detection and coding of correlations may play a role in the establishment of stereoscopic vision.

AXONS IN THE CORTEX OF THE MOUSE REPRESENT INBORN CONSTRAINTS TO LEARNING

In our studies of young mice we were surprised to find that much of the intracortical axonal population, in contrast to basal dendrites, is present very early in life. Moreover, we found that axon collaterals leave the axons of pyramidal cells in a very regular fashion and then traverse the neuropil in a fairly straight course, leaving little over of the idea that their growth course is being determined by functional activities within the nerve net. A paper by Steffen (1975) analyzes some of these points in a quantitative fashion. Among other things, Steffen found a reproducible variation of the length of axon collaterals in different regions of the cortex of the mouse. This is in good agreement with older descriptions of "myeloarchitectonics" in higher mammals, which also seem to indicate regional and laminar variations of the density of intracortical fibers, related to different functional specializations (Braitenberg, 1962). If the junction between an axon collateral and a basal dendrite can incorporate the effects of experience, it would follow that the distribution of axon collaterals around a pyramidal cell, being established before any learning takes place, predetermines the extent to which new connections may be made with a set of neighboring pyramidal cells.

CONCLUSIONS

We strongly urge nerve net theorists to incorporate available anatomical knowledge into their constructs, and even to request that certain new facts be obtained. The relevant data which could determine crucial differences between one theory and the other, may well be expressed in such perhaps seemingly trivial things as: length of axon collaterals, growth of dendrites, number and type of synapses visible under the electron microscope, or geometry of the nerve fiber patterns.

REFERENCES

Autrum, H.J. and Wiedmann, I. (1962) Versuche über den Strahlengang im Insektenauge (Appositionsauge). *Z. Naturforsch.*, 17: 480–482.

Altman, J. (1967) Postnatal growth and differentiation of the mammalian brain, with implications for a morphological theory of memory. In *The Neurosciences*, G.C. Quarton, Th. Melnechuk and F.O. Schmitt (Eds.), The Rockefeller University Press, New York, pp. 723–743.

Boschek, C.B. (1971) On the fine structure of the peripheral retina and lamina ganglionaris of the fly *Musca domestica. Z. Zellforsch.*, 118: 369–409.

Braitenberg, V. (1962) A note on myeloarchitectonics. *J. comp. Neurol.*, 118: 141.

Braitenberg, V. (1967) Patterns of projection in the visual system of the fly. 1. Retina-lamina projection. *Exp. Brain Res*, 3: 271–298.

Braitenberg, V. (1970) Ordnung und Orientierung der Elemente im Sehsystem der Fliege. *Kybernetik*, 7: 235–242.

Braitenberg, V. (1973) *Gehirngespinste: Neuroanatomie für Kybernetisch Interessierte.* Springer, Berlin, 137 pp.

Braitenberg, V. and Burkhardt, W. (1976) Beyond the wiring diagram of the lamina ganglionaris of the fly. In *Neural Principles in Vision*, F. Zettler and R. Weiler (Eds.), in press.

Braitenberg, V. and Debbage, P. (1974) A regular net of reciprocal synapses in the visual system of the fly, *Musca domestica. J. comp. Physiol.*, 90: 25–31.

Burkhardt, W. and Braitenberg, V. (1976) Some peculiar synaptic complexes in the first visual ganglion of the fly. In preparation.

Cajal, S. Ramón y (1909) Nota sobre la retina de la mosca (*M. vomitoria* L.). *Trab. Lab. Invest. biol. Univ. Madrid*, 7: 217–257.

Cajal, S. Ramón y y Sanchez, D. (1915) Contribucion al conocimiento de los centros nerviosos de los insectos. Parte 1. Retina y centros opticos. *Trab. Lab. Invest. biol. Univ. Madrid,* 13: 1–168.

Globus, A. (1971) Neuronal ontogeny: its use in tracing connectivity. In *Brain Development and Behavior,* M. Sterman, D. McGinty and A. Adinolfi (Eds.), Academic Press, New York, pp. 253–264.

Götz, K.G. (1968) Flight control in *Drosophila* by visual perception of motion. *Kybernetik,* 4: 199–208.

Hassenstein, B. und Reichardt, W. (1953) Der Schluss von Reiz-Reaktionsfunktionen auf Systemstrukturen. *Z. Naturforsch.,* 8: 518.

Horridge, G.A. and Meinertzhagen, I.A. (1970) The accuracy of the patterns of connexions of the first- and second-order neurons of the visual system of *Calliphora. Proc. roy. Soc. B,* 175: 69–82.

Hubel, D.H. and Wiesel, T.N. (1965) Binocular interaction in striate cortex of kittens reared with artificial squint. *J. Neurophysiol.,* 28: 1041–1059.

Kirschfeld, K. (1967) Die Projektion der optischen Umwelt auf das Raster der Rhabdomere im Komplexauge von *Musca. Exp. Brain Res.,* 3: 248–270.

Mark, R. (1974) *Memory and Nerve Cell Connections.* Oxford University Press, London, 156 pp.

Reichardt, W. (1957) Autokorrelations-Auswertung als Funktionsprinzip des Zentralnerven-systems. *Z. Naturforsch.,* 12: 448–457.

Rosenzweig, M.R., Bennett, E.L. and Diamond, M.C. (1972) Brain changes in response to experience. *Sci. Amer.,* 226/2: 22.

Schüz, A. (1976) Pyramidal cells with different densities of dendritic spines in the cortex of the mouse. *Z. Naturforsch.,* 31c: 319–323.

Steffen, H. (1975) *Quantitative Untersuchungen der Axon-Kollateralen der Pyramidenzellen in der Gehirnrinde der Maus.* Master's thesis. University of Tübingen.

Strausfeld, N.J. (1970) Golgi studies in insects. Part II: The optic lobes of Diptera. *Phil. Trans. B,* 258: 135–223.

Strausfeld, N.J. (1971) The organization of the insect visual system (light microscopy). I. Projections and arrangements of neurons in the lamina ganglionaris of Diptera. *Z. Zellforsch.,* 121: 377–441.

Trujillo-Cenóz, O. (1965) Some aspects of the structural organization of the intermediate retina of Dipterans. *J. ultrastruct. Res.,* 13: 1–33.

Wiesel, T.N. and Hubel, D.H. (1965) Comparison of the effects of unilateral and bilateral eye closure on cortical unit responses in kittens. *J. Neurophysiol.,* 28: 1029–1040.

DISCUSSION

H. UYLINGS: Concerning the spines: have you separated the various parts of the dendritic tree, for comparison of the basal dendritic spines against the apical dendritic spines?

V. BRAITENBERG: What I showed was the average of the entire basal dendritic tree, compared to the average of the apical dendritic tree. But in all cases Miss Schuez has counted spines in many places on the same neuron, and then you can see that the variance for one neuron is smaller than the variance of the whole population.

M.A. CORNER: Did I see correctly that in the Golgi picture of the very immature mouse cortex there was some indication of innervation of those superficial apical dendrites? Work on the prenatal sheep showed very gradual ingrowth of axon collaterals from the subcortical zone into the cortical plate, and I thought that the stage at which the first sensory driving of cortical evoked potentials occurred in the mouse was more advanced than these very primitive stages that you showed. It would be very interesting to have physiological evidence in this material that at these early stages there was really an afferent input. If there were not, then although the functional activity generated in these axon collaterals may well be having an effect upon the growth of basal dendrites, this "plastic" response will be a result of *endogenously* generated neuronal excitation. As such, it would have quite a different developmental significance than if it were *afferent* stimulation which were the important factor for growth of the nerve cell processes.

V. BRAITENBERG: Molliver and Van der Loos counted synapses in the newborn dog, and found that the highest density of synapses is up there in the most superficial layer. Tactile evoked potentials can be demonstrated in the young animal already at the time of birth; a surface negativity has been observed in many different species.

M.A. CORNER: Spine development in the "cortex" of the chick embryo occurs very explosively at about two days before the animal hatches. This takes place within a very short period of time, and it is related to the appearance of spontaneous "paradoxical" episodes of electroencephalographic arousal in the predominantly slow wave pattern of activity. In the couple of weeks of postnatal development that we followed it, you don't see any further obvious changes in spine development. So, certainly the major periods of spine development don't appear in the chick embryo to be at all correlated with what you would expect if they were being determined largely by extrauterine experiential type of stimulation.

S.P.R. ROSE: I was disturbed in the second part of Dr. Braitenberg's paper where he was talking about plasticity and, showing the development of spines during the early neonatal period in the mouse cortex, he used the phrase that the enrichment in spines was probably related to learning. He cited as an example of this, furthermore, the fact that in sensory deprivation you can get a decrease in spine number, while with enriched versus impoverished environments you can also get corresponding changes in spine number and dendritic branching. Now I am worried about that: simply because in particular circumstances where learning occurs you also get a change in dendritic branching, or changes in synapse and spine number, it does not follow that changes in the spines are necessarily a consequence of, or even related to, learning processes. All you really know is that there are certain situations in which you effectuate a change in spine number, for example, in different stages of sexual development.

V. BRAITENBERG: Where a correlation has been established, you don't have to conclude that there is a causal connection, but of course it is always very tempting to do so.

Problems of Understanding
the Substructure of Synapses

E.G. GRAY

Department of Anatomy, University College London,
London (Great Britain)

INTRODUCTION

This brief review is restricted to morphological aspects of synapses thought to have a chemical mode of transmission. It will include recent observations of the author, using a new albumin technique which, it is hoped, will bring a new understanding to the normal and pathological fine structure of the synapse. But first a few introductory remarks about trends in recent synaptology. The contradictions and anomalies make generalizations hazardous, to say the least, but the subject is becoming so complex that one must have some sort of scheme to hold on to whilst threading one's way through the literature. For further details the following reviews should be consulted: Gray and Guillery, 1966; Gray, 1966, 1969, 1971, 1974, 1975a; Akert and Waser, 1969; Bloom, et al., 1970; Peters, et al., 1970; Sotelo, 1971; Pappas and Purpura, 1972; Pfenninger, 1973; Cotman and Banker, 1974; Kornguth, 1974; Palay and Chan-Palay, 1974; Uchizono, 1975. Krnjević (1974) has recently reviewed the chemical nature of transmission in vertebrates.

THEORETICAL BACKGROUND

Classification of synapses

My Type 1 and Type 2 classification based on synaptic cleft morphology, and in several CNS sites related to excitatory and inhibitory chemical transmission (see Eccles, 1964), still needs much more detailed investigation (see Gray, 1974). There are, furthermore, many locations where the classification is not meaningful at present, e.g., spinal cord, peripheral (autonomic) nervous system and invertebrate synapses in general. We need, of course, a much better understanding of the nature of the presynaptic dense projections, cleft material and postsynaptic thickening (see below). In 1965, Uchizono gave a new impetus to synaptology, when he showed that after suitable aldehyde treatment, known excitatory synapses in the cerebellar cortex showed a preponderance of round synaptic vesicles whereas at inhibitory synapses the vesicles took on flattened or polymorphic shapes (see also Uchizono, 1975). Thus, the Type 1–round vesicle–excitation and Type 2–flat vesicle–inhibition correlations were established, and then extended from the cerebellar cortex to other CNS sites. The flattening of synaptic vesicles has usually been assumed to be a tonicity or osmotic effect (see Korneliussen, 1972) but this remains unproven. More recently Gray (1975a, see below) has suggested an alternative hypothesis based on observations that the cytoproteins in the inhibitory synapses precipitate into a net-like *stereoframework* during fixation and processing, and that the stereoframework imposes its contours on the vesicles causing them to assume a flattened shape. This hypothesis has certain advantages over the osmolarity one, one of which, although perhaps somewhat tenuous, is that the flat vesicle–Type 2 cleft relationships can be linked to the common factor of the presence of protein complexes (Gray, 1975a).

As a working hypothesis it has been suggested that some Type 1–round vesicled–known or presumed excitatory synapses may utilize glutamic acid as a transmitter, while some Type 2–flat vesicled–known or presumed inhibitory synapses may utilize GABA or glycine (Gray, 1974; Iversen et al., 1973). To test this hypothesis further we need more refined electron microscopic (EM) histochemical methods for localizing these different transmitter substances in situ. Matus and Dennison (1972), using EM autoradiography, made a significant advance when they showed that labeled glycine was preferentially taken up by flat-vesicled synapses in incubated spinal cord slices. EM visualization of GABA and glutamate sites present more difficult problems. It must always be borne in mind, of course, that it is the nature of the receptors on the postsynaptic membrane that determines excitation and inhibition, rather than the transmitter per se (for review see Krnjević, 1974, for further details of vertebrate transmitters).

Detection of GABA uptake by synapses using EM autoradiography presents problems because of ready uptake also by neuroglia. Promising results have been obtained by using $[^3H]DABA$ (L-2,4-diaminobutyric acid) as an analogue (and hence a competitive inhibitor) for GABA (Schon and Kelly, 1974a,b; Dick and Kelly, 1975). DABA is much more readily taken up by nerve terminals than by glial processes.

Localization of specific cholinergic synapses, particularly within the central nervous system, presents a variety of problems. Vertebrate motor endplates are readily recognizable of course, but the junctional cleft — with its linear rather than triagonal dense projections (see below), and its wide gap (up to 60 nm) containing a basement lamina and junctional folds — is organized rather differently from the synapse, and the Type 1 and Type 2 classification cannot be applied. Certainly, the vesicles are usually round rather than flat after aldehyde initial fixation (Korneliussen, 1972), but there is no specific marker for EM identification of cholinergic synapses. One has to rely exclusively on the indirect method of demonstrating the presence of cholinesterase (Lewis and Shute, 1967; Shute and Lewis, 1967) and this has disadvantages (Burt and Silver, 1973). What is really needed is a specific EM marker for the presence of choline acetyltransferase (choline acetylase) (Kása et al., 1970; Burt, 1971; Kása, 1971). It is perhaps not generally realized that the cholinergic synapses on Renshaw cells have not yet been localized with the electron microscope

(Gray, 1974). Thus, until we can identify central cholinergic synapses with the EM we cannot say whether the clefts are Type 1 or 2 and whether the vesicles are round or flat.

Monoaminergic synapses are, without doubt, the best characterized synapses at present (Dahlström, 1973); the detection of the amine by means of fluorescence microscopy, the presence of a dense core in a percentage of the relatively small synaptic vesicles, the depletion or prevention of uptake of the amine by a variety of drugs, the uptake of false transmitters, 5- and 6-hydroxydopamine (the latter causing specific degeneration; Thoenen and Tranzer, 1971), and uptake of tritiated noradrenaline which can be detected by EM autoradiography, all provide important clues for identification. There is no evidence, however, that the synaptic clefts of aminergic synapses can be classified into Types 1 or 2, or into any other categories, nor has the shape of the (often granulated) synaptic vesicles been related to the round/flat classification. The vesicles usually appear round in aldehyde preparations.

Purinergic synapses, where ATP is thought to be the transmitter, can be recognized in the autonomic nervous system by their complement of large vesicles with dense contents (Burnstock, 1972), but more morphological data are required, especially regarding the distribution and morphology of such synapses in the vertebrate central nervous system.

It must be emphasized that while it is an important advantage to be able to use EM morphological clues to reveal the nature of the transmitter and/or the excitatory or inhibitory sign of the synapse, such clues play an equally important role in the unravelling of connections for an understanding of circuitry. For this we rely, of course, on an extension of the Dale principle. But can we be sure that, in general, all endings from a given neuron will have the same type of cleft and the same shape of synaptic vesicle (see Lieberman and Webster, 1974)?

Formation of synaptic vesicles

The questions of whether the transmitter is contained within the synaptic vesicle, whether there is an additional store of transmitter in the presynaptic cytoplasm outside the vesicle (cf. Whittaker, pp. 45–65 in this volume), where the vesicle is formed, and at what point in its formation it becomes charged with transmitter, are all highly debatable points at present.

One theory is that synaptic vesicles are formed in the cell body, perhaps from the Golgi apparatus (see Gray, 1970; Holtzman et al., 1973), and travel down the axon by fast or slow axoplasmal flow or related mechanisms (Schmitt and Samson, 1968; Jeffrey and Austin, 1974; and see below). Another is that they are budded off by a process of endocytosis from the wall of the presynaptic bag into the presynaptic cytoplasm. Kanaseki and Kadota (1969) have proposed that endocytosis is induced by the formation of a coat formed from a proteinaceous network of polygonal subunits. This becomes the coated vesicle, which migrates into the presynaptic cytoplasm. The vesicle emerges from the coat, the fragments of which can be seen in the cytoplasm with the now denuded synaptic vesicles. Heuser and Reese (1973), in stimulation experiments of the motor endplate, give support to this theory. However, the theory that synaptic vesicles are formed from coated vesicles leaves many observations unaccounted for (Gray, 1972, 1973, 1974, 1975a; Paula-Barbosa and Gray, 1974). One source of evidence is that exogenous horseradish peroxidase is taken up by endocytotic vesicles that appear indistinguishable from synaptic vesicles (see Turner and Harris, 1973, 1974; Holtzman et al., 1973). However, foreign proteins might well stimulate endocytosis so that this need not be the normal mechanism for synaptic vesicle formation. The mode of migration of the synaptic vesicle to the terminal membrane will be considered further below. Also considered below will be a third possible mechanism for synaptic vesicle formation, namely that synaptic vesicles are formed not by proliferation (budding off, endocytosis) from pre-existing membrane, but are formed de novo in the presynaptic cytoplasm.

Release of transmitter from the vesicle

Morphological evidence for this will also be considered further below, but one or two points will be discussed here. Synaptic vesicles, apparently opening on to the synaptic cleft are very rarely seen with the EM (see Couteaux and Pécot-Dechavassine, 1970; Uchizono, 1975; Gray, 1975a — his Fig. 14). (This will be considered further below.) Yet there are now quite a number of studies that have related transmitter release to vesicle depletion by various agents, e.g., electrical stimulation, suitable ions and spider venom (Jones and Kwanbun-bumpen, 1970; Ceccarelli et al., 1973; Clark et al., 1972; Heuser and Reese, 1973; Birks, 1974; Pysh and Wiley, 1974). The most popular theory is that the vesicle, after liberating the transmitter, fuses with, and is incorporated into, the surface membrane and reforms by endocytosis from the wall of the presynaptic bag so that constant recycling takes place (but see Birks, 1974). However, if a vesicle discharges its transmitter (following a stimulation) only once and then is incorporated into the presynaptic membrane, the recycling must be an extremely rapid process. What is needed is a technique for attaching a marker to the membrane of the synaptic vesicle. Then, if the vesicle membrane is incorporated without change into the presynaptic membrane the latter should also show markers to match the number of incorporated vesicles. For example, Gray and Paula-Barbosa (1974) have shown dense particles on the inside of the synaptic vesicle membrane in brain fixed with acid-aldehyde. However, no accumulations of such particles are apparent on the presynaptic membrane (neither cleft nor lateral wall region). This would suggest either that synaptic vesicle membrane is not incorporated into the presynaptic membrane (see below) or that, if it is, then the lipoprotein structure of the synaptic vesicle has changed. Whittaker (1966) and Lepetina et al. (1968) have, in fact, shown a different chemical composition between the two sorts of membrane.

Further evidence for the possible mechanism of transmitter release has come from freeze-fracture-etching studies. These will be discussed below.

RECENT EXPERIMENTAL WORK

What are the dense projections? In 1958 (Gray, 1959) I used alcoholic phosphotungstic acid, which is an electron-dense stain with an affinity for intra- and extracellular protein complexes (see Pfenninger, 1973), to study brain and spinal cord. I was struck by the appearance of dense spike-like bodies forming hexagonal arrays on the cytoplasmic side of the presynaptic membrane and around which the synaptic vesicles formed clusters. I termed these bodies "dense projections" (Gray, 1963). They varied greatly in appearance with different preparative procedures, often appearing more prominent in badly fixed tissue. Their consistent presence on the presynaptic membrane of vertebrate synapses and their marked regularity of spacing (particularly in en face sections) led to the statement, "they might play a role in guiding synaptic vesicles to special localities of the presynaptic membrane" (Gray, 1966, p. 167). As we shall see, this indeed might well be the case.

From the outset, it became clear that the small dimensions of the dense projection meant that it was usually wholly enclosed within the thickness of the section and that tilting and stereoscopic (3-D) EM observations were essential for the analysis of its substructure. This led to a detailed investigation of problems of 3-D EM visualization in tissue sections (Gray and Willis, 1968).

At about the same time, the concept of the presynaptic grid was developed on the basis of various experimental procedures, including freeze-fracture methods. The spacing of the dense projections was sufficient to accommodate up to 6 synaptic vesicles around each, the vesicles lying adjacent to the "accessible" presynaptic membrane. Freeze-fracturing showed dimples or "synaptopores" in the membrane with a hexagonal spacing corresponding to the vesicle sites, while the dense projections were now recognized to have a triagonal spacing. The role of the synaptopores in presumed transmitter extrusion from the synaptic vesicles is currently a major field for discussion, and is beyond the scope of this article (Akert et al., 1969, 1972; Pfenninger et al., 1969, 1971, 1972). Incidentally, the synaptopores have more recently been termed VAS (for "vesicle attachment sites") (see Pfenninger and Rovainen, 1974; Landis and Reese, 1974). However, the question, "What are the dense projections?" remains.

The stereoframework concept

Several years of exhaustive observations on literally hundreds of high resolution stereopairs of electron micrographs, showing dense projections cut in all conceivable planes and using a variety of fixing and staining methods, failed to reveal their nature. At the outset they were thought to be small tufts of filaments, possibly actin, particularly since Berl et al. (1973) had described actin- and myosin-like proteins in brain synaptosome fractions. However, the 3-D observations showed that the dense projections were composed neither of membrane fragments, filaments, microtubules nor granules. The 3-D observations were extended to various intra- and extracellular organelles, and, to cut a long story short, the *stereoframework* concept was evolved (Gray, 1975a). The term *cytonet* was used originally (Gray, 1972, 1973) for cytoplasmic "networks", but then the concept was extended to intranuclear and extracellular protein "precipitates", so that the more general term of stereoframework (to indicate a 3-D foam-like framework containing polyhedral lacunae) was adopted. Problems of analyzing the substructure of the stereoframework along with difficulties in its visualization in 3-D pairs of stereomicrographs, have been considered elsewhere (Gray, 1975a). Suffice it here to say that the two-dimensional appearance of a stereoframework is net-like, with a small or large mesh of irregular (but sometimes regular) polygons. The conclusion was reached that the stereoframework is actually an artifact of fixation and/or processing of protein complexes but, as such, it can be regarded as a useful marker for high concentrations of protein complexes. However, any attempt to relate the stereoframework substructure to the true protein architecture was futile, since it was simply a coarse precipitate. Further evidence was given (Gray, 1975a) that stereoframework formation during fixation could distort or destroy delicate organelles. Thus, it was postulated that fine actin filaments or metastable microtubules could well be present in the presynaptic bag, but that under conventional EM fixing and processing they would be obliterated by precipitation of the agglomerations of various protein complexes known to be present in the presynaptic bag. More specifically, the dense projections were recognized as blobs of stereoframework, while the other structures (e.g., coats of coated vesicles, synaptic cleft substance (extracellular) and postsynaptic density, microfilamentous network of growth cones, glycoprotein surface coats (extracellular), EM-fixed blood plasma (extracellular), initial segment and node of Ranvier subsurface coats, nuclear pore complexes and even the nuclear chromatin itself) were all considered to be stereoframework precipitates.

The Schmitt sliding-vesicle model

Let us now go back to 1968, when the role of microtubules as agents involved in the intracellular translocation of organelles (e.g., chromosomes and melanin granules) was first coming into prominence. Schmitt (1968) was particularly interested in axoplasmic transport mechanisms, and since microtubules are commonly seen in axons he proposed that synaptic vesicles might be translocated down axons, right up to the release points on the presynaptic membrane, by sliding along the surfaces of microtubules (and possibly also along neurofilaments) (Fig. 1). Microtubules (either as doublets or singlets) are undoubtedly involved in generating force for cilia or flagellar movement, but here they have recognizable side arms and central spokes, which contain an ATPase called dynein (Gibbons, 1966) and probably the sliding of microtubules with respect to one another is involved (see Warner and Satir, 1974). There are several important features to note about Schmitt's model (Fig. 1). (1) Dynein side-arms are not seen on the axonal and preterminal microtubules (with the possible exception of axonal initial segments), so Schmitt proposed a binding and unbinding of vesicle membrane subunits to protein subunits of the (stationary) microtubules, involving ATPase activity analogous to the actin and myosin sliding interaction of muscle; (2) from Schmitt's diagram, it can be seen that he postulated microtubules to (a) run right up to the presynaptic membrane and (b) have synaptic vesicles closely associated with the surfaces of the microtubules (Schmitt, 1970); and (3) Schmitt made no mention of the presynaptic dense projections, and so did not include them in his scheme. Understandably, at the time, Schmitt's model was

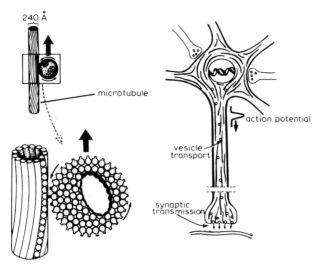

Fig. 1. Hypothetical sliding-vesicle model involving microtubules proposed by Schmitt (1968). Reproduced by kind permission of the author. (For a key to the figures and a list of abbreviations for this and all subsequent figures see p. 229.)

regarded as strictly hypothetical since electron micrographs showed that microtubules usually ended in the preterminal axon without entering the presynaptic bag (en passant synapses are often an exception to this rule). Even when they did so, they petered out before approaching the presumed "active zone" of the presynaptic membrane where aggregates of synaptic vesicles can be seen. Nor could any close association be observed between the synaptic vesicles and the preterminal microtubules.

Schmitt's hypothesis became somewhat strengthened (Fig. 2) when Smith et al. (1970) and Smith (1971) showed clear associations between regular arrays of synaptic vesicles and axonal microtubules. Smith et al. (1970) stated, however, "within a synaptic focus, immediately adjoining the presynaptic membrane, vesicles are randomly arranged and are not associated with microtubules" (Fig. 2). Thus, the problem of how the synaptic vesicles reached and formed clusters at the specialized zone of the presynaptic membrane, remained unsolved. Also in the illustration of Smith et al. (Fig. 2) the presynaptic dense projections can be seen (x), but they were neither labeled nor referred to, and hence not given any functional consideration.

Meanwhile, my continued observations on adult and neonatal rat brain mentioned above, reinforced the hypothesis that metastable filamentous organelles such as actin filaments and/or microtubules might well fail to be preserved in regions rich in cytoproteins, such as the presynaptic bag. This would then fit in with the biochemical evidence for synaptosomal actomyosin (see Berl et al., 1973) (and the less strong morphological evidence — see Metuzals and Mushynski, 1974; Lebeux and Willemot, 1975). Also there is biochemical evidence for synaptosome tubulin, the basic subunit protein of the microtubules (Feit and Barondes, 1970; Feit et al., 1971; Lagnado et al., 1971; Kadota et al., 1975). Berl et al. (1973) implicated the actomyosin in the

214

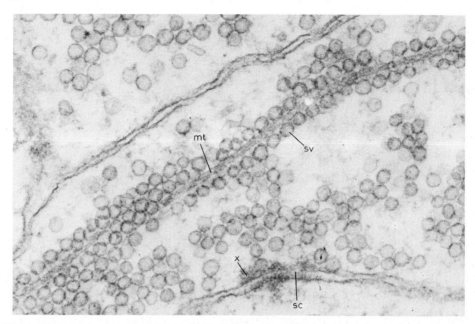

Fig. 2. Synapse in the spinal cord of the lamprey larva showing synaptic vesicles associated with microtubules (mt). (From Smith et al., 1970; reproduced by kind permission of the authors.)

mechanism of transmitter extrusion following Ca^{2+} entry into the presynaptic bag in response to stimulation. Berl et al., did not take into account the possibility that actomyosin plays a role in the translocation of the synaptic vesicles up to the presynaptic membrane, nor did they mention the dense projections.

Having decided that, in spite of a large volume of literature suggesting otherwise, a complex system of labile actomyosin filaments and/or

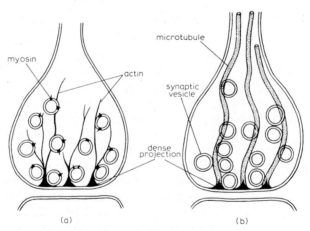

Fig. 3. Alternative hypothetical models (a) and (b) to account for the concentrations of synaptic vesicles close to the presynaptic membrane, and to account for the presence of dense projections.

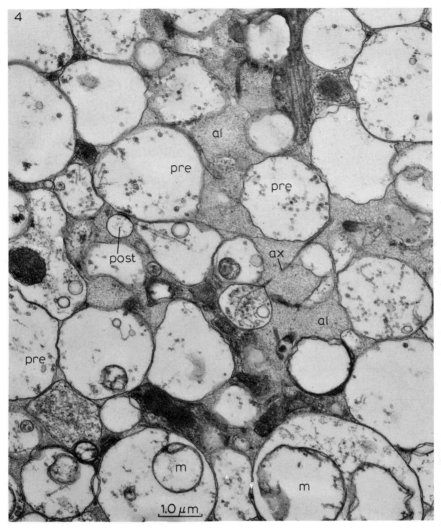

Fig. 4. Rat occipital cerebral cortex after albumin treatment. The region is about 20 μm from the edge of the tissue fragment.

microtubules might well be present in vivo in the presynaptic bag, I proposed that the dense projections could be the focal or anchoring points for actin filaments or microtubules (Gray, 1975a) with the synaptic vesicles moving along their surfaces (Fig. 3a, b). If so, then myosin would presumably be situated in the wall of the synaptic vesicle (Gray and Paula-Barbosa, 1974).

To test my hypothesis, I decided to subject fresh unfixed brain fragments to high protein ·concentrations to see whether this would deform or obliterate microtubules (and other sensitive organelles), the logic being that they could be seen well preserved in axons and dendrites, because the cytoregions they occupied contained much less concentrated cytoproteins than the presynaptic bags. A 20–25% solution of bovine serum albumin (Sigma) in distilled water was chosen for no special reason other than its solubility and availability. Four

216

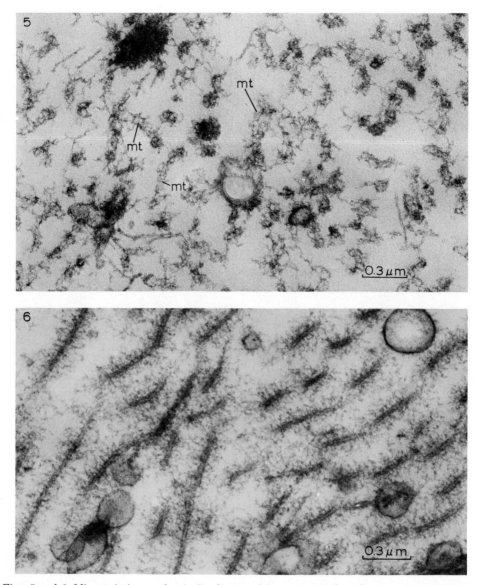

Figs. 5 and 6. Microtubules mechanically disrupted by teasing before fixation show a net-like (stereoframework) substructure (Fig. 5). Microtubules treated with albumin become stabilized and resist disruption. (Rat cerebral cortex.)

per cent unbuffered osmium tetroxide followed by 12% unbuffered glutaraldehyde were used for fixation (Kanaseki and Kadota, 1969). Experiments underway suggest that this may be an essential part of the technique. To date, the following tissues have been investigated by this method in *rat* cerebral and cerebellar cortices and posterior pituitary, and *frog* forebrain, retina, spinal cord and motor endplate. The observations were first mentioned in a footnote (Gray, 1975a) and then in a short paper (Gray, 1975b). Fig. 4 shows the marginal region of a fragment of rat cerebral cortex at low magnification. The albumin (al) can be seen between the apparently swollen presynaptic bags (pre) and sometimes a postsynaptic profile (spine head or dendrite-post) can be seen as in synaptosomal preparations. Previous work (Gray, 1973, 1975a) had shown that mechanical trauma to microtubules before fixation (Fig. 5, mt) causes them to disintegrate into a net-like (stereoframework) substructure. However, in the albumin preparations at present under consideration, unexpectedly, microtubules could be seen in the albumin (Fig. 6) extruded from the dendrites and remarkably intact in spite of the teasing.

Attention was then turned to the synapses. Quite surprisingly, microtubules (mt) "clothed" in synaptic vesicles could be seen running out of the preterminal axon and sweeping down to the "active zone" of the presynaptic membrane where they appeared to be anchored by the dense projections (Figs. 7–10). En face sections taken close to and parallel with the presynaptic

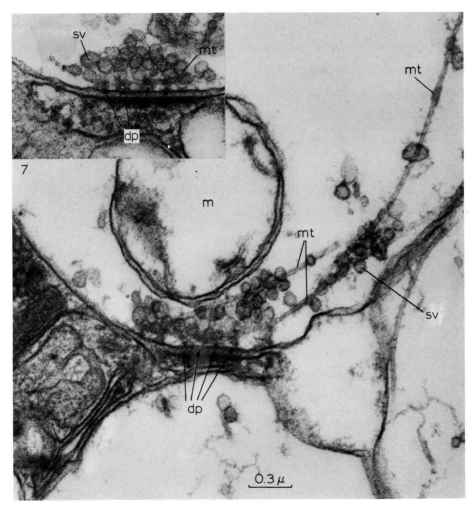

Fig. 7. Albuminized synapse in frog (*Rana temporaria*) forebrain. Inset: "active zone" of another frog synapse from forebrain.

218

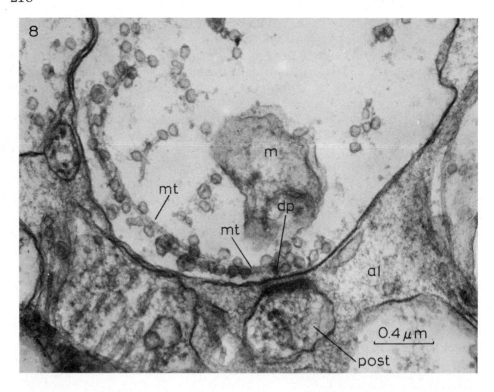

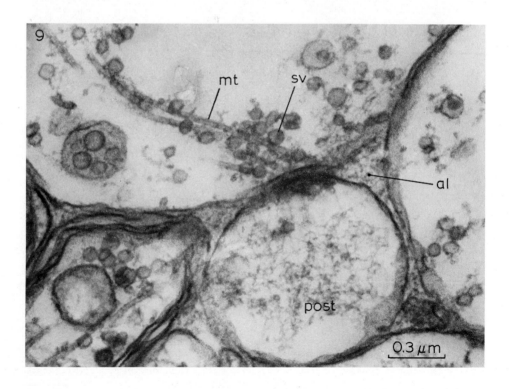

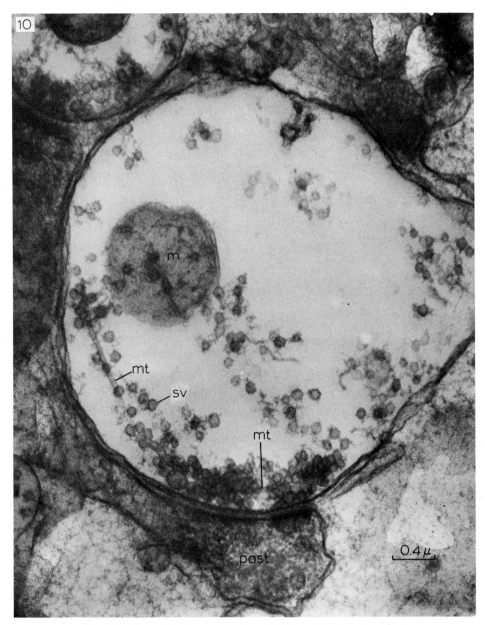

Fig. 10. Albuminized synapse in occipital cerebral cortex of rat.

membrane (Fig. 11) reveal up to 8 or more microtubules (arrows) criss-crossing. Somehow the regular spacing of the dense projections is determined by the spacing and arrangements of the microtubules (or vice-versa!). This is at present under further investigation. Figs. 12–14 show the close relationships between the microtubules and the synaptic vesicles, just as described by Smith et al. (1970 — compare with Fig. 2). Fig. 13 (arrows) shows apparent contact "bridges" (see Smith, 1971, for detailed discussion).

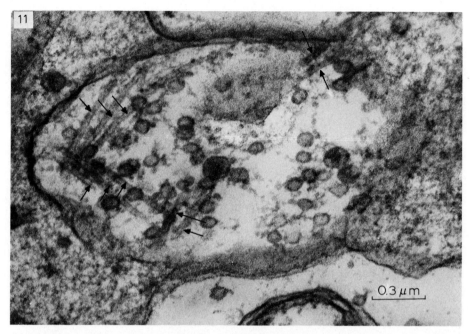

Fig. 11. Albuminized synapse in frog forebrain. En face view of "active zone".

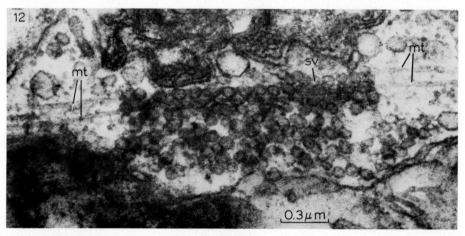

Fig. 12. Albuminized synapse (en passant varicosity) in frog spinal cord showing closely packed and hence regularly arranged synaptic vesicles associated with microtubules.

Only a few sections from albuminized rat posterior pituitary have yet been examined (Fig. 15). Microtubules (mt) can be seen apparently anchored to the surface membrane by the dense projections (dp). However, no dramatic close association between the neurosecretory vesicles (nv) and the microtubules has been seen, although the small agranular vesicles (av) sometimes lie close to the microtubules.

In the albuminized retina, microtubules (mt) can be seen running right up to and parallel with the synaptic ribbon (Figs. 16 and 18, sr) of the bipolar and

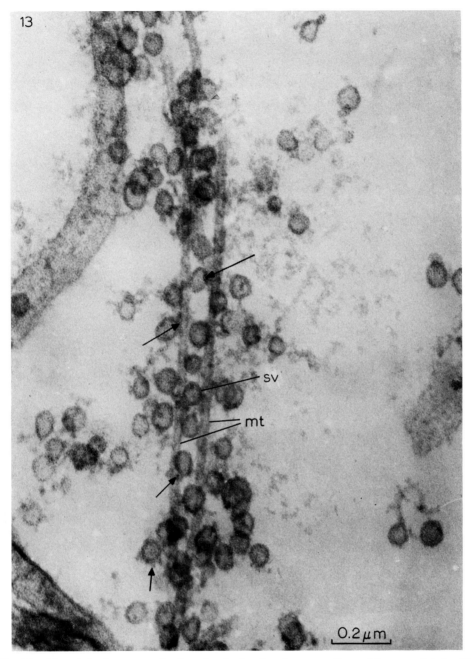

Fig. 13. Albuminized synapse in frog forebrain showing synaptic vesicles associated with microtubules.

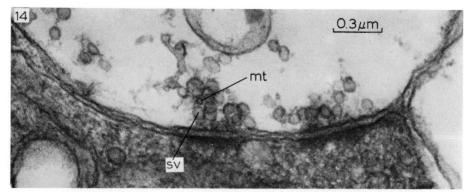

Fig. 14. As Fig. 13 showing a microtubule (in transverse section) with associated synaptic vesicles.

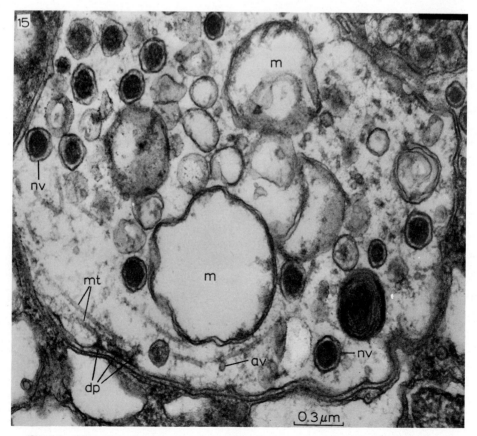

Fig. 15. Albuminized neurosecretory ending in pars nervosa of rat pituitary gland.

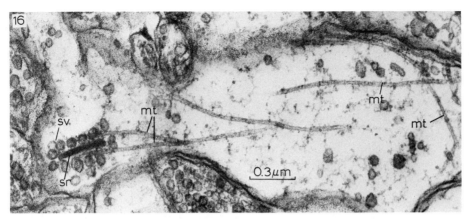

Fig. 16. Albuminized ribbon synapse in inner plexiform layer of frog retina.

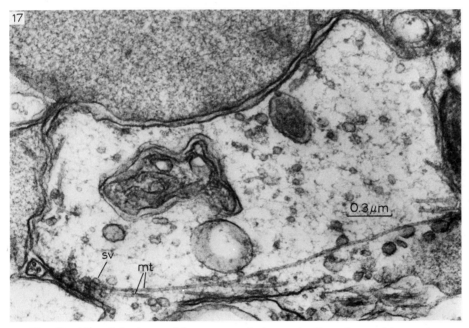

Fig. 17. Albuminized non-ribbon synapse in inner plexiform layer of frog retina.

receptor synapses. In the inner plexiform layer, microtubules (Fig. 17, mt) can be seen focused on the "active zone" in non-ribbon synapses.

In the albuminized motor endplate, microtubules (mt) "clothed" in synaptic vesicles can be seen sweeping down towards the terminal membrane (Fig. 19). It remains to be seen whether or not the microtubules are anchored to the presynaptic membrane dense zones, first described by Birks et al. (1960), which would account for the aggregations of synaptic vesicles seen at the dense zones by these authors.

224

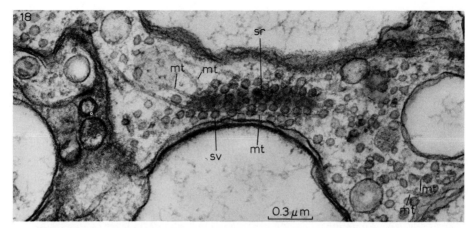

Fig. 18. Albuminized receptor synapse in outer plexiform layer of frog retina.

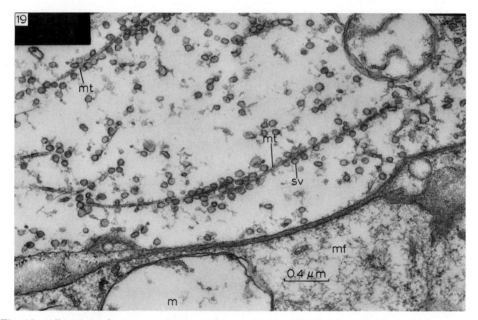

Fig. 19. Albuminized motor endplate in frog striated muscle (extensor longus digitorum 4).

DISCUSSION

It will be recalled that I had previously suggested (Gray, 1975a) that local high concentrations of cytoproteins, as in axon terminals, might be responsible for the disintegration, during fixation, of labile microtubules or actin filaments that might be present in vivo. To test this hypothesis, brain fragments were teased in concentrated protein (albumin) solution before fixation for electron microscopy, anticipating the disappearance of these structures from the sections. Contrary to such expectations, microtubules showed remarkably good preservation and could be seen, clothed in synaptic vesicles, running out of the preterminal axon and up to the presynaptic membrane. Here they contacted, and appeared to be anchored by, the dense projections (Gray, 1975b).

In spite of numerous experiments, it is not at all clear at present why the albumin technique should preserve the presynaptic microtubules. Certainly, contrary to the statement made in Gray (1975b), fixation with the 4% unbuffered osmium tetroxide, followed by postfixation with 12% glutaraldehyde and aqueous uranyl staining (Kanaseki and Kadota, 1969), is an *essential* part of the technique (how important the glutaraldehyde postfixation and/or the aqueous uranyl treatment is, has not yet been ascertained). Indeed, re-examination of micrographs and sections of rat cerebral cortex which had been immersion-fixed directly by this method even without albumin pretreatment revealed a few synapses where microtubules could vaguely be seen running right up to the presynaptic membrane.

At an early stage it was thought that the albumin was possibly chelating Ca^{2+}, which might otherwise enter the presynaptic bag during fixation and interfere with the preservation of the microtubules (see Weisenberg, 1972). This led to the re-examination of EDTA-treated rat cortex fragments, prepared in collaboration with Drs. K. and T. Kadota in studies on coated vesicles. The material had, incidentally (but now significantly!), been fixed by the Kanaseki and Kadota (1969) method. Some of the endings did, in fact, show vesicle-associated presynaptic tubules. However, further experiments using various hypotonic media, including distilled water, for pretreatment gave similar results, although the albumin method has given the best results so far. So, at present, in spite of numerous experiments, the mechanism of the procedure remains obscure. The essential steps seem to be a brief exposure of the brain fragments to a hypotonic medium, followed by fixation with 4% unbuffered osmium tetroxide. The hypotonic medium swells the presynaptic bag and at the same time highly dilutes the extracellular ions. The albumin may, in addition, have a special role not understood at present. The 4% unbuffered osmium is also hypotonic. Hence the swollen presynaptic bags might fix with no change in size. Certainly the 4% osmium acts much more quickly (judged by the speed of darkening of the tissue) than the conventional 1%. Thus, mechanical and ionic effects have been implicated, but many other factors need to be considered.

It is too early to speculate further about whether or not the microtubules are really involved in the transport of synaptic vesicles (cf. Droz et al., 1975). The vesicles may become artifactually applied to the surfaces of the microtubules during fixation. However, since the vesicles become applied to the surfaces of microtubules (when present in the same synapse), but not to agranular endoplasmic reticulum, neurofilaments, or surfaces of the mitochondria, the preference of the vesicles for microtubules would have to be explained.

The presence of synaptic vesicles at the surfaces of microtubules suggests the possibility (in addition to other theories of synaptic vesicle formation) that synaptic vesicles may be forming de novo as "bubbles" of phospholipid in the cytoplasm, the microtubules somehow catalyzing this formation. There is, in fact, recent evidence for the association of phospholipid with microtubule protein (Daleo et al., 1974).

The cytonet described in presynaptic bags (Gray, 1972, 1973), later called the stereoframework (Gray, 1975a), was considered to be an artifactual fixation material derived from regions rich in cytoproteins. It now seems that at least part of the presynaptic stereoframework may be derived from the protein of microtubules that are intact.

It was further postulated that, in aldehyde-fixed material, stereoframework formation could somehow distort the shape of the synaptic vesicles so that they became flattened at certain synapses (in some cases known to be inhibitory, Uchizono, 1965). Quite frequently, in albuminized synapses, synaptic vesicles can be seen sandwiched (and hence flattened) between two microtubules. Hence, vesicle-flattening could indeed be caused by the microtubules pulling closer together during the aldehyde fixation. The flattening thus would result from the intact protein microtubules rather than from the stereoframework. The microtubules themselves are, of course, not visualized in the conventional aldehyde-fixed material, only their presumed remnants: the stereoframework.

The present results give strong support to Schmitt's (1968) original hypothesis (although in the 1970 diagram he showed the microtubules stopping short of the presynaptic membrane) that synaptic vesicles slide along the microtubules and so arrive at the "active zone" of the presynaptic membrane. We now, therefore, have a morphological explanation (lacking for so long) of the clustering of synaptic vesicles at the appropriate zone of the presynaptic membrane for transmitter release. Fig. 20a and b illustrate this point; (b) shows

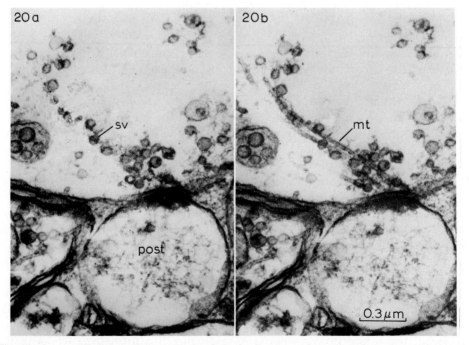

Fig. 20. b: an albuminized synapse in frog forebrain with microtubules present. a: the picture has been retouched to remove the microtubules showing the "mysterious" aggregation of synaptic vesicles at the "active zone" characteristic of previous investigations.

an albuminized synapse with the microtubules present, while in (a) the micrograph has been retouched to eliminate the microtubules and rephotographed. It is now also possible to understand the appearance commonly seen in conventional micrographs, and which has long puzzled the author, of chains of synaptic vesicles, apparently "descending" on the "active zone". The vesicles have in fact retained linear arrays in relationship to the microtubules, assumed to be present in vivo.

Finally, back to the question that has puzzled the author for 15 years, viz. "what are the dense projections?", and which the author suggested (Gray, 1966) might somehow play a role in guiding the vesicles to the presynaptic membrane. It now seems likely that they are bodies that attach or anchor the microtubules to the presynaptic membrane. The dense projections are probably proteinaceous (see Pfenninger, 1973), but their precise substructure still remains to be determined. Their regular array on the presynaptic membrane is probably determined by the orientation and spacing of the microtubules (up to 8 in some presynaptic bags) — or vice versa! Fig. 21a shows a model of the manner in which the microtubules may be distributed in the presynaptic bag (whether the microtubules end blindly or loop back up into the axon still remains to be determined). The dense projections have been omitted. The microtubules appear to cross over each other, and the crossing points may be the sites of the dense projections. Fig. 21b and c show two possible arrangements. In (b) the dense projection is simply visualized as an amorphous blob of protein that encases the crossing point of the microtubules (presumably anchoring them to the presynaptic membrane). In (c) the dense projection is visualized as a more discrete, peg-like structure. In Fig. 21d the dense projection is shown as first described (Gray, 1963). It has a net-like appearance

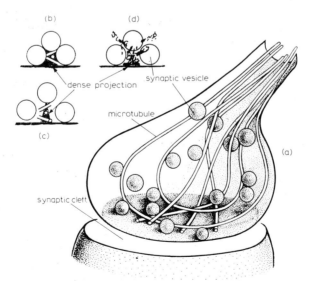

Fig. 21. a: model based on observations showing the probable relationships of microtubules (with associated synaptic vesicles) to the dense projections. b and c: alternative interpretations of the structure of the dense projection. d: appearance of dense projection seen in the past in conventional preparations.

228

— the stereoframework precipitation from in vivo protein. Thus, the dense projection will now be considered to consist, in part, of overlapping microtubules (converted by conventional fixation methods into stereoframework debris) and in part of a proteinaceous attachment body. The arrangement predicted in Gray (1975a), and shown in Fig. 3b of this paper, is now given experimental support, i.e., that the dense projections are related to microtubules approaching the terminal membrane. However, it would now seem that the microtubules sweep past the dense projections, rather than terminating there.

SUMMARY

Using special prefixation and fixation techniques on synapses of rat central nervous system (cerebral and cerebellar cortices) and posterior pituitary endings, and frog forebrain, retina and motor endplate, microtubules can be observed focused on the terminal membrane. Synaptic vesicles can usually be observed associated with the microtubules (except in the rat pituitary and frog retina).

ADDENDUM

While this paper was in press, further observations have shown that in the presynaptic bag, in addition to synaptic vesicles, agranular reticulum is often seen associated with the microtubules. It is often wrapped round the microtubules between the vesicles and the presynaptic membrane. Since such an arrangement would appear to prevent the movement of synaptic vesicles to

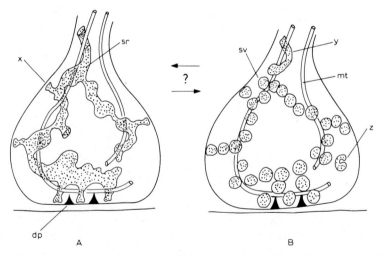

Fig. 22. A: diagrams to show the postulated in vivo relationships of the presynaptic smooth endoplasmic reticulum (sr) to microtubules (mt). B: during fixation the sr is thought to fragment into the characteristic synaptic vesicles (sv). dp, dense projection; x, "end-feet" made by sr on the surface membrane; y and z, profiles suggesting derivation of sv's from sr.

the presynaptic membrane, the theory that microtubules are involved in moving the vesicles along appears less attractive. Recent experiments by the author suggest that presynaptic agranular endoplasmic reticulum (sr) (Fig. 22A) is extremely labile and breaks down artifactually into synaptic vesicles during fixation (Fig. 22B). This would explain the apparent association of synaptic vesicles with microtubules. It can now be postulated that microtubules play a role in directing the growth of sr towards the presynaptic membrane. A full account of experiments suggesting that synaptic vesicles are artifacts will be published elsewhere.

ACKNOWLEDGEMENTS

I am indebted to Professor Sir Bernard Katz, F.R.S. and Drs. A. Matus and J. Lagnado for advice, to Mrs. H. Samson for skilled technical assistance and to the Medical Research Council for financial support.

KEY TO FIGURES

All material has been fixed with 4% unbuffered osmium tetroxide and 12% unbuffered glutaraldehyde with aqueous block uranyl staining and lead on the section. Abbreviations are:

al,	albumin in extracellular space;
av,	agranular vesicle;
ax,	unmyelinated axon (usually shrunken);
dp,	dense projections;
m,	mitochondrion (usually swollen);
mt,	microtubules;
mf,	muscle fiber;
nv,	neurosecretory vesicle;
post,	postsynaptic process (dendrite or its spine);
pre,	presynaptic bag;
sc,	synaptic cleft;
sr,	synaptic ribbon;
sv,	synaptic vesicles; and
x,	dense projection(s) unlabeled in the original publication of Smith et al. (1970).

REFERENCES

Akert, K. and Waser, P.G. (Eds.) (1969) *Mechanisms of Synaptic Transmission, Progress in Brain Research, Vol. 31*, Elsevier, Amsterdam.

Akert, K., Moor, H., Pfenninger, K. and Sandri, C. (1969) Contributions of new impregnation methods and freeze etching to the problems of synaptic fine structure. In *Mechanisms of Synaptic Transmission, Progress in Brain Research, Vol. 31*, K. Akert and P.G. Waser (Eds.), Elsevier, Amsterdam, pp. 223–240.

Akert, K., Pfenninger, K., Sandri, C. and Moor, H. (1972) Freeze-etching and cytochemistry of vesicles and membrane complexes in synapses of the central nervous system. In *Structure and Function of Synapses*, G.O. Pappas and D.P. Purpura (Eds.), North-Holland Publishing Co., Amsterdam, pp. 3–86.

Berl, S., Puszkin, S. and Nicklas, W.J. (1973) Actomyosin-like protein in brain. *Science*, 179: 441–446.

Birks, R.I. (1974) The relationship of transmitter release and storage to fine structure in a sympathetic ganglion. *J. Neurocytol.*, 3: 133–160.

Birks, R.I., Huxley, H.E. and Katz, B. (1960) The fine structure of the neuromuscular junction of the frog. *J. Physiol. (Lond.)*, 150: 134–144.

Bloom, F.E., Iversen, L.L. and Schmitt, F.O. (1970) Macromolecules in synaptic function. *Neurosci. Res. Progr. Bull.*, 8: 325–455.

Burnstock, G. (1972) Purinergic nerves. *Pharmacol. Rev.*, 24: 509–581.

Burt, A.M. (1971) A histochemical localization of choline acetyltransferase. In *Histochemistry of Nervous Transmission, Progress in Brain Research, Vol. 34*, O. Eränkö (Ed.), Elsevier, Amsterdam, pp. 327–336.

Burt, A.M. and Silver, A. (1973) Histochemistry of choline acetyltransferase: a critical analysis. *Brain Res.*, 62: 509–516.

Ceccarelli, B., Hurlbut, W.P. and Mauro, A. (1973) Turnover of transmitter and synaptic vesicles at the frog neuromuscular junction. *J. Cell Biol.*, 57: 499–524.

Clark, A.W., Hurlbut, W.P. and Mauro, A. (1972) Changes in fine structure of the neuromuscular junction of the frog caused by black widow spider venom. *J. Cell Biol.*, 52: 1–31.

Cotman, C.W. and Banker, G.A. (1974) The making of a synapse. *Rev. Neurosci.*, 1: 1–62.

Couteaux, R. et Pécot-Dechavassine, M. (1970) Vésicules synaptiques et poches au niveau des "zones actives" de la jonction neuromusculaire. *C.R. Acad. Sci. (Paris)*, 271: 2346–2349.

Dahlström, A. (1973) Aminergic transmission. *Brain Res.*, 62: 441–460.

Daleo, G.R., Piras, M.M. and Piras, R. (1974) The presence of phospholipids and diglyceride kinase activity in microtubules from different tissues. *Biochem. biophys. Res. Commun.*, 61: 1043–50.

Dick, F. and Kelly, J.S. (1975) L-2,4-diaminobutyric acid (L-DABA) as a selective marker for inhibitory terminals in rat brain. *Brit. J. Pharmacol.*, 53: 439.

Droz, B., Rambourg, A. and Koenig, H.L. (1975) The smooth endoplasmic reticulum: structure and role in renewal of axon membrane and synaptic vesicles by fast axonal transport. *Brain Res.*, 93: 1–13.

Eccles, J.C. (1964) *The Physiology of Synapses.*, Springer, Berlin.

Feit, H.G. and Barondes, S.H. (1970) Colchicine-binding activity in particulate fractions of mouse brain. *J. Neurochem.*, 17: 1355–1364.

Feit, H.G., Dutton, S.H., Barondes, S.H. and Shelanski, M.L. (1971) Microtubule protein. Identification in and transport in nerve endings. *J. Cell Biol.*, 51: 138–147.

Gibbons, I.R. (1966) Studies on the ATPase activity of 14S and 30S dynein from cilia of *Tetrahymena. J. biol. Chem.*, 241: 5590–5596.

Gray, E.G. (1959) Axosomatic and axodendritic synapses of the cerebral cortex: an electron microscope study. *J. Anat. (Lond.)*, 93: 420–433.

Gray, E.G. (1963) Electron microscopy of presynaptic organelles of the spinal cord. *J. Anat. (Lond.)*, 97: 101–106.

Gray, E.G. (1966) Problems of interpreting the fine structure of vertebrate and invertebrate synapses. *Int. Rev. gen. exp. Zool.*, 2: 139–170.

Gray, E.G. (1969) Electron microscopy of excitatory and inhibitory synapses: a brief review. In *Mechanisms of Synaptic Transmission, Progress in Brain Research, Vol. 31*, K. Akert and P.G. Waser (Eds.), Elsevier, Amsterdam, pp. 141–155.

Gray, E.G. (1970) The question of relationships between Golgi vesicles and synaptic vesicles in *Octopus* neurons. *J. Cell Sci.*, 7: 189–202.

Gray, E.G. (1971) The fine structural characterisation of different types of synapse. In *Histochemistry of Nervous Transmission, Progress in Brain Research, Vol. 34*, O. Eränkö (Ed.), Elsevier, Amsterdam, pp. 149–160.

Gray, E.G. (1972) Are the coats of coated vesicles artifacts? *J. Neurocytol.*, 1: 363–382.

Gray, E.G. (1973) The cytonet, plain and coated vesicles, reticulosomes, multivesicular bodies and nuclear pores. *Brain Res.*, 62: 392–435.

Gray, E.G. (1974) Synaptic morphology with special reference to microneurons. In *Essays on the Nervous System — A Festchrift for Professor J.Z. Young*, R. Bellairs and E.G. Gray (Eds.), Clarendon Press, Oxford, pp. 155–178.

Gray, E.G. (1975a) Synaptic fine structure and nuclear, cytoplasmic and extracellular networks. *J. Neurocytol.*, 4: 315–339.

Gray, E.G. (1975b) Presynaptic microtubules and their association with synaptic vesicles. *Proc. roy. Soc. B*, 190: 369–372.

Gray, E.G. and Guillery, R.W. (1966) Synaptic morphology in the normal and degenerating nervous system. *Int. Rev. Cytol.*, 19: 111–182.

Gray, E.G. and Paula-Barbosa, M. (1974) Dense particles within synaptic vesicles fixed with acid-aldehyde. *J. Neurocytol.*, 3: 487–496.

Gray, E.G. and Willis, R.A. (1968) Problems of electron stereoscopy of biological tissues. *J. Cell Sci.*, 3: 309–326.

Heuser, J.E. and Reese, T.S. (1973) Evidence for recycling of synaptic vesicle membrane during release at the frog neuro-muscular junction. *J. Cell Biol.*, 57: 315–344.

Holtzman, E., Teichberg, S., Abrahams, S.J., Citkowitz, E., Crain, S.M., Kawai, N. and Peterson, E.R. (1973) Notes on synaptic vesicles and related structures. *J. Histochem. Cytochem.*, 21: 349–385.

Iversen, L.L., Kelly, J.S., Mirchin, M., Schon, F. and Snodgrass, S.R. (1973) Role of amino acids and peptides in synaptic transmission. *Brain Res.*, 62: 567–576.

Jeffrey, P.L. and Austin, L. (1974) Axoplasmic transport. *Progr. Neurobiol.*, 2: 205–255.

Jones, S.F. and Kwanbunbumpen, S. (1970) The effects of nerve stimulation and hemicholinium on synaptic vesicles at the mammalian neuromuscular junction. *J. Physiol. (Lond.)*, 207: 31–50.

Kadota, T., Kadota, K. and Gray, E.G. (1975) Coated vesicle shells, particle-chain material and tubulin in brain synaptosomes: an electron microscopic and biochemical study. *J. Cell Biol.*, in press.

Kanaseki, T. and Kadota, K. (1969) The vesicle in a basket. *J. Cell Biol.*, 42: 202–220.

Kása, P. (1971) Ultrastructural localisation of choline acetyltransferase and acetylcholinesterase in central and peripheral nervous tissue. In *Histochemistry of Nervous Transmission, Progress in Brain Research, Vol. 34*, O. Eränkö (Ed.), Elsevier, Amsterdam, pp. 337–344.

Kása, P., Mann, S.P. and Hebb, C. (1970) Localization of choline acetyltransferase. *Nature (Lond.)*, 226: 812–816.

Korneliussen, H. (1972) Elongated profiles of synaptic vesicles in motor end-plates. Morphological effects of fixative variations. *J. Neurocytol.*, 1: 279–296.

Kornguth, S.E. (1974) The synapse: a perspective from in situ and in vivo studies. *Rev. Neurosci.*, 1: 63–114.

Krnjévić, K. (1974) Chemical nature of synaptic transmission in vertebrates. *Physiol. Rev.*, 54: 418–540.

Lagnado, J.R., Lyons, C. and Wickremasinghe, G. (1971) The subcellular distribution of colchicine-binding protein ("microtubule protein") in rat brain. *FEBS Lett.*, 15: 254–259.

Landis, D.M. and Reese, T.S. (1974) Differences in membrane structure between excitatory and inhibitory synapses in the cerebellar cortex. *J. comp. Neurol.*, 155: 93–126.

Lebeux, Y.J. and Willemot, J.G. (1975) Identification at the ultrastructural level of actin-like filaments in rat brain neurons by means of HMM labelling, *Anat. Rec.*, 181: 407.

Lepetina, E.G., Soto, E.F. and De Robertis, E. (1968) Lipids and proteolipids in isolated subcellular membranes of rat brain cortex. *J. Neurochem.*, 15: 437–445.

Lewis, P.R. and Shute, C.C.D. (1967) The cholinergic limbic system: projections to hippocampal formation, medial cortex, nuclei of the ascending cholinergic reticular system, and the subformical organ and supra-optic crest. *Brain*, 90: 521–540.

Lieberman, A.R. and Webster, K.E. (1974) Aspects of the synaptic organization of intrinsic neurons in the dorsal lateral geniculate nucleus. *J. Neurocytol.*, 3: 677–710.

Matus, A.I. and Dennison, M.E. (1972) An autoradiographic study of uptake of exogenous glycine by vertebrate spinal cord slices in vitro. *J. Neurocytol.*, 1: 27–34.

Metuzals, J. and Mushynski, W.E. (1974) Electron microscope and experimental investigations of the neurofilamentous network in Deiters neurons. *J. Cell Biol.*, 61: 701–722.

Palay, S.L. and Chan-Palay, V. (1974) *Cerebellar Cortex — Cytology and Organization.* Springer, Berlin, 348 pp.

Pappas, G.D. and Purpura, D.P. (1972) *Structure and Function of Synapses.* Raven Press, New York.

Paula-Barbosa, M. and Gray, E.G. (1974) The effects of various fixatives at different pH on synaptic coated vesicles and cytonets. *J. Neurocytol.*, 3: 471–486.

Peters, A., Palay, S.L. and Webster, H. deF. (1970) *The Fine Structure of the Nervous System.* Harper and Row, New York.

Pfenninger, K.H. (1973) Synaptic morphology and cytochemistry. *Progr. Histochem. Cytochem.*, 5: 1–86.

Pfenninger, K. and Rovainen, C.M. (1974) Stimulation- and calcium-dependence of vesicle attachment sites in the presynaptic membrane: a freeze-cleave study of the lamprey spinal cord. *Brain Res.*, 72: 1–23.

Pfenninger, K., Sandri, C., Akert, K. and Eugster, C.H. (1969) Contribution to the problem of structural organization of the presynaptic area. *Brain Res.*, 12: 10–18.

Pfenninger, K., Akert, K., Moor, H. and Sandri, C. (1971) Freeze-fracturing of presynaptic membranes of the central nervous system. *Phil. Trans. B*, 261: 387.

Pfenninger, K., Akert, K., Moor, H. and Sandri, C. (1972) The fine structure of freeze-fractured synaptic membranes. *J. Neurocytol.*, 1: 129–149.

Pysh, J.J. and Wiley, R.G. (1974) Synaptic vesicle depletion and recovery in cat sympathetic ganglia electrically stimulated in vivo. *J. Cell Biol.*, 60: 365–374.

Schmitt, F.O. (1968) The molecular biology of neuronal fibrous proteins. *Neurosci. Res. Progr. Bull.*, 6: 119–144.

Schmitt, F.O. (1970) In Macromolecules in Synaptic Function, F.E. Bloom, L.L. Iversen and F.O. Schmitt (Eds.), *Neurosci. Res. Progr. Bull.*, 8: 329–332.

Schmitt, F.O. and Samson, F.E. (1968) Neuronal fibrous proteins. *Neurosci. Res. Progr. Bull.*, 6: 113–219.

Schon, F. and Kelly, J.S. (1974a) Autoradiographic localization of [^{3}H]GABA and [^{3}H]glutamate over satellite glial cells. *Brain Res.*, 66: 275–288.

Schon, F. and Kelly, J.S. (1974b) The characterization of [^{3}H]GABA uptake into the satellite glial cells of rat sensory ganglia. *Brain Res.*, 66: 289–300.

Shute, C.C.D. and Lewis, P.R. (1967) The ascending cholinergic reticular system: neocortical, olfactory and subcortical projections. *Brain*, 90: 497–520.

Smith, D.S. (1971) On the significance of cross-bridges between microtubules and synaptic vesicles. *Phil. Trans. B*, 261: 395–405.

Smith, D.S., Järlfors, U. and Beránek, R. (1970) The organisation of synaptic axoplasm in the lamprey (*Petromyzon marinus*) central nervous system. *J. Cell Biol.*, 46: 199–219.

Sotelo, C. (1971) General features of the synaptic organisation of the CNS. In *Chemistry and Brain Development*, R. Paoletti and A.N. Davison (Eds.), Plenum, New York, pp. 239–286.

Thoenen, H. and Tranzer, J.P. (1971) Functional importance of subcellular distribution of false adrenergic transmitters. In *Histochemistry of Nervous Transmission, Progress in Brain Research, Vol. 34*, O. Eränkö (Ed.), Elsevier, Amsterdam, pp. 223–236.

Turner, P.T. and Harris, A.B. (1973) Ultrastructure of synaptic vesicle formation in cerebral cortex. *Nature (Lond.)*, 242: 57–59.

Turner, P.I. and Harris, A.B. (1974) Ultrastructure of exogenous peroxidase in cerebral cortex. *Brain Res.*, 74: 305–326.

Uchizono, K. (1965) Characteristics of excitatory and inhibitory synapses in the central nervous system of the cat. *Nature (Lond.)*, 207: 642–643.

Uchizono, K. (1975) *Excitation and Inhibition Synaptic Morphology* Shoin, Tokyo.

Warner, F.D. and Satir, P. (1974) The structural basis of ciliary bend formation. *J. Cell Biol.*, 63: 35–63.

Weisenberg, R.C. (1972) Microtubule formation in vitro in solutions containing low calcium concentrations. *Science*, 177: 1104–1105.

Whittaker, V.P. (1966) Some properties of synaptic membranes isolated from the central nervous system. *Ann. N.Y. Acad Sci.*, 137: 982–998.

DISCUSSION

V.P. WHITTAKER: It is well known that, in order to isolate microtubules you have your centrifuge running at 30–37 degrees, since microtubules disintegrate and depolymerize in the cold. I wonder, therefore, whether you have studied the effect of fixation at different temperatures?

E.G. GRAY: Indeed, fixation at low temperatures is not the right thing to do if one wants to preserve microtubules. About ten years ago we stopped fixation at low temperatures and since then we have been doing it at room temperature. The present work has all been carried out at room temperature.

S.P.R. ROSE: Did you select those pictures that you have shown, or did all synapses show the microtubule structure?

E.G. GRAY: Oh yes, these pictures were certainly selected. The presynaptic microtubules can only be seen in sections taken through the margin of the brain fragment — usually 10–20 μm in. In the more central regions, the synapses all have the more familiar appearance of microtubules apparently petering out where the preterminal axon expands into the presynaptic bag.

S.P.R. ROSE: Could one not suggest that in some way albumin would precipitate out along the synaptic vesicles in some sort of way, to make a trap that looked like a tubule?

E.G. GRAY: No reply. (*Note added in proof*: as stated in the above paper, the effect can be produced without albumin.)

B.T. PICKERING: You talked about the origin of the vesicles and said that they could either be transported from the perikaryon, or arrive by endocytosis. Now do you feel that these possibilities are mutually exclusive?

E.G. GRAY: No, we are still not sure how synaptic vesicles form. They may form at the Golgi apparatus and be transported down the axon, or they may form locally either by endocytosis from the wall of the presynaptic bag or from the local agranular reticulum. I am adding a fourth possibility, namely, that the synaptic vesicles may form de novo in the presynaptic bag as "bubbles" of phospholipid. They may form at the surfaces of the microtubules, which somehow play an organizing or catalyzing role.

V. BRAITENBERG: From most of their course, it seemed to me that the microtubules are running, like two railway lines, to the dense projections.

E.G. GRAY: They seem to follow round the contours of the walls of the presynaptic bag and eventually reach the dense projections.

E. MEISAMI: What is the evidence that the vesicles move in the direction of the presynaptic membrane? Or could they also go in the other direction?

E.G. GRAY: I agree this is still a problem. It is not yet possible to visualize a synaptic vesicle in living tissue and we should not, of course, presume dynamic events from static pictures alone.

E. MEISAMI: My second question is whether you have any morphological evidence that these tubules actually come into the membrane. Or do they just end within the vesicle projection? Because with freeze-etching, we see these little holes in the membranes.

E.G. GRAY: My impression is that the microtubules are anchored by the dense projections. They seem to sweep past them and I wonder if they loop back up the axon. It is very difficult to tell whether a microtubule is ending, or is simply going out of the plane of section.

R. STOECKART: You did not mention coated vesicles at all. Do they fit in somewhere in your story?

E.G. GRAY: It has been suggested that the vesicle invaginates and the coat forms around it, as on a template. The then coated vesicle moves into the presynaptic bag, and the vesicle comes out of the coat, but one may still see the debris of the coat. There is a sequential series which is suggestive, but the proposition that the synaptic vesicles come from coated vesicles is still very much under debate.

H. GRUNDFEST: There are conditions under which one can evacuate the vesicles by giving drugs or by continued functional activity. Would you still be able to see tubules in these cases?

E.G. GRAY: I don't know anything about what the vesicles would do, assuming they in fact form on the surface of the tubules. Could Dr. Whittaker say anything about the vesicles' discharge?

V.P. WHITTAKER: In our studies with electric tissue it is possible to get a depletion of vesicle numbers by intensive stimulation. Then there seems to be a very rapid part of the recovery phase which involves the formation of empty vesicles. It's not clear whether or not the final and complete recovery of the synapse involves the reacquisition of transmitter by these empty vesicles, or whether they just represent a salvage operation. If you get an increase in the surface area of the external membrane as a result of the exocytosis, you must, provided there is a physiological recovery, have a taking-in of external membrane, and that would appear in the cytoplasm as vesicles. The question is whether those vesicles have to be returned to the cell body for reprocessing or reconstitution, or whether they can be completely reconstituted as fully competent vesicles in the terminals. This is one of the basic problems of the system, and the answer may be different for different synapses.

The Nerve Growth Factor:
Its Role in Growth, Differentiation and Function of the Sympathetic Adrenergic Neuron

RITA LEVI-MONTALCINI

Laboratory of Cell Biology, Rome (Italy) and Department of Biology, Washington University, St. Louis, Mo. (U.S.A.)

THE SYMPATHETIC NERVE CELL: A BRIEF BIOGRAPHIC SKETCH

In the course of divergence of cell lineages among the 10–12 billions of nerve cells which build the vertebrate nervous system, the sympathetic nerve cell is the first to acquire structural and biochemical differentiative marks. In the 3-day chick embryo or in the 6-week, 1-cm-long human embryo, two thin bands of undifferentiated cells migrate from their site of origin, the neural crest, and move along the sides of the diminutive, still open, neural tube into the underlying mesenchymal tissue. A few of these cells assemble as two strands and segregate from other neural crest derivatives which give origin to sensory neurons, neural supporting elements, pigment, cartilage and connective tissue. The two cellular strands consist of loosely packed cells with no differentiating marks and may already be designated as the primary sympathetic trunks. They segregate in turn into two components: one of these moves in a dorsolateral direction and gives rise to the segmentally arranged paravertebral ganglia, which settle in close apposition to the motor roots of the spinal nerves; the other migrates in a ventromedial direction in the pre-aortal region and forms the prevertebral sympathetic ganglia which extend from the thoracic to the pelvic region.

A cellular contingent from the same source becomes transformed into chromaffin cells of the adrenal medulla, and into the extra-adrenal chromaffin tissue (which also includes some scattered cells intermingled with sympathetic neurons in para- and prevertebral ganglia). Proliferative and differentiative processes take place in all ganglia during embryonic and early postnatal life. Axonal elongation and establishment of synaptic connections with end tissues occur during the first and second postnatal week in rodents (the most extensively explored mammalian species), that is, at a time when other nerve cells in the same ganglia are still in the process of dividing.

Long before the sympathetic adrenergic neurons have established morphological and functional connections with their effector organs, the developing nerve cells have acquired a biochemical differentiation which permits one to recognize them among all the billions of non-adrenergic neurons. The Falck-Hillarp fluorescence technique showed, in fact, that in the 3·5-day chick embryo these nerve cells, though at a still incipient stage of differentiation, exhibit a green fluorescence to ultraviolet light. This is indicative of the presence, within the cell cytoplasm, and also in the outgrowing axon, of noradrenaline (NA), the humoral agent by means of which the sympathetic adrenergic neuron stimulates or inhibits a vast array of other neuronal or non-neuronal cells (Burnstock and Costa, 1975).

It was this property of the sympathetic neuron to release, upon activation, a humoral agent strikingly similar to the adrenal medullarly hormone, adrenaline, which first led to the identification of the neurotransmitter. Then, as more sophisticated techniques became available, it offered a sort of Ariadne thread for probing inside the cell to unravel the mechanisms of synthesis, storage and release of the neurotransmitter (Blaschko, 1972). The adrenergic neuron thus became, thanks to this invaluable biochemical marker (NA), the most extensively explored and better known of all nerve cells. These studies paved the way for the development of an ever growing list of compounds which interfere with the synthesis, storage, release and reuptake of the neurotransmitter. The well known results of these investigations have made it possible to control the functioning of these nerve cells, which in turn exert control over a wide spectrum of body functions.

EXPERIMENTAL ANALYSIS OF THE SYMPATHETIC NERVE CELL: THE NERVE GROWTH FACTOR

While these studies were in progress, the same neuron came to the forefront of research in an entirely different area of investigation, viz, that dealing with growth, differentiation and cellular interactions during neurogenesis. These problems were explored in the first half of the century with rather crude tools and techniques developed in the field of experimental embryology, consisting of surgical ablation or implantation of additional limb or organ primordia in amphibian, avian and mammalian embryos.

The discovery that certain mouse tumors grafted into the body wall of 3-day chick embryos called forth a marked volume increase of sensory (Bueker, 1948) and sympathetic ganglia (Levi-Montalcini and Hamburger, 1951) adjacent to the implanted tumor, and providing its innervation, was the starting point of an investigation which was to give definitive evidence for the outstanding role played by extrinsic factors in growth and differentiation of nerve cells, and, more importantly, succeeded in identifying one of these factors. The long and tortuous route which led to the isolation and characterization of this factor has been described many times and does not need to be recounted here (Levi-Montalicni, 1975). We shall only mention some early findings, which gain significance when viewed in retrospect, against the background of a recent more sophisticated approach.

The first evidence that the growth effect elicited by two mouse tumors known as sarcomas 180 and 37 is due to a factor released by the tumoral cells came from experiments of transplantation of one or the other tumor onto the chorioallantoic membrane of 4–6-day chick embryos. In such a position, the tumor and the embryonic tissues share the circulation but no direct contact is established between neoplastic and embryonic tissues. The finding that the sympathetic ganglia in embryos bearing these transplants were greatly enlarged, and most of the viscera were invaded by nerve fibers growing out from these ganglia, was taken as indicative of the release from these tumors of a humoral growth factor. Even more revealing, was the observation that sympathetic fiber bundles gained access to the inside of large and small veins, where they floated freely or formed large neuromas inside the cavity of the blood vessels (Levi-Montalcini, 1952). This most unusual event suggested that sympathetic nerve fibers do not grow out in a random direction but follow a concentration gradient of the growth factor produced and released by the tumor. A high concentration of this agent (at that time still unidentified) was possibly also the reason why the sympathetic nerve fibers produced in large number by hypertrophic and hyperplastic sympathetic ganglia, built a fibrillar plexus of much higher density in an excretory organ such as the mesonephros than in other embryonic viscera (Levi-Montalcini and Hamburger, 1953). The hypothesis of a neurotropic effect of the nerve growth factor (NGF) has since received strong support from recent studies to be considered in a following section.

An in vitro bioassay devised in 1953 (Levi-Montalcini et al., 1954) opened the way for the study of other morphological and biochemical parameters of the responses elicited by the tumoral agent in its target cells. More importantly, it made possible the characterization of this molecule, which in 1954 was tentatively identified in a nucleoprotein tumoral fraction and christened with the name of nerve growth factor (NGF; Cohen et al., 1954). This test, which has been performed without substantial modifications in the subsequent years, consisted in the explantation in a semi-solid medium of embryonic sensory or sympathetic ganglia of chick embryos in combination with small fragments of one or the other of the two mouse sarcomas which elicited the striking in vivo effects. In control cultures the ganglia were combined with normal embryonic tissues or tumors which did not produce the growth effect when implanted in the chick embryo. As reported in all previous articles, ganglia facing fragments of mouse sarcomas 180 or 37 produced a dense fibrillar halo in a 6–10 hr period. The same effect was obtained by replacing the tumors with their cell-free extract.

This simple and rapid in vitro bioassay made possible the screening of other tissues and biological fluids as potential sources of NGF. These studies led to the discovery, respectively in 1956 and 1958, that snake venom and mouse salivary glands produce and release a molecule endowed with biological properties identical with those of the two mouse sarcomas (Cohen and Levi-Montalcini, 1956; Cohen, 1958; Levi-Montalcini, 1958). A most important difference is that the NGF molecule is present at a concentration 1000 times higher in snake venom and mouse salivary glands than in mouse sarcomas. The striking similarity in the chemical properties of the snake venom and salivary NGFs, and their antigenic relatedness, were taken as evidence that two very closely related molecules elicit the growth response from the target nerve cells. Definitive proof that the snake venom and salivary NGFs are indeed very similar proteins was recently obtained by more sophisticated techniques (Hogue Angeletti, 1971; Hogue Angeletti et al., 1973, 1976; Server et al., 1976).

In 1971 the primary structure of the salivary NGF was elucidated by Hogue

Angeletti and Bradshaw (1971) and a few months ago the same molecule was crystallized by another group (Wlodawer et al., 1975). These two achievements bring our knowledge of NGF to the same level as that of protein hormones such as insulin and ACTH which have been under investigation for a much longer time than NGF. Although these studies have advanced at a remarkably fast pace, our knowledge of many other features of the NGF-target cell interaction still lags behind. Among these are: (a) the source or sources of origin, and regulatory mechanisms, of NGF production in the organism; (b) its mechanism of action at the molecular level; (c) its effect on the immature and fully developed sympathetic nerve cell and (d) its way of access to this cell. Only these last two aspects will be considered in the following sections.

NGF EFFECTS ON SYMPATHETIC NERVE CELL PRECURSORS

The neural crest derivatives: an in vitro approach

The problem of whether the NGF molecule gains access and elicits a response from cells which still have not acquired any differentiating marks, and thus do not differ by morphological criteria from precursors of other cell lines which originate from the neural crest, was recently studied by Bjerre and Björklund (1973). Cranial and trunk level segments of chick embryos, explanted in vitro between the stage of formation of the neural plate and the early migration of neural crest derivatives, were cultured in nutrient liquid media with or without NGF for an 8-day period. The cultures were then fixed and processed according to a modification of the Falck-Hillarp original technique and examined under the ultraviolet microscope for the presence of fluorescent catecholamine-containing cells. A marked increase in the number of these cells was seen in the experimental cultures, and was well documented by the microphotographic illustrations. The authors proposed the hypothesis that this effect might be due to: (1) an inductive NGF effect on neural crest cells leading to an increased recruitment of uncommitted cells; (2) an NGF effect on mitotic activity in catecholamine (CA)-containing cells, or in their immediate precursors; (3) an accelerative NGF effect on the in vitro differentiation of CA-containing cells, or (4) a preservative role of NGF which would favor survival and further development of CA-containing cells. Bjerre and Björklund favor this last alternative. Whatever the actual cause of the marked increase in adrenergic nerve cells in NGF-treated cultures, it gives evidence for an effect of this factor on neural crest derivatives prior to their differentiation, as stated by the authors, "from the stage of labile neural crest cells and onwards" (1973, p. 160).

The dividing sympathetic nerve cells: an in vivo study

Subcutaneous injection of the salivary NGF in neonatal rodents during a 1–2 week period produces a marked hyperplastic effect. The neuronal population in NGF-injected and control littermate mice, determined by cell counts at the end of the first week, gave evidence for a 2- or 2·5-fold increase in the number of nerve cells in experimental ganglia (Levi-Montalcini and Booker, 1960). Two alternative mechanisms were considered: either an increase of mitotic activity or the production of a larger number of sympathetic nerve cells at the expense of germinal or pluripotential cells. Counts of mitotic figures in control and experimental ganglia during the first 10 postnatal days showed a sharp increase in these figures in experimental ganglia between 3 and 7 days, with a peak at 5 days (a finding which clearly favored the first alternative). However, the reliability of criteria followed in this study was questioned by Jacobson (1970), on the basis of the difficulty of ascertaining whether the dividing cells were neuronal or non-neuronal. Other authors offered the hypothesis that multipotential cells "may be diverted into a variety of mature cells according to the type of stimulus they receive" (Zaimis, 1972, p. 68), or that the apparent hyperplastic effects may result from the "decreased number of normally developmental programmed cell death" (Herrup et al., 1974, p. 382). Neither of these two alternative mechanisms, however, was the object of studies which would provide convincing evidence for their implication in determining the final size of the nerve cell population in experimental and control ganglia.

We reinvestigated this problem in pulse labeling experiments performed in the first postnatal week in NGF-treated and control mice and rats. Tritiated thymidine was injected at day 3, 4 or 5. Since the labeled nucleotide remains available for only 1–3 hr, only the nuclei of sympathetic or other non-neuronal cell which had engaged in DNA synthesis at the time of the injection of [^{3}H]thymidine, will be heavily labeled in ganglia examined at later developmental stages (depending on whether this was the final division or the cell divided again before undergoing differentiation). Autoradiographic studies performed in two-week-old mice and rats (a time when neuronal cells differ by virtue of their larger size and certain specific morphological features, from satellite cells), showed a marked increase in heavily labeled nerve cells in the experimental ganglia. This gives convincing support to the hypothesis submitted earlier of a direct NGF effect on mitotic activity in sympathetic nerve cell precursors (Menesini Chen et al., unpublished results).

NGF EFFECTS ON DIFFERENTIATING SYMPATHETIC NERVE CELLS

The growth response of sympathetic nerve cells to the salivary NGF prior to their establishment of synaptic connections with end organs, and the attainment of the status of fully differentiated cells, has been the main object of studies on NGF-target cell interaction ever since this effect was first described in 1960 (Levi-Montalcini and Booker). It is sufficient to recall here that daily injection of 10 μg/g of body weight of NGF in neonatal rodents for a two-week period results in a volume increase in the superior cervical ganglia (evidence was obtained that all other sympathetic ganglia of the para- and prevertebral chains undergo the same increase) of 6–9 times that of control ganglia. The considerable fluctuation in the degree of enlargement produced by NGF treatment depends on the purity and potency of the NGF preparation, as well as on the length of the treatment. In recent studies, volume determination of the SCG in rats injected with NGF from the day of birth to the end of the third week showed that the ganglia were 10 times larger than those of control littermates (Aloe et al., 1976).

The most relevant features of the growth response studied at the ultrastructural level are: massive increase in neurotubules and neurofilaments which fill all available space in the cell cytoplasm; rise in free and membrane-bound ribosomes, and marked enlargement of the Golgi complex (Angeletti et al., 1971; Levi-Montalcini et al., 1968). Metabolic studies performed mainly in vitro, gave evidence for increases in RNA, protein and lipid syntheses and glucose utilization (Angeletti et al., 1968). The stimulatory effect of NGF on sympathetic nerve cells has also been demonstrated for the pathway which distinguishes their functional activity, i.e., the synthesis of the adrenergic neurotransmitter itself. Studies of the enzymes of the noradrenaline (NA) pathway by Thoenen et al. showed, in fact, that tyrosine hydroxylase activity is 15–20-fold greater in NGF-treated ganglia with a concomitant 3–4-fold apparent increase in specific activity of this key enzyme in the NA synthetic pathway (Thoenen et al., 1971). The total content of NA in sympathetic ganglia was found in earlier studies to be greatly increased by NGF treatment (Crain and Wiegrand, 1961).

It has become customary to describe the plurifold structural and biochemical effects elicited by NGF under the general term of "trophic effects", a designation which does not do full justice to the role of NGF in the life of sympathetic nerve cells. Evidence that this protein molecule not only enhances the differentiation of immature nerve cells and the maintenance of fully differentiated sympathetic neurons, but also is endowed with a much more important and vital function in the life of these cells (particularly during their early developmental stages) will be presented in a following section. Another much less extensively explored aspect of the NGF-sympathetic nerve cell interactions, namely, a directing role of NGF on growing adrenergic nerve fibers, will be considered here since it provides evidence for a much debated, and generally refuted, property of developing nerve fibers to respond to chemical signals issued by end organs during neurogenesis.

The neurotropic role of NGF

The early findings that sympathetic nerve fibers hyperneurotize the viscera of chick embryos bearing transplants of mouse sarcomas 180 or 37, and that a contingent of these fibers gains access inside the veins of the host, was taken as indicative of a neurotropic effect of this factor which at that time was not yet identified (Levi-Montalcini, 1952; Levi-Montalcini and Hamburger, 1953). Experiments performed two decades later, with the much more highly purified salivary NGF, provided what seems to be more compelling evidence for such an effect. In view of the interest of these findings, which have a direct bearing on one of the most important and still unsolved problems of developmental neurobiology, namely, the role of chemical signals in the formation of neuronal circuits, we shall consider in some detail the results of both in vitro and in vivo experiments.

Studies on the in vitro directing role of NGF on sensory and sympathetic nerve fibers

The problem of a possible chemotaxic effect of NGF was explored by Charlwood et al. (1972) by comparing the length and the pattern of nerve fiber outgrowth from sensory ganglia of 8-day chick embryos cultured on collagen in liquid medium, in the presence of a localized NGF source. For this purpose a glass capillary, filled with an aqueous NGF solution, was fixed horizontally on the bottom of the culture dishes, with the open tip at 2 mm distance from the ganglia. In control experiments the capillary was filled with heat-inactivated NGF or with saline solution. Fibers emerging from the side of the ganglia facing the active NGF source were markedly longer and denser than from other sides and a number of fibers even gained access to the inside of the capillary. These results were considered as being indicative of an orientating effect produced by a NGF concentration gradient. More extensive and detailed studies (Chamley et al., 1973; Chamley and Dowel, 1975) provided additional evidence for an in vitro NGF neurotropic effect. Sympathetic ganglia from midterm to two-day-old rats were cultured in modified Rose chambers between explants of normally densely innervated tissues such as vas deferens and atrium, or normally sparsely innervated tissues such as kidneys, adrenal medulla, uterus, ureter and lung. Nerve fibers grew more readily and in larger number towards the first than towards the second set of explants. The hypothesis that this differential axonal growth is due to attraction by a specific chemical substance received support from the demonstration that NGF is present at higher levels in densely innervated than in sparsely innervated tissues (Johnson et al., 1971), and that the same NGF is synthetized and released in vitro by tissues such as the iris, which is characterized by a dense adrenergic nerve plexus (Johnson et al., 1972).

An in vivo NGF neurotropic effect

The experiments to be reported below were not aimed at the study of possible NGF neurotropic effects. They were prompted by the report of Swedish investigators that intracerebrally injected NGF enhances regenerative growth and profuse branching from axotomized monoaminergic neurons located in the cerebrospinal axis (Bjerre et al., 1973). No evidence, however, was ever produced by these or other investigators for a growth-promoting effect of NGF on monoamine-containing neurons located in the CNS. In order to study this problem, we injected NGF daily with a micropipette inserted through the soft head tissues into the rhombencephalon of newborn rats for a 7–10-day period at 20 µg/g/body weight, while littermates received the same amount of physiological saline solution. The brain and spinal cord, with attached cephalic and spinal roots, sensory and sympathetic ganglia, were dissected out in both groups at the end of the injection period, processed according to the histofluorescence technique, sectioned serially and examined under the ultraviolet microscope. The results to be considered below are based on the study of 200 experimental and 200 control rats (Levi-Montalcini et al., 1974a; Menesini Chen, unpublished data).

All experimental cases showed markedly larger and more intensely fluorescent sympathetic ganglia than controls and large and strongly fluorescent fiber bundles in the dorsal funiculi of the spinal cord and in the lateral and central aspects of the medulla oblongata. This latter finding seemed at first to lend support to the hypothesis of a growth effect elicited by NGF on the central monoamine neurons. Comparative studies of the locus coeruleus and other smaller noradrenergic cell aggregates in the brain stem of experimental and control littermates showed, however, no apparent size differences in these centers. Also, there was no topographical relationship between the fluorescent fiber bundles and the monoamine neurons of the locus coeruleus and other nuclei. The origin of these fibers from sympathetic ganglia became apparent from the inspection of the entire neural tube and adjacent structures.

Fibers emerging from these ganglia, and easily recognizable as adrenergic fibers on account of their intense green fluorescence, invaded the spinal roots in large numbers. Those which entered the ventral roots innervated blood vessels in the choroid and subarachnoid space in much larger number than in controls. An even more striking deviation from normality was apparent in dorsal roots. These roots are barely discernible in controls under the ultraviolet illumination due to two exceedingly thin fluorescent fiber bundles lining the non-fluorescent sensory fibers, which form the main bulk of the roots. In NGF-injected animals, they appear instead intensely fluorescent as a result of the large number of noradrenergic fibers which enter these roots soon after their emergence from the adjacent sympathetic ganglia (Fig. 1c). The fluorescent fibers run across the sensory ganglia, where they lose their compactness and spread all over the neuronal cell population; they reassemble again as they leave the ganglia and enter into the spinal cord, where they take up a position in the posterior and lateral funiculi (Fig. 1d). Serial studies of the entire spinal cord and adjacent ganglia showed the same features at all levels, as illustrated in Fig. 2. Once inside the spinal cord the fluorescent fiber bundles become ascendant and reach the rostral cervical levels and the brain stem, where they are joined by other adrenergic fibers entering into the neuronal tube with the cephalic nerves. The origin of these later fibers was traced to the superior cervical ganglion. All along their course in the posterior and lateral funiculi, large collaterals or stem fibers detach from the main ascendant fiber tracts and enter deeply in the neural tube in close apposition to blood vessels. A similar system is not apparent in controls (Figs. 1a, b and 2).

At the level of the brain stem, the adrenergic fiber tract (which in the spinal cord formed a unique dorsolateral system) segregates into two dorsolateral and ventrolateral funiculi, which decrease progressively in size. They end a short distance from the locus coeruleus without, however, establishing connections either with it or with adjacent fluorescent or non-fluorescent systems (Figs. 2 and 3). Discontinuation of the intracerebral NGF injections results in the progressive fading away and complete disappearance of these fiber bundles; a result which suggests that these fibers do not belong, nor find acceptance in the CNS, where they are ignored as intruders by intrinsic neuronal systems. The same fiber tracts persist, however, indefinitely if NGF is continuously supplied by either intracerebral or even the systemic route. It is of interest in fact to note that, while subcutaneous NGF injections do not enable the penetration of adrenergic fibers inside the neural tube, they do permit their survival once this

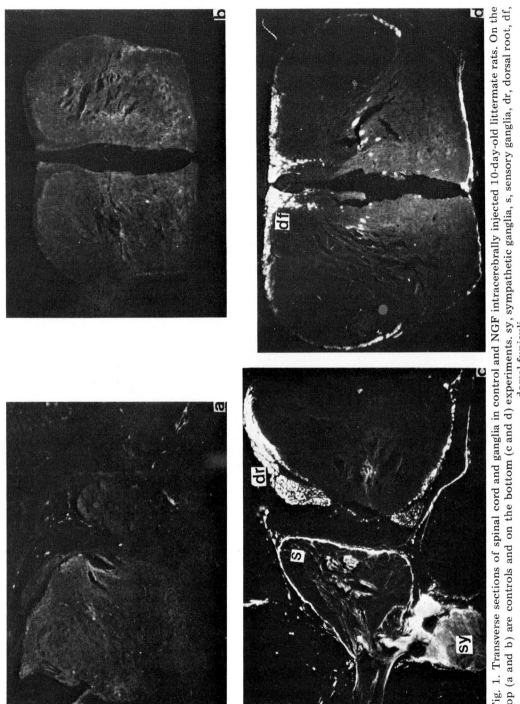

Fig. 1. Transverse sections of spinal cord and ganglia in control and NGF intracerebrally injected 10-day-old littermate rats. On the top (a and b) are controls and on the bottom (c and d) experiments. sy, sympathetic ganglia, s, sensory ganglia, dr, dorsal root, df, dorsal funiculi.

244

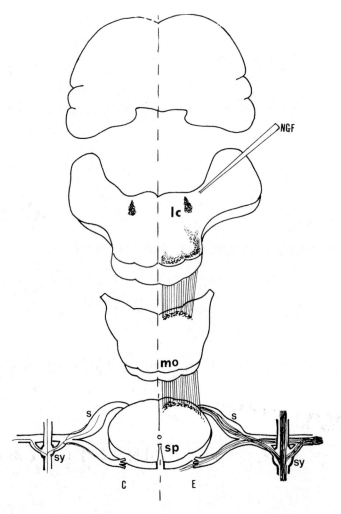

Fig. 2 Diagrammatic representation of sympathetic fiber bundles which enter into the spinal cord and medulla oblongata from adjacent sympathetic ganglia in intracerebrally NGF injected neonatal rats. Left half: control (C). Right half: experimental (E) case. NGF, site of injection of NGF into the floor of the fourth ventricle; lc, locus coeruleus; mo, medulla oblongata; sp, spinal cord; s, sensory ganglia; sy, sympathetic ganglia. Sympathetic fibers run across the sensory ganglion and enter into the neural tube with the dorsal roots.

system has come into existence in NGF intracerebrally injected neonatal rats. In the confined area of the dorsal funiculi and lateral fiber tracts, the adrenergic sympathetic system persists as an apparently non-functional system, as long as the cells of origin in the sympathetic ganglia are supplied with exogenous NGF. Studies to be reported in detail elsewhere provided evidence for the presence of considerable amounts of NGF inside the neural tube, even after discontinuation of the intracerebral injections. This would support the hypothesis that the sympathetic fibers were being routed inside the CNS by a NGF diffusion gradient. The problem whether the "NGF trail"

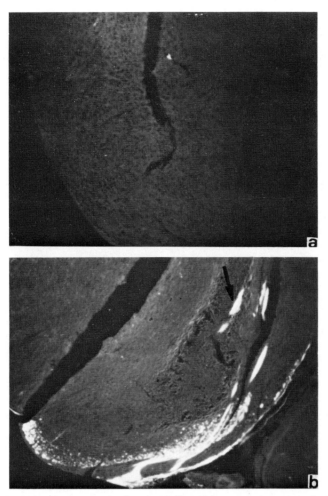

Fig. 3. Ventrolateral sections of the medulla oblongata in control (a) and NGF intracerebrally injected 10-day-old rats (b). Histofluorescence technique. Some large fibers enter deeply into the medulla oblongata (arrow) together with blood vessels.

results from binding of this molecule to a substrate or rather from NGF trapped inside the dense texture of the neural tube but free from connections with endogenous nerve structures or supporting cells, is now under investigation.

NGF EFFECTS ON FULLY DIFFERENTIATED SYMPATHETIC NEURONS

Evidence that the fully differentiated sympathetic nerve cells undergo a marked hypertrophy following NGF injections in adult rodents was already presented in 1960 (Levi-Montalcini and Booker, 1960). A 1975 report that the size of mature nerve cells is never exceeded in NGF-treated adult mice, can only be attributed either to the use of a weak and inefficient NGF preparation, or to a too short treatment time (Banks et al., 1975). The size difference in NGF-treated and control sympathetic nerve cells of the superior cervical ganglia of adult rats is illustrated in Fig. 4. Here we shall consider two of the most recent studies of NGF effects in the mature sympathetic neurons, since they focus attention upon problems of general interest, namely, the ability of the fully differentiated intact nerve cell to produce additional collateral branches and its competence to respond to axonal or non-axonal mediated chemical signals.

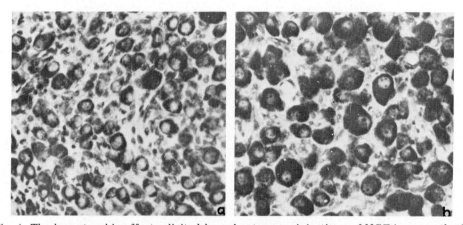

Fig. 4. The hypertrophic effects elicited by subcutaneous injections of NGF in sympathetic nerve cells of adult mice. (a): transverse section of superior cervical ganglion of 45-day-old mouse. (b) transverse section of superior cervical ganglion of littermate mouse injected daily from the 33rd to the 45th day with NGF at doses of 7 μg/g of body weight (× 384).

Collateral sprouting and hyperneurotization of end organs upon NGF injections in adult mice

Systemic NGF injections in young and adult mice call forth a marked increase in the density and fluorescence of the adrenergic plexuses in terminal organs, and in a parallel increase in endogenous NA levels (Bjerre et al., 1975). The hypothesis submitted by these authors, that this effect is due to collateral sprouting from the intact adrenergic neurons under the action of exogenous NGF, seems most plausible and is in line with previous observations on collateral sprouting from nerve cells confronted with denervated peripheral fields (Raisman and Field, 1973). Although in the present situation the periphery has not been modified, the metabolic and synthetic cell processes have been markedly enhanced by NGF which has gained access to the cells, either through accumulation in the peripheral end organs or by direct binding to cell membrane receptors. These results prove that the growth potentialities of sympathetic nerve cells do not materialize in full in the adult organism but can be reactivated and enhanced when additional fields of innervation are made available or sympathetic nerve cells are supplied with excessive doses of NGF. The similarity of the effects produced by these two different procedures suggests that in both instances the cells respond to the same agent whether artificially injected or naturally released by end organs. Further evidence in favor of this hypothesis will be presented in the last two sections.

The selective retrograde NGF transport in the fully differentiated sympathetic nerve cell

The demonstration of the retrograde axonal transport of labeled amino acids along a nerve trunk from peripheral muscles (Kerkut et al., 1967) and of the accumulation of fluorochrome-labeled albumin in spinal motor neurons following injections of this protein into the gastrocnemius of suckling mice (Kristensson, 1970), suggested that a retrograde axonal transport system may fulfill the role of conveying chemical messages from end organs back to the innervating nerve cells (Kristensson and Olsson, 1971). Studies performed in these last two years with iodine-labeled NGF have provided strong evidence in favor of this hypothesis, and at the same time have indicated that NGF is the trophic factor released by end organs to be selectively taken up by sympathetic nerve endings. The selectivity of the uptake and transport system of labeled NGF from end organs to the cells of origin in the superior cervical ganglia was documented in an extensive series of investigations in which the kinetics of transport and of accumulation of [^{125}I] NGF in the cell perikarya were studied with different methodologies and under different experimental conditions (Hendry et al., 1974a, b; Iversen et al., 1975; Paravicini et al., 1975; Stoeckel et al., 1974, 1976). Other protein molecules which share many physicochemical properties in common with NGF, but do not display any biological function on the sympathetic nerve cells, are not retrogradely transported into the cell bodies. Heat or chemically inactivated NGF preparations likewise lose this property (Hendry et al., 1974a). Additional evidence for the functional role of the NGF (moiety), which reaches the cell through retrograde axonal transport, was obtained in determination studies of the level of tyrosine hydroxylase in the superior cervical ganglia following unilateral injections of labeled NGF into two of its main end organs: the eye and the submaxillary salivary glands (Paravicini et al., 1975). The decidedly higher level of this enzyme in the ganglion of the injected side provides perhaps the most convincing proof of the biological role of exogenous NGF, and of its retrograde transport from end organs to the innervating sympathetic cells.

A DUAL NGF TRANSPORT SYSTEM

The demonstration of an axonal retrograde transport of NGF from peripheral tissues to the sympathetic cell perikarya gives strong support to the hypothesis that this molecule mediates trophic effects of end organs on the nerve cells which provide their innervation, and that it does so through the highly selective transport system represented by the nerve fiber. These findings do not, however, exclude the alternative way of access through the membrane which envelops the cell perikaryon. In fact this is the way of course in which hormones and other humoral factors gain access to their target *non-neuronal* cells.

Evidence that embryonic sympathetic cells are receptive to the growth promoting activity of NGF, even before developing an axonal process has already been presented (p. 239), and will be considered again in the last section dealing with the response to NGF of surgically and chemically axotomized sympathetic nerve cells. Studies performed in these last two years (Hendry and Iversen, 1973) confirmed earlier reports on the presence of NGF in circulating blood (Caramia et al., 1962; Levi-Montalcini and Booker, 1960), a finding which suggests that this molecule may reach its target cell also through humoral channels, namely, via the fluid which bathes the cell surface. In favor of this hypothesis is the unequivocal evidence obtained by several groups of the presence of specific NGF binding sites on the surface of NGF target cells: the embryonic sensory cells and the embryonic or mature sympathetic nerve cells (Banerjee et al., 1973; Frazier et al., 1973; Herrup and Shooter, 1973; Levi-Montalcini et al., 1974b; Snyder et al., 1974). A neoplastic cell, the neuroblastoma cell, which shares the origin and other properties in common with the sympathetic cell, also possesses specific NGF receptors on its outer membrane (Revoltella et al., 1974). The physiological role of NGF membrane binding sites in the NGF-target cell interaction is also indicated by the demonstration that the affinity constant for binding (about 0.2 nM) is similar to the plasma levels of NGF (Banerjee et al., 1975). The problem of whether NGF reaches the target cell solely through retrograde axonal transport or, under given physiological or experimental conditions, also through humoral channels, will be considered again in the next and last section.

NGF EFFECTS ON CHEMICALLY OR SURGICALLY AXOTOMIZED SYMPATHETIC NERVE CELLS

An outstanding difference between immature and mature nerve cells is their differential response to deprivation of their peripheral field of innervation achieved either through ablation of these fields prior to their innervation or through axotomy of the growing or fully developed axon. Differentiating nerve cells prevented from establishing connections with their end organs, by one or the other procedure, undergo irreversible regressive changes leading to their degeneration and death. Mature nerve cells, on the other hand, suffer only moderate regressive changes which disappear as soon as the lesioned axons have regenerated and re-established connections with their end organs. These different effects, long known to neuroembryologists (Hamburger, 1934), came even more sharply into focus in experiments performed some years ago with 6-hydroxydopamine (6-OHDA), a dopamine derivative which produces destruction of adrenergic nerve endings in both mature and immature sympathetic nerve cells. The result of this treatment is a temporary block of the transmission of the nerve impulse from the fully differentiated nerve cells to end organs. Return of function ensues following regeneration of the chemically lesioned adrenergic ending during a 6–8 week period (Thoenen and Tranzer, 1968). Injections of 6-OHDA in newborn rodents produce, instead, irreversible damage and destruction of 95% of the sympathetic nerve cell population. This process, which became known as chemical sympathectomy (Angeletti and Levi-Montalcini, 1970), seemed at first to indicate that the much more severe effects called forth by 6-OHDA in the immature sympathetic nerve cells as compared with the fully differentiated neuron, were due to a more efficient amine group in the former than in the latter. This would account for the rapid diffusion of the noxious agent from the nerve ending to the cell perikarya of the immature but not of the mature cells (Thoenen, 1971).

More recent studies have called for a revision of this hypothesis. It was shown that the simultaneous treatment of newborn rodents with 6-OHDA and NGF results in the compartmentalization of the two opposite effects: on the one hand, destruction of adrenergic nerve endings to the same extent as caused by injection of the dopamine derivative alone; and on the other hand, hypertrophic and hyperplastic changes of the neuronal cell population comparable to those called forth by NGF (Levi-Montalcini et al., 1975). In addition to the increase in size and number of nerve cells, the dual combined treatment results in a volume increase of sympathetic ganglia much more pronounced in fact than that of ganglia submitted to the treatment of NGF alone. At 21 days the superior cervical ganglia of rats injected since birth with NGF plus 6-OHDA are about 30 times larger than controls, and 2·5 times larger than those of littermates injected with NGF alone (Fig. 5) (Aloe et al., 1976). This paradoxical volume increase is due only in part to the already mentioned hypertrophic and hyperplastic effects called forth by NGF in nerve cells. To a much larger extent it is due to massive de novo production of axonal material which accumulates inside the ganglion in the form of tangled masses of nerve fibers, and around the ganglion as a dense fibrillar capsule which encircles the nerve cell population and increases progressively in thickness in animals submitted to longer treatments. Ultrastructural studies showed that nerve fibers agglomerated in disorganized bundles inside the ganglia, or else stacked in orderly superimposed layers within the capsule, are exceedingly thin fibers of 0·1–0·2 μm in cross-section.

These findings suggest that adrenergic nerve cells prevented from establishing connections with end organs by the destructive effects of 6-OHDA of the nerve end terminals, but geared to a higher than normal metabolic activity by NGF, produce an extraordinarily large amount of neurofibrillar material which is routed into collateral branches along the entire course of the axon. Evidence for the excellent state and enhanced function of cells submitted to this dual treatment was obtained from determinations of tyrosine hydroxylase in ganglia of littermates injected with 6-OHDA and NGF, versus NGF alone. The enzyme level was much higher in ganglia of the first than of the second group, a result of considerable interest since it proves that NGF calls forth an increase in the synthesis of the neurotransmitter even when the release of NA is impeded by the destruction of the adrenergic endings (Levi-Montalcini et al., 1975).

Effects similar to those produced by chemical axotomy were elicited by surgical transection of postganglionic roots of the superior cervical ganglia combined with simultaneous NGF injections in newborn mice and rats. Surgical axotomy alone, performed in the first few postnatal days, results in massive death of the immature sympathetic nerve cells (Hendry, 1975a, b). Supply of exogenous NGF calls forth a growth response very similar to that described

250

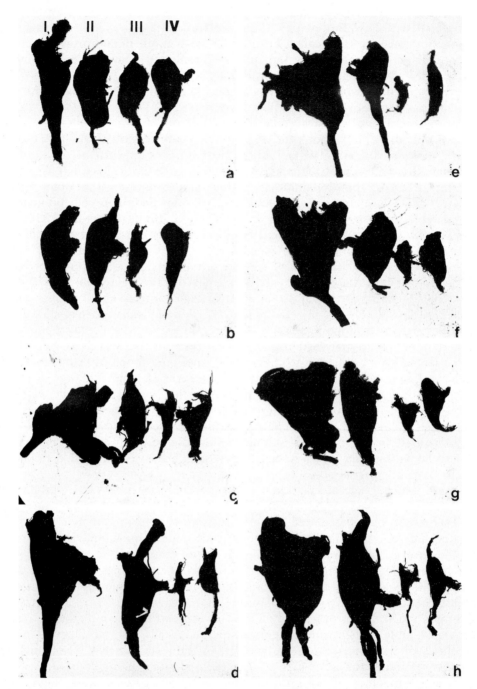

Fig. 5. Whole mounts of superior cervical ganglia of rats sacrificed respectively at 4 days (a), 6 days (b), 8 days (c), 10 days (d), 12 days (e), 19 days (f), 21 days (g) and 26 days (h). Type of treatment is indicated in (a) with roman figures: I, NGF and 6-OHDA; II, NGF; III, 6-OHDA; IV, saline. a and b × 12; c–h × 8 (From Aloe et al., 1975.)

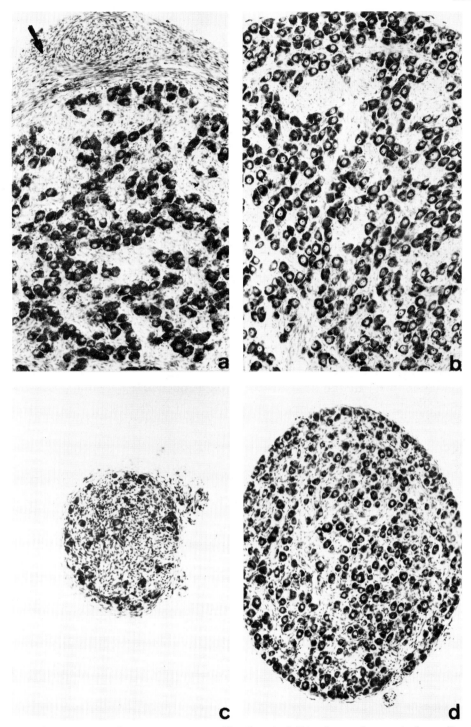

Fig. 6. Transverse sections at same magnification (x 240) of superior cervical ganglia of 32-day-old littermate rats injected daily since birth with 6-OHDA and NGF (a), NGF alone (b), 6-OHDA (c) or physiological solution (d). Toluidine stain. Note the fibrillar capsule in a indicated with arrow and the size increase of nerve cells in both sections (a and b) as compared to control. c and d show the largest sections of atrophic (c) and control (d) ganglia.

above for ganglia submitted to dual NGF and 6-OHDA treatment. Electron microscopic studies of the neuronal cell population and of nerve fibers showed that the similarity between the effects called forth by the two combined treatments also extends to the subcellular level (Aloe and Levi-Montalcini, unpublished data).

The similarity of chemically and of surgically axotomized nerve cells in their growth response to NGF suggests that, in both instances, the NGF molecule produces its effects through binding to the membrane receptors. The severe lesions which develop at the distal end of the axon make it most unlikely that NGF can gain access, and then be retrogradely transported to the cell perikarya. This leaves as the only alternative its access through the intact cell surface. It seems conceivable, therefore, that both transport systems co-exist but that one or the other is utilized preferentially at different times, or under different physiological or experimental conditions during the life cycle of the sympathetic nerve cell. When the most recently developed, and possibly most efficient retrograde transport system, is abolished by means of surgical or chemical procedures, the alternate route provided by the membrane receptors remains available and permits not only survival but even overgrowth of cells supplied with exogenous NGF. Discontinuation of the NGF and 6-OHDA treatment results in the progressive atrophy of the axotomized nerve cells. The entire nerve cell population is wiped out within a few days (Aloe and Levi-Montalcini, unpublished results). These findings testify to the unique role of this protein molecule in the life of the sympathetic nerve cell, whether it gains access through the axonal ending or through the membrane receptors. The evidence is all in favor of the hypothesis that the trophic functions displayed by the peripheral end organs are due to the release of this factor.

CONCLUDING REMARKS

It was the aim of this article to comment upon those aspects of the NGF-sympathetic nerve cell interaction which give evidence for the multiple and diversified roles played by this molecule in the life of the sympathetic nerve cell, from its early inception right through full maturity.

In reviewing the work on NGF in his 1970 essay on developmental neurobiology (p. 233), Jacobson wrote: "To state that a substance of such great potency must surely have an important biological function is merely a declaration of faith". This assertion (which was hardly justified even 5 years ago, when the evidence for a biological function for NGF was already apparent to most investigators and outside observers) would have been appropriate two decades earlier, when we were indeed puzzled by the magnitude and strangeness of the growth effects elicited by two mouse sarcomas on the sympathetic system of the developing chick embryo. The faith referred to by Jacobson was at that time the driving force which directed all the studies, long before the identification of the growth promoting factor as a protein molecule made possible a more precise approach to the problem of studying and defining its biological function.

It will be recalled that the sympathetic nerve cell in the not too remote past, had already moved to the forefront of research, when it provided evidence for the chemical basis of the synaptic transmission of the nerve impulse. More recently, the same cell offered an ideal object for exploring the sequence of events leading to the biosynthesis, release and inactivation of the neuro-transmitter. Without this most favorable model, it is likely that much information of utmost importance for the understanding of nerve cell function would never have been attained. The belief that the sympathetic nerve cell may play an equally important role in the field of neurogenesis is based upon results already achieved, thanks to the discovery of NGF and of its interaction with this nerve cell, which mimics to a remarkable degree the interaction between the same cell and its end organs.

Thus, the trophic function of these organs and the directing role of humoral factors in the building of neuronal circuits and establishment of synaptic connections, two vague concepts with no clear-cut evidence in favor of the former nor decisive proof against the latter, are now amenable to a more precise experimental analysis than in the past. An equally valuable contribution of these studies is to have broadened the field of investigation, and erased the demarcation lines between problems in neurogenesis and in neurobiology, in this way making available more sophisticated tools and techniques, currently used in neighboring fields, for the study of the developing nervous system.

In closing with another "declaration of faith", we believe that in spite of the large unfilled gaps in our knowledge of the NGF-target cell interaction, this system is likely to play an increasingly important role in the study of structure and function of nerve cells and neuronal circuits.

ACKNOWLEDGEMENT

This work was partially supported by grants from the National Institutes of Health (NS-03777 and MH-24604).

REFERENCES

Aloe, L., Mugnaini, E. and Levi-Montalcini, R. (1975) Light electron microscopic studies on the excessive growth of sympathetic ganglia in rats injected daily from birth with 6-OHDA and NGF. *Arch. ital. Biol.*, 113: 326–353.

Angeletti, P.U. and Levi-Montalcini, R. (1970) Sympathetic nerve cell destruction in newborn mammals by 6-hydroxydopamine. *Proc. nat. Acad. Sci. (Wash.)*, 65: 114–121.

Angeletti, P.U., Levi-Montalcini, R. and Calissano, P. (1968) The nerve growth factor: chemical properties and metabolic effects. *Advanc. Enzymol.*, 31: 51–75.

Angeletti, P.U., Levi-Montalcini, R. and Caramia, F. (1971) Ultrastructural changes in sympathetic neurons of newborn and adult mice treated with nerve growth factor. *J. ultrastruct. Res.*, 36: 24–36.

Banerjee, S.P., Snyder, S.H., Cuatrecasas, P. and Greene, L.A. (1973) Binding of nerve growth factor receptor in sympathetic ganglia. *Proc. nat. Acad. Sci. (Wash.)*, 70: 2519–2523.

Banerjee, S.P., Cuatrecasas, P. and Snyder, S.H. (1975) Nerve growth factor receptor binding. *J. biol. Chem.*, 259: 1427–1433.

Banks, B.E.C., Charlwood, K.A., Edwards, D.C., Vernon, C.A. and Walter, S.J. (1975) Effects of nerve growth factor from mouse salivary glands and snake venom on the sympathetic ganglia of neonatal and developing mice. *J. Physiol. (Lond.)*, 247: 289–298.

Bjerre, B. and Björklund, A. (1973) The production of catecholamine-containing cells in vitro by young chick embryos. Effects of nerve growth factor (NGF) and its antiserum. *Neurobiology*, 3: 140–161.

Bjerre, B., Björklund, A. and Stenevi, U. (1973) Stimulation of growth of new axonal sprouts from lesioned monoamine neurons in adult rat brain by nerve growth factor. *Brain Res.*, 60: 171–176.

Bjerre, B., Björklund, A., Mobley, W. and Rosengreen, E. (1975) Short- and long-term effects of nerve growth factor on the sympathetic nervous system in the adult mouse. *Brain Res.*, 94: 261–277.

Blaschko, H. (1972) In *Catecholamines*, H. Blaschko and E. Muscholl (Eds.), Springer Verlag, Berlin, pp. 1–15.

Bueker, E.D. (1948) Implantation of tumors in the hind limb field of the embryonic chick and developmental response of the lumbo-sacral nervous system. *Anat. Rec.*, 102: 369–390.

Burnstock, G. and Costa, M. (1975) *Adrenergic neurons: their organization, function and development in the peripheral nervous system.* Chapman and Hall, London.

Caramia, F., Angeletti, P.U. and Levi-Montalcini, R. (1962) Experimental analysis of the mouse submaxillary salivary gland in relationship to its nerve growth factor content. *Endocrinology*, 70: 915–922.

Chamely, J.H. and Dowel, J.J. (1975) Specificity of nerve fiber "attraction" to autonomic effector organs in tissue culture. *Cell Res.*, 90: 1–7.

Chamley, J.H., Goller, J. and Burnstock, G. (1973) Selective growth of sympathetic nerve fibers to explants of normally densely innervated autonomic effector organs in tissue culture. *Develop. Biol.*, 31: 362–379.

Charlwood, K.A., Lamont, D.M. and Banks, B.E.C. (1972) In *Nerve Growth Factor and its Antiserum,* E. Zaimis and J. Knight (Eds.), Athlone Press, London, pp. 102–107.

Cohen, S. (1958) In *Chemical Basis of Development*, W.D. McElroy and B. Glass (Eds.), The Johns Hopkins Press, Baltimore, Md., pp. 665–676.

Cohen, S. and Levi-Montalcini, R. (1956) A nerve growth stimulating factor isolated from snake venom. *Proc. nat. Acad. Sci. (Wash.)*, 42: 571–574.

Cohen, S., Levi-Montalcini, R. and Hamburger, V. (1954) A nerve growth stimulating factor isolated from sarcomas 37 and 180. *Proc. nat. Acad. Sci. (Wash.)*, 40: 1014–1018.

Crain, S.M. and Wiegand, R.G. (1961) Catecholamine levels of mouse sympathetic ganglia following hypertrophy produced by salivary nerve growth factor. *Proc. soc. exp. Biol. (N.Y.)*, 107: 663–665.

Frazier, W.A., Forrest Boyd, L. and Bradshaw, R.A. (1973) Interaction of nerve growth factor with surface membrane: biological competence of insolubilized nerve growth factor. *Proc. nat. Acad. Sci (Wash.)*, 70: 2931–2935.

Hamburger, V. (1934) The effects of wing bud extirpation on the development of the central nervous system in chick embryos. *J. exp. Zool.*, 68: 449–494.

Hendry, I.A. (1975a) The response of adrenergic neurons to axotomy and nerve growth factor. *Brain Res.*, 94: 87–97.

Hendry, I.A. (1975b) The effects of axotomy on the development of the rat superior cervical ganglion. *Brain Res.*, 90: 235–244.

Hendry, I.A. and Iversen, L.L. (1973) Changes in tissue and plasma concentrations of nerve growth factor following removal of the submaxillary glands in adult mice and their effects on the sympathetic nervous system. *Nature (Lond.)*, 243: 500–504.

Hendry, I.A. and Thoenen, H. (1974) Changes of enzyme pattern in the sympathetic nervous system of adult mice after submaxillary gland removal; response to exogenous nerve growth factor. *J. Neurochem.*, 22: 999–1004.

Hendry, I.A., Stach, R. and Herrup, K. (1974a) Characteristics of the retrograde axonal transport system for nerve growth factor in the sympathetic nervous system. *Brain Res.*, 82: 117–128.

Hendry, I.A., Stoeckel, K., Thoenen, H. and Iversen, I.L. (1974b) Retrograde axonal transport of the nerve growth factor. *Brain Res.*, 68: 103–121.

Herrup, K. and Shooter, E.M. (1973) Properties of the nerve growth factor receptor of avian dorsal root ganglia. *Proc. nat. Acad. Sci. (Wash.)*, 70: 3884–3888.

Herrup, K., Stickgold, R. and Shooter, E.M. (1974) The role of the nerve growth factor in the development of sensory and sympathetic ganglia. *Ann. N.Y. Acad. Sci.*, 228: 381–392.

Hogue Angeletti, R. (1971) Immunological relatedness of nerve growth factors. *Brain Res.*, 25: 424–427.

Hogue Angeletti, R. and Bradshaw, R.A. (1971) Nerve growth factor from mouse submaxillary gland: amino acids sequence. *Proc. nat. Acad. Sci. (Wash.)*, 68: 2417–2420.

Hogue Angeletti, R., Angeletti, P.U. and Levi-Montalcini, R. (1973) In *Humoral Control of Growth and Differentiation, Vol. 1*, J. LoBue and A.S. Gordon (Eds.), Academic Press, New York, pp. 229–247.

Hogue Angeletti, R., Frazier, W.A., Jacobs, J.W., Niall, R.D. and Bradshaw, R.A. (1976) Purification, characterization and partial amino acid sequence of nerve growth factor from cobra venom. *Biochemistry*, in press.

Iversen, L.L., Stoeckel, K. and Thoenen, H. (1975) Autoradiographic studies of the retrograde transport of nerve growth factor in mouse sympathetic neurons. *Brain Res.*, 88: 37–43.

Jacobson, M. (1970) *Developmental Neurobiology*. Holt, Rinehart and Winston.

Johnson, D.G., Gordon, P. and Kopin, I.J. (1971) A sensitive radio-immunoassay for 7S nerve growth factor antigens in serum and tissues. *J. Neurochem.*, 18: 2355–2362.

Johnson, D.G., Silberstein, S.D., Hanbauer, I. and Kopin, I.J. (1972) The role of nerve growth factor in the ramification of sympathetic nerve fibers into the rat iris in organ culture. *J. Neurochem.*, 19: 2025–2029.

Kerkut, G.A., Shapira, A. and Walker, R.J. (1967) The transport of ^{14}C-labeled material from CNS-muscle along a nerve trunk. *Comp. Biochem. Physiol.*, 23: 729–748.

Kristensson, K. (1970) Transport of fluorescent protein tracer to peripheral nerves. *Acta neuropath. (Berl.)*, 16: 293–300.

Kristensson, K. and Olsson, Y. (1971) Retrograde axonal transport of protein. *Brain Res.*, 29: 363–365.

Levi-Montalcini, R. (1952) Effects of mouse tumor transplantation on the nervous system. *Ann. N.Y. Acad. Sci.*, 55: 330–343.

Levi-Montalcini, R. (1958) In *Chemical Basis of Development*, W.D. McElroy and B. Glass (Eds.), The Johns Hopkins Press, Baltimore, Md., pp. 646–664.

Levi-Montalcini, R. (1975) In *The Neurosciences: Paths of Discovery*, MIT Press, Cambridge, Mass., pp. 243–265.

Levi-Montalcini, R. and Booker, B. (1960) Excessive growth of the sympathetic ganglia evoked by a protein isolated from mouse salivary glands. *Proc. nat. Acad. Sci. (Wash.)*, 46: 373–384.

Levi-Montalcini, R. and Hamburger, V. (1951) Selective growth stimulating effect of mouse sarcoma on the sensory and sympathetic nervous system of the chick embryo. *J. exp. Zool.*, 116: 321–362.

Levi-Montalcini, R. and Hamburger, V. (1953) A diffusible agent of mouse sarcoma producing hyperplasia of sympathetic ganglia and hyperneurotization of the chick embryo. *J. exp. Zool.*, 123: 233–288.

Levi-Montalcini, R., Meyer, H. and Hamburger, V. (1954) In vitro experiments on the effects of mouse sarcomas 180 and 37 on the spinal and sympathetic ganglia of the chick embryo. *Cancer Res.*, 14: 49–57.

Levi-Montalcini, R., Caramia, F., Luse, S.A. and Angeletti, P.U. (1968) In vitro effects of the nerve growth factor on the fine structure of the sensory nerve cells. *Brain Res.*, 8: 347–362.

Levi-Montalcini, R., Chen, M.G. and Chen, J.S.(1974a) Effects of intracerebral NGF injections in newborn rodents. *Soc. Neurosci. 4th Annu. Meet., St. Louis, Mo.*, abstract, p. 305.

Levi-Montalcini, R., Revoltella, R. and Calissano, P. (1974b) In *Recent Progress in Hormone Research*, R.O. Greep (Ed.), Academic Press, New York, pp. 635–669.

Levi-Montalcini, R., Aloe, L., Mugnaini, E., Oesch, F. and Thoenen, H. (1975) Nerve growth factor induces volume increase and enhances tyrosine hydroxylase synthesis in chemically axotomized sympathetic ganglia of newborn rats. *Proc. nat. Acad. Sci. (Wash.)*, 72: 595–599.

Paravicini, U., Stoeckel, K. and Thoenen, H. (1975) Biological importance of retrograde axonal transport of nerve growth factor in adrenergic neurons. *Brain Res.*, 84: 279–291.

Raisman, G. and Field, P.M. (1973) A quantitative investigation of the development of collateral reinnervation after partial deafferentation of the septal nuclei. *Brain Res.*, 50: 241–264.

Revoltella, R., Bertolini, L., Pediconi, M. and Vigneti, E. (1974) Specific binding of nerve growth factor by murine C 1300 neuroblastoma cells. *J. exp. Med.*, 140: 437–451.

Server, A.C., Herrup, K. and Shooter, E.M. (1976) Comparison of the nerve growth factor proteins from cobra venom (*Naja naja*) and mouse submaxillary gland. *Biochemistry*, in press.

Snyder, S.H., Banerjee, S.P., Cuatrecasas, P. and Greene, L.A. (1974) In *Dynamics of Degeneration and Growth in Neurons*, K. Fuxe, L. Olson and Y. Zotterman (Eds.), Pergamon Press, Oxford, pp. 347–357.

Stoeckel, K. and Thoenen, H. (1975) Retrograde axonal transport of nerve growth factor: specificity and biological importance. *Brain Res.*, 85: 337–341.

Stoeckel, K., Paravicini, U. and Thoenen, H. (1974) Specificity of the retrograde axonal transport of nerve growth factor. *Brain Res.*, 76: 413–421.

Stoeckel, K., Guroff, G., Schwab, M. and Thoenen, H. (1976) The significance of retrograde axonal transport for the accumulation of systematically administered nerve growth factor (NGF) in the rat superior cervical ganglion. *Brain Res.*, in press.

Thoenen, H. (1971) In *6-Hydroxydopamine and Catecholamine Research*, T. Malmfors and H. Thoenen (Eds.), North-Holland Publ. Comp., Amsterdam, pp. 75–85.

Thoenen, H. and Tranzer, J.P. (1968) Chemical sympathectomy by selective destruction of adrenergic nerve endings with 6-hydroxydopamine. *Naunyn-Schmiedeberg's Arch. exp. Path. Pharmak.*, 261: 271–288.

Thoenen, H., Angeletti, P.U., Levi-Montalcini, R. and Kettler, R. (1971) Selective induction by nerve growth factor of tyrosine hydroxylase and dopamine β-hydroxylase in the rat superior cervical ganglia. *Proc. nat. Acad. Sci. (Wash.)*, 68: 1598–1602.

Wlodawer, A., Hodson, K.O. and Shooter, E.M. (1975) Crystallization of nerve growth factor from mouse submaxillary glands. *Proc. nat. Acad. Sci. (Wash.)*, 72: 777–779.

Zaimis, E. (1972) In *Nerve Growth Factor and its Antiserum*, E. Zaimis (Ed.), Athlone Press, London, pp. 59–70.

DISCUSSION

R.M. GAZE: You suggested that there is a release of this substance (NGF) which you injected into the brain. I would expect you to find diminishing concentrations of the substance in progressively posterior regions of the brain. Can you demonstrate this?

R. LEVI-MONTALCINI: As a first approach to this problem, we assayed cell-free homogenates of the entire neural tube and brain for the presence of NGF at time intervals after discontinuation of the treatment, and following repeated washing in order to remove free NGF. These experiments gave evidence for the presence of substantial amounts of bound NGF in the CNS of experimental but not of control animals. Studies now in progress are aimed at determining the NGF levels in different segments of the neural tube in NGF-injected rodents. I would expect, as you suggest, a decrease of these levels in a rostrocaudal direction, that is, at progressively longer distances from the site of injection.

R.M. GAZE: A second point is: do you think that this is mechanically going down between the fibers, or is it being transported inside axons?

R. LEVI-MONTALCINI: An NGF retrograde axonal transport has been demonstrated for sympathetic and sensory fibers, but there is no evidence that it also occurs in other axonal systems. It therefore seems unlikely that the injected NGF would be conveyed along the neural tube in this way, and more plausible is the alternative suggestion, viz, that NGF is transported in a rostrocaudal direction by the trail provided by nerve fibers of dorsal and lateral funiculi.

E.G. GRAY: A very exciting example of experimental chemotaxis! Presumably, if you put some now on the peripheral nerve you would also get the fibers to grow peripherally, as well as back into the central nervous system.

R. LEVI-MONTALCINI: The only evidence for a neurotropic effect produced by a peripheral circumscribed NGF source was obtained in early experiments of transplantation of mouse sarcomas into the body wall of chick embryos. The massive invasion of these two NGF-producing and releasing tumors, by sensory and sympathetic fibers of the host, was taken as being indicative of an NGF neurotropic effect. It is, however, much more difficult to obtain the same evidence with the purified salivary NGF, since one cannot prevent its diffusion into surrounding tissues. The CNS is secluded from other organs by the blood-brain barrier. Furthermore, its dense texture favors a slow diffusion of the NGF, but I agree with you that additional proof for an NGF neurotropic effect should come from the demonstration that sympathetic nerve fibers also converge towards a restricted NGF peripheral source. This demonstration has so far been obtained in vitro but not in vivo.

M.A. CORNER: Dr Balázs showed a novel experimental way of demonstrating the dependence of nerve cell differentiation, or maintenance, upon some kind of feedback from their target cells; namely, the experimental Purkinje cell reduction in the cerebellum, with a consequent loss of the granule cells. In an attempt to integrate some of the other known examples of dependence of nerve cell maintenance upon their end organs with what Dr. Levi-Montalcini talked about, concerning the possible *tropic* effect of NGF, I wonder if you cannot work towards the following working hypothesis: that the dependence of a given neuron upon the integrity of its end organ innervation is due to a similar type of NGF dependence, a *specific* NGF dependence for that particular type which has not yet been demonstrated, which is then in a retrograde way imposed upon the presynaptic neuron by its end organ. This gives at one and the same time a mechanism for explaining the trophic dependence as well as the "tropic" effect which was illustrated. Here you would have this substance upon which the neuron is ultimately dependent, also diffusing out and impregnating the substrate along a gradient, which would then assist fibers in finding the proper direction. With respect to the sympathetic neuron and its differentiation, if the foregoing were true, you would then expect that in the immunosympathectomy experiments the reason for the disappearance of the sympathetic nervous system would *not* be an effect operating upon the initial differentiation, but rather something analogous to the experiments of removal of the periphery. Thus, there would be an initial neuronal differentiation, and subsequently (because of the immunosympathectomy) a loss equivalent to that occurring when the target tissues are absent. How does this idea square with the facts?

R. LEVI-MONTALCINI: I agree with you that the trophic and tropic effects of the NGF molecule may possibly best be considered as two different aspects of the same stimulus-response system: the NGF and its target sympathetic nerve cell. You also submitted the hypothesis that the destructive effects produced by antibodies to the NGF molecule on the developing sympathetic nerve cells (immunosympathectomy) and those produced by removal of the peripheral field of innervation on the same immature nerve cells, may be due in both instances to depletion of NGF. In favor of this hypothesis is the finding that disruption of the normal connections of nerve fibers with their end organs, by surgical or chemical axotomy performed in neonatal rodents, calls forth the same destructive effects as does immunosympathectomy. In the case of surgical or chemical axotomy, the lethal effects are prevented by exogenous supply of NGF; these findings give additional support to the viewpoint that NGF is the trophic factor released by end organs.

M.A. CORNER: Concerning the "tropic" orienting pattern emerging from the NGF experiments, even if there were no peripheral orientation one way or the other, but rather some fibers going one way and some the other way, or even if most fibers were branching and going both ways, you would still see a tendency of some fibers to grow in the direction of the brain. Before one would really be very satisfied that this is a tropic effect, there would need to be an indication that already at the single fiber level there is preferential growth in that direction. Has that in fact been demonstrated? Secondly, what would be the extent to which, by altering the position in the brain where you inject the NGF, you can move this whole ingrowing pathway around at will?

R. LEVI-MONTALCINI: The massive penetration of sympathetic nerve fibers in the neural tube of neonatal rats, injected intracerebrally with NGF, does not represent a preferential distribution of these fibers into the spinal cord and brain stem, rather than in the peripheral tissues; but it does show an entirely novel pattern of nerve fiber outgrowth, which does not occur in controls nor in littermate rats injected systematically with NGF. These ectopic fiber bundles are reabsorbed as soon as the intracerebral injections are discontinued. It seems difficult, therefore, to conceive of their formation and intracentral location as being a case of chance, and not an oriented direction along an NGF diffusion gradient. However, I must admit that we still have not succeeded in changing the distribution of sympathetic nerve fibers inside the CNS by changing the site of injection of the NGF.

T.D. KERNELL: Have you tried to inject the NGF into the spinal cord?

R. LEVI-MONTALCINI: We did not try this, since it is difficult to inject into the spinal cord of newborn rodents in view of its very small size, and also in view of the fact that NGF would probably diffuse in a rostrocaudal and caudorostral direction, and therefore also reach sympathetic ganglia above and below the level of injection.

Neuronal Circuitry and its Development*

H. VAN DER LOOS

*Institut d'Anatomie, Université de Lausanne.
1011 Lausanne (Switzerland)*

INTRODUCTION

I will submit neuronal circuitry to three levels of consideration. Although there are more such levels, and some of them may be more significant than the ones I shall talk about, I limit myself to the things I have until now studied and which, together with my collaborators, I will continue to study. I hope to convince you that neuroanatomy — looking at the brain, usually after a bit of tampering and always with some kind of microscope — is a worthwhile discipline, one that must be kept alive as a vital part of neuroscience.

At each of these three levels, I will describe an area of activity of our laboratories (first at Johns Hopkins and now in Lausanne) that provided an outcome and that offers an *Ausblick*, and in which work is continuing (or planned) in operational terms. My collaborators to whose work I will allude are, in order of appearance, E.M. Glaser, M.E. Molliver, I. Kostović, P.P. Giorgi, T.A. Woolsey, F.L. Rice, D. Jeanmonod, E.L. White, M.T. Shipley and E. Perentes.

Because of limitations of space certain lines of inquiry will be mentioned but not dwelt upon. The reported work is largely on cerebral neocortex. The parts to this presentation are:

(i) *Small circuits*, the basis of local signal processing; the role of chance in cortex development.

(ii) *Circuit formation*, pertaining to both small circuitry and trunk connections; the role of intrinsic and extrinsic directive factors in cortex development.

(iii) *Trunk connections* and their topological relations; the role of the periphery in cortex development.

Sections (i) and (iii) both end with a general comment.

(i) SMALL CIRCUITS

Only at the turn of the last century — when the concepts "neuron" and "neuronal connectivity" were developed — did it become possible even to talk

---

* Dedicated to Professor David Bodian.

260

~1850–~1885	~1885–~1890	~1890–~1900
The period of cell continuity: junctions of proximal dendrites and of plexus, first dendritic, then axonal.	Declaration of Independence of the neuron.	Development of the concepts "synapse" and "law of dynamic polarization".
Key figures: WAGNER, GERLACH, GOLGI	Key figures: HIS, FOREL, CAJAL	Key figures: CAJAL, VAN GEHUCHTEN, M. LENHOSSEK

Fig. 1. Summary of the three periods in the ideogenesis of neuronal connectivity. For full "flow chart" see Fig. 36 in Van der Loos (1974).

about small circuits. This development was interesting, emotional and complex.

There was a period of plexuses: dendritic, then axonal; cells interacted by means of structural continuity. Subsequently, the notions of interaction through contiguity, and that of chains of neurons were born. Finally, the idea was formulated, mainly by Cajal, that in neurons signals flow in one direction; where information is negotiated between cells an outstanding contact point exists: the synapse, or "articulation" as Cajal would have it. Fig. 1 summarizes this ideogenesis. The ideas had still to be developed that (a) signals in an individual nerve cell are of two distinct kinds, and (b) that the translation from one (the local potential) into the other (the action potential) takes place either at the first node of Ranvier or at the initial axon segment (see Fig. 2). The same holds true for the fact that the unidirectionality of signal flow is caused by properties of the synaptic junction rather than by properties of the length of neuron lying between two synapses.

Cajal developed the idea of unidirectional signal flow in neurons from the inspection of Golgi preparations in physiologically transparent situations. From an analysis, for example, of the olfactory paths (Fig. 3, taken from Cajal, 1891) — where the signal flow is clear: the nose is *not* an effector organ — he deduced that axons conduct away from their point of origin and dendrites towards the point of axon origin. Then he generalized his awakening idea to practically all

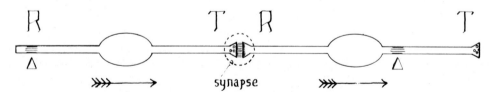

Fig. 2. Two bare neurons in interactive relationship. The neuron on the left is a primary sensory neuron of the somatosensory system. The neuron on the right is an intercalated neuron or a motor neuron. R and T refer, respectively, to the cell's receptor and transmitter zones. Cajalian arrows symbolize the "law of dynamic polarization". We now know that these arrows are caused by — in most cases — secretory events at the synapse. The arrowheads indicate sites of analogue-to-digital conversion of signals. Postsynaptic potentials are translated there into action potentials. The left arrowhead is placed at the first node of Ranvier, the right one at the initial axon segment. Ultrastructural differentiations have been discerned at both sites (Andres, 1966; and Palay et al., 1968, respectively).

stainable bits of nervous tissue*. *This was Cajal's greatness.* In cerebral cortex, however, Cajal (1892) got stuck; his realistic diagrams (Cajalian arrows and all) remained tentative (Cajal, 1911). We are still far from knowing the construction of small cortical circuits. I suspect that such circuits, if indeed they ever will be grasped, will turn out to be more complex than logical variations on the present neuronal-chain theme admit.

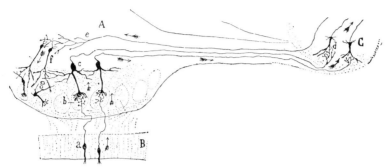

Fig. 3. Cajal's legends speak for themselves. Illustration accompanies proceedings of the Congreso médico de Valencia in June 1891, which became a historic event for neuroscientists. Note Cajalian arrows that were to permeate the Iberian neurobiological literature. (From Cajal, 1891.)

There are, besides axosomatic and axodendritic synapses, axoaxonal and dendrodendritic synapses and junctions. They constitute one of the lines of inquiry that I shall not develop here (see Van der Loos, 1964, 1968). I will dwell only upon the connections between axons and dendrites of the same cell, which we called "autapses" (Van der Loos and Glaser, 1972). We analyzed individual neurons in Golgi preparations of neocortex, using a high resolution computer-microscope that Glaser and I designed (Glaser and Van der Loos, 1965). We traced all visible axon branches of each cell, plus all the dendrites with which they made contacts. In so doing, for half the number of axonal trees analyzed, these dendrites belonged to the cell that gave rise to the axon (Fig. 4).

Brushing aside momentarily the serious caution that one must have when analyzing circuits with Golgi methods (is a contact a synapse?) we ask: what could such an arrangement, by no means rare, mean? We propose that it is a gating mechanism: part of the neuron's input is put under the influence of the cell's own output, i.e. excitatory inputs from other cells on the dendrite segment distal to an autapse would have their influence at the neuron's impulse generating zone modified by that autapse. Other inputs, on other dendrite segments and dendrites, would not. We assume that autapses are inhibitory contacts.

The observation of autapses, although independently made, shared a fate with many current observations in neurobiology: it was already reported before

---

* Thus, his thoughts on the cerebellar cortex (from which no a priori idea about signal flow can be extracted), which initially were at best vague (Cajal, 1888), crystallized quickly into the clear and popular wiring diagram we still embrace (e.g., see Cajal, 1911, Figs. 103 and 104). His idea was formulated as a "law", the law of dynamic polarization, of which the final version appeared in Cajal (1897).

262

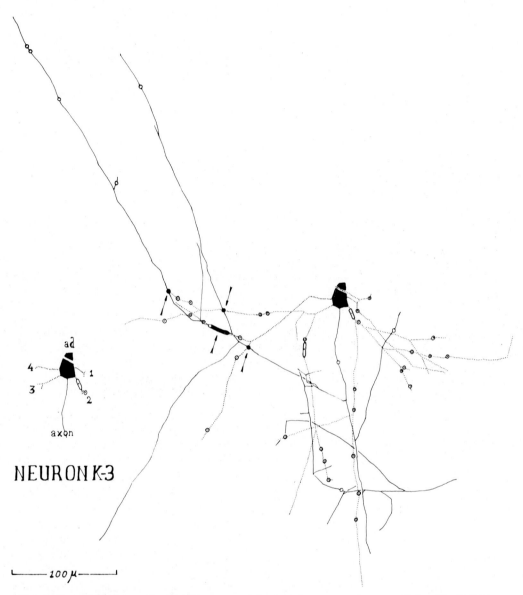

NEURON K-3

└───── *100 μ* ─────┘

Fig. 4. Computer trace of a Golgi-impregnated autaptic neuron (a pyramidal cell) of rabbit neocortex. For key, see insert; ad is apical dendrite (not analyzed); 1 to 4 are basal dendrites; the axon is represented by a continuous line. ⊙ are presumed synapses between this cell's dendrites and Golgi-impregnated axons of other cells; ○ are presumed synapses between this cell's axon and other neurons' dendrites. While the circles are "punctiform" contacts, the elongated structures of the same diameter are climbing fiber arrangements.

Arrows point to autapses (blackened symbols). (From Van der Loos and Glaser, 1972.)

1900. Held (1897) in his ample and very interesting "Beiträge zur Structur der Nervenzellen und ihrer Fortsätze" described that Purkinje cells bear "autocelluläre Collateralen" and he speculated on their significance*. Cajal did not like them, though, and his deserved authority effectively killed this type of connection. We plan to further investigate the autaptic cells by means of several techniques; Procion brown injection of individual neurons (Christensen, 1973) would make their offshoots traceable in serial thin sections, while the ultrastructure remains decipherable. Likewise, methylene blue intravital staining (Richardson, 1969) and a Golgi technique recently developed by Blackstad (1975) do not attack the electron microscopic features of a synapse. I like to stress that, until such studies are made, the inferences drawn so far from the analysis of autapses are of a highly speculative nature.

How are autaptic connections made? Do the two poles of the cell, the transmitter zone and the receptor zone, have a special attraction for each other? If that were so, there should be many more autapses than in fact there are. Why so few then? Because the two poles of the cell shun each other? If that were so, then we should not see these contacts at all. Or are they, perhaps, an accident of geometry? Some have used the latter thought to bolster their disbelief in the possible significance of the autapse.

But — and this is the general comment I should like to make at this point — is there any relationship between accident and significance? I propose that there is not. Everyone (myself included) is a center of the cosmos and, so placed, is not without significance. I am an accident. My grandmother on my mother's side once broke the lace of one of her ice skates. She was a girl then, and a young man skated by and, conforming to Dutch couleur locale, asked if he might not tie the pieces. After a reasonable latency period my mother was born. I am an accident, a consequence of a broken skate lace. I propose that in smaller cosmoi the consequences of this reasoning hold: an accident, for example one of geometry, may yet well be of significance, for example in the sense of functional significance.

(ii) CIRCUIT FORMATION

Since about 90% of a neuron's receptive surface is dendritic (Sholl, 1955, 1956), and since in general by far the most synapses are upon dendrites, it cannot be very wrong to say that circuit formation is largely due to the outgrowth of, and the encounter between, axons and dendrites of neuron sets. (Of course, this is not to say that the migration of neuroblasts in toto plays no role!).

Growing axons make synapses (Bodian, 1966) and growing dendrites do (Vaughn et al., 1974). In the cerebral cortex, synapses appear to be formed on the more mature elements of a dendrite population in a developing piece of

---

* It is of interest, and in line with our assumption that autaptic cells are inhibitory, that Purkinje cells indeed have been shown to be inhibitory (Eccles et al., 1967).

gray matter. Molliver, Kostović and I reached that conclusion after laminar analyses of synaptogenesis in the developing cortex of dog and man, combining results obtained by the study of electron micrographs and of Golgi preparations (e.g., Molliver and Van der Loos, 1970). That study is one of a series, and one of our principal aims is to analogize the stages of cortex development in different species so that data from, say, mouse, rat, dog and man can be integrated: each of these species has different types of data to contribute to the overall developmental picture of neocortex. This is, again, one of the lines of inquiry that, for lack of space, I will not develop any further here. At this point, I should like to discuss the *directedness* of processes as they are spun out by growing nerve cells.

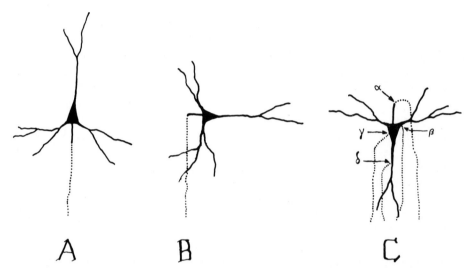

Fig. 5. Cell bodies of neocortical pyramids are represented by triangles. (Parts of) processes whose direction is governed by factors intrinsic to the cell are drawn in continuous lines: the dendrites and the initial segment of the axon. The direction in which the rest of the axon (stippled) grows is governed by extrinsic factors. A: properly oriented cell. What is governed by intrinsic and what by extrinsic factors is deduced from the geometries portrayed in B and C. B: a sideways-oriented cell. C: an inverted pyramidal cell. Points α, β, γ and δ are points of axon emanation as seen in *different* inverted pyramids.

For axons, *chemotaxis* (see Sperry, 1951, for his views and a review) and *contact guidance* (see Weiss, 1955, for his views and review) have been invoked. Hamburger (1962) tried to reconcile these concepts by proposing a "biochemical infiltration of the substrate over considerable range, perhaps in gradient fashion". Dendrites have not been considered much.

I put forward the thesis that the nature of the factors which work upon axons is different from the nature of the factors which work upon dendrites. I arrived at that conclusion while worrying about the geometry of "improperly" oriented pyramidal cells in cerebral neocortex. Pyramidal cells pathognomonic for this part of the brain, are characterized by a pyramid-shaped cell body, by a set of basal dendrites, and by an apical dendrite. The axon leaves from the base of the cell body, or from a basal dendrite near the base (see Fig. 5A). These neurons sit, when they sit properly, with their apex directed towards the pial surface. I propose that, at least in the case of pyramidal cells, the directedness of growth both of dendrites and of the initial axon segment is primarily governed by factors intrinsic to the cell, whereas the axon beyond its initial segment grows under the auspices of factors extrinsic to the cell (Van der Loos, 1965). Why?

If and when certain pyramids[§] come to be improperly oriented during migration — during that period the pallium is a veritable neurodrome — their geometries are as shown in Fig. 5B and C. The dendrites are disobedient to the overall dendrite orientation but in accordance with the disobedience of the cell bodies. The axons may either (1) initially behave likewise and then re-think (Fig. 5B, and α in Fig. 5C); (2) follow their instincts about what is proper right away (β in Fig. 5C) or (3) impatiently overdo things and grow from the cell body's side (γ in Fig. 5C) and even from the apical dendrite (δ in Fig. 5C); cases γ and δ are never seen in properly oriented pyramids[*].

The question that we are now re-asking is: *what makes an axon go where it goes*? It seems that a growing offshoot of this sort has two problems to solve: (1) where does it direct itself upon emergence? and (2) where does it terminate when it has arrived at its approximate destination? The latter question has been asked by many investigators, who used as a sample of nature particularly the fish and amphibian tectum (for a review see Keating and Gaze, 1970). The concept "neuronal specificity" arose to a large extent from work done to answer this (latter) question. This concept owes much of its power to the insistence of retinal axons that come from specific places in the retina to grow into specific places in the tectum. But the question: "where does an axon look when it starts out fresh in the world, in search of a destination?" is not so often posed. It is as with the Pilgrim Fathers' voyage: they first decided to go to the New World; questions about who would live where in their settlement were to be solved not while on the Mayflower, but only after they arrived at their approximate destination. P.P. Giorgi of the Institut d'Anatomie in Lausanne and I have made a start at this question by putting eyes in odd places near the spinal cord of *Xenopus* larvae. Our questions are: where will the axons grow? When they reach the cord, where will they turn? Transplanting is done at the tail-bud stage, the animals are killed at the mid-larval stage.

So far we have found that, given certain experimental conditions, the fibers leave the third eye in such a manner that the optic disc is grossly eccentric and displaced towards the brain, while normally the point of emergence of the nerve is placed axially in the back of the eye (i.e., also towards the brain). Results obtained from serially cut, reduced-silver preparations show that the axons enter the spinal cord and then appear to travel towards the brain. Now, radioactive proline has been injected into the ectopic eyes of a new set of larvae; autoradiography of the material after transport down the axons may provide better evidence in support of these first observations.

[§] About 10%; I made the observations mainly in rabbit.
[*] See the following figures of Van der Loos (1965) for documentation of the various cases of improper cell orientation as shown in Fig. 5: figure 5 for the case depicted in B, figure 11 for case α depicted in C, figure 9 for cases β and γ, and figure 10 for case δ.

266

(iii) TRUNK CONNECTIONS

That many functional units of the brain are related to the periphery in a topologically homeomorphic manner is well established. (In what follows I refer to this relationship as a "topological relationship".) The idea is old, and it is interesting that the telencephalon figured so early in its formulation.

In the 1660s, Descartes proposed that the visual periphery makes it to the brain in topological fashion (Descartes, 1664). See, in Fig. 6, periphery A, B, C — via the 1, 3 and 5s in the eyes — projected as 2, 4, 6s upon the visual cortex, conveniently placed in the frontal lobes. In the experimental vein, Munk, in the 1880s, extirpated various pieces of cortex from trained dogs and observed specific gaps in the learned performance of his animals. He found a visual

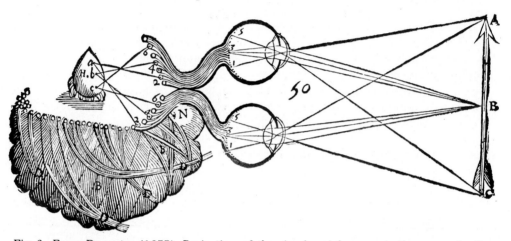

Fig. 6. From Descartes (1677). Projection of the visual periphery — via the eyes — to the brain. We do not consider here this author's notion that the mind, residing in the pineal gland — the pine-cone placed in the center of the brain — is at liberty to scrutinize the "visual cortex".

cortex, an auditory cortex and a somatosensory cortex. In the latter he distinguished a head, an arm, and a leg region (Munk, 1881). Our emphasis, here, will be on somatosensory cortex.

Through trunk connections from the periphery the somatosensory cortex maintains, through at least two synaptic relay stations, a topological relationship with the periphery. This concept has withstood analysis at high resolution. At the highest resolution, the homeomorphic representation of the periphery consists of sets of cortical columns (Werner and Whitsel, 1968). These functional columns — functional because they were defined by physiological means — were first described by Mountcastle (1957). This discovery was an extremely important one. The columns are small areas extending from pia to white matter, with diameters smaller than 0.5 mm. In such a column all, or most, cells have the same modality and carry the same local sign.

Another still valid concept is old: that of the basic structural organization of neocortex — an organization in layers. Baillarger (1840) carefully inspected the cortex with the naked eye and presented his findings accompanied by an unusual illustration (Fig. 7A) to the Académie Royale de Médecine (Paris). About 20 years later, Berlin (1858) produced an Inauguralabhandlung in which he gave this layering a cellular basis (Fig. 7B). Parenthetically, he also gave the cortex three cell types, among which were the "Pyramidenförmige Zellen". There is an odd discrepancy: *functionally*, the cortex is columnar and, considered tangentially, discontinuous with a periodicity of between 0·1 and 0·5 mm; *structurally*, however, the cortex is layered and, considered tangentially, continuous.

In part of the mouse somatosensory cortex (SI) things are quite different. Woolsey and I found that one layer, layer IV, is *not* continuous and in the discontinuity — it has a period ranging from 0.1 to 0.5 mm — we may have the substrate of place-columns (Woolsey and Van der Loos, 1970). At the appropriate depth, a tangential cut through the cortex reveals a characteristic grouping of neurons. We called these cell groups "barrels"; they are cylinder-like, have a "hollow" and a "side", and are separated by "septa". Hollows, as well as the septa, have a lower packing density of perikarya than do the sides. The "barrelfield" lies on the lateral, convex aspect of the cerebral hemisphere. It is best seen in brains cut at an odd plane: starting from the horizontal, the anterior end of the hemisphere needs to be tipped down by 10°, the lateral side by 30°. The configuration of the barrel assembly is remarkably constant from one mouse to the next (see Fig. 14 in Woolsey and Van der Loos, 1970). The barrelfield consists of two parts. One part contains 35 large oblong barrels, arranged in 5 rows; this is the PosteroMedial Barrel SubField (PMBSF) and is portrayed in Fig. 8A. The other part, located anterior to the PMBSF, contains about 150 small cylindrical barrels. In the present paper, I consider only the assembly of the large oblong barrels. A fortunate section of the PMBSF is shown in Fig. 8B. In each large barrel there are about 2000 neurons (Lee and Woolsey, 1975). Once one knows what to look for one sees, in a cut perpendicular to the pial surface, that the barrels and the septa between them extend throughout the thickness of layer IV. A non-random distribution of perikarya in layer IV of this region of cortex has been noted before (cf., Woolsey and Van der Loos, 1970, Table II). It is odd that barrels and barrelfield have not been picked up earlier.

To what part of the periphery is this cortex topologically related, if at all? How do we know it is somatosensory? The PMBSF is related to the whiskerpad on the animal's muzzle. This whiskerpad is, for mice, a most important sense organ. *One* whisker is related to *one* barrel. How do we know?

(a) Woolsey (1967), combining surface evoked response recording with histological inspection of the underlying cortex, concluded that a cortical area exhibiting a "cell-dense net" (which was later to be called the barrelfield) contains the whisker projection.

(b) The approximately 35 largest vibrissae are part of as many complex tactile receptor organs. The large papillae contain a wealth of receptors (Andres, 1966), and from each papilla leads a "vibrissal nerve" containing about 200 myelinated fibers (Lee and Woolsey, 1975). In the cortex, the 35 or so oblong barrels are the largest of the barrelfield as a whole.

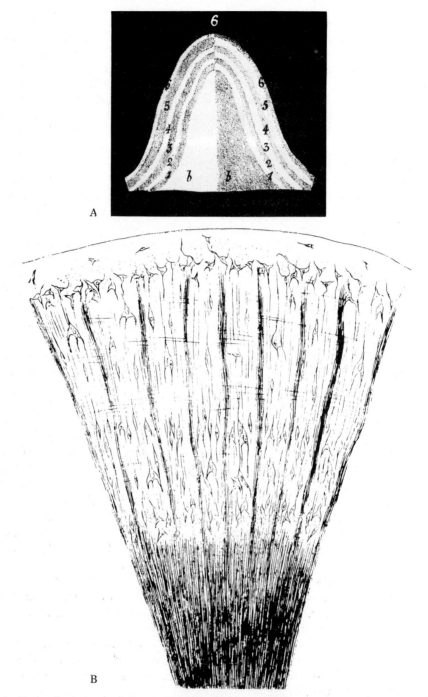

Fig. 7. Early depictions of the layered organization of (human) cortex. A: taken from Planche I of Baillarger's (1840) communication. The left half of the gyrus is viewed with incident light: the white matter core is white; going towards the pia one meets successively gray and white layers of cortex; Baillarger counted them "backwards". The right half is transilluminated. The (opaque) white matter (b) is dark; in the cortex are, in succession, relatively translucent and relatively opaque layers. B: taken from Tafel I of Berlin's (1858)

(c) The large vibrissae stand in a characteristic array: 5 rows, with 4 "straddling" barrels at the rows' ends. The pattern of barrels in the cortex is much the same: 5 rows plus 4 straddlers (Woolsey and Van der Loos, 1970). Compare Fig. 8A with 8H and 8G.

(d) Welker (1971) found, through the systematic mapping of driveable units and unit-clusters in the SI face-area of the rat, that each large vibrissa projects separately to an area of cortex of about 0.3 to 0.6 sq. mm. She determined that, in a field that contains barrels, caudal vibrissae project medially and rostral vibrissae project laterally. Allowing for species differences, the rat cortex whisker map fits our mouse barrelfield quite well. Similar experiments are now being conducted on mice (Axelrad and Verley, personal communication, 1974; Shipley, Frost and Rice, personal communication, 1975).

(e) Finally, the topological relationship between whisker array and barrel pattern, as well as the single whisker-to-single barrel connection, are borne out by a set of experiments performed by Woolsey and myself (Van der Loos and Woolsey, 1973). I shall briefly report them here. As importantly, the experiments also show how the cortex can be profoundly disturbed when the periphery is tampered with during the appropriate "critical" period.

Deprive a newborn mouse of its whiskers, or of some of its whiskers, and the adolescent or adult individual (12- and 43-day-old respectively) will not bear the corresponding barrels in its contralateral barrel cortex. The barrel arrangement can be disrupted in any desired pattern simply by damaging various arrays of whiskers. Two types of insults are portrayed in Fig. 8I and J, and in Fig. 8K and L, respectively. In the former, all but whisker-row C and straddler β were removed; in the latter, row C and β were the only whiskers removed. "Removed" means that the whiskers are pulled out and the follicles cauterized (I and J) or electrolytically damaged by a small metal electrode at $-6 \cdot 5$ V (K and L). The results of these experiments are illustrated in Fig. 8B and E, and 8C and F, respectively. The experimentally produced barrelless domain in Fig. 8C and F is smaller than it would have been had barrels been there. The privileged barrels shown in Fig. 8B and E are bigger than their control counterparts shown in 8A and D.

A few questions are forced immediately upon the experimenter. What part of the periphery projects to the new barrelless land — if the periphery projects there at all? How is it that the barrelless land, adjacent to intact barrels, is bordered by what appears to be a barrel-side, and why is it separated from them by what looks like a normal septum? Is it lack of input signals or lack of

---

Inauguralabhandlung. The subcortical white matter (bottom) is packed with radially arranged nerve fibers (note the bundles that continue into the cortex) while the cortex exhibits layers of neurons. From white matter to pia, Berlin — he also used the "inverse" numbering system — distinguished 6 layers; all contain, among other cell types, pyramidal cells. Layers 1 and 3 (our layers VI and IV) contain many middle-sized cells; in layers 2 and 4 (our layers V and III) cells are less densely packed, while large cells outnumber middle sized ones; layer 5 (our layer II) is very densely packed, all cells "remind one of the pyramid form"; the outer cells send processes into layer 6 (our layer I) which constituted for Berlin no gray matter; it contains mainly "intercellular substance" and cell processes, and only a few pyramids of smallest size.

270

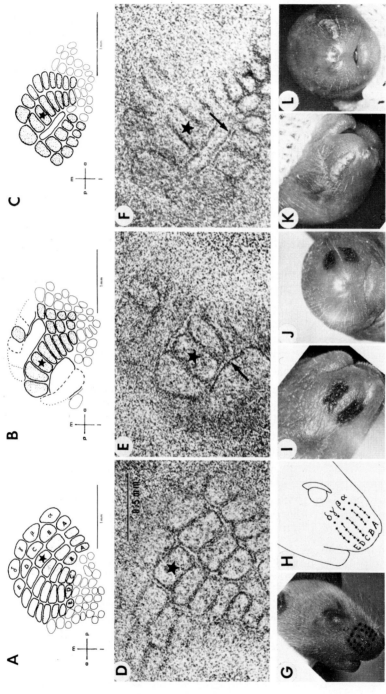

Fig. 8. A–C are reconstructions from serial, tangential sections through layer IV of adult mouse posteromedial barrel subfield (PMBSF). a = anterior, p = posterior, m = medial and l = lateral. The bars are 1 mm. In A, A–E are the barrel rows and α–δ the straddlers. A represents a control field in a left hemisphere and B and C, right fields of which the periphery was damaged at birth (see text). D–F are choice cuts that contributed to the reconstructions. Asterisks match asterisks in A, B and C. G–L show muzzles. In G and H a right normal whiskerpad of a 6-day-old mouse is shown: a photograph taken after light cosmetic treatment (India ink applied to the follicles), and a drawing that bears the names of the rows and of the straddlers. Orientation matches that of A. In I and J, a newborn mouse's face is shown with, on the left side, all papillae except of the C-row injured. In K and L the papillae of β and of the C-row are injured. (From Van der Loos and Woolsey, 1973.)

some trophic factor that is responsible for the observed changes (after all, the papillae in question are damaged)? The elementary point to be made here is that we have demonstrated a transsynaptically induced alteration of a mechanism or mechanisms, leading to a normal cortex. *What* mechanisms? The following alternatives come to mind:

(a) There is an alteration in the proliferation of neuroblasts destined for barrels.

(b) There is a modification of the pattern of migration and of the pattern of intracortical cell rearrangement.

(c) There is an altered pattern of developmental cell death.

In these cases, the missing barrels were never there. Two further alternatives include the notion that barrels related to damaged papillae exist at some period, but then disintegrate through lack of some critical factor that, at a given stage of development, is necessary for their maintenance.

(d) Barrels exist at birth and the peripheral insult makes them disappear.

(e) Barrels form some time after the lesion is made but, because of the missing factor, they subsequently disappear.

Answers to these questions about the formation of somatosensory cortex and the influence upon that formation from distant sites in afferent pathways, may help to elucidate something about the general nature of interdependence of bits of the developing nervous system, that can be several synaptic stations removed from one another. The most important question of course is: are options (a)–(e) the most valuable ones to consider?

Some answers have been forthcoming with respect to these problems. My collaborator Rice showed that neurons destined for barrels are born 4 and 5 days before birth (Rice, 1975a, b). A lesion made at birth cannot therefore influence proliferation of prospective barrel neurons. It was also found that barrels do not appear before the 4th postnatal day (Rice, 1973, 1975b; Rice and Van der Loos, 1976). Thus, while barrels might form and then, in the absence of a relevant periphery, disappear, this reversible modeling would have to take place between birth and adolescence (0 and 12 days, respectively). At birth, neuroblasts destined for layers II and III are still en route (Rice, 1975a, b). Deeper cortex, already laid down and including layer IV, serves as neurodrome. A lesion at that time could have a disturbing effect on barrel formation, although the neuronal logistics for travel and lodging are not clear.

Jeanmonod together with Rice and myself are presently engaged in an effort to test the possibility that, after lesioning the receptors at birth, barrels first form and then disintegrate. Also, we are working at a better definition of the critical period during which a peripheral lesion has an effect on cortex architecture. Weller and Johnson (1975), who confirmed for two species of mice that a lesion at birth leads to the absence of barrels in the adult animal, found that a lesion made at day 5 has no qualitative effect.

White, in Lausanne, made a quantitative electron microscopic study of the synapse-rich barrel neuropil. He designed an ingenious method by which it was possible to pick out a barrel under light microscopic control and select small regions from it for the production of ribbons of up to 100 serial sections. He distinguished 4 types of synapses that are rather evenly distributed through the barrel neuropil (White, 1975, and 1976). Now, in an attempt to unravel barrel circuitry, Shipley and he are collaborating to define the synapses that deliver the signals from the ventrobasal complex (VB) of thalamus to the barrel.

And what about septa? Work by Perentes (also in Lausanne) shows that this term, coined by Woolsey and myself, has no more than descriptive value: it is no less superficial than "cortex" (= bark) and "thalamus" (= bedroom) and so many other terms affixed to bits and pieces of the CNS. By using techniques similar to those of White, Perentes found a synapse-rich neuropil and no structural signs of biological efforts to keep barrels apart, such as glial sheets. What projects then to these septa? Ordinary skin between the whiskers? That would be contrary to the finding that in the SI face-area of the rat, no units could be driven from the ordinary hairy skin of the whiskerpad (Welker, 1971) and Killackey (1973), also in rat and using Fink and Heimer's method, found little degeneration in septa upon making large lesions in VB of thalamus, while the degeneration appeared particularly sparse when small lesions were made. Are septa, then, places where signals from individual barrels are integrated? But, if so, where would the whiskerpad's hairy skin project?

I like to believe — I cannot do much more at this point — that the whisker-to-barrel path represents a *special sense*, and is therefore entitled to *its own* cortical field, topologically as unconnected with the rest of SI as the visual, auditory and olfactory cortices are. If so, the existing cortical somatosensory *muscululi* (Woolsey, 1967; Woolsey and Van der Loos, 1970) must be redrawn, after a fitting place is found for the banal afferents from the hairy skin of the whiskerpad.

At this point I should like to make my second general comment. It touches upon something that has bothered me since I realized I was engaged in science. The point — or, rather, the question — is: when hitting upon an unexpected observation, how do we know it has value beyond the unexpectedness?

How do we know that it is not just an exception to a rule — in the case of the barrels, an exception to a rule that governs cortical organization? In that case, the unexpected observation would better be ignored and left to detail-biters.

Alternatively, *how do we know that it is not an exaggeration (and, therefore, part) of a general principle* — in the case of the barrels, a general principle of cortical circuit organization? In that case the observation should better be jumped upon as a means to get closer to that general principle.

I think I can clarify the question: "how do we know that an unexpected observation has value?" by describing two cartoons. Both are by Charles Addams, (1950 and 1957, respectively). In the first, we see an audience that is viewing a motion picture. The film (we do not see the scene) moves everybody to tears. We make an unexpected observation: there is one happy man laughing his head off. He forms an exception to a general rule, the rule that a certain film has a given effect on an audience.

One may use this observation to reinvestigate that rule. Whether one *does* or *does not* depends on the investigator's whim.

In the second cartoon, we see a barber's shop with its classic arrangement of mirrors: one frontally, one occipitally placed with respect to the client, who thus sees himself front-back-front-back . . . . . ad infinitum. We make an unexpected observation: the fifth reflection is that of a demon's head; reflections 6, 7, and so forth are of the client's head again. *This* observation, I suggest, must lead to a complete overhaul of optical physics. Whether it *does* or *does not* depends on the investigator's astuteness or obtuseness, respectively.

Our challenge and our trouble are that in biology — particularly in neurobiology — we cannot know whether we are in a cinema or in a barber's shop.

SUMMARY

In this paper, I discuss (i) the role of chance, (ii) the role of directive factors, and (iii) the role of the periphery, in the development of neuronal circuitry.

Part (i) deals with small circuits. Among the various types of interneuronal connections in several areas of central nervous system gray matter are "autapses": synapses between a neuron's axon and its own dendrites. They may come about by *chance*, but that does not diminish their possible significance.

Part (ii) deals with circuit formation in general, which is largely caused by the outgrowth of, and the encounter between, axons and dendrites of neuron sets. The course of the axon is determined by the influence of *directive factors* intrinsic and extrinsic to the parent cell, whereas dendrites are guided by intrinsic directive factors alone. This hypothesis was inspired by the geometry of "improperly" oriented pyramidal cells of cerebral neocortex.

Part (iii) deals with trunk connections. The whiskerpad-to-barrelfield path in small rodents facilitates the analysis of topological relations in the nervous system. If proper, point-to-point correspondence between *periphery* and cortex is to develop, the periphery must be intact during a given critical period.

ACKNOWLEDGEMENTS

I thank my wife for assistance in all phases of the work reported, and my friends Drs. Laurence J. Garey and Frank L. Rice for many helpful comments on the manuscript.

The work at Johns Hopkins was supported by Grant NS 04012 from the United States Public Health Service and by grants from the Joseph P. Kennedy, Jr., Memorial Foundation, and the work in Lausanne was supported by Grant 3.1350.73 from the Fonds national suisse de la recherche scientifique.

REFERENCES

Addams, Ch. (1950) *Monster Rally.* Simon and Schuster, New York.
Addams, Ch. (1957) *Night Crawlers.* Simon and Schuster, New York.
Andres, K.H. (1966) Über die Feinstruktur der Rezeptoren an Sinushaaren. *Z. Zellforsch.*, 75: 339–365.

Baillarger, J.G.F. (1840) Recherches sur la structure de la couche corticale des circonvolutions du cerveau. *Mém. Acad. Méd. (Paris)*, 8: 149–183.

Berlin, R. (1858) *Beitrag zur Structurlehre der Grosshirnwindungen. Inauguralabhandlung*, Erlangen, 27 pp.

Blackstad, T.W. (1975) Electron microscopy of experimental axonal degeneration in photochemically modified Golgi preparations: a procedure for precise mapping of nervous connections. *Brain Res.*, 95: 191–210.

Bodian, D. (1966) Development of fine structure of spinal cord in monkey fetuses. I. The motoneuron neuropil at the time of onset of reflex activity. *Bull. Johns Hopk. Hosp.*, 119: 129–149.

Cajal, S. Ramón y (1888) Estructura de los centros nerviosos de las aves. *Rev. trim. Histol. norm. patol.*, 1º de Mayo, 1888.

Cajal, S. Ramón y (1891) Significación fisiológica de las expansiones protoplasmáticas y nerviosas de las células de la sustancia gris. *Rev. Cienc. méd. (Barcelona)*, 22–23: pp. 15.

Cajal, S. Ramón y (1892) Nuevo concepto de la histología de los centros nerviosos. *Rev. Cienc. méd. (Barcelona)*, 18: 89–124.

Cajal, S. Ramón y (1897) Leyes de la morfología y dinamismo de las células nerviosas. *Rev. trim. microgr.*, 2: 1–28.

Cajal. S. Ramón y (1911) *Histologie du Système Nerveux de l'Homme et des Vertébrés. Tome II.* Maloine, Paris, 993 pp. (1955 Edition, Consejo Superior de Investigaciones Científicas, Madrid.)

Christensen, B.N. (1973) Procion brown: an intracellular dye for light and electron microscopy. *Science*, 182: 1255–1256.

Descartes, R. (1664) *L'Homme.* Angot, Paris. (Second Edition, 1677, 511 pp., Girard, Paris.)

Eccles, J.C., Ito, M. and Szentágothai, J. (1967) *The Cerebellum as a Neuronal Machine.* Springer-Verlag, New York, 335 pp.

Glaser, E.M. and Van der Loos, H. (1965) A semi-automatic computer-microscope for the analysis of neuronal morphology. *IEEE Trans. biomed. Engng*, BME-12: 22–31.

Hamburger, V. (1962) Specificity in neurogenesis. *J. cell. comp. Physiol.*, 60: 81–92.

Held, H. (1897) Beiträge zur Structur der Nervenzellen und ihrer Fortsätze, 2. Abh., *Arch. Anat. Physiol. (Lpz.)*, 204–294.

Keating, M.J. and Gaze, R.M. (1970) Rigidity and plasticity in the amphibian visual system. *Brain Behav. Evol.*, 3: 102–120.

Killackey, H.P. (1973) Anatomical evidence for cortical subdivisions based on vertically discrete thalamic projections from the ventral posterior nucleus to cortical barrels in the rat. *Brain Res.*, 51: 326–331.

Lee, K.J. and Woolsey, T.A. (1975) A proportional relationship between peripheral innervation density and cortical neuron number in the somatosensory system of the mouse. *Brain Res.*, 99: 349–353.

Molliver, M.E. and Van der Loos, H. (1970) The ontogenesis of cortical circuitry: the spatial distribution of synapses in somesthetic cortex of newborn dog. *Ergebn. Anat. Entwickl.-Gesch.*, 42: 1–54.

Mountcastle, V.B. (1957) Modality and topographic properties of single neurons of cat's somatic sensory cortex. *J. Neurophysiol.*, 20: 408–434.

Munk, H. (1881) *Über die Funktionen der Grosshirnrinde*, 3te Mitteilung, Hirschwald, Berlin, pp. 28–53. (English translation in G. von Bonin, *The Cerebral Cortex*, Thomas, Springfield, Ill., pp. 97–117.)

Palay, S.L., Sotelo, C., Peters, A. and Orkand, P.M. (1968) The axon hillock and the initial segment. *J. Cell Biol.*, 38: 193–201.

Rice, F.L. (1973) Somatosensory cortex of the mouse: development of barrels and of barrel field. *Anat. Rec.*, 175: 423–424.

Rice, F.L. (1975a) Neuroblasts destined for the barrels of mouse somatosensory cortex: time of origin and pattern of postnatal migration: a quantitative autoradiographic analysis. *Exp. Brain Res.*, 23: Suppl., 174.

Rice, F.L. (1975b) *The Development of the Primary Somatosensory Cortex in the Mouse: (1) A Nissl Study of the Ontogenesis of the Barrels and the Barrel Field, (2) A*

Quantitative Autoradiographic Study of the Time of Origin and Pattern of Postnatal Migration of Neuroblasts in Area SI. Ph.D. Thesis, Johns Hopkins University, Baltimore, Md., pp. 337.

Rice, F.L. and Van der Loos, H. (1976) The development of the primary somatosensory cortex in the mouse. An analysis of the developing barrels and barrel field. In preparation.

Richardson, K.C. (1969) The fine structure of autonomic nerves after vital staining with methylene blue. *Anat. Rec.*, 164: 359–378.

Sholl, D.A. (1955) The surface area of cortical neurons. *J. Anat. (Lond.)*, 89: 571–572.

Sholl, D.A. (1956) The measurable parameters of the cerebral cortex and their significance in its organization. In *Progress in Neurobiology*, J. Ariëns Kappers (Ed.), Elsevier, Amsterdam, pp. 324–333.

Sperry, R.W. (1951) Mechanisms of neural maturation. In *Handbook of Experimental Psychology*, S.S. Stevens (Ed.), Wiley, New York, pp. 236–280.

Van der Loos, H. (1964) Similarities and dissimilarities in submicroscopical morphology of interneuronal contact sites of presumably different functional character. In *Topics in Basic Neurology, Progress in Brain Research, Vol. 6*, W. Bargmann and J.P. Schadé (Eds.), Elsevier, Amsterdam, pp. 43–58.

Van der Loos, H. (1965) The "improperly" oriented pyramidal cell in the cerebral cortex and its possible bearing on problems of neuronal growth and cell orientation. *Bull. Johns Hopk. Hosp.*, 117: 228–250.

Van der Loos, H. (1968) Anatomic and physiologic considerations. In *The Biologic Basis of Pediatric Practice, Section 16, Regulating Systems — Nervous*, R.E. Cooke (Ed.), McGraw-Hill, New York, pp. 1177–1200.

Van der Loos, H. (1974) Dendrodendritic junctions. In Dynamic Patterns of Brain Cell Assemblies, Report of NRP Work Session, May 14–16, 1972, A.K. Katchalsky, V. Rowland and R. Blumenthal (Eds.), *Neurosci, Res. Prog. Bull.*, 12: 86–90.

Van der Loos, H. and Glaser, E.M. (1972) Autapses in neocortex cerebri: synapses between a pyramidal cell's axon and its own dendrites. *Brain Res.*, 48: 355–360.

Van der Loos, H. and Woolsey, T.A. (1973) Somatosensory cortex: Structural alterations following early injury to sense organs. *Science*, 179: 395–398.

Vaughn, J.E., Henrikson, C.K. and Grieshaber, J.A. (1974) A quantitative study of synapses on motor neuron dendritic growth cones in developing mouse spinal cord. *J. Cell Biol.*, 60: 664–672.

Weiss, P. (1955) Special vertebrate organogenesis. Nervous system (neurogenesis). In *Analysis of Development*, B.H. Willier, P. Weiss and V. Hamburger (Eds.), Saunders, Philadelphia, Pa., pp. 346–401.

Welker, C. (1971) Microelectrode delineation of fine grain somatotopic organization of SmI cerebral neocortex in albino rat. *Brain Res.*, 26: 259–275.

Weller, W.L. and Johnson, J.I. (1975) Barrels in cerebral cortex altered by receptor disruption in newborn, but not in five-day-old mice (Cricetidae and Muridae). *Brain Res.*, 83: 504–508.

Werner, G. and Whitsel, B.L. (1968) Topology of the body representation in somatosensory area I of primates. *J. Neurophysiol.*, 31: 856–869.

White, E.L. (1975) Ultrastructural aspects of circuitry in barrels of mouse SI cortex. *Anat. Rec.*, 181: 508.

White, E.L. (1976) Ultrastructure and synaptic connections in barrels of mouse SI cortex. *Brain Res.*, 105: 229–251.

Woolsey, T.A. (1967) Somatosensory, auditory and visual cortical areas of the mouse. *Johns Hopk. med. J.*, 121: 91–112.

Woolsey, T.A. and Van der Loos, H. (1970) The structural organization of layer IV in the somatosensory region (SI) of mouse cerebral cortex. The description of a cortical field composed of discrete cytoarchitectonic units. *Brain Res.*, 17: 205–242.

DISCUSSION

V. BRAITENBERG: I have something to say about your point of view that the dendritic organization in the cerebral cortex is "intrinsically" determined, whereas the axonal orientation is governed by the milieu into which they grow. This is exactly the contrary of my own impression that the dendritic tree, especially in the basal dendrites, is sensitive to functional activity within the cortex. I only assume this, of course, for the time when these dendrites are actually growing, which is during the first two weeks of life in the mouse. Of course, I put it as a hypothesis: that some of the cell structure embodies experience, that different experiences will lead to different structures despite identical initial conditions. But, is this more a property of axons or of dendrites? I favor the latter for the following reason: the axons contain much more regularity in their layout, the collaterals often appearing in certain highly regular sequences. Furthermore, many of these axon collaterals are strikingly straight, which makes me think that they could not be directed by the bioelectric activity of the internets. Dendrites are much less straight, on the other hand, or branching in a more irregular way.

H. VAN DER LOOS: I do not think that there is an antithesis between what you say and what I said. In fact, I think our views complement each other. With respect to dendrites, it is the direction in which they grow that is intrinsically determined. Local, playful variations should not be ruled out, and these variations may well be the consequence of modifications in the animal's environment, brought to the notice of the growing cortical dendrites via the afferent systems that link that environment with the cortex. With respect to the axon, it appears that there are two distinct things going on: *first*, the cell expresses its drive to spin out an axon; *then* comes the problem: where does it go? The drive to grow at all must reside within the cell; it may be stimulated by some extrinsic factors: factors generated in the cell's local environment, or factors produced far away (hormones, for example). *In what direction* the axon will grow (beyond its initial segment, or immediately upon its emanation) is determined by extrinsic, directive factors. In the same vein: where collaterals emanate and in what direction (i.e., at what angle from the axon-stem) they'd initially grow, would be intrinsically commanded, but where they would turn subsequently, would be determined by directive factors that are extrinsic with respect to the parent-neurons. These axon-directing extrinsic factors may well be insensitive — but how are we to know? — to variations in functional activity in the cortex, which, in turn, is influenced by variations in the animal's environment.

V. BRAITENBERG: I would also like to make a comment on the "autapses" in your Golgi preparations: when a neuron has an autapse you will always see it, but when a neuron innervates another neuron, you will of course see it only if they have both been stained. The autapses may in fact be a very rare affair, simply a consequence of the growing axon collaterals establishing contacts with all the dendrites they meet on their course.

H. VAN DER LOOS: I agree with your comment about the chance of staining an autapse versus that of staining a synapse. There are many geometrical problems that one will have to deal with before being able to make a pronouncement about the actual ratio between synapses and autapses (provided one dares indeed draw conclusions from Golgi-stained material: is a contact between an axon swelling and, for example, a spine, a synapse or an autapse, as the case may be?). A practical consideration is that in our sections ($100 \ \mu$m) one sees but 50% of the total basal dendrite length (Van der Loos, 1960). An estimate for the length of axon caught in a $100 \ \mu$m section cannot be made at present, but 50% is not an unreasonable guess. Thus, it is unfortunately not true that an autaptic neuron always identifies itself as such (serial reconstruction of complete dendrite and axon arborizations from serial Golgi sections is exceedingly difficult). Autapses are not rare: half the neurons analyzed had them. Per neuron, they may be rare, say 2–4 autapses per 1000 synapses, but that need not indicate they are insignificant: particularly those relatively close to the cell body may gate a lot of signals impinging upon the dendrites distal to the autapse. About their being "simply a consequence of the growing axon collaterals establishing contacts with all the dendrites they meet on their course", see the parable about my own family tree.

O.D. CREUTZFELDT: The barrels seem to be concentrated in the fourth layer as a continuous structured pattern, but are there connections among different barrels? It may really be that the barrel is a sort of localized projection field within that one layer, but that its actual function would be represented in the whole barrel extension, which is lost in the upper and in the lower areas of the cortex.

V. BRAITENBERG: Yes, but the actual question is: are there any connections between neighboring barrels?

H. VAN DER LOOS: Dr. Creutzfeldt's remark touches a general neurophilosophical point: can one define the actual function of an isolated, particular bit of nervous tissue — say, a barrel? In fact, I think one cannot. Barrels, I bet, intimately interact with the other cortical layers — where the "punctiformness" of the barrel pattern seems to get lost. Through this arrangement, the sensory sheet — in casu the whisker-array — may be reconstituted at the cortical level. Recently I saw in your (Braitenberg's) laboratory some interesting Golgi preparations. If I remember well, these contained, and not so rarely, neurons in layer IV of the barrelfield, cells that have axons that grow into more than one barrel. There are also cells with dendrites that penetrate more than one barrel.

H. GRUNDFEST: Have you looked also at the hippocampus (because there are local spikes generated in the dendritic tree, which points to connections)?

H. VAN DER LOOS: Yes, I have indeed seen autapses in hippocampus.

F. LOPES DA SILVA: When you are talking about barrels, it is again a question of how you look at it: you could talk about a grid instead of a barrel. Actually, what you see is that the cells are more dense. If you look at sections of the cortex, it is quite obvious that there are layers where you have more cell somata, and layers where you have more fibers. How does this horizontal plane grid and the vertical plane grid actually interact with each other?

V.P. WHITTAKER: Can you produce any physical basis for a physical reality of these barrels by applying very gently sheer forces to the whole structure? I mean, it is very easy for the eye to make patterns; but I am not convinced that there really are two rows of cells, the one belonging functionally to one barrel and the other belonging to the other.

H. VAN DER LOOS: Layer IV in the mouse barrelfield, considered as a sheet parallel to the pial surface, consists of three domains: one is continuous, the other two discontinuous. The continuous domain is one of low perikaryon packing-density; it consists of the ensemble of the septa. One of the discontinuous domains is of high perikaryon density; it consists of the barrel sides. The other discontinuous domain is of low perikaryon density; it consists of the barrel hollows. One side plus one hollow make a barrel. One hollow is in contact with one side. The septum domain is in contact with all sides. Septa are not in contact with hollows. Septa *do* exist; they may, in a given preparation, not be outstandingly visible everywhere: when one cuts through them not perfectly perpendicularly, the sides, by their high perikaryon density, obscure the septa. (I assume that, in your comment "the cells are more dense", you mean "the cells in the sides are *more densely packed*". In any case, the cells in the sides are, individually, *not* more intensely stained.) In résumé, septa may be considered as a grid, sides may not. Above and below layer IV lie layers III and V, respectively. I have not much to say about the perikaryon distribution in those layers. Impressionistically viewed, cell dispersion is random, except at the layer III-IV interface: mouse barrels appear to have "lids" of high perikaryon packing density. With respect to "fibers", from various sources we can give the following data (some must be regarded as tentative). Thalamic axons enter the barrels from below and branch prolifically within the hollows. Collaterals from barrel neurons do the same but may leave the axon also at the level of layer IV. Lateral

278

(= basal?) dendrites of any barrel neuron commonly are confined to the hollow of its own barrel. Assemblies of myelinated axons and clusters of layer V pyramids run preponderantly in septa and in sides. The suggestion to separate barrels by applying sheer force is interesting. I have not tried that. Attempts (I must admit: meager attempts) at microdissection have been without results. But I should add that even when two sides would cling to a septum (as pre- and postsynaptic elements may cling to synaptic cleft substance at the business-end of a synaptosome), that would not take away from the argument that barrels are "physical realities" and functional units. Since Perentes (unpublished data) found in septa a synapse-rich neuropil that is, a prima vista, hard to distinguish from that in hollows, I don't dare to predict where the barrelfield would crack up under the impact of physical forces of whatever nature.

D.F. SWAAB: You were speaking about the formation of barrels in terms of a critical period. Could you please specify this critical period? I am asking this because there are other systems that have such a critical period in their development. For instance the development of the male or female reproductive patterns depends on the presence of certain sex hormones during a critical phase. The events during this period also give rise to neuroanatomical changes during the course of development. Is it a determined stage in the development of a neuron that is very sensitive to stimuli, and is it always the same stimulus for which the given area is sensitive in adults, that causes the changes during this period? In other words, is this a general principle in brain development?

H. VAN DER LOOS: At present, Jeanmonod, Rice and I are attempting to define more precisely the critical period during which the periphery has to be intact for proper cortex architecture to emerge. Also, we are trying different kinds of deprivation: we like to know what it is in the periphery that must be there during the critical period in order for a proper cortex to come about. This touches upon the second point you raise (one of more general significance): need the pertinent "stimuli" be the same throughout life? I do not know. All we can say is that when we deprive the trigeminal periphery of its input in the way we did (a coarse way from the mouse's point of view no doubt) *right after birth*, there are no barrels in the adult. This same operation when carried out *at a later date* — which may well result in the abolishment of another set of "stimuli" — does *not* seem to interfere with normal structure, at least when layer IV is impressionistically analyzed, as both we and Weller and Johnson (1975) did.

REFERENCES

Van der Loos, H. (1960) In *Structure and Function of the Cerebral Cortex*, D.B. Tower and J.P. Schadé (Eds.), Elsevier, Amsterdam, pp. 36–42.
Weller, W.L. and Johnson, J.I. (1975) Barrels in cerebral cortex altered by receptor disruption in newborn, but not in five-day-old mice (Cricetidae and Muridae). *Brain Res.*, 83: 504–508.

SESSION V

THE BRAIN AS A FUNCTIONAL SYSTEM

Models of Neuronal Populations: The Basic Mechanisms of Rhythmicity

F.H. LOPES da SILVA, A. VAN ROTTERDAM, P. BARTS, E. VAN HEUSDEN
and W. BURR

Brain Research Group, Institute of Medical Physics TNO, Utrecht (The Netherlands)

GENERAL FRAMEWORK

From a neurophysiological point of view there is a general interest in the problem of how the nervous system processes information and controls behavior. In order to tackle this problem one usually follows an analytical approach, which at the limit involves the study of functional properties of single cells. In this way a good deal of our knowledge of the basic characteristics of the nervous system has been gained. However, the nervous system is not simply made up of *isolated* elementary units, the neurons. It is important to emphasize that neurons are organized in networks which are, as such, responsible for more or less well defined functional properties. Our present knowledge of this organization depends mainly upon neurohistology, but it can only advance if this knowledge is integrated with functional concepts. This problem is complex and very difficult to tackle using exclusively experimental methods. Indeed, it is not possible to record simultaneously from all single neurons which are related to each other within a certain structure. Similarly, it is not easy to interpret the field potentials generated by a large group of neurons which are active more or less synchronously.

In order to make progress in this field it is necessary to develop conceptual models of interaction patterns of neural networks. Therefore it is necessary to employ both *analytical* and *synthetic* methods. We may add: it is essential to employ both approaches in a *dialectic* way. The experimental data, obtained through histological and/or physiological analytical methods, has to be put together just as pieces of a puzzle are assembled. However, our knowledge of most neurophysiological systems is rather limited. The puzzle is far from ready and very often the relationship between the different pieces is still unclear. It is at this level that a synthetic approach becomes extremely helpful. The point is then to put together the available data in such a way as to form the most likely pattern which can be conceived. In this way a model of a neurophysiological system can be constructed. Such a model can contribute to advancing our knowledge of the system in two respects: (a) it provides a possibility for testing the influence of different types of inputs, or of changing some of the properties of the constituting elements, upon the output of the system (in this way the model helps to systematize our understanding of the system's behavior and to clarify our own thoughts); and (b) it implies the formulation of hypotheses concerning new elementary properties, relationships and overall behavior (it may thus predict new properties of the system, raise new questions and suggest new experiments to explore these hypotheses). In this way the dialectic interplay between experimentation and theory can become reality. As Harmon (1964) once stated, it is in suggesting functional relationships between the activity of single neurons and the behavior of groups of neurons that theoretical neurophysiology may be most potent.

In the present article we shall try to demonstrate the potentialities of this approach by following the argument according to three steps: (1) firstly, we shall present a concrete example by means of which models of different parts of the olfactory system have led to a deeper understanding of the functional interactions between the neuronal populations in this system; (2) secondly, a step towards a more general view of the problem of interaction between different neuronal populations will be discussed: some recent attempts to formulate a general theory will be elaborated upon; and (3) thirdly, a series of concrete cases where the main question concerns the origin of rhythmic activity in neuronal populations, such as reflected in the electroencephalogram, will be presented. In this way we will travel from the particular to the general case and back again towards some particular problems.

TERMINOLOGY

In any field of scientific endeavor it is common to find a relatively confusing terminology when it is still poorly developed. This also applies to the topic under discussion here. Very often one finds references to neural nets, or networks or populations, meaning in general some more or less vaguely defined groups of neurons. It is worthwhile to introduce some form of systematization into this nomenclature. The attempts of Freeman (1972, 1974a, 1975) in this sense merit particular attention. He defined some useful terms as regards interactive sets of neurons. His description of these sets, called K-sets, follows a hierarchical order.

Aggregates are those groups of neurons which are placed in parallel and without anatomical interconnections; these are called KO sets: they are not interactive.

Populations are groups of neurons with mutual interactions which are either excitatory or inhibitory; these are called KI sets: the interactions may be excitatory (KIe) or inhibitory (KIi) sets.

Cartels are groups of two interacting populations of neurons; these are called KII sets: they are formed by the interaction of a KIe set with a KIi set. Further, KIII sets can be defined which are formed by interaction between two KII sets. These sets form the basic components which permit an analysis of the activity of a neural mass.

Neural mass — groups of neurons and their interconnections occupying a few sq. mm of cortical surface or a few cu. mm of nuclear volume in the brain stem or spinal cord. Typically a neural mass would consist of approximately 10^4 to 10^7 neurons.

Neural networks — groups of relatively small numbers of neurons (10 to 10^4) such as occurs in well-defined parts of invertebrate nervous systems and in sensorimotor relays of the vertebrate spinal cord.

Systems are those assemblies of aggregates, populations and cartels which correspond to a well defined functional level.

It should be added that the term *neural networks*, as well as neural nets is also frequently used at another level of abstraction, in the sense of sets of interconnected neurons in analogy with the nets or networks of electronic components which form the basic modules of computers. At this level of abstraction these terms have often been employed by theoreticians or modelers, sometimes with the underlying assumption that such groups of neurons resemble in their functional properties those of digital computers. In a simplified view the neurons are considered as elements capable of carrying out binary logic operations. In this sense it is assumed that the capabilities of information processing of the nervous system are akin to those of digital computers. In an extreme statement it may even be stated that "the brain *is* a computer". Such a statement implies not only a similarity in physical organization but also in the way of function. However, the resemblance is more illusory than real. Some functions of the nervous system can be imitated, or modeled, by computers but the way in which both accomplish such functions is, in general, quite different. One may add that the most interesting functions of the nervous system are exactly those which can hardly be mimicked at all by existing computers, such as one-trial learning or motivated behavior.

A STUDY OF A MODEL: THE NEURONAL POPULATIONS OF THE OLFACTORY SYSTEM

Interactions between neuronal populations have been intensively studied in the olfactory system, and they have been the object of intensive and illuminating studies by Freeman (for review see 1975). These investigations have led to comprehensive models of the most important neuron populations which constitute the olfactory system. This work offers an excellent opportunity to understand how neuron population models can contribute to a better understanding of neurophysiological phenomena. Therefore we shall deal with these models in some detail.

General anatomical organization

For a good understanding of the following it is useful to give a brief review of the general organization of the olfactory system.

The olfactory system consists of 3 main stages: the sensory transducer in the *nasal mucosa,* the *olfactory bulb* (OB) and the *prepyriform cortex* (PPC). The first stage is the sensory transducer, which consists of a surface array of receptor neurons, the axons of which form the primary olfactory nerve (PON). These axons form an array of parallel channels without any interconnections. The second stage is the olfactory bulb. The PON axons terminate on the surface of the olfactory bulb in the layer of the glomeruli (gl): these consist of

284

synaptic endings of PON axons and periglomerular neurons (P). The output of this layer is fed to the layer of the mitral (M) and tufted (T) neurons, which two groups have important interconnections. These neuron groups both project into the underlying layer formed by the granule cells (gr). It should be added that the periglomerular neurons also form receiving and transmitting dendrodendritic synapses with mitral-tufted apical dendrites (Pinching and Powell, 1971; Reese and Shepherd, 1972; Freeman, 1974b). The output of the OB is constituted by axons of the mitral cells, which make up the lateral olfactory tract (LOT). The third stage is the prepyriform cortex, which forms a neural mass. The axons of the LOT terminate on the superficial pyramidal neurons (A), which make synaptic contacts with the granule cells (B) and the

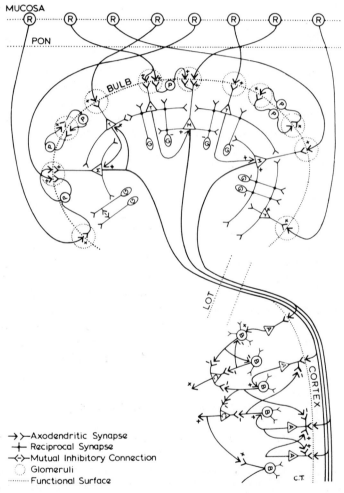

Fig. 1. Diagram of the neuron populations of the olfactory system according to Freeman (1973). Symbols: +, excitatory interaction; —, inhibitory interaction; R, receptors; PON, primary olfactory nerve; OB, olfactory bulb; P, periglomerular neuron; M, mitral neuron; T, tufted neuron; G, glomerular neuron; LOT, lateral olfactory tract; prepyriform cortex; A, superficial pyramidal neuron; B, short axon (cortical granule) neuron; C, deep pyramidal neuron.

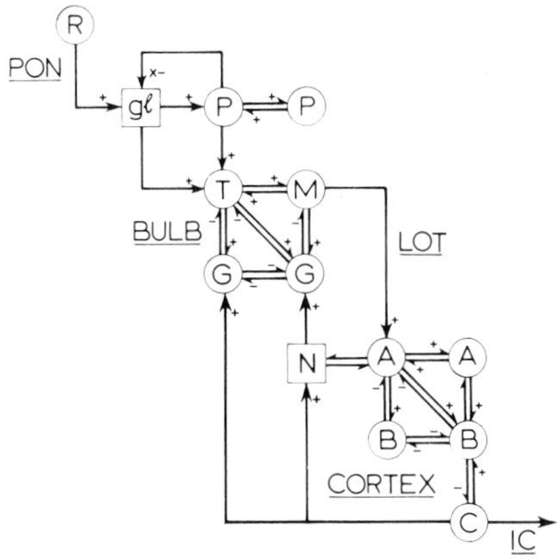

Fig. 2. Lumped circuit diagram of the two cartels in the olfactory bulb and cortex following Freeman (1973). Symbols: gl, glomeruli; N, anterior olfactory nucleus; IC, external capsule; X —, multiplicative inhibition (related to presynaptic inhibition). The other symbols are those of Fig. 1.

latter in turn terminate on deep pyramidal neurons (C). The axons of these last neurons constitute the output of the PPC, which forms a divergent set of channels projecting upon several structures of the basal forebrain. They also feed back onto the OB.

The concatenation of these different neuronal structures is shown as an anatomical diagram in Fig. 1. By means of recordings of single neuron activity and of field potentials it was possible to determine the type of synaptic interactions among the different cell groups and layers of the olfactory system. A scheme of the proposed interactions is shown in Fig. 2. In this scheme the different types of neurons are represented as *lumped systems*, since they are considered to have, on average, similar properties and reciprocal connections within the population. Freeman's basic methodology of study of those neural masses has been to follow a *linear systems analysis* approach. For linear analysis to be justifiable the system under consideration must obey the superposition principle, which states that when the input is multiplied by a constant, k, the system's response must be multiplied by the same constant. It has been shown by Freeman (1964, 1972) that, within determined limits of input amplitude, the responses of the olfactory system's neural masses do in fact obey the *principle of superposition*. This fundamental property is not unique within the central nervous system. It has also been shown to hold in the case of other types of sensory evoked potentials, for example, in the visual system, by van der Tweel (1961), Spekreijse and van der Tweel (1970), Lopes da Silva et al. (1970), Regan (1968); for a review see Regan (1972). According to this approach the output signal of the neural mass is a holistic event, a *field potential*, the amplitude of which is proportional to the input. In conjunction with the field potentials, *poststimulus time histograms* of single neurons have been recorded and analyzed in a similar fashion. The fundamental aspects of the olfactory system which form the essence of the model can be summarized as follows.

Basic modules

Aggregates. The input transducer consists of an *aggregate* because they have no anatomical synaptic interconnections.

Populations. The modules of the olfactory system consist of *five neuronal populations*, which are formed by those groups of neurons which have a common type of output (exclusively excitatory or inhibitory) and a common afferent source. It should be noted that from a functional viewpoint it is more important to be able to make such a statement than it is to define the different groups of neurons in terms of their actual histological appearance. The 5 populations are the following.

The periglomerular neurons which probably form an excitatory population; this is an interesting controversial point, since Shepherd (1972) has considered the periglomerular neurons to provide inhibition. Experimental and model studies of Freeman (1974b, c) support the excitatory hypothesis, but recent experiments by Getchell and Shepherd (1975) cast doubt on this point.

The mitral-tufted neuron population, which is also excitatory.

The granule neuronal population, which is inhibitory.

The surface pyramidal neuron population of the PPC, which is excitatory.

The granule neuron population of the PPC, which is inhibitory.

Cartels. There are several cartels in the system, such as that formed by the interaction between the periglomerular and the mitral-tufted neuron populations; this interaction is probably mutually excitatory (Freeman, 1974b). The interaction between the tufted-mitral and the granule neuron populations forms an inhibitory feedback loop. The interaction between the surface pyramidal and the granule neuron populations in the PPC also forms an inhibitory feedback loop.

Feedback loops

The importance of feedback loops in the neuron cartels emerges from this type of analysis. The basic constants which allow a mathematical description of a neuronal feedback loop are 3: (i) the membrane time constants; (ii) the length constants, i.e., the distances of the interactions; and (iii) the gain factors, i.e., the strength of interactions. If one thinks in terms of neural plasticity, it is worth emphasizing that it is likely that it is these gain factors which are the most modifiable parameters within a neural mass. Two types of loops should be distinguished: the inhibitory and the excitatory feedback loops. We shall consider one example below.

It should be noted that the terms negative and positive feedback, are often used in a rather loose way to characterize the interactions between neuron populations. However, the sign of feedback is defined in an exact way by comparing the overall gain modulus of the system with feedback (closed loop gain: $|Y_0(j\omega)|$) and without feedback (open loop gain: $|Y_1(j\omega)|$). The feedback is said to be negative if $|Y_0(j\omega)| < |Y_1(j\omega)|$ and positive in the opposite case (e.g., Hammond, 1958). The exact sign of feedback in the interaction between neuron populations is in most cases not known. It therefore seems to us preferable to use, in general terms, the terms excitatory and inhibitory feedback in order to define the main synaptic type of interaction between neuron populations. This will be considered from the reference point of the "main" population (usually the population which receives the input from another source and/or sends its output to another structure).

Freeman has described an inhibitory feedback loop in the OB cartel between the mitral-tufted and granule neuron populations. Excitation of the mitral-tufted (M-T) neurons leads to excitation of the granule (G) neurons, and to feedback inhibition of the M-T neurons. Therefore, the G neurons are disexcited and the M-T neurons disinhibited, so that they may become excited again, and the whole process can be described as oscillatory. Indeed, the average evoked potential of the neural mass (generated by the G neurons) and the poststimulus time histogram of mitral neurons both display this oscillatory character (Fig. 3). The basic oscillation is at about 40 Hz (Freeman, 1972), which is also seen as a spectral peak in the EEG of the OB of the cat. It is important to note that, in this sense, the field potential revealed in the EEG is not a necessary part of the mechanisms of the cartel. The EEG as well as the average evoked potential are to be viewed as electrical epiphenomena that permit observation of events in the neural mass (Katchalsky et al., 1974).

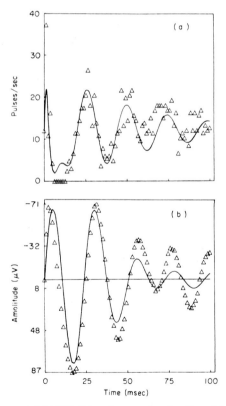

Fig. 3. Average evoked potential (AEP) (b) and poststimulus time histogram (PSTH of mitral neurons) (a) recorded in the olfactory bulb in response to LOT stimulation (see Fig. 1). The triangles are experimental points; the curves were obtained using the lumped model. (From Freeman, 1973.)

A similar type of inhibitory feedback loop occurs in the PPC cartel, where the surface pyramidal neuron population excites the cortical granule cell population, which in turn inhibits the former. Without entering into details of the mathematical analysis (e.g., Freeman, 1972) it is interesting to note that this type of model can be used to relate changes of the average evoked potential, recorded in different behavioral states, to interactions between different neuron populations in well defined layers of the PPC. For instance, by introducing selective attention to the evoking stimulus (a shock to the PON), a change in the average evoked potential was obtained. This change could be modeled by a change in the gain factor (strength of interaction) in the superficial pyramidal population (i.e., in the excitatory layer). In a situation where a non-specific arousal factor was introduced changes in the average evoked potential were observed which could be interpreted, in terms of Freeman's model, as being related to changes in the gain factor in the cortical granule neuron population (i.e., in the inhibitory layer). These are clear examples of how a model can be used in order to interpret experimental results in terms of underlying neuronal properties.

Surface distributions

The input to the olfactory system which comes from the olfactory transducers presents divergence and convergence at each relay stage. Therefore, there is a spatiotemporal transformation of the input. The important quantities for the processing of olfactory information may be exactly contained in the surface distributions of neural activity over the different neuron populations. In this sense, as Freeman points out (1973), the activity of a single neuron has no meaning in itself, but only as it specifies the value at a point of the surface function for the whole population.

"NEURAL MASSES" MODEL FOR THE GENERATION OF RHYTHMIC ACTIVITY

A current view in neurophysiology is that the origin of certain rhythmic electrical activity seen in the EEG, namely that characteristic of some thalamic nuclei and cortical areas after administration of a barbiturate (Andersen and Andersson, 1968; Andersen et al., 1967), and possibly also that occurring spontaneously (mainly at eye closure: alpha rhythm) (Lopes da Silva et al., 1974), is to be found in a cartel of neurons characterized by the interaction between excitatory and inhibitory neuronal populations. Essentially the same applies to the EEG of the olfactory bulb's cartel as shown by Freeman and discussed in the previous section. This hypothesis has direct implications for the origin of some important features of the electroencephalogram, or "EEG"; it may turn out to be of paramount interest for clinical neurophysiologists, considering the widespread use of the EEG in the assessment of brain diseases and behavioral states, but the remarkable lack of understanding of its nature. In order to evaluate the above-mentioned hypothesis, it is useful to develop models which may lead to tests of the validity of some assumptions, and to formulate new experiments.

A distributed model of alpha rhythm

We have proposed recently (Lopes da Silva et al., 1974) a model which incorporates the main physiological and histological assumptions necessary to explain the generation of the alpha rhythm, i.e., the EEG stochastic signal which lies in the frequency range of 8–13 Hz; this appears mainly at eye closure, and can be recorded best from the posterior regions of the skull in humans. A similar type of activity has also been recorded at the visual cortex and some thalamic nuclei in dogs (Lopes da Silva et al., 1973) and cats (Lanoir, 1972). The model consists of a set of simulated neurons, thalamocortical relay cells (TCR) and interneurons (IN). In contrast with the lumped models (of which we have given some examples above, for the olfactory system) this model is a *distributed* one in the sense that each neuron is modeled individually: it occupies a specific position within a matrix of neurons. Such a distributed model offers some special possibilities for theoretical studies which are not easily available in lumped models such as those of Freeman.

Without entering here into great detail about the alpha rhythm distributed model, which has been described elsewhere (Lopes da Silva et al., 1974), it is of interest to point out some of its characteristics. To start with, it is necessary to state that the *structure* of the distributed model consists of 144 TCR neurons and 36 INs; the 32 TCR neurons which surround one IN are responsible for its

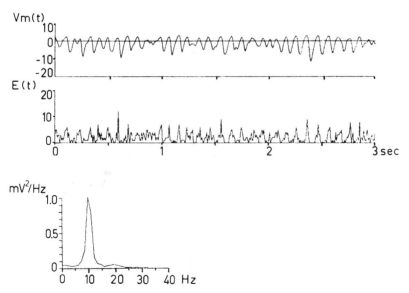

Fig. 4. Output of the standard distributed model of alpha rhythm where each interneuron (IN) is excited by the surrounding 32 thalamocortical relay (TCR) cells; on its turn each IN inhibits the 12 TCR neurons around it. $V_m(t)$: summed membrane potentials of all TCR neurons (scale in mV); E(t): impulse density (number of action potentials) produced by all TCR neurons. Lower curve: power spectrum of the signal $V_m(t)$ estimated by ensemble averaging. Note the alpha frequency peak and the smaller peak at the second harmonic frequency.

excitation, while each IN is responsible for the inhibition of the 12 TCRs around it. The excitation and inhibition are represented by time functions which give an approximation to the wave forms of EPSPs and IPSPs respectively. The matrix of neurons should be viewed as lying at the surface of a torus. Furthermore, each neuron fires whenever the membrane potential exceeds a simple threshold; a short refractory period then follows. A basic characteristic of this model is that the input, received by each TCR neuron, is

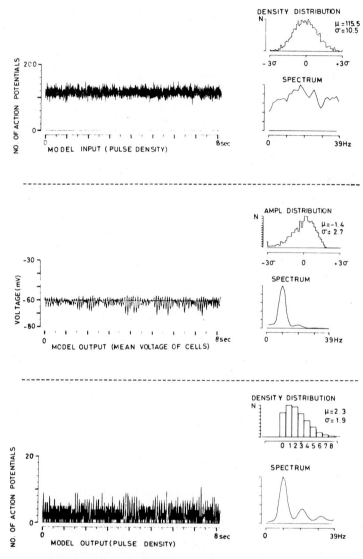

Fig. 5. Input and output signals of the distributed model of alpha rhythm. Upper part: impulse density of the input to all thalamocortical relay (TCR) neurons. Middle part: summed membrane potentials of all TCR neurons. Lower part: impulse density of all TCR neurons. At the right-hand side the amplitude distributions and the power spectra of the three signals are shown. Note the apparent waxing and waning of the alpha rhythm, and the dominant alpha frequency. (From Lopes da Silva et al., 1974.)

in the form of a series of pulses (action potentials) which have a Poisson distribution; the inputs to the individual TCR neurons are uncorrelated. The model's output signal is the sum of the membrane potential fluctuations of all TCR neurons. This output signal simulates very closely an alpha rhythm, provided that: (a) the postsynaptic potentials have the appropriate time constants (small EPSPs lasting about 20 msec and larger IPSPs lasting about 100 msec); (b) the input has sufficient strength (about 20 imp./sec per axon, and a convergence of 10 axons upon one TCR neuron) and (c) the matrix of the two populations has the dimensions indicated above. This result is illustrated in Figs. 4 and 5.

One interesting possibility offered by the distributed model is to elucidate the *relationship among the activity of single units, and between unit activity and the whole population's "EEG"*. This type of problem is not easy to tackle either experimentally (because simultaneous measurements of the activity of even a few neurons is difficult to realize in practice) nor in a lumped model, for fairly obvious reasons. It has been generally observed that the electrical activity of single neurons can vary considerably even when the units are closely packed together and when there is a clear field potential (e.g., rhythmic EEG activity) which can be recorded from their neighborhood. This finding has puzzled many experimentalists, and it has even helped to cast doubts on the neuronal origin of such EEG activity. With the help of the distributed model it is possible to demonstrate that a clear field potential (the sum of all membrane potentials in the model TCR neurons) with a rhythmic component is in fact compatible with quite a low degree of correlation among closely spaced population units. This is illustrated in Fig. 6. In this figure, the fluctuations of the membrane potential of 6 neurons are shown; these neurons form a closed

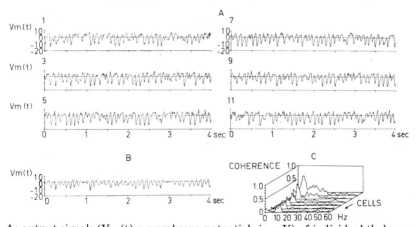

Fig. 6. A: output signals ($V_m(t)$ = membrane potentials in mV) of individual thalamocortical relay (TCR) neurons in the *standard* distributed model which generated the signals presented in Fig. 4. The cells lie on a diagonal of the lattice in a close ring because the sides of the lattice are assumed to be continuous. B: summed membrane potentials of 12 neurons on the diagonal. C: coherence (squared function) between the $V_m(t)$ of neuron 1 in the ring and the $V_m(t)$ of the neighbors (3, 5 . . .), as a function of frequency and distance. The coherence is estimated by means of ensemble averaging. Notwithstanding the closeness between the model neurons there is considerable variability between the different signals. The coherence decreases rapidly with distance (no volume conduction effect is allowed in the model).

292

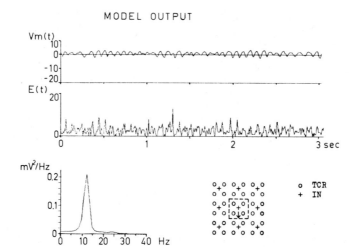

Fig. 7. Output signals and power spectrum of all thalamocortical relay (TCR) neurons in the distributed model with a *smaller* inhibitory area than the standard model as in Fig. 4: here one interneuron (IN) inhibits only 4 TCR neurons as shown in the inset V_m (t), E(t) and power spectrum as in Fig. 4. Note that the intensity of the alpha peak is weaker than that of the standard model (Fig. 4) and that the bandwidth is larger.

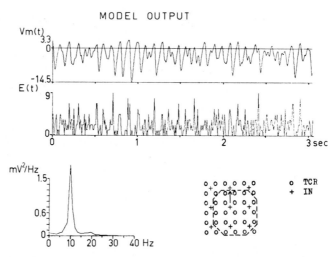

Fig. 8. Output signals and power spectrum of all thalamocortical relay (TCR) neurons in the distributed model with a *larger* inhibitory area than the standard model as in Fig. 4: here one interneuron (IN) inhibits 21 TCR neurons (inset). Note that the intensity of the alpha peak is larger and the bandwidth smaller in comparison with the model of Fig. 4.

ring on the surface of the torus. It can be seen that the time fluctuations of the potential in individual neurons show considerable variations. The progressive decrease of coherence coefficient (in the alpha frequency range) computed between the neuron in position 1 and the other neurons in the ring, up to the most distant, reveals in quantitative terms that the correlation between slow wave activity in two neurons depends greatly upon the distance between them.

In the distributed model it is also easy to investigate the *result of changing the range of excitatory and inhibitory influence* of, respectively, TCRs and INs. In the case of Fig. 4, there were 12 TCR neurons which were inhibited by one IN, which is the common situation; the effects of reducing this number to 4 and of increasing it to 21 are shown in Figs. 7 and 8. Reduction of the inhibitory area of influence of an IN results in a decrease of the spectral peak amplitude (alpha frequency) and an increase in band width; an increase in the inhibitory area has the opposite effects. These are some of the phenomena which can be studied using a distributed neuronal model of rhythmic activity. However, this type of model has one main theoretical disadvantage: it is difficult to treat it analytically in a general way. Therefore, we needed to develop a lumped model which would take into account the main characteristics of the distributed model. A lumped model of the same type as those of Freeman (described above) would lead to a more general treatment of the activity of neuronal populations.

A lumped model of rhythmic activity

The development of the lumped model in analytical terms included, of course, the step of translating the properties of the discrete matrix of neurons into a simplified system such as depicted in Fig. 9. Essentially, the neural mass (here thalamic nucleus) of which the EEG is of interest, forms a cartel (KII set) which is constituted by the interaction of an excitatory and an inhibitory population (KIe and KIi sets). In order to introduce the analytic simplification of the distributed model it is also useful to consider the general *model of Wilson and Cowan* (1972), who have formulated a set of equations that describe the overall activity (not specifically the EEG) in a cartel of excitatory

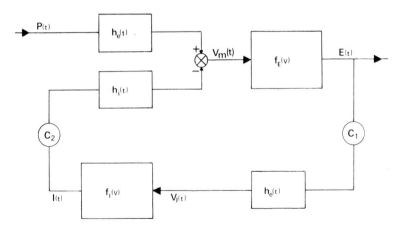

Fig. 9. Block diagram of the lumped model for rhythmic activity or simplified alpha rhythm model. The thalamocortical relay (TCR) neurons are represented by two linear systems having impulse responses simulating an EPSP ($h_e(t)$) and an IPSP ($h_i(t)$) respectively together with the static non-linearity ($f_E(V)$) representing the spike generating process. The interneurons (IN cells) are represented by one linear system ($h_e(t)$) and a non-linearity ($f_I(V)$). C_1 represents the number of INs to which one TCR neuron projects, C_2 represents the number of TCRs to which one IN projects. (From Lopes da Silva et al., 1974.)

and inhibitory neurons having a large number of interconnections. In this model it is assumed that all types of interactions are possible, not only between excitatory and inhibitory neurons, but also within the same population.

Zetterberg (1973) has made use of this formulation in order to simplify the distributed model of alpha rhythm. Two quantities, E(t) and I(t), have to be introduced which represent, respectively, the proportion of excitatory neurons and of inhibitory neurons firing per unit of time at instant t. The expression for the average level of excitation generation in an excitatory neuron can be given in terms of (1) the external input P(t) to the excitatory population and (2) the constants C_3 and C_2 which represent the average number of, respectively, excitatory and inhibitory synapses at the input of the excitatory population:

$$V_m(t) = \int_0^\infty [C_3 E(t-t') - C_2 I(t-t') + P(t-t')]\, \alpha\,(t')\, dt' \tag{1}$$

where the time course of the decay of the stimulation effect is given by $\alpha(t)$. A similar expression can be written for the inhibitory population, with Q(t) as external input, C_1 as the number of excitatory synapses, and C_4 of inhibitory synapses at the input of this population.

$$V_i(t) = \int_0^\infty [C_1 E(t-t') - C_4 I(t-t') + Q(t-t')]\, \alpha\,(t')\, dt' \tag{2}$$

Wilson and Cowan eventually arrive at the following pair of equations to describe the overall neuronal activity at time $t + \tau$:

$$E(t + \tau) = \left[1 - \int_{t-r_e}^t E(t')\, dt'\right] \cdot f_E\,[V_m(t)]$$

$$\tag{3}$$

$$I(t + \tau) = \left[1 - \int_{t-r_i}^t I(t')\, dt'\right] \cdot f_I\,[V_i(t)]$$

The expression

$$\left[1 - \int_{t-r_e}^t E(t', dt')\right]$$

gives the proportion of excitatory neurons that are sensitive at time t, where r_e denotes the absolute refractory period for the excitatory neurons (r_i for the inhibitory). The two sigmoid functions, $f_E(x)$ and $f_I(x)$, play of course a crucial role. They may be viewed as representing the distribution of thresholds within the population.

Elaborating on this theory, Zetterberg (1973) has adapated equations (1) and (2) in order to obtain the analytical description of the distributed model of EEG (alpha) activity. An essential aspect is the introduction of the time functions, $h_e(t)$ and $h_i(t)$ (see also Fig. 9) which represent the EPSP (excitatory postsynaptic potential) and the IPSP (inhibitory postsynaptic potential) respectively; these functions will substitute for the function $\alpha(t)$ in equations

(1) and (2). Another modification consists in changing the "average level of excitation" into "average membrane potential" in the neuronal population; with these modifications equations (1) and (2) become:

$$V_m(t) = \int_0^\infty [C_3 E(t-t') + P(t-t')]\, h_e(t')\, dt' - \int_0^\infty C_2 I(t-t')\, h_i(t')\, dt'$$

$$V_i(t) = \int_0^\infty [C_1 E(t-t') + Q(t-t')]\, h_e(t')\, dt' - \int_0^\infty C_4 I(t-t')\, h_i(t')\, dt'$$

(4)

In order to write a simplified expression for the number of neurons firing at a given time, as given in equation 3, Zetterberg (1973) disregarded the influence of the refractory period, and assumed the following expressions:

$$E(t) = f_E\{V_m(t)\}$$
$$I(t) = f_I\{V_i(t)\}$$

(5)

in which $E(t)$ and $I(t)$ are equivalent to the impulse density of the populations of excitatory and inhibitory neurons. The system given in Fig. 9 is described by equations (4) and (5), considering that $Q(t) = 0$, $C_3 = 0$, and $C_4 = 0$. In this way we do not assume any explicit interactions within the populations themselves nor any external input upon the inhibitory interneurons. This for the sake of simplicity.

Linear analysis

To test whether or not the lumped model would be appropriate, it was considered that the basic objective was to simulate the power spectrum of the alpha rhythm as recorded under physiological conditions. This was done first by using a linear approximation of the lumped model; the main objective here was to obtain a simulated EEG, the spectrum of which would present a peak within the alpha frequency band.

The variables $V_m(t)$, $V_i(t)$, $E(t)$ and $I(t)$ in equations (4) and (5) were assumed to be stationary, and they were described in terms of the fluctuations around their respective mean values.

At a certain mean input level, $\bar{P}$, the relations between $\bar{E}$ and $\bar{I}$ can be given by substituting in (4) and (5):

$$(C_3 \bar{E} + \bar{P})\, H_e - C_2 \bar{I}\, H_i = f_E^{-1}(\bar{E})$$
$$(C_1 \bar{E} + \bar{Q})\, H_e - C_4 \bar{I}\, H_i = f_I^{-1}(\bar{I})$$

(6)

setting $H_e = \int_0^\infty h_e(t)\, dt$ and $H_i = \int_0^\infty h_i(t)\, dt$

The membrane potentials, $V_m(t)$ and $V_i(t)$, are described around their means

$$\bar{V}_m = f_E^{-1}(\bar{E}) \quad \text{and} \quad \bar{V}_i = f_I^{-1}(\bar{I}); \quad f_E^{-1} \quad \text{and} \quad f_I^{-1}$$

are developed in a Taylor series, but only the linear terms will be considered here; in the following "Non-linear analysis" section we shall take into account the contribution of the non-linear terms:

$$V_m(t) = f_E^{-1}(E) \approx f_E^{-1}(\bar{E}) + a_{e1}(E - \bar{E})$$
$$V_i(t) = f_I^{-1}(I) \approx f_I^{-1}(\bar{I}) + a_{i1}(I - \bar{I}) \tag{7}$$

Therefore, the following relationships apply:

$$v_m(t) = V_m(t) - \bar{V}_m;$$
$$v_i(t) = V_i(t) - \bar{V}_i;$$
$$p(t) = P(t) - \bar{P};$$
$$i(t) = \bar{I}(t) - \bar{I}.$$

And from equation (7):

$$v_m(t) = a_{e1} e(t);$$
$$v_i(t) = a_{i1} i(t).$$

By putting $C_3 = 0$, $Q = 0$, and $C_4 = 0$, the equations (4) can now be written as follows:

$$v_m(t) = \int_0^\infty h_e(t') p(t-t') dt' - C_2 \int_0^\infty h_i(t') i(t-t') dt'$$

$$v_i(t) = \int_0^\infty C_1 h_e(t') e(t-t') dt' \tag{8}$$

These expressions correspond to the diagram of Fig. 9. Transforming into the Laplace domain, the expression for the input $P(s)$/output $V_m(s)$ transfer function becomes:

$$\frac{V_m(s)}{P(s)} = \frac{H_e(s)}{1 + \dfrac{C_1 C_2}{a_{e1} a_{i1}} H_e(s) H_i(s)} \tag{9}$$

One EPSP and one IPSP can be approximated by the following expressions:

$$H_e(s) = \frac{(a_2 - a_1) A}{(s + a_1)(s + a_2)} \qquad H_i(s) = \frac{(C_2 - C_1) B}{(s + b_1)(s + b_2)} \tag{10}$$

In order to investigate the spectral properties of the $V_m(s)$, Zetterberg (1973) modified (9) into

$$V_m(s) = \frac{(a_2 - a_1) A (s + b_1)(s + b_2)}{(s + a_1)(s + a_2)(s + b_1)(s + b_2) + K} \cdot P(s) \tag{11}$$

where

$$K = \frac{C_1 C_2 (a_2 - a_1)(b_2 - b_1) AB}{a_{e1} a_{i1}}$$

The spectrum of p(t) is considered as being equal to unity, considering that p(t) is a random process with a flat spectrum. Expression (9) represents the transfer function of a 4th order linear system. The power spectrum of V_m (s) can be directly computed by

$$R(f) = | V_m (2\pi jf) |^2 \times cst \qquad (12)$$

The following numerical parameters were used in computation of the spectrum:

$a_1 = 55 \sec^{-1}$; $a_2 = 605 \sec^{-1}$; $b_1 = 27\cdot5 \sec^{-1}$; $b_2 = 55 \sec^{-1}$; $C_2 = 3$;

$C_1 = 32$; $A = 1\cdot65$ mV; $B = 32$ mV; $1/a_{e1} = 2130$ mV^{-1} sec^{-1};

$1/a_{i1} = 2130$ mV^{-1} sec^{-1}

The spectrum $R(f)$ indeed shows a peak around 10 Hz, as was expected (Fig. 10). The band width and the peak frequency both depend upon the coefficient K. Up to a point, a larger K will cause an increase in the frequency of the rhythmic activity, but too large a K will cause instability. K is also proportional to the derivatives, $1/a_{e1}$ and $1/a_{i1}$ of the sigmoid functions in their working point, which in turn is determined by the mean input pulse density $\bar{P}$. The peak frequency will increase and the bandwidth decrease with an increase of the coupling constants, C_2 and C_1, i.e., with an increase in synaptic interactions within the neuronal cartel.

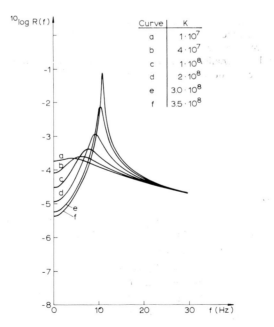

Fig. 10. The influence of the feedback factor K (for explanation see text) on the power spectrum of the output signal of the lumped model of Fig. 9. Note that if K is small the spectrum is that of a low-pass filter; as K increases the spectrum acquires a clear selectivity at the alpha frequency. (From Lopes da Silva et al., 1974.)

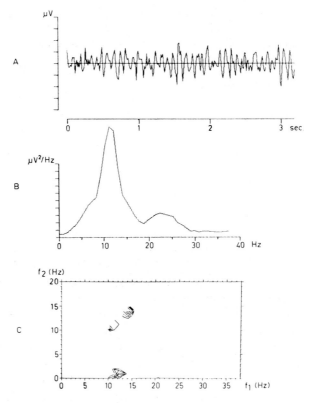

Fig. 11. An epoch of alpha rhythm (A) experimentally recorded from the visual cortex of the dog (technique as used in Lopes da Silva et al., 1973). The power spectrum (B) and the bicoherence (C) were obtained by ensemble averaging. Note the peak in the power spectrum at about 10 Hz and the smaller peak at the second harmonic frequency, which are related to each other as the bicoherence shows. A: experimentally recorded alpha rhythm (arbitrary scale). B: power spectrum (arbitrary scale). C: bicoherence limits 99% at 0·119, 95% at 0·096, 5 lines from 0·18 until 0·26.

Non-linear analysis

The linear analysis of the preceding section only gives a first approximation to the spectral characteristics of the alpha rhythm, both experimentally measured and simulated. The spectrum of the experimentally measured alpha rhythm also presents a clear component at the second harmonic of the peak frequency (Fig. 11). It can be demonstrated by means of bispectral analysis that this component is indeed a second harmonic of the peak frequency. This fact implies that important non-linear properties have also to be taken into account. It is necessary to state more precisely in what consists bispectral analysis. The bispectrum of a stochastic signal, x(t), is defined as:

$$B_{xxx}(f_1, f_2) = E\{X(f_1)X(f_2)X^*(f_1 + f_2)\} \tag{13}$$

BICOHERENCE MODEL OUTPUT

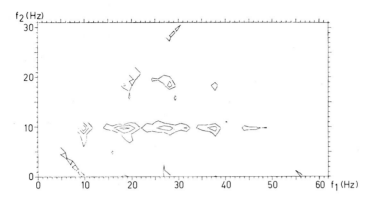

Fig. 12. Bicoherence of the lumped model output ($V_m(t)$) as a function of the frequencies f_1 and f_2. Lines are drawn between coordinates having the same bicoherence values (iso-value lines). Three sets of lines are drawn at values 0·2, 0·3 and 0·4 respectively. This analysis is done by means of averaging over 4 epochs which gives confidence limits of 0·187 (99%) or 0·151 (95%). Thus in the closed regions the hypothesis that there is no relation between the different frequency components can be rejected.

where $X(f)$ represents the Fourier component at frequency f; $E\{---\}$ represents the averaging procedure. The normalized bispectrum (also called auto-bicoherence) is defined as:

$$C_{xxx}(f_1, f_2) = \frac{|B_{xxx}(f_1, f_2)|^2}{S_{xx}(f_1) \, S_{xx}(f_2) \, S_{xx}(f_1 + f_2)} \qquad (14)$$

where $S_{xx}(f)$ is the estimate of the power spectrum of $X(t)$; in case the system were to possess non-linearities, by means of which higher harmonics would be introduced, the normalized bispectrum would be significantly different from zero. In particular, when there occurs both a fundamental frequency component and a second harmonic in the system's output a peak will appear in the bispectrum at the intersection of f_1 and f_2. This is what happens both for the experimentally recorded and for the simulated alpha rhythms, as shown in Figs. 11 and 12.

This non-linear behavior of the system depends upon the characteristics of the sigmoid relationships between pulse density and membrane potential. These sigmoid functions have been introduced in expressions (7) as linear approximations around the operating point. However, in order to understand the non-linear behavior of the system, in particular the generation of second harmonics, higher order terms have to be taken into account. Thus, expressions (7) should be expanded at least until the second order term, as follows:

$$f_E^{-1}(E) \approx f_E^{-1}(\bar{E}) + a_{e1}(E - \bar{E}) + a_{e2}(E - \bar{E})^2 \qquad (15)$$

300

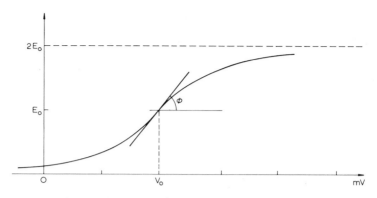

Fig. 13. The sigmoid shape static non-linearity of the lumped model for rhythmic activity. The function $f_E(V)$ which is given by the two exponential functions in the text (equation 16) describes the relation between the membrane potential V (abscissa) and the impulse density E (ordinate). In the linear approximation the non-linearity is replaced by an amplification factor $1/a_{el} = arctg(\phi)$. (From Van Heusden, 1975.)

and similarly for $f_I^{-1}(I)$. In the lumped model, the functions $f_E(V)$ and $f_I(V)$ have been approximated by two exponentials, as shown in Fig. 13:

$$f_E(V) = f_I(V) = E_o \exp\{-b(V_o - V)\} \qquad V \leqslant V_o$$
$$f_E(V) = f_I(V) = E_o [2 - \exp\{-b(V - V_o)\}] \qquad V > V_0 \tag{16}$$

Using expressions (15), it is possible to perform a non-linear analysis of the lumped model by means of a Kernel description. In this way the output of the system is expanded in a Volterra series. A thorough treatment of the non-linear transfer function of the model can be found in van Heusden (1975).

EXTENSION OF THE MODEL OF RHYTHMIC ACTIVITY TO INCLUDE EXCITATORY AND INHIBITORY FEEDBACK

The basic model analyzed so far should in fact be more complex in order to embrace more recent physiological data. It was suggested by Andersson et al. (1971) that the input not only excites a TCR neuron but also leads to inhibition of the interneurons IN, through an intermediate neuron (inhibitory feedforward). Furthermore, it is also reasonable to consider that the INs receive inputs which have their origin outside the matrix; these inputs may be either excitatory or inhibitory. The cartel of neurons which includes all these new aspects is indicated schematically in Fig. 14. (Note that in this scheme an excitatory feedback loop is also incorporated, but for the results discussed at this stage this loop is not active: i.e., $C_3 = 0$, $C_4 = 0$.) These extra inputs which affect the INs may be called *modulating influences*, because they influence the main cartel of neurons in the sense of a rein-control system.

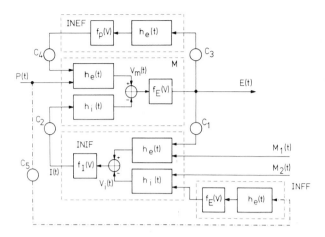

Fig. 14. Block diagram of the lumped model for rhythmic activity with a possibility of modulation of inhibitory feedback and excitatory feedback. The cartel consists of four populations. M: main cells with input and output impulse density, respectively P(t) and E(t) and membrane potential $V_m(t)$; spike generation non-linearity: $f_E(V)$. INIF: inhibitory population with membrane potential $V_i(t)$ and modulating inputs: excitatory by means of $M_1(t)$ and inhibitory by means of $M_2(t)$, spike generation with sigmoid $f_1(V)$. INFF: excitatory population driven by the main input P(t) inhibiting the inhibitory population INIF. INEF: excitatory population feeding back on to the main population; spike generation sigmoid $f_p(V)$. The interconnectivity constants giving the number of cells of one population projecting to one cell of the other population are C_1 and C_2 for the inhibitory feedback and C_3 and C_4 for the excitatory feedback. C_5 represents the number of cells of the INFF population, excited by one input fiber (feedforward).

An example is shown in Fig. 15: here it can be seen that an inhibitory modulating influence upon the INs will lead to a very low output of the IN, so that the gain of the feedback loop is very low and the resulting EEG signal is rather irregular; an excitatory input upon the INs leads progressively to a more or less complete inhibition of the whole cartel. It will be evident that the existence of these modulating influences, impinging onto different cartels of neurons which occupy different brain areas, will lead to the simultaneous appearance or disappearance of rhythmic activity in those cartels. They thus work as a *gating mechanism*, which may project to many thalamic and cortical areas. The correlation or coherence between the EEGs generated in these cartels will be determined by the degree of correlation between the respective inputs/outputs (Lopes da Silva et al., 1974); however, even if the correlation is low, bursts of rhythmic activity may tend to occur simultaneously as a consequence of common gating mechanisms. This type of mechanism would be able to explain the fact that, although alpha rhythms (Lopes da Silva et al., 1973) and barbiturate spindles (Gánes and Andersen, 1975) both tend to occur at the same time in different thalamic and cortical areas, the coherence or correlation between the activity recorded from several such areas, is often only moderate; e.g., similar experimentally obtained coherence values (the

302

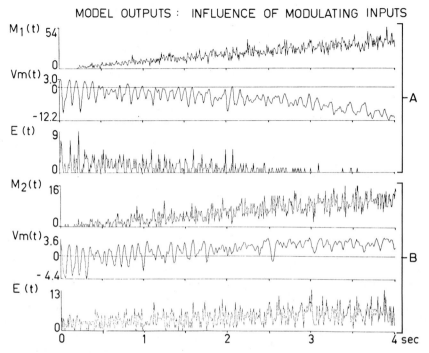

MODEL OUTPUTS : INFLUENCE OF MODULATING INPUTS

Fig. 15. The effect of modulating inputs of the summed membrane fluctuations of all main cells of the model of Fig. 14. The modulating inputs $M_1(t)$ and $M_2(t)$ are in the form of impulses, the density of which increases as a ramp function. A: the model output signals $V_m(t)$ (mV) and $E(t)$ (imp./sec) change in the course of time due to the modulating influence of a steadily increasing noisy impulse density $M_1(t)$ (imp./sec), exciting the inhibitory population. B: the same output signals $V_m(t)$ and $E(t)$ were influenced by a steadily increasing inhibition of the inhibitory population by means of $M_2(t)$. Note that in case A the rhythmicity characteristic of the alpha mode of response of the model (seen in the first 0·5 sec) decreases and the DC level moves to the hyperpolarization side. In B there is also a decrease in alpha rhythmicity, but the DC level changes in the opposite direction.

coherence equals a squared correlation coefficient) have been reported for thalamocortical α rhythms and barbiturate spindles by Lopes da Silva et al. (1973) and Ganes and Andersen (1975), respectively, although quite different recording methods were used by the two groups.

In several cases it has been suggested that, besides inhibitory feedback, also excitatory feedback can play an essential role in neuronal cartels. Freeman has shown this, as was discussed in the above "Feedback loops" section for the olfactory system. It has also been suggested for the hippocampus (Dichter and Spencer, 1969) and for the system which is "pacing" the hippocampal theta rhythm, as can be deduced from the work of McLennan and Miller (1974). While we ourselves were trying to simulate the hippocampal theta rhythm, the importance of excitatory feedback also emerged from the model studies. In this case the model structure which we propose corresponds to the complete schema shown in Fig. 14, but here we shall only consider the linear case. The linear transfer function is similar to that of expression (9), but now including the elements corresponding to the excitatory feedback loop (a_{p1}, C3, C4, $H_e(s)$):

$$V_m(s) = \frac{H_e(s)}{1 - \dfrac{C_3 C_4}{a_{e1} a_{p1}} H_e^2(s) + H_i(s) H_e(s) \dfrac{C_1 C_2}{a_{e1} a_{i1}}} \cdot P(s) \tag{17}$$

substituting expressions (10) in (17) and setting

$$K^- = \frac{C_1 C_2}{a_{e1} a_{i1}} \cdot (a_2 - a_1)(b_2 - b_1) \cdot A \cdot B \tag{18}$$

and

$$K^+ = \frac{C_3 C_4}{a_{e1} a_{p1}} \cdot (a_2 - a_1)^2 \cdot A^2 \tag{19}$$

we obtain

$$V_m(s) = \frac{A(a_2 - a_1)(s + a_1)(s + a_2)(s + b_1)(s + b_2)P(s)}{(s + b_1)(s + b_2)(s + a_1)^2(s + a_2)^2 + K^-(s + a_1)(s + a_2) - K^+(s + b_1)(s + b_2)} \tag{20}$$

K^+ and K^- can be considered to be the factors determining the influence of the excitatory and inhibitory feedback loops. It is interesting to note how the introduction of excitatory feedback influences the peak frequency and the bandwidth of the simulated EEG. This was investigated using the same constants for the IPSP and EPSP as indicated in the above "Linear analysis" section, although any other values may, of course, be employed in the same way. Fig. 16 shows the dependence of peak frequency and bandwidth of the rhythmic activity upon K^+ and K^-.

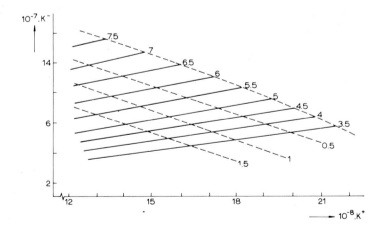

Fig. 16. Generalization of the effect of different combinations of excitatory and inhibitory feedback on peak frequency and bandwidth of the model output (V(t)). ————, lines with equal peak frequencies; — — — —, lines with equal bandwidths. Above the zero bandwidth line the system is unstable.

LIMIT CYCLE BEHAVIOR

The models discussed in the preceding sections may exhibit unstable behavior; for example, the range of instability of the model with excitatory and inhibitory feedback can be easily deduced from Fig. 16. This type of instability may well be of general interest, but the most interesting thing to investigate is how far such models can show oscillatory behavior independently of the initial input signal. This type of behavior would be of particular importance considering that, in real neuron cartels, it is possible to obtain oscillations which appear to be independent of the input conditions, such as in the case of epileptic seizures. A useful way to investigate this problem is to use phase-plane analysis, i.e., by analyzing the trajectories in the plane whose coordinates are $V_m(t)$ and $dV(t)/dt$.

For example, a linear oscillatory system with damping will have as a trajectory in the phase plane a spiral which, with increasing time, tends towards the origin. When closed trajectories exist it is said that there are limit cycles: they are a unique property of non-linear systems (Fig. 17).

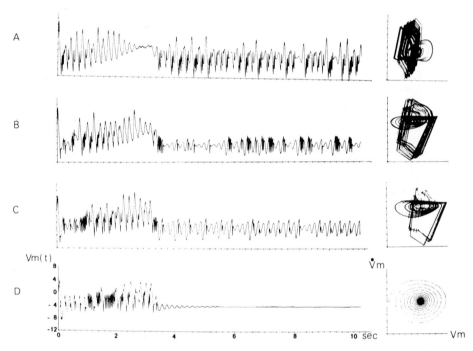

Fig. 17. Output ($V_m(t)$) of the model of Fig. 14 under 4 different conditions. In all cases the input (P(t)) is a ramp increasing from 0 to 2 units from $t = 0$ to $t = 3 \cdot 2$ sec and then decreasing down to zero in $0 \cdot 32$ sec. D: V_0 of the sigmoid function (Fig. 13) set at 6 mV. Note that the oscillations are damped and no free oscillations occur. C, B and A: the behavior of the model for decreasing values of V_0 (C, $V_0 = 5$ mV; B, $V_0 = 4$ mV; A, $V_0 = 3$ mV). Note that at this lower level of V_0 the system presents free oscillations with spike-and-wave patterns. Note also the limit cycles shown in phase planes on the right-hand side.

We have started an investigation of the conditions under which the model discussed under "Extensions of the model of rhythmic activity to include excitatory and inhibitory feedback" would produce limit cycles. The idea was that this might give us some insight as regards the properties of neurons, and/or populations, which are important for changing the mode of a stable neuron cartel into an unstable one, as in the case of epilepsy. This problem is being currently analyzed, and preliminary results are shown in Fig. 17. This figure shows that, under certain conditions, the model which has been excited by a ramp (linear increase of the pulse density) is capable of producing self-oscillations even after removal of the input. In this case, the necessary condition is a reduction of V_0 (see Fig. 13) by 1 mV from the value encountered in the stable case. This implies a decrease of the mean threshold of the neuron population. It is truly remarkable that the wave form of the self-oscillation so closely resembles that found in real EEGs recorded during epileptic seizures.

DISCUSSION AND CONCLUSIONS

In the introduction we quoted the statement of Harmon (1964), who suggested that theoretical neurophysiology may be particularly useful in suggesting functional relationships between the activity of single neurons and the behavior of populations. We think that the studies reviewed above support this statement. The main purpose of this type of theoretical study is precisely to bridge the gap between the two domains of neurophysiology: on the one hand the single neuron, and on the other the neuron population or, better said, the neural mass in the sense used by Freeman (1975). The central problem is that in order to understand the brain processes which control behavior it is necessary to grasp the functional interactions between neuronal populations. These interactions cannot easily be deduced by simply juxtaposing the properties of single neurons.

Besides this general aspect, the models presented here have allowed us to advance in the understanding of the neural mechanisms underlying certain types of field potentials revealed in the EEG, particularly the generation of alpha or theta rhythms, and of epileptic paroxysms. The importance of this aspect to general neurophysiology may be secondary, however, considering the fact that the field potential does not form an essential element of the activity of neuron populations. However, it appeared very relevant to us, in view of the paramount importance of the EEG in clinical neurophysiology. In this respect, it should be noted that the EEG is still the neurophysiological signal most widely employed in order to evaluate normal and pathological human brain activity. The models of alpha and theta rhythms presented here should not be considered as *the* models of *the* EEG, however. They may well be relevant only for particular aspects of EEG signals; the EEG as recorded from the scalp includes a variety of phenomena about which we do not yet have sufficient basic information, so that exact models are for the time being precluded. An exception may be the case of paroxysmal activity characteristic of epileptic foci.

The fact that our extended model, which included both excitatory and inhibitory feedback, generates limit cycles is of general interest and merits further discussion according to two basic questions: (a) do the limit cycles form a general mechanism as regards the origin of the EEG recorded in normal circumstances; or rather (b) do the limit cycles correspond to a particular mode of EEG activity, characteristic of an abnormal state such as epilepsy? Before we deal with these questions it is necessary to consider more explicitly what we do mean by limit cycles. In system analysis the term limit cycles is used to denote periodic oscillations of a non-linear system, with an external forcing function equal to zero, i.e., free oscillations. Limit cycles may be stable or unstable, although only the former have any physical significance (see Hammond, 1958). A stable limit cycle returns to the original state after being perturbed. Question (a) has been answered positively in several ways: Dewan (1964) has proposed that non-linear oscillations of the limit cycle type may explain certain EEG phenomena; Wilson and Cowan (1972) have shown that, in their model of interaction between excitatory and inhibitory neuron populations, limit cycles occur (although they do not explicitly propose this model as a basis for EEG generation); Freeman (1975) has interpreted the origin of the EEG waves recorded from the olfactory bulb (frequency range about 40 Hz; see also the "Feedback loops" section) in terms of a limit cycle. According to Freeman (1975), during each inspiration the burst of action potentials from the receptors increases the background activity of the mitral-tufted and granule neurons of the bulb; this would lead to an increase in the feedback gains in the cartel (KII set); if this increase were sufficiently large the activity of the cartel would switch into a stable limit cycle state. This would be the origin of the oscillatory burst of EEG waves appearing with inspiration.

A positive reply to the first question mentioned above thus appears to be supported by several good arguments. However, we should like to stress that, although limit cycles may form a good model for some of the EEG phenomena which occur in physiological circumstances, they are not necessary to account for certain other typical EEG features, such as alpha and theta rhythms. These may be viewed as oscillations occurring in non-linear systems of neurons when submitted to a (more or less) random input. The energy source for such driven oscillators may be found in the noisy activity of neural channels, for example, the typical dark discharge in the optic pathway (see Lopes da Silva et al., 1974) or the activity in the mesencephalic reticular formation (Skvaril et al., 1971). At the present stage of our knowledge it seems to us a reasonable proposal to accept that oscillatory phenomena in the EEG can occur either in the form of filtered noise (the neural filters being non-linear, however), or in the form of stable limit cycles.

The reply to the second question (b) also appears to be positive. Indeed, our model studies show that the changes occurring in the EEG of an epileptic focus may be modeled by modifications of parameters of the neuron populations such that limit cycles become possible. These modifications could be in the form of changes either in threshold or in coupling constants, determined for example by an extracellular accumulation of K^+ ions (e.g., Katchalsky et al., 1974).

Our general conclusion is that the formulation in terms of mathematical models of the modes of interaction among neuronal populations can provide a most promising step towards a better understanding of many brain phenomena. Furthermore, and perhaps of equal importance. it leads to an assessment in clear terms of the strong and weak points in our experimental knowledge.

ACKNOWLEDGEMENT

We thank Drs. W. Freeman, L.H. Zetterberg and L.H. van der Tweel for reading the manuscript and for their valuable suggestions and criticisms.

REFERENCES

Andersen, P and Andersson, S.A. (1968) *Physiological Basis of Alpha Rhythm.* Appleton-Century-Crofts, New York.

Andersen, P., Andersson, S.A. and Lømo, T. (1967) Nature of thalamocortical relations during spontaneous barbiturate spindle activity. *J. Physiol. (Lond.)*, 192: 283–307.

Andersson, S.A., Holmgren, E. and Manson, S.R. (1971) Localized thalamic rhythmicity induced by spinal and cortical lesions. *Electroenceph. clin. Neurophysiol.*, 31: 347–356.

Dewan, E.M. (1964) Nonlinear oscillations and electroencephalography. *J. theoret. Biol.*, 7: 141–155.

Dichter, M. and Spencer, W.A. (1969) Penicillin-induced interictal discharges from the cat hippocampus. II. Mechanisms underlying origin and restriction. *J. Neurophysiol.*, 32: 663–687.

Freeman, W.J. (1964) A linear distributed feedback model for prepyriform cortex. *Exp. Neurol.*, 10: 525–547.

Freeman, W.J. (1972) Linear analysis of the dynamics of neural masses. *Ann. Rev. Biophys. Bioeng.*, 1: 225–256.

Freeman, W.J. (1973) A model of the olfactory system. In *Neural Modeling*, M.A.B. Brazier, Walter and Schneider (Eds.), Brain Information Service, University of Los Angeles. Res. Report 1.

Freeman, W.J. (1974a) Measurement of transmission distance from mitral-tufted to granule cells in olfactory bulb. *Electroenceph. clin. Neurophysiol.*, 36: 609.

Freeman, W.J. (1974b) A model for mutual excitation in a neuron population in olfactory bulb. *IEEE Trans. biomed. Engng.*, BME-21: 350–358.

Freeman, W.J. (1974c) Stability characteristics of positive feedback in a neural population. *IEEE Trans. biomed. Engng.*, BME-21: 358–364.

Freeman, W.J. (1975) *Mass Action in the Nervous System.* Academic Press, New York.

Ganes, T. and Andersen, P. (1975) Barbiturate spindle activity in functionally corresponding thalamic and cortical somato-sensory areas in the cat. *Brain Res.*, 98: 457–472.

Getchell, T.V. and Shepherd, G.M. (1975) Short-axon cells in the olfactory bulb, dendrodendritic synpatic interactions. *J. Physiol. (Lond.)*, 251: 523–548.

Hammond, P.H. (1958) *Feedback Theory and its Applications.* English University Press, London.

Harmon, L.D. (1964) Problems in neural modeling. In *Neural Theory and Modeling, Proceedings of the 1962 OGAI Symposium*, R.F. Reiss (Ed.), Stanford University Press, Stanford, Calif.

Heusden, E. van (1975) *Model of the Septal Pacemaker.* Report Department Bio-Informatics, Technical University Twente, The Netherlands.

Katchalsky, A., Rowland, V. and Blumenthal, R. (1974) Dynamic patterns of brain cell assemblies. *Neurosci. Res. Prog. Bull.*, 12: 3.

Lanoir, J. (1972) *Etude électrocorticografique de la veille et du sommeil chez le chat, Organisation du cycle nycthérméral, Rôle du thalamus.* Thèse doct. Sci., Centre Régional du recherche et de documentation Pédagogiques, Marseille.

Lopes da Silva, F.H., Rotterdam, A. van, Storm van Leeuwen, W. and Tielen, A.M. (1970) Dynamic characteristics of visual EP's in the dog. I. Cortical and subcortical potentials evoked by sine wave modulated light. *Electroenceph. clin. Neurophysiol.*, 29: 246–259.

Lopes da Silva, F.H., Liertop, T.H.M.T. van, Schrijer, C.F. and Storm van Leeuwen, W. (1973) Organization of the thalamic and cortical alpha rhythms: spectra and coherences. *Electroenceph. clin. Neurophysiol.*, 35: 627–639.

Lopes da Silva, F.H., Hoeks, A. and Zetterberg, L.H. (1974) Model of brain rhythmic activity, the alpha-rhythm of the thalamus. *Kybernetik*, 15: 27–37.

McLennan, H. and Miller, J.J. (1974) The hippocampal control of neuronal discharge in the septum of the rat. *J. Physiol. (Lond.)*, 237: 607–624.

Pinching, A.J. and Powell, T.P.S. (1971) The neuron types of the glomerular layer of the olfactory bulb. *J. Cell. Sci.*, 9: 305–345.

Reese, T.S. and Shepherd, G.M. (1972) Dendrodendritic synapses in the central nervous system. In *Structure and Function of Synapses*, G.D. Pappas and D.P. Purpura (Eds.), Raven, New York, pp. 121–136.

Regan, D.A. (1968) A high frequency mechanism which underlies visual evoked potentials. *Electroenceph. Clin. Neurophysiol.*, 25: 231–237.

Regan, D.A. (1972) *Evoked Potentials in Psychology, Sensory Physiology and Clinical Medicine*. Chapman and Hall Ltd. London.

Shepherd, G.M. (1972) Synaptic organization of the mammalian olfactory bulb. *Physiol. Rev.*, 52: 864–917.

Skvaril, J., Radil-Weiss, T., Bohdanecky, Z. and Syka, J. (1971) Spontaneous discharge patterns of mesencephalic neurons: internal histogram and mean interval relationship. *Kybernetik*, 9: 11–15.

Spekreijse, H. and Tweel, L.H. van der (1970) System analysis of linear and non-linear processes in electrophysiology of the visual system. In *Introduction to Biocybernetics*, M. Clynes, Yates and Milsum (Eds.), John Wiley, New York.

Tweel, L.H. van der (1961) Some problems in vision regarded with respect to linearity and frequency response. *Ann. N.Y. Acad. Sci.*, 89: 829–856.

Wilson, H.R. and Cowan, J.D. (1972) Excitatory and inhibitory interaction in localized populations of model neurons. *Biophys. J.*, 12: 1–23.

Zetterberg, L.H. (1973) *Stochastic Activity in a Population of Neurons — A System Analysis Approach*. Report Inst. Med. Physics, TNO, Utrecht, 1: 153.

Organization of Spontaneous Electrical Activity in the Neocortex

J. SCHERRER

Physiology Laboratory, Faculté de Médecine
Pitié-Salpêtrière, Paris (France)

INTRODUCTION

It is possible to recognize four different levels of bioelectrical activity in the cerebral cortex. The first level is the *elementary* one: what cellular phenomena are related to the EEG waves first registered by Berger, and later by many physiologists and electroencephalographers. The second level concerns the *organization* of the elementary processes: a certain synchronization of events on the cellular level has to take place in order to record them by scalp or cortical gross electrodes. As the cortical EEG activity is related to inputs coming from deep structures and afferent nerve fibers, so the third level of our knowledge *integrates* the cortex with the functioning of the central and peripheral nervous systems. The fourth and last level consists of the relationship between the electrocortical activity and events in the *environment*: how does this cortical activity reflect the animal's behavior?

This presentation will essentially consider the second level of our knowledge, *the intrinsic organization of cortical activity.* Of course, it will be necessary to consider briefly some elementary events related to EEG activity, as well as to make reference to the role of deep cerebral or encephalic structures in EEG activity. Only spontaneous electrical activity will be examined. Due to the author's specialization, the biochemical aspect of the cortical activity will not be discussed, nor will morphology, cellular biophysics or behavior be considered in any detail.

The whole subject of the physiological basis of EEG was thoroughly reviewed by Creutzfeldt (1974) in Rémond's textbook of EEG. The symposium organized and published by Petsche and Brazier (1972) summarizes in turn our present knowledge of synchronization mechanisms in the central nervous system. Schematically, it is possible to admit that several points regarding the bioelectrical cortical activity are now well established. This is the case for the neuronal (not glial) origin of the EEG activity, for the particular importance of pyramidal cells, and for the fact that the recorded waves are related to postsynaptic potentials (PSPs). Two important points of central bioelectrical organization are still under discussion: the precise relationship of EEG waves to the depolarization or hyperpolarization of cortical neurons, and the displacement of these waves on the cortical surface. Finally, despite much excellent work, the precise synchronizing mechanisms of corticothalamic function are still unknown.

ELEMENTARY PHENOMENA IN CORTICAL ACTIVITY

The glia problem

The possibility for glia to generate wave-type electrical activity (see Cohen, 1974, for a general review) is a relatively new but now well-established fact. The b wave of the electroretinogram, for instance, is probably related to electrical events originating in the retinal glial cells. Now the problem of a role of cortical glial cells in the EEG activity may be considered. It is possible that changes in glial cells' membrane potential may account for some of the long-lasting potential modifications recorded by the DC recording technique, but it seems extremely unlikely that the usual EEG phenomena could be related to a glial generator. Among other arguments against such an hypothesis, the results of stratigraphic cortical analysis and, particularly, the results of intracellular recordings should be mentioned.

Priority for the pyramidal cells

The cerebral cortex contains different types of neurons, and it is possible a priori to consider that the EEG activity may be related either to the functioning of all of the types or of any single type. A quick look at the schematic representation of the different types of cortical neurons shows that the orientation of dendrites and axons very strongly suggest that electrical phenomena recorded on the surface of the cortex and even on the scalp must be largely generated by a population of neurons having a similar orientation, acting in an open field. That is the case for the pyramidal cells, almost all of them having definite radial (vertical) orientation. The exceptions (inverted and oblique neurons) are not numerous enough to change this statistical situation. Non-pyramidal neurons often have a closed field geometry, and it is difficult to imagine how the potential differences generated by them may effectively summate. It is possible, and even likely, that other types of neurons are activated simultaneously with the pyramidal cells, but the cortical waves are unlikely to reflect their activity. Still another fact which must be taken into account here is that pyramidal cells represent, according to different anatomists, 80–90% of all cortical neurons.

Postsynaptic potentials and EEG

The third established point regarding bioelectrical cortical organization is the relationship between EEG waves and neuronal postsynaptic potentials. For many years the possibility was stressed that the waves registered on the cortex might be related to the action potentials generated by cortical neurons. Such an assumption was discarded on two bases: (1) negative findings regarding the role of cellular spike discharges, and (2) a better knowledge of the neuronal membrane fluctuation in the cortical neurons.

There are two major arguments against the role of cell firing in generating EEG waves. Biophysical studies have shown that the spike-like phenomena decrease very rapidly in the volume conductor represented by the cerebral cortex (Humphrey, 1968). Secondly, there is the fact that even when spike discharges are suppressed under different conditions the cortical wave activity persists (see Creutzfeldt, 1974).

Positive arguments concerning *the role of PSPs in EEG activity have mostly come from intracellular recordings*, which have also yielded important facts concerning neuronal elementary properties. It is evidently impossible to summarize all the data obtained in this field here. Figs. 1 and 2, one of Purpura

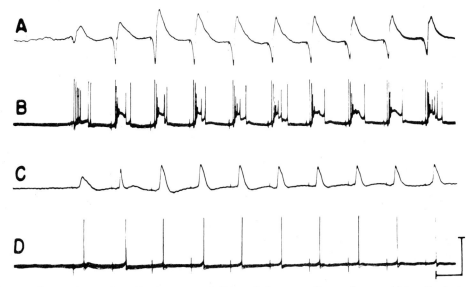

Fig. 1. Comparison of cortical waves and intracellular recordings of pyramidal cells during augmenting (A and B) and recruiting (C and D) responses evoked by thalamic stimulation. Note the duration of the EPSP, and the lack of any simple relationship between extracellular and intracellular recordings. Calibrations; 100 msec and 50 mV. (From Purpura et al., 1964.)

et al. (1964) the other of Creutzfeldt et al. (1966a, b), stress some crucial points. Depolarization and hyperpolarization of the synaptic type are present in cortical neurons, the former frequently accompanied by action potentials, the latter evoking inhibition of cell firing. The PSPs are relatively long-lasting phenomena, particularly the IPSP, whose duration can exceed 100 msec. There are some data which indicate that for EPSPs the site of synaptic transmission might be mainly on the dendrites. It is therefore possible that for cortical neurons, as for other central synapses (see Eccles et al., 1967), depolarization is initiated primarily in dendrites, whereas hyperpolarization would be largely somatic in origin.

The manner in which *PSPs located in pyramidal cells could be registered on the cortex* was first clearly discussed by Eccles (1951); an excellent summary of the studies published since that initial paper is to be found in Creutzfeldt

312

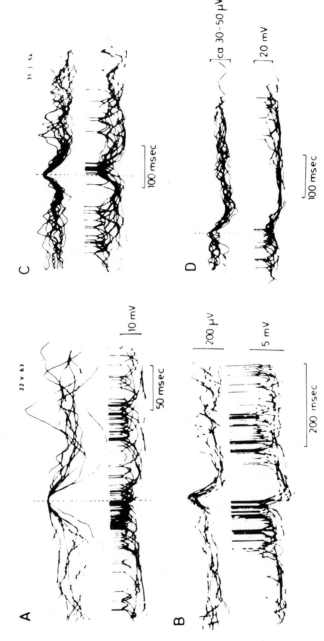

Fig. 2. Superimposed line drawings of the two types of EEG waves and the corresponding cellular record. EEG waves were collected according to shape. A and C: with surface-negative waves of symmetrical shape, only excitation (EPSPs and discharges) is seen in the cellular record. B and D: synchronized IPSPs together with surface-positive potentials are seen, preceded by cellular excitation and surface-negative potentials. (From Creutzfeldt et al., 1966a, b.)

(1974). The general basis of the interpretation is simple: in the case of hyperpolarization with inhibition, the cell body will act as the source and the dendrites as a sink; the reverse will occur during depolarization with excitation (see Llinás and Nicholson, 1974). For the cerebral cortex, three additional factors must be considered: (1) in some cases dendrites might be the site of depolarization, (2) the membrane potential change could either first be located in the soma and only later in the dendrites, or vice versa, and (3) different cortical cellular layers may not necessarily be simultaneously activated. In fact, most of the authors performing intracellular recordings did not find a general rule relating cellular PSPs and cortical waves. However, as will be seen later, a clear-cut relationship can in fact be established between definite cortical waves and PSPs.

The geometrical arrangement of pyramidal cells with apical and basilar dendrites would predict a potential gradient simultaneously oriented in vertical (radial) and horizontal (tangential) directions for a single cell or for a column of pyramidal cells. In some cases the tangential dipole is predominant (Raabe and Lux, 1972). In experiments done in our laboratory (Fig. 3) the vertically oriented dipole was the larger of the two: for bipolar recordings with an interelectrode distance of 1–1·5 mm, the wave phenomenon had an amplitude 5–10 times larger for a bipolar transcortical recording (surface cortical − intracortical) than for a bipolar recording on the surface of the cortex. The differences between our results and those of Raabe and Lux are probably explained by the extension of the area of activated pyramidal cells. If the area is large, the horizontal intermingling of dendrites may diminish the tangential dipole recorded by two electrodes situated in the active area (Scherrer, 1965).

RELATION OF CORTICAL WAVES TO NEURONAL UNIT FIRING PATTERNS

Simultaneous EEG wave and action potential recording method

An indirect approach to the relationship between hyperpolarization or depolarization of cortical cells and EEG waves is suggested by *simultaneous wave and action potential recordings*. This type of technique has been used in our laboratory on cats for almost 15 years and has yielded some interesting results. Wave recording is done between a superficial electrode and intracortical electrodes situated at different depths. The electrodes are frequently platinum semi-microelectrodes. The depth electrode is situated at 1000 μm from the surface (partial transcortical recording) or at 2000 μm (total transcortical recording). In addition, a micropipette can be used to obtain unitary action potentials (Fig. 3). Wave phenomena and action potentials are nowadays compared on a statistical basis. A pattern recognition programme developed on a Linc 8 Computer selects EEG waves of definite polarity, duration and amplitude from periods of spontaneous activity. Usually 50–100 such waves are selected and averaged. Averaging of the concomitant action potentials is simultaneously performed.

314

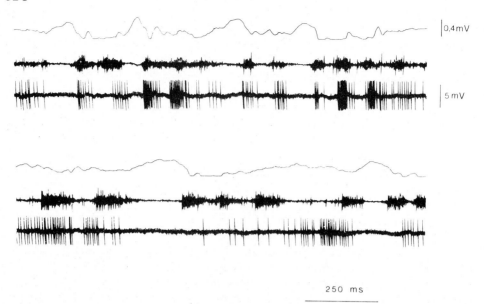

0,4 mV

5 mV

250 ms

Fig. 3. Simultaneous recording of wave activity and cell discharges in the suprasylvian gyrus of the cat (chronic preparation). Wave activity is recorded between two vertically aligned glass-insulated platinum electrodes. One electrode is on the surface of the cortex, the other one at a depth of 1200 μm. The depth electrode also functions as a semi-microelectrode for recording multiple spike discharges. A micropipette situated close to the 1200 μm depth electrode records the isolated unitary activity.

The generators of spontaneous electrocortical activity

Utilizing these techniques it was possible to consider EEG activity as being primarily the result of three different generators (Fig. 4; Calvet et al., 1964; Scherrer and Calvet, 1972). Generator A is located within the upper 500 μm, i.e., the superficial layers of the cortex, and underlies the purely surface-negative phenomena. When generator B is active, on the other hand, two partial dipoles can be observed. One is superficial and reaches down to approximately 1000 μm; the other has the opposite sign and is found between 1000 and 2000 μm below the surface. The negativities of both of these dipoles are maximal at a depth of about 1000 μm. Since the potential difference produced by the deeper dipole is smaller than the one produced by the more superficial one, a transcortical derivation over the entire cortical depth (thus algebraically summing up the effects of both dipoles) will result in an electropositive phenomenon from the cortex whenever generator B is active. Generator C results in a positivity of the cortical layers at 800–1000 μm with respect to both its surface and deeper layers. In this case again (since the partial superficial dipole produces larger potentials than the deep one), the total dipole resulting from the addition of the two partial dipoles will cause surface-negative events.

When generator A is active, there is no obvious interference with any cellular discharges. In contrast, there is a remarkable relation between cellular discharges and waves caused by generators B and C; with surface-positive waves

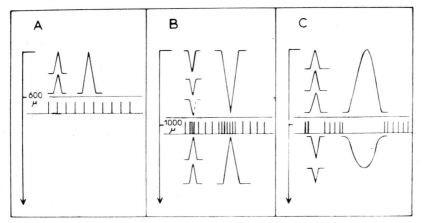

Fig. 4. Cortical levels of each generator. Generator A, registered in the upper 600 μm, is surface-negative. Generators B and C each have a double dipole. Cell firing increases during B generator activity, decreases for C, and remains constant for A. (From Calvet et al., 1964.)

(generator B) an increase of spike discharges is found, whereas with the activity of generator C the opposite phenomenon is observed. Fig. 5 shows the relationship between (1) a spontaneous surface-negative wave and the concomitant suppression of discharges, and (2) a surface-positive wave associated with an increase in firing.

The location of the depolarization, with the increase in spike discharges, permits the assumption that *generator B reflects a depolarization of neuronal somata*; this would mean that the surface-positive wave reflects the summation of EPSPs. Similar arguments may explain the surface-negative waves which result from generator C in terms of a *hyper*polarization of neuronal somata, i.e., a summation of IPSPs. Even if these conclusions are not absolutely substantiated, their credibility at least is sufficiently well established. The interpretation proposed by Calvet et al. (1964) and supported by Fig. 5 is in

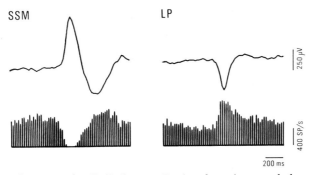

Fig. 5. Averaging of wave and cell discharges. During drowsiness and sleep: 64 spontaneous surface-negative waves averaged from the medial part of the suprasylvian gyrus (SSM), after selection by pattern recognition (see text). The cell discharges were averaged for the same waves. Note the inhibition of cell firing, and the postinhibitory rebound concomitant with the surface-positive wave. During paradoxical sleep: 102 spontaneous surface-positive waves and concomitant cell discharges, averaged by identical procedures from the lateral posterior gyrus (LP). Note the definite increase of cell firing without any rebound. (An unpublished figure of Calvet et al.)

316

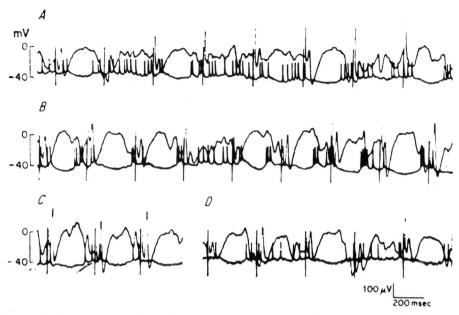

Fig. 6. Simultaneous recording of cortical waves and intracellular potential changes during thalamic stimulation at 3/sec. A and B: when surface-negative wave drops out, IPSPs are usually absent. C: no drop-out. D: two exceptional instances when a surface-negative wave was *not* accompanied by comparable IPSPs. (From Pollen, 1964.)

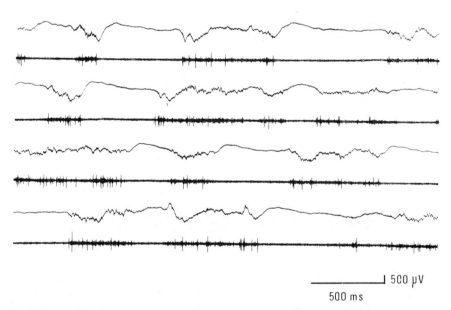

Fig. 7. Relationship between waves and unit discharges during spontaneous activity in isolated cortex. Wave activity (upper trace) and unit activity (lower trace) on a continuous record obtained from a chronic neuronally isolated suprasylvian cat gyrus. Note the clear increase in cell firing during surface-positive waves (downwards deflection).

agreement with the experimental findings and theoretical development postulated by Holmes and Houchin (1967) and by Pollen (1964). The sink and source schema of the former accounts for the activity of the B generator, while emphasizing the necessity of using transcortical recording electrodes. Fig. 6 (from Pollen, 1964) demonstrates a clear relationship between somatic hyperpolarization and cortical surface-negative wave.

The spike-to-wave relationship established for spontaneous activity in a chronic preparation has been observed in other experimental conditions, although without the same thorough statistical analysis. During ontogenetic development in the cat and the rabbit, the slow negative sleep waves, which appear at the age of two or three weeks are already concomitants of the diminution or total suppression of spontaneous cell discharges (Garma and Verley, 1967). In an isolated gyrus (Fig. 7) the surface-negative waves have the same effect (Hirsch, 1975). During epileptiform cortical activity in the cat, the same relationship is observed at the beginning and at the end of a seizure but not during its paroxysmal phase (Jami, 1972); this relationship has also been seen in the human cortex (Hirsch et al., 1966).

Comparison of extracellular and intracellular methods

The discrepancy between certain results obtained by the intracellular technique, versus those obtained by the method of comparing EEG waves and spike activity, might be explained by several factors. For recording intracellular potentials a general anesthetic must be used. Very often the authors who developed the intracellular technique examined not only spontaneous but also evoked activity, for which the wave and discharge relationship seems to be more complicated. The primary reason, however, might simply be the wave recording technique employed (Fourment et al., 1965). As will be seen later, the extension of an EEG wave can be quite important. When this is true the reference electrode used is sometimes not neutral, and "sees" the activated cortical area under a large solid angle (Jami et al., 1968). The misleading results of the monopolar method may be increased if the activated cortical area is in fact a double dipolar layer. Then the best comparison of the action potentials is done on the activity of the superficial cortical dipolar layer (between 0 and 1200 μm), that is, grossly speaking, between apical dendrites and the soma. As a matter of fact, the bipolar transcortical technique itself may also be criticized on both theoretical and practical grounds (Creutzfeldt, 1974).

EXTENSION OF CORTICAL WAVES

Measurement of the extension

Due to the nature of the relationship between the wave-type phenomena and the cortical cell discharges, it seems worthwhile to study the magnitude of the cortical surface occupied by a given wave during spontaneous activity. The following technique is used: a simultaneous continuous recording on magnetic tape of waves and cortical cellular discharges is performed in several regions of

318

the neocortex, most often in 7 different areas (Fig. 8). The record of one of the registered areas is then analyzed on a Linc 8 computer by a wave pattern recognition programme. In this way, using the technique already mentioned, the averaging of a selected wave is performed simultaneously with the averaging of intracortical action potential discharges. The peak of the first averaged wave is then used as a time signal for averaging the electrical phenomena recorded by the 6 other cortical leads. If, in a given area, an electrical event is time-locked with this signal, the averaging technique will be equally efficient for wave phenomena and for cellular increase or decrease in firing. Usually a continuous recording of one or two minutes is submitted to the pattern recognition technique and for subsequent averaging.

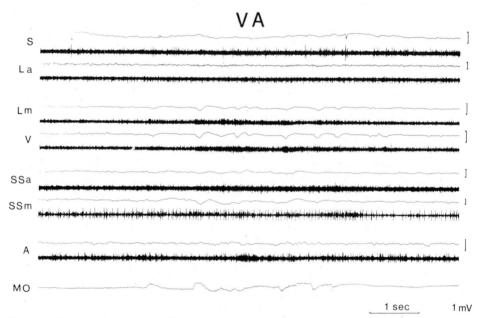

Fig. 8. Simultaneous recording of 7 different cortical regions in cat during active wakefulness. Somesthetic, S; lateral anterior, La; lateral medial, Lm; suprasylvian anterior, SSa, and medial, SSm; visual, V, auditory, A, areas; eye movements, MO. For each region, concomitant recording of wave activity (upper trace) and cell discharges (lower trace).

Two types of waves were studied, the surface-negative wave (of the C type) during which cortical cell firing is diminished or even suppressed, and the surface-positive wave (of the B type) during which firing increases (see Fig. 4).

The surface-negative wave

Surface-negative waves are recorded during drowsiness, when they appear irregularly, and during slow wave sleep, where they constitute the major part of EEG activity (Fig. 9). The duration of the surface-negative waves varies somewhat with the amplitude, but most frequently they are quite long-lasting, 200 or 300 msec. Positive rebound often follows the negative phenomenon. It is interesting to mention the fact that surface-negative waves have been

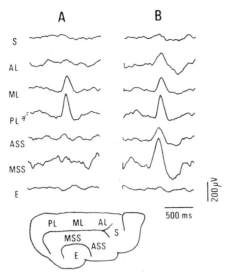

Fig. 9. Averaging of surface-negative waves during a period of 85 sec. A: 27 waves summated during an initial period of slow wave sleep. B: 25 waves summated during a later phase of slow wave sleep. Pattern recognition of the surface-negative wave is from the visual region. The peak of the recognized and averaged wave is used to average the 6 other regions. Note the extension of the sector invaded by the surface-negative wave.

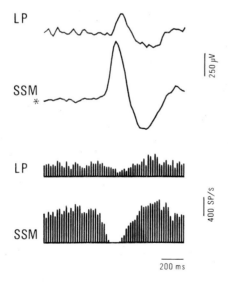

Fig. 10. Averaged wave and cell discharges in two distant cortical areas. Wave recognition was performed on the medial part of the suprasylvian gyrus (SSM), followed by averaging of 64 waves and simultaneous cell discharges in this region. Averaging in lateral posterior gyrus (LP) involved the same technique as in Fig. 5. Note the time delay between waves (and related cell discharge inhibition) in SSM and LP areas.

320

successfully averaged on all the explored sites of the neocortex, but have a larger amplitude in the suprasylvian gyrus than in the primary sensory projection areas. This is probably related to the fact that, whereas in the primary sensory areas the surface-negative wave only partially diminishes the cortical cell firing, in the non-primary areas action potential activity may be completely suppressed (Calvet et al., 1973).

The cortical sector occupied at any given time by a surface-negative wave is variable in extent but usually more than one cortical lead is occupied by this type of activity. When the territory is restricted, the surface-negative wave is found only in the suprasylvian gyrus. This is the case in drowsiness. During slow wave sleep (particularly after several minutes of this type of sleep) the negative wave extension is maximal, any one wave occupying several gyri. In this case there is no perfect simultaneity for the different areas. The occipital regions typically lag around 50 msec behind the suprasylvian gyrus (Fig. 10).

The surface-positive wave

The surface-positive wave is detected in the cat in two different states, viz., during full wakefulness and during paradoxical sleep (Fig. 11). It is evoked in both cases by eye movements, although the precise relationship is not easy to characterize. In paradoxical sleep the surface-positive potential may also be associated with the classical ponto-geniculo-occipital wave phenomenon. During wakefulness the eye movement may be part of an orientation response.

The amplitude of the surface-positive wave, as well as its duration, seem to be less variable than for the surface-negative wave. Typical figures would be 100–200 μV and 100 msec, respectively. There is a rather wide sector occupied

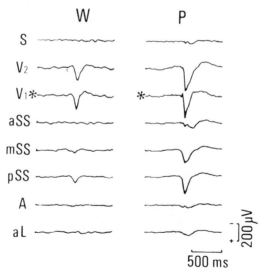

Fig. 11. Averaging of surface-positive waves. During wakefulness (W) 130 waves were averaged, and 113 during paradoxical sleep (P). In both cases wave recognition was done in the primary visual area (V_1). Averaging of the other areas by same technique as in Figs. 5 and 10. S, somesthetic; V_2, medial lateral; a, m and pSS, anterior, medial and posterior suprasylvian; A, auditory; aL, anterior lateral.

by the surface-positive wave, which differs during wakefulness and slow wave sleep. Simultaneity of the phenomenon in the different regions seems excellent, but very small delays would not be seen with the type of averaging used.

Mechanisms of wave formation

To sum up the facts presented above, it appears that a wave phenomenon in the cerebral cortex implies the simultaneous, or almost simultaneous, depolarization or hyperpolarization of a population of pyramidal cells in either a limited or a large sector. The major problem, therefore, is to localize and to analyze the mechanism which underlies the synchronized membrane changes within a pool of cortical neurons.

Studies on the chronically isolated gyrus confirm the already known fact that surface-negative or surface-positive waves may arise without any thalamic input. As seen above, the usual relation of these waves with the neuronal action potentials is still valid. So the functional substrate is present within the cortex to synchronize the activity of a large number of neurons. It seems likely, however, that in the intact brain this cortical mechanism is usually triggered from some deep structures. The major importance of such structures is stressed by the fact that, despite some contrary evidence (see Hirsch, 1975), no typical rhythmic activity is recorded from an isolated gyrus, and also by a body of other arguments developed since Dempsey and Morison's initial experiments (see Andersen and Andersson, 1968). Unfortunately, however, the interplay between cortical and deep structures is outside the scope of the present paper.

SUMMARY

There is general agreement about several aspects of the cortical bioelectrical organization. It is admitted, for instance, that the EEG waves are related chiefly to postsynaptic potentials generated in pyramidal cells. These potentials are of a long-lasting type, particularly the inhibitory ones. It is unlikely that changes in glial membrane potential act as a generator for the usual EEG waves. Except in certain situations, intracellular recordings do not show a general relationship between the polarity of EEG waves and, respectively, depolarization or hyperpolarization of the cortical neurons. However, by taking into account action potential discharges during spontaneous EEG activity it becomes possible to demonstrate a clear-cut statistical relationship between several types of waves and elementary cellular phenomena. This relationship is preserved in an experimentally isolated cortical gyrus, and has also been established for the human cortex.

The presence of an EEG wave implies synchronous and largely homogenous activity in a population of pyramidal cells. The amplitude of the wave is related then to the number of neurons simultaneously invaded by the same postsynaptic phenomenon. Another property of a given EEG wave is to occupy a definite surface area of the cortex. This involvement of a cortical sector may be virtually simultaneous, or else a small delay can separate the occurrence of the wave in different cortical regions. Mechanisms underlying cortical slow wave synchronization are located at least partially within the cortex itself, although the role of thalamic nuclei is firmly established for other types of rhythmic bioelectric activities.

ACKNOWLEDGEMENTS

Some of the data and figures presented in this paper were obtained in the Laboratoire de Recherches Neurophysiologiques de l'INSERM et de l'Association Claude Bernard (Paris) from ongoing research by J. Calvet, M. Thieffry, A. Fourment, J. Hirsch and Y. Burnod. Part of this research is already published.

REFERENCES

Andersen, P. and Andersson, A. (1968) In *Physiological Basis of the Alpha Rhythm*, A. Towe, (Ed.), Appleton-Century-Crofts, New York.

Calvet, J., Calvet, M.-C. et Scherrer, J. (1964) Etude stratigraphique de l'activité EEG spontanée. *Electroenceph. clin. Neurophysiol.*, 17: 109–125.

Calvet, J., Fourment, A. and Thieffry, M. (1973) Electrical activity in neocortical projection and association areas during slow wave sleep. *Brain Res.*, 52: 173–187.

Cohen, M.W. (1974) Glial potentials and their contribution to extracellular recordings. In *Handbook of Electroencephalography and Clinical Neurophysiology, Vol. 2, Sect. III*, A. Rémond (Ed.), Elsevier, Amsterdam, pp. 2B-43–59.

Creutzfeldt, O. (1974) Neuronal basis of EEG-Waves. In *Handbook of Electroencephalography and Clinical Neurophysiology, Vol. 2, Sect. I*, A. Rémond (Ed.), Elsevier, Amsterdam, pp. 2C 5–53.

Creutzfeldt, O., Watanabe, S. and Lux, H.D. (1966a) Relations between EEG phenomena and potentials of single cortical cells. I. Evoked responses after thalamic and epicortical stimulation. *Electroenceph. clin. Neurophysiol.*, 20: 1–18.

Creutzfeldt, O., Watanabe, S. and Lux, H.D. (1966b) Relations between EEG-phenomena and potentials of single cortical cells. II. Spontaneous and convulsoid activity. *Electroenceph. clin. Neurophysiol.*, 20: 19–37.

Eccles, J.C. (1951) Interpretation of action potentials evoked in the cerebral cortex. *Electroenceph. clin. Neurophysiol.*, 3: 449–464.

Eccles, J.C., Llinás, R. and Szentágothai, J. (1967) *The Cerebellum as a Neuronal Machine.* Springer, New York.

Fourment, A., Jami, L., Calvet, J. et Scherrer, J. (1965) Comparaison de l'EEG recueilli sur le scalp avec l'activité élémentaire des dipoles corticaux radiaires. *Electroenceph. clin. Neurophysiol.*, 19: 217–229.

Garma, L. et Verley, R. (1967) Activités cellulaires corticales étudiées par électrodes implantées chez le lapin nouveau-né. *J. Physiol. (Paris)*, 59: 357–376.

Hirsch, J. (1975) *Contribution à l'Etude de l'Activité Spontanée et Paroxystique d'un Gyrus Cortical Isolé.* Thèse Doct.-ès-Sci., Université Paris VI, 236 pp.

Hirsch, J.F., Buisson-Ferey, J., Sachs, M., Hirsch, J.C. et Scherrer, J. (1966) Electrocorticogramme et activités unitaires lors de processus expansifs chez l'Homme. *Electroenceph. clin. Neurophysiol.*, 21: 417–428.

Holmes, O. and Houchin, J. (1967) A model of the potential evoked from the cerebral cortex by afferent stimulation. *J. Physiol. (Lond.)*, 191: 3–4P.

Humphrey, D.R. (1968) Re-analysis of the antidromic cortical response. II. On the contribution of cell discharge and PSPs to the evoked potentials. *Electroenceph. clin. Neurophysiol.*, 25: 421–442.

Jami, L. (1972) Patterns of cortical population discharges during metrazol induced seizures in cats. *Electroenceph. clin. Neurophysiol.*, 32: 641–654.

Jami, L., Fourment, A., Calvet, J. et Thieffry, M. (1968) Etude sur modèle des méthodes de détection EEG. *Electroenceph. clin. Neurophysiol.*, 24: 130–145.

Llinás, R. and Nicholson, C. (1974) Analysis of field potentials in the central nervous system. In *Handbook of Electroencephalography and Clinical Neurophysiology, Vol. 2, Sect. IV*, A. Rémond (Ed.), Elsevier, Amsterdam, pp. 2B 61–92.

Petsche, H. and Brazier, M.A.B. (1972) (Eds.) *Synchronization of EEG activity in Epilepsies.* Springer, Berlin, 431 pp.

Pollen, D.A. (1964) Intracellular studies of cortical neurons during thalamic induced wave and spike. *Electroenceph. clin. Neurophysiol.*, 17: 398–404.

Purpura, D.P., Shofer, R.J. and Musgrave, F.S. (1964) Cortical intracellular potentials during augmenting and recruiting responses. II. Patterns of synaptic activities in pyramidal and nonpyramidal tract neurons. *J. Neurophysiol.*, 27: 133–151.

Raabe, W. and Lux, H.D. (1972) Studies on extracellular potentials generated by synaptic activity on single cat motor cortex neurons. In *Synchronization of EEG Activity in Epilepsies*, Springer, Berlin, pp. 46–58.

Scherrer, J. (1965) Analyse de l'activité électrocorticale spontanée. *Actualités neuro-physiol.*, 6: 201–221.

Scherrer, J. and Calvet, J. (1972) Normal and epileptic synchronization at the cortical level in the animal. In *Synchronization of EEG Activity in Epilepsies*, H. Petsche and M.A.B. Brazier (Eds.), Springer Verlag, Berlin, pp. 112–132.

DISCUSSION

C.V. DE BLÉCOURT: There is an opinion that hippocampal theta activity may be conducted to the cortex by volume conduction, so that what we actually record during physiological arousal is a mixture of volume-conducted synchronized hippocampal theta activity along with the "desynchronized" cortical activity. We found in our own experiments, in which the EEG and cortical blood flow were registered simultaneously in the visual cortex of the rabbit, a highly significant correlation between the theta band activity of the analyzed EEG and cortical blood flow. But in view of the foregoing, we hesitate to interpret this as a direct causal relationship because the recorded EEG may be only the reflection of a subcortical instead of a cortical event. I want to ask you if you think that there is any experimental evidence for a volume-conductor theory regarding the origin of cortical recorded synchronized activity.

J. SCHERRER: In recording conditions such as ours we are not going to register any activities which originate outside the cortex, and that is one of the reasons why we are using this type of transcortical electrode, with relatively small intertip distances. In the monopolar situation, on the other hand, there is very often a large degree of contamination from activity arising at quite some distance from the recording electrode.

P.B. BRADLEY: You showed cells which were always discharging action potentials. But if the EEG is dependent upon summated EPSPs and IPSPs, is it really necessary for individual neurons to be continuously firing?

J. SCHERRER: For this statistical analysis we were using a semi-microelectrode, and statistically you always have some neurons which are discharging. If we had used micropipettes only, that would not have shown the same thing, because what is true for a population of 50 or 60 cells is no longer true for each individual cell.

J. OLDS: Dr. Scherrer, I have noticed that when you recorded both with a glass pipette and with the small semi-microelectrode, there was rather poor correlation between your glass pipette and the multiple unit activity. I have seen that in other laboratories too, and I wonder if it is possible that they are in fact biased to different families of cells, rather than the one simply being a subfamily of the other?

J. SCHERRER: That is a very difficult question to answer. It is quite possible that the micropipette makes a selection of these neurons from which it is recording. For instance, we hoped to find some cells which discharged out of phase from the other ones, e.g., interneurons which would be generating the inhibition which follows the recorded excitatory waves, but we have been unable to find any.

O. CREUTZFELDT: I would like to stimulate you to speculate a little bit more about the proposed increase of neuronal synchronization during slow-wave sleep, and also to ask one specific question: how far does this concept also hold for the spindle waves; are they too more synchronized? Andersson thinks that the actual projection of rhythmic activity from the specific thalamic nuclei to cortical points is very limited, and he even thinks in terms of different thalamic oscillators, more or less dependent of each other, each one serving an area of only 100–200 μm in diameter.

J. SCHERRER: Andersson worked mostly on barbiturate spindles, not on spindles of the type which one could register during wakefulness without any anesthesia. Moreover, we did not study the area in which only a single spindle wave was present, nor did we make the same type of analysis for spindle activity as we did for the surface-positive and -negative cortical slow waves. I have the impression that there is a relationship between the amplitude of the wave and its extension over the cortex. Since spindle waves are very small, we suppose that the area occupied by a given spindle wave will be a modest one, which would fit in nicely with Andersson's study. But one really has to consider not only the individual waves within the spindle but also the entire spindle activity, and the cortical surface covered by a whole spindle certainly exceeds the surface activated during one wave.

F.H. LOPES DA SILVA: I want to put a question to Dr. Scherrer about the glial potentials, which he did not think would contribute much to the electroencephalogram. Now this has been a controversial point for some time, and it depends first of all upon how you define the electroencephalogram. If you define it as everything you can record from the brain, or from the skull, then it is a question of difference in band frequency as well, because you have a low frequency band which may cause the so-called infra-slow potentials. There is some evidence that the very slow potential oscillations indeed represent the membrane activity of glial cells. Although the membrane resistance of the glial cell is relatively low, it *can* give rise to potential changes if the depolarizations are sufficiently localized.

J. SCHERRER: I quite agree. I spoke only about the usual EEG, meaning the frequency range from 1 or 2 Hz to 40 or 50 Hz. For these frequencies, for which we have some good comparisons with intracellular recordings from neurons, I think there is no problem anymore. On the other hand, for the slower frequencies and for the potentials which are usually called DC-potential fluctuations, there is undoubtedly a relationship with glial membrane phenomena, and also with the potassium stores.

M.A. CORNER: I wonder if I could pick up a very striking observation (in Prof. Scherrer's presention), to see what implication this might have for model constructions for generation of the EEG: that is, these "type B" and "type C" generators. It is very striking that the type B generators, i.e., the excitatory kind, can be related preferentially to the specific states of paradoxical sleep and waking, whereas you can show that generator C, the inhibitory one, is a slow-wave sleep phenomenon. Both of these are undoubtedly different types of synaptic input onto a common population of cortical neurons, the pyramidal cells. At the same time, they have a very striking phenomenological similarity to the spike and wave components, respectively excitatory and inhibitory, in the classical epileptiform type of discharge. It might be a good working hypothesis that what happens in the epileptic situation is that, by virtue of some kind of artificially intense driving type B generators, each B-discharge triggers an inhibitory C discharge (with possibly a rebound hyperexcitability, so as to sustain the discharges). In other words: there would be an abnormal linking within a specific, albeit pathological, state of two types of neuronal "generators" which normally are each specifically related to quite distinct physiological states. How would one deal with this phenomenon in a neuronal network model: you have one particular type of output cell which, under specific circumstances, can have quite different types of output patterns: excitatory at one frequency, versus inhibitory at quite a slower frequency? And, under what circumstances could you put these two together, so as to get a very abnormal stereotyped complex paroxysmal discharge?

F.H. LOPES DA SILVA: In order to make a useful model you must know something about the different neuronal populations and how they interact. It is not sufficient to say: we have this type of cell or that type of cell; you must also know something about the interconnectivity among these cells. In the case where there are excitatory and inhibitory feedback groups, you can easily drive the system into a certain limit cycle which will then be self-oscillatory, and where the potentials generated by even a small assembly may look very much like the spike and wave patterns you have mentioned. But to relate the cortical generator types A, B and C to known cell types in the cortex seems impossible at present, because we need to know much more about the interconnectivity among such cells.

J. SCHERRER: The surface negative wave in the spike and wave epileptic discharge is very definitely an inhibitory phenomenon, which we could verify using our techniques. But the rest of the epileptic waveform does not correlate as well with the generators which were postulated for the spontaneous synchronized excitatory activity. Therefore, there are probably still other "generators", which we don't know about at this time.

A. MIODONSKI: Are there differences in the EEG recorded from the gyral as opposed to the sulcal cortex? After all, only about 30% of the cortex is at the external surface.

J. SCHERRER: I can't answer you, unfortunately, because we had enough trouble in studying the cortex which was on the surface, not to try also to study the cortex which is deep inside the gyri. I don't see any reason a priori, however, why gyral cortex would generate a different EEG pattern from that of the cortex which lies at the surface, but this is only a guess.

The Formation of
Continuously Ordered Mappings

R.M. GAZE and R.A. HOPE

National Institute for Medical Research, London (Great Britain)

INTRODUCTION

In this paper we discuss the mechanisms that may be required to account for the formation of ordered nerve connections; in particular, of continuously ordered projections. It was originally suggested to us that the title of the paper should be "Membrane Matching"; the reference is to the role of matching chemoaffinities in the development of neural connections. We feel, however, that this title would rather put the cart before the horse, since it has yet to be established that membrane matching in fact occurs in these situations.

The emergence of pattern in the developing organism is perhaps the central problem in biology today. The question is that of the origin of the increasing, and ordered, cellular diversity seen in ontogenesis. One cell, the fertilized egg, eventually gives rise to all the many cell types found in the adult. And since embryonic development is highly non-random, is in fact remarkably consistent from one animal to another, we must conclude that the cells of the early embryo contain sufficient information to permit their progeny, when interacting with a normal environment, to manifest the organized diversity seen in the adult. It is obviously nonsense to suppose that early embryonic cells each contain a plan of the adult, and it has been argued (Apter and Wolpert, 1965) that what the cells contain in their genetic material is merely a set of instructions: it may well be very much simpler, and require less information, to specify how to make something than to specify the thing itself.

Even at first sight it would seem that, complex as these unsolved problems of embryology are, the problems associated specifically with the development of the nervous system are even more so. The nervous system, more than most parts of the body, is highly dependent on the spatial ordering of its components for its proper function. Spatial order is, of course, important elsewhere in the organism; but the nervous system has more of it, and the result of function of a cell here will depend critically on where it is and what it is connected to. The complexity of spatial ordering in the mature nervous system is many times greater than in any other part of the body; this adds to our difficulties in trying to envisage how the system develops.

In the morphological development of the nervous system we may consider the situation on three levels — as three interrelated problems. Firstly there is the general differentiation and morphogenesis of the various major subdivisions of the system; secondly there is the emergence of the various cell types and cell populations that characterize the mature system; and thirdly there is the problem, seemingly the most intractable of all, of how the various parts and cells become connected up. We say most intractable because it seems that the first two classes of phenomena can more easily be fitted into our general framework of embryological mechanisms — ideas involving gradients, positional information, inductive interactions and so forth. It is in this sense not too difficult to envisage how the various parts of the nervous system, and its various cell types, might come into being.

But it is quite otherwise with the problem of neural connectivity. Here, it is probably fair to say that our level of understanding is still very elementary indeed. In this field we are largely making guesses, and one of the main reasons for this is that we do not know the *extent* of the phenomenon we are trying to account for. We do not know what nerve connections actually exist, and we do not know what constraints there are on the development of these connections — how tightly it is all controlled.

This paper is concerned particularly with the problem of the formation of continuously ordered nerve connections, or mappings, between neuronal arrays. A continuously ordered mapping is one in which, by and large, neurons which are neighbors in one array project to or receive from neurons which are neighbors in the other array. In formal terms, such a mapping is termed a homeomorphism, as both the map and its inverse are continuous. A perfectly ordered mapping of this sort would be one in which these conditions are met without exception, and an example of this is the retinotectal system in lower vertebrates (Gaze, 1970). In addition there are many neural projections which conform with these conditions in the main but not exactly, and much of what we say will, we hope, apply to such mappings.

The problem of the formation of continuously ordered mappings (referred to henceforth as ordered mappings or projections) is not of limited interest only, since such mappings are a common feature in the nervous system. In the visual system there is an ordered mapping of the retina not only on the optic tectum or its mammalian homologue, the superior colliculus, but also on the lateral geniculate nucleus and the visual cortex. In the auditory system the cochlear nerve cells project in an ordered fashion to both the dorsal and the ventral cochlear nuclei. This ordered projection is maintained at the level of the inferior colliculus and as far as the ventral portion of the medial geniculate. There is an essentially ordered mapping of the surface of the body in the somatosensory pathway at the dorsal column nuclei, the thalamus and the three areas of the somatosensory cortex, although these pathways do show fascinating discontinuities, discussed in detail by Werner and Whitsel (1973). Ordered mappings are found not only in sensory systems but also in motor systems. Wyman (1973) has recently suggested that nerves descending in the spinal cord project in a manner which preserves topological order rather than each nerve selecting its particular motor neuron on the basis of the muscle that it innervates.

We will concentrate in this paper on the formation of continuously ordered mappings, without prejudice to the possibility that there may be other forms of ordering in the nervous system, and even connections with no ordering at all. Consideration of the history of neuroanatomy, suggests the generalization that the random nerve connections of yesterday are the ordered connections (or perhaps even the continuously ordered projections) of today or tomorrow; here, much depends on what techniques are used, and how well, and we would agree with Kennedy et al. (1969) that, since we cannot distinguish formally between alleged randomness of connections and our own ignorance about them, the matter will have to await further investigation.

POSSIBLE BIOLOGICAL MECHANISMS FOR THE PRODUCTION OF ORDERED MAPPINGS

For the purposes of our further argument, we will consider theories to account for the development of ordered mappings under three general headings:

(a) time-position mechanisms;
(b) target affinity mechanisms; and
(c) fiber-sorting mechanisms.

These three classes are related, in that each uses, to a greater or lesser extent, elements taken from the others.

(a) *Time-position mechanisms*. We refer here to the idea that if cell division, axon growth and differentiation of the neuron arrays occur at carefully controlled relative times, then the ordered connections could result without need for any but the simplest additional rules governing axon growth and the formation of synaptic connections.

Such a theory may, for example, postulate that different neurons will mature at different times. Axonal outgrowth could also take place at different times and at different rates. On this model, these timing differences are major factors in the control of the formation of the pattern of connections.

(b) *Target affinity mechanisms*. The earliest and most widely accepted version of an affinity mechanism is the chemoaffinity hypothesis of neuronal specificity, first proposed by Sperry (1943, 1944, 1945, 1951, 1963, 1965). The idea in its most general form is that there are differences in the affinity of one fiber in the presynaptic array for cells in the postsynaptic array and vice versa. These differences then account for the formation of the map between the arrays. In this paper we are concerned with the distributions of such affinities rather than with the question of whether they are based on chemical differences, electrical phenomena, or whatever.

(c) *Fiber-sorting mechanisms*. Fiber-sorting models, as treated in this paper, differ from affinity models in denying that there need be variations in the affinities of fibers for different postsynaptic cells, or vice versa. They do not necessarily deny, however, that presynaptic fibers make use of certain information present on the postsynaptic cells. The map is ordered by the fibers sorting themselves out into the correct patterns.

TIME-POSITION MECHANISMS

In this section we will be mainly concerned with invertebrate neurobiology, for it is here that the strongest support for a time-position mechanism is to be found. Precise information on the interconnections between two cells presupposes the ability to identify and investigate these cells. Among vertebrates, however, the only neuron that can be identified with certainty is the Mauthner cell; all other neurons are only identifiable as classes of cells. In certain invertebrates the situation is different and one can choose animals with very small nervous systems where it may be possible, at least in principle, to obtain a complete description of the entire system. This is an approach that is being used with considerable success by Brenner and his colleagues (Ward et al., 1975), who map the entire nervous system in the nematode *Caenorhabditis elegans* by computer-aided reconstruction from serial electron microscope sections. Of even more immediate interest from our present point of view are the observations of Lopresti et al. (1973), who have used comparable methods of analysis on the visual system of developing *Daphnia.* The remarkable degree of cell constancy and fiber constancy that these and other studies are revealing in certain invertebrates is just the sort of information that we need if we are to ask useful questions about how the connections are formed. And the situation in these invertebrates serves to accentuate the inadequacy of our information about the vertebrates.

Thus, one of the most exciting contributions to the investigation of neural connectivity to appear recently is a study of the connections and development of the eye of *Daphnia magna* (Macagno et al., 1973; Lopresti et al., 1973). *Daphnia* is a small crustacean which can reproduce parthenogenetically and can thus produce a population with a fixed genome. The compound eye of *Daphnia* consists of 22 ommatidia, each containing 8 receptor cells. The eye of the adult is cyclopean but it is derived from two precursor regions, symmetrically located about the midplane of the animal. In the adult, the receptor cells are arranged in an accurate mirror-symmetric fashion about the midline and there are thus 11 ommatidia on each side. The optic nerve contains the 176 fibers coming from the receptor cells, divided into 22 fascicles, one for each ommatidium. The fascicles travel to the optic ganglion where the first optic synapses are found and form an ordered mapping. The optic ganglion is a two-lobed structure, with fused lobes symmetrically located about the midline. The anterior cell group, or lamina, contains 110 neurons, 5 of which associate with each fascicle of optic nerve fibers. The posterior cell group is the medulla, which contains over 200 neurons. In the lamina, each cell is identifiable on the basis of shape, position and connectivity pattern.

It is concluded by Macagno et al. (1973) that, as long as the position of cell bodies and the branching and synaptic patterns of the nerve fibers are recorded to a resolution of only a few micrometers, great similarities are observed between animals of the same clone, and bilateral symmetry is seen between corresponding cells in the two sides of the same animal. If the branching and synaptic patterns are examined at levels of resolution ranging from a few tenths to a micron or two, however, variations are found among animals and between the two sides of any one animal. The authors think that, since the genomes of the animals are presumably identical, the small variations represent the noise level of the genetic control of structure.

Having established an anatomical baseline, the authors then went on to study the development of the visual connections in *Daphnia* (Lopresti et al., 1973). Analyses were made of a closely timed series of embryos and the authors conclude that a well-defined temporal sequence of growth and migration can account for most, if not all, of the spatial specificity of the nerve fibers that are establishing connections between the eye and the ganglion. Thus, early in development, all 5 lamina cells that will eventually make up an optic "cartridge", in collaboration with the 8 receptor cell axons from one ommatidium, are located at different anteroposterior levels. With maturation, and as the cells are sequentially contacted by the lead axon of the 8, the cells come to lie in the same plane. Ingrowth of optic axons occurs near the midline, and when a cartridge has been formed by the association of 8 retinular axons with 5 lamina cells, the cartridge moves laterally as a whole and a new sequence of these events takes place medially. Of the 8 retinular axons which go to form a cartridge, only one, the lead axon, has a growth cone; and contact between this lead axon and the lamina cells is associated with the onset of differentiation and axon outgrowth in the latter.

Lopresti et al. (1973) suggest that, although the visual system of adult *Daphnia* has a well-defined three-dimensional geometry, it is possible to design a model for the events that occur during the establishment of neural connections that only requires cells or fibers to receive very limited signals to determine their position or appropriate targets for connections, together with precise timing of axon ingrowth. In particular, they suggest that the only positional information the axons require is an indication as to whether or not they are near the midplane, and which positions are anterior and which are posterior.

The authors argue that, if we assume that only morphologically undifferentiated neuroblasts can act as axonal targets, the eventual three-dimensional relationships could be determined if cell behavior were simply controlled by: (i) contact with some midline-determining landmark, and (ii) a somewhat stereotyped response of a neuroblast when it is touched by the growth cone of a lead axon.

Such a model for the establishment of ordered nerve connections implies that the active role is played by the lead axon, which recruits whatever undifferentiated neuroblasts it happens to hit, until the proper number of 5 have coalesced to form a cartridge. As the authors have it, the song of the axons would be: "I touched you, you're mine"; very different from a Sperry-type mechanism where the cells would sing "I'm yours, come and get me".

A good prima facie case has thus been presented for the major significance of timing, together with a small amount of positional information (Wolpert, 1969) to indicate the extremities of the two-dimensional array, in the formation of the visual map in *Daphnia*. In no case, however, is it possible to identify the mechanism of connection formation by mere study of the end product; for this purpose we must perturb the developing system appropriately and observe the consequences. Thus, if the mode of development of this system is as suggested

332

by Lopresti et al. (1973), one might hope to be able to delete one or more ommatidia at a particular stage of development without inconveniencing the formation of connections in the lamina, which would merely accept the next group of optic fibers to arrive, in place of those deleted. Thus with a Sperry-type mechanism (Attardi and Sperry, 1963; Meyer and Sperry, 1973) one might expect deletion of ommatidia 3, 4, 5 to give the result shown in Fig. 1a; whereas the mechanism proposed by Lopresti et al. ought to give that shown in Fig. 1b. Variations on the chemoaffinity theme might predict still other results.

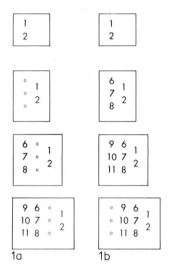

Fig. 1. a: the numbers and relative positions of developing optic cartridges present in one lobe of the optic lamina at various stages of development, on the basis of a Sperry-type of selective affinity mechanism, and assuming that ommatidia 3, 4, 5 have been deleted. Each rectangle represents the lobe of the lamina, at stages, from above downwards, of 29 hr, 32 hr, 35 hr and 37·5 hr. The open circles indicate "vacant" cartridges. b: as 1a, but on the time-position assumptions of Lopresti et al. (1973). For explanation, see text.

Or again, since the first group of optic fibers to grow into the lamina is near the midline, it would similarly be of interest to observe the result of reversing the mediolateral arrangement within the eye.

If the suggested mode of development in *Daphnia* is what actually happens, it is difficult to envisage how the rest of the nervous system becomes connected. Lamina neurons are supposed to be specified (in the sense of being given a name and an address) by contact with a particular optic axon. But lamina neurons themselves contact other neurons, serially, and eventually the chain of contacts will lead to the effector organs. There are other receptor systems apart from the eye, however, and if each were to use the same method of connectivity development, chaos could easily result.

Essentially, the same type of problem faces the presynaptic modulation theory of Weiss (1936) if it is extended right through the nervous system. Thus a muscle may modulate its motor neuron, which in turn may modulate an interneuron, which in turn may modulate an interneuron further up the path until we find ourselves deep within the nervous system; and, starting from the other end, a retinal ganglion cell may modulate a tectal cell, which in turn may modulate a cell further down the line and so forth. The problem, of course, is to make the two chains meet, as they must in the real nervous system.

Thus, in relation to the observations on *Daphnia*, we can say that, somewhere in the system, *some* form of adjustment would probably be required, to permit the various chains of neurons to link up. This type of difficulty is not unique to the nervous system. Users of keyboard instruments have long known that in tuning the instruments one runs into trouble if one starts with a low note and tunes upwards in octaves and perfect fifths — because if one then repeats the performance, but this time starting at the top note reached and progressing downwards, using the same principles, one does not arrive back at the starting point. The developing nervous system, like a keyboard instrument, cannot usefully be "tuned" in perfect intervals: equal temperament is required.

The observations of Levinthal and his co-workers (Lopresti and Macagno op. cit.) were made on the normally developing visual system in *Daphnia*. Experiments involving regeneration of the optic axons in locusts have also been performed (Horridge, 1968). When the retina was rotated $180°$ in second instar nymphs and then allowed to regenerate its central connections, normal visuomotor behavior was seen in the adult. The interpretation of these experiments is complicated, however, by the fact that at the time of operation less than half the adult number of ommatidia was present, while the rest were recruited later from unrotated head epidermis. This system, which would seem to offer great possibilities, is being further investigated (Meinertzhagen, 1973). It has been suggested that the ordered retinolamina projection found in the locust probably cannot arise in conditions of synchronous axon regrowth, i.e., without the sequential growth of ommatidial axon bundles that occurs in normal development (Meinertzhagen, 1973). This suggestion thus would be in accord with the tentative conclusions of Lopresti et al. (1973).

In vertebrates, observations compatible with a time-position mechanism come from the work of Gottlieb and Cowan (1972) on the development of the rat hippocampus. Dendrites of granule cells in the dentate gyrus receive synaptic input from axons coming from cells in the hippocampal CA3 region, and the input to these granule cells is from the same region in both ipsilateral and contralateral CA3. The cells of the dentate gyrus are formed in sequence, with those lying laterally in its dorsal blade being formed first, the cells in the medial part of the dorsal blade being formed later, and the cells in the ventral blade being formed last. Thus, if temporal factors are critical in establishing the relative numbers of synapses from the hippocampus on the two sides, the ratio of the two inputs (ipsi:contra) would be expected to vary systematically along the axis of generation of the cells. If, on the other hand, a chemoaffinity mechanism were operative in enabling the granule cell dendrites to recognize the contributions of crossed and uncrossed fibers, one might not expect the ratio between inputs to vary significantly from one region of the gyrus to another. In fact, there do turn out to be clear differences in the relative number of afferents from the two sources in the dorsal and ventral blades of the gyrus. Thus, the ipsi : contra ratio is 3 : 1 at that part of the gyrus which forms first,

2 : 1 at the next part to form, and approximately 1 : 1 at the part of the gyrus that forms last. It could be, therefore, that the dentate neurons accept inputs as they mature, but that only ipsilateral inputs are available when the cells first mature. It must be emphasized, of course, that while these observations are compatible with a time-position mechanism, they are not compelling evidence for one.

If carefully controlled timing of outgrowth of fibers is to be considered a major part of the mechanism of formation of ordered connections, to upset the timing should upset the connection pattern. The observations of Palka and Edwards (1974) have relevance here. They showed that accurate regeneration of cercal nerves in the cricket can occur even after a period of deprivation that occupies at least two-thirds of the period of postembryonic development. In this case, gross disturbance of the normal timing of ingrowth has not prevented the formation of properly patterned connections. We may note, however, that only the overall timing of ingrowth of the entire array of cercal nerves has necessarily been upset. Since cercal regeneration appears to go through stages that recapitulate the normal sequence of development, it is possible that the orderliness of timing *within* the array of cercal nerves is maintained; this could then be very important for the establishment of proper connections.

The likelihood of timing being involved as the main mechanism in the formation of ordered connections in all types of nervous system, or in all parts of the nervous system is also lessened by observations made on a very different structure, the vertebrate retinotectal projection. Here too it is possible to interfere with the timing of arrival of the nerve fibers without apparently upsetting the pattern of projection that is formed. Thus, optic nerve fibers innervating a virgin tectum after metamorphosis (Feldman et al., 1971) can give a normal retinotectal map; furthermore, it is possible to grow the optic nerve back to the tectum via the oculomotor nerve root (Gaze, 1959; Hibbard, 1967), which will presumably upset the timing of arrival of the fibers by causing them to take a longer than normal path; here again the evidence, scanty though it is, suggests that a normal projection pattern is formed.

Other studies on the regeneration of optic nerve fibers in adult *Rana temporaria* (Gaze and Jacobson, 1963) and in *Xenopus laevis* tadpoles (Gaze and Grant, 1975) support the view that timing of fiber ingrowth is inadequate as an explanation for the restoration of an orderly projection between eye and tectum. Thus, in normal development in *Xenopus*, the eye establishes synaptic connections with the tectum from approximately stage 43/45 (Chung et al., 1974). At this early stage the eye is very small, and it continues growing until after metamorphosis. The mode of growth of the retina involves the serial addition of rings of cells at the ciliary margin (Straznicky and Gaze, 1971). The retinal cells which first form connections with the tectum, therefore, are those cells close to the optic nerve head which, in the adult, comprise central retinal fundus. The *rest* of the retina is added, normally over a period of 4–6 weeks. Comparison of the mode of growth of the retina (which grows in rings; Straznicky and Gaze, 1971) and the tectum (which grows in a curvilinear fashion, from rostroventral to caudomedial; Straznicky and Gaze, 1972) with the mode of expansion of the retinotectal projection (Gaze et al., 1974; Scott, 1974) suggests strongly that, during development, there occurs a continual shift of synaptic connections between individual retinal axons and individual tectal units.

This continuing shift of synaptic connections with development would, by itself, argue strongly against timing as a mechanism in the ordered formation of selective retinotectal connections. At any one time in larval life in *Xenopus*, fibers are growing simultaneously from retina to tectum, from new ganglion cells at both the nasal and the temporal edges of the retina. Yet these two sets of newly arriving axons distribute themselves at opposite ends of the tectum; temporal fibers ending mainly in rostral tectum while nasal fibers go to caudal tectum. When the optic nerve regenerates to the tectum in *Rana*, the earliest responses found as the fibers return to the tectum are abnormal in their distribution (Gaze and Jacobson, 1963). Animals with early regeneration tend to show "pattern 1" maps, where one or two regions at the edges of the retina project in a disorganized fashion over large areas of tectum. The point is that the first responses tend to come from peripheral retina, whereas during initial development presumptive central retina (i.e., what is to be central retina in the adult) is the first part to connect (Chung et al., 1974). When optic nerves regenerate in mid-larval *Xenopus*, the earliest tectal responses found also come from peripheral retina and not central retina (Gaze and Grant, 1975). Thus, studies of optic nerve regeneration, in both larval and adult amphibians, offer no support for the hypothesis that the establishment of the normal map is dependent upon closely controlled timing of ingrowth of the fibers.

Lastly, we can say that the most permanent alteration of timing is achieved by removing part of the array of neurons giving rise to a projection; in this case the missing axons will never arrive, since their cells of origin have disappeared. When such an operation is performed on the retinotectal projection of goldfish, and the optic nerve is cut and allowed to regenerate, the fibers from the residual retina form (initially, at least) a normal partial projection. In one such experimental situation, fibers from residual nasal retina were seen to grow right across "empty" rostral tectum to arborize in caudal tectum (Attardi and Sperry, 1963), and this is indeed where nasal retinal fibers normally arborize.

Other invertebrate systems that have been investigated include sensory and interneuronal regeneration in the leech (Baylor and Nicholls, 1968, 1971; Jansen and Nicholls, 1972) and the regeneration of chromatophore nerves in octopus (Sanders and Young, 1974).

The work on octopus and on leech cutaneous input shows that in these situations, peripheral nerves appear to be able to reform their proper connections. In addition, section of a ganglion connective in leech may be followed by "correct" regeneration in that the interconnections regenerated between identified cells in ganglia on each side of the lesion were modality-specific and location-specific (Baylor and Nicholls, 1971), although slightly less so than in normal animals. One particularly intriguing result which accentuates the great complexity of the functional interconnections between neurons in even so comparatively simple an animal as a leech, is the observation (Jansen and Nicholls, 1972) that, even though the spatial and modality specificity of neural interconnection is restored after regeneration of a ganglionic connective, the normal balance of excitation and inhibition between cells is not restored. This abnormality is not confined to the operated region but shows itself elsewhere, in that cells linked between ganglia, distant from the lesion, also manifest altered excitatory-inhibitory patterns.

TARGET AFFINITY MECHANISMS

The studies on invertebrates mentioned above have so far revealed the remarkable constancy of certain neuronal positions and patterns of connectivity and have demonstrated that, during regeneration, the normal connectivity patterns may be largely restored. These studies have not, up to the present time, applied experimental tests capable of distinguishing between the various mechanisms which could be responsible for the *formation* of the ordered connections seen. At present we can only speculate as to whether precisely controlled timing and spatial positioning might be able to account for the findings, or whether we have to postulate some other mechanism. For the result of more analytical experiments we have to look to the vertebrates, where many transplantation experiments have been performed. It is experiments in these systems that have led to the postulation of the various affinity hypotheses. Unfortunately, while the nature of the operations performed on vertebrates has been more useful to date, we have to trade this advantage for the disadvantage of being unable in most cases to identify individual neurons with certainty.

Until fairly recently, most types of experiment on the development and regeneration of neuronal connections had been performed exclusively on lower vertebrates — amphibia and fishes. Although these are still the animals most extensively studied in this sort of work, it is now known that some of the main classes of phenomena previously reported for the visual system in lower vertebrates (e.g., compression or side-to-side transposition of a projection) are also to be found in young mammals (see below). Thus some of the phenomena to be accounted for are probably universally present in vertebrates; at least as a first approximation, therefore, observations made and mechanisms suggested for lower vertebrates may be expected to have a general relevance for vertebrates, and probably for invertebrates as well.

It will, we hope, be of some help to the reader in following our arguments if we now list the main types of phenomena that have been found in experimental work on the lower vertebrate visual system. Some of the phenomena we will mention have also been reported for the mammalian visual system. This list is presented for purposes of general orientation, and several of the classes of result mentioned are not considered further in this paper.

(a) The setting up in development of orderly projections.

(b) The regeneration of orderly projections, following section of the optic nerve, with and without rotation of the eye. This has been demonstrated in amphibians and fishes (see Gaze, 1970).

(c) Transposition of projections from their proper territory to a bilaterally symmetrical territory on the opposite side of the midline, with preservation of polarity and internal ordering. This has been demonstrated in anurans, after section of one optic nerve close to the chiasma (Gaze and Jacobson, 1963) or after uncrossing the chiasma (Straznicky et al., 1971); in goldfish, after removal of one tectum (Sharma, 1973); and in fetal rats, after removal of one colliculus (Miller and Lund, 1975).

(d) Translocation of a partial projection to an inappropriate part of the proper territory on the same side of the midline, with preservation of polarity and internal ordering. This has been shown to occur in goldfish, where the partial projection from a nasal half-retina may give an ordered map across an inappropriate residual rostral half-tectum (Horder, 1971; Yoon, 1972).

(e) Compression of the projection from one neuronal array onto a surgically diminished array of receptor neurons. In this situation, fibers from an intact retina form a compressed but normally ordered and orientated, map across a residual half-tectum. This phenomenon, originally reported in adult goldfish (Gaze and Sharma, 1970; Yoon, 1971), has recently been found in anurans (Gaze and MacDonald, in preparation) and has also been shown to occur in young hamsters (Jhaveri and Schneider, 1974).

(f) Expansion of the projection from a surgically diminished neuronal array onto a complete array of receptor neurons. This phenomenon was first reported in experiments on "compound eyes" in *Xenopus* (Gaze et al., 1963; but see below) and has since been described in adult goldfish (Horder, 1971; Yoon, 1972), where a surgically formed residual half-retina has been found to expand, in order, across the whole tectum.

(g) Subdivision of territory between populations of axons. In newborn hamsters (Schneider, 1973) destruction of the superficial layers of one superior colliculus results in axons from the eye contralateral to the damaged area forming an abnormal decussation and ending in the undamaged colliculus. Axons from the two eyes subdivide this colliculus between them, for they terminate in a non-overlapping manner; further, if axons from the eye contralateral to the normal colliculus are eliminated at birth, the anomalous recrossing axons from the other eye then spread out over the entire colliculus on the "wrong" side of the brain.

This situation in hamsters, where fibers from the two eyes subdivide the territory between them, contrasts with the finding in amphibia (Straznicky et al., 1971) that each eye may map independently to the whole of one tectum. Subdivision of territory has been reported in goldfish, however (Cronly-Dillon and Glaizner, 1974).

In connection with the subdivision of territory between two eyes, we may mention the somewhat different case described by Lund and Lund (1971) in young rats. In these animals the uncrossed retinocollicular projection is sparse and localized. If the contralateral eye is removed at birth, the ipsilateral projection is later found to have spread virtually across the entire colliculus, whereas if the contralateral eye is removed on the fifth postnatal day, the ipsilateral projection only spreads across approximately one-third of the colliculus. A comparable, though less dramatic, spreading of the ipsilateral retinocollicular projection is seen following early eye enucleation in the rabbit (Chow et al., 1973).

(h) Rotation of part of the map following rotation of a tectal graft (Sharma and Gaze, 1971; Yoon, 1973; Levine and Jacobson, 1974).

(i) Translocation of part of the map, following tectal graft translocation.

This phenomenon has been found in frogs (Jacobson and Levine, 1975) and in fish (Hope et al., 1976).

The first and most important affinity mechanism to be proposed was put forward by Sperry in his chemoaffinity theory (1943, 1944, 1945, 1951, 1963, 1965). He cut the optic nerve in newts, rotated the eye by 180°, and investigated the behavior of the animals after the nerve had regenerated. His observations showed that the animal's visuomotor reactions, through that eye, were then reversed. He suggested that this was because the fibers had reformed connections with their original central sites. In searching for a mechanism to account for how the fibers could have found their proper terminal sites, Sperry discounted mechanical guidance since it was difficult to see how the fibers could have found their original pathways beyond the scar formed at the site of the lesion in the nerve. He therefore postulated that the retinal ganglion cells differ intrinsically from each other, as the tectal cells would also have to do. Meyer and Sperry have recently summarized this view as follows: ". . . during development the cells of the retina and tectum acquire individual position-dependent cytochemical specificities which determine optic fiber outgrowth patterns, and enable central synaptic connections to be formed in topographic order on the basis of preferential chemical affinities between matching retinal and tectal loci" (Meyer and Sperry, 1973).

This theory, which holds that connections are determined by a matching of presynaptic and postsynaptic elements is, as will become clear in the next section, by no means the only way of accounting for an ordered mapping, even if we reject mechanical guidance or timing mechanisms. Furthermore, it is not at all clear precisely how the theory is to be understood; recent experimental work has led to the hypothesis being differently interpreted by different investigators, as is evidenced by some recent debates (Meyer and Sperry, 1973, 1974; Hunt and Jacobson, 1974). Such differences of opinion are due not to a sudden interest in the history of neuronal specificity, nor to a delight in the minutiae of historical interpretation, but to recent experimental results which require for their interpretation a more thoroughly worked out theoretical basis. Such debates, as historical interpretation, are empty; because the distinctions which are now being made were not considered at the time Sperry proposed his theory. The debates are important, however, in as much as they lead to more distinctions being made, which enable us to interpret these experimental findings more satisfactorily. Sperry's theory was distinct from various alternatives current at the time (resonance theory, mechanical guidance), and this was enough to generate many interesting new experiments. It is a central purpose of this paper to argue that theoretical work in this field has resulted only from the pressure of experimental results, and that at the present time there has arisen a great requirement for improved theoretical analysis.

Early experiments on optic nerve regeneration involved observation of the results of allowing an intact eye to reconnect with an intact tectum (see Gaze, 1970). The recovery of vision which occurred in these circumstances, and also the restoration of the fiber projection that has been demonstrated by many investigators, could undoubtedly result from the mechanism proposed in Sperry's hypothesis. Recovery in such cases, however, could perhaps also have been accounted for by other mechanisms, for instance involving timing as a main factor. It was partly in response to such considerations that a different kind of experiment was devised: the mismatch experiment (Attardi and Sperry, 1963). In this class of experiment, part of the retina is removed, the optic nerve is cut and the projection is assayed following regeneration of fibers from the residual retina; alternatively, part of the optic tectum is removed, the optic nerve is cut and the regeneration of fibers from the intact eye to the residual tectum is studied. If the retinotectal map is formed by a rigid matching of retinal and tectal cells, one might predict that half a retina would project to only half of the tectum, i.e., to those tectal sites which match the half-retina. Similarly, half a tectum might be expected to accept fibers from only half of an intact retina.

The first results indeed confirmed these expectations (Attardi and Sperry, 1963; Jacobson and Gaze, 1965) but there was one rather curious exception. In 1963, Gaze, Jacobson and Székely made what they called a "compound eye" in *Xenopus*. Half of the eye was removed at an early developmental stage, before any retinal fibers had reached the tectum. It was then replaced by a half-eye from another animal. The first such compound eyes to be made consisted of either two nasal or two temporal half-eyes. Electrophysiological recordings from these animals, after metamorphosis, showed that each half-eye projected to the whole tectum (Fig. 2). In other words, every part of the tectum received input from two points in the retina — the two points being mirror-symmetrical about the vertical midline.

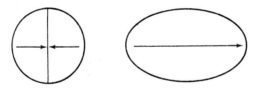

Fig. 2. Compound eye projection. The circle represents the retina and the ellipse the tectum. The arrow on the tectum represents a row of tectal points, while the arrows on the retina indicate the functionally corresponding retinal points.

One might have expected each half-retina to project only to its corresponding half-tectum. A compound eye would then have projected as in Fig. 3.

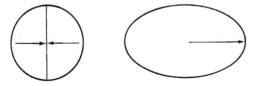

Fig. 3. The predicted projection of a compound eye to the tectum, on the assumptions that each half of the compound eye contains only its appropriate half set of specificities (i.e., retinal pattern regulation has not occurred), and that the tectum has not regulated its specificity structure, and that a normal rule of matching specificities operates. Conventions as in Fig. 2.

It was the difference between prediction and the result in this situation that forced a more detailed look at the postulated mechanisms underlying the formation of retinotectal connections. If a particular retinal fiber can make contact only with a tectal site which has a corresponding label, then these results can be accounted for only by supposing either that each half retina now possesses a full complement of labels (i.e., has undergone pattern regulation), or that the tectum has only half its normal complement of labels, but spread out over the whole tectum.

Two main theoretical points were brought out by this result. Sperry's theory, or indeed any theory of retinotectal mapping, will make three assertions (Straznicky et al., 1971).

(a) It will say something about the properties of retinal ganglion cells and their fibers.

(b) It will say something about the properties of tectal cells.

(c) It will give the mapping rules which determine how the retinal fibers will use their own properties plus the properties of the target neurons in order to order themselves on the tectum.

The first theoretical point is this: in assaying the retinotectal map, one is seeing the result of (a), (b) and (c), and it is impossible to experimentally separate these three parts. In the particular case of the compound eye map, the result at first sight appears to contradict the mapping rule, viz., each retinal fiber has a label, and will make contact only with the tectal site that has a corresponding label; but this mapping rule would be saved if one supposed that the retinal or tectal labels had changed. In general it could be argued, therefore, that no rules for mapping can ever be tested, since any result can be made compatible with the rules by postulating some change in the state of the retina or of the tectum. Nor, indeed, can one say anything about the state of the retina or of the tectum, for to do so would be to presuppose the mapping rules (Chung and Feldman, 1974; Hunt and Jacobson, 1974).

This argument constitutes a serious challenge: if correct, then there is really no point to any of the experiments performed in this field. The argument in this strong form, however, would indeed be sufficient to induce total scepticism about the whole of *any* field of scientific enterprise, since any theory can be saved, whatever the experimental evidence, if one makes sufficient ad hoc assumptions. While the validity of such scepticism can be debated, and indeed is central to the philosophy of science, we do not intend to debate it here.

In its weaker form viz., that there can never be a good reason for deciding whether or not labels have changed, independently of holding a theory about the mapping rule, the argument is false. For example, in a situation where some fibers from a limited part of a complete retina project to one entire tectum, and yet the complete retina also projects normally to the other tectum (Feldman et al., 1975), it seems unreasonable to suppose that the aberrant fibers possess a complete complement of labels. A mapping rule which could account for the result in such a situation without such a supposition is to be preferred over one which would necessitate it.

The second theoretical point to emerge from the compound eye results is more positive. In order to retain "the mapping rule" of precise and exclusive connections between complementary labels in the retina and the tectum, it was necessary to suppose that the labels in either the retina or the tectum had changed. Such an alteration in the cellular labels would amount to a form of "regulation"; and, since the compound eye operation had indeed been performed at embryonic stages, it was entirely reasonable to propose retinal pattern regulation as the explanation of the results. However, in 1970, Gaze and Sharma described experiments on adult goldfish in which they found that, after removal of the caudal half of the tectum, the whole eye eventually projected to the remaining rostral half of the tectum to form a compressed but otherwise normal map. This phenomenon has since been confirmed (Yoon, 1971) and the complementary phenomenon of expansion of a half-retinal projection over a whole tectum in adult goldfish has also been described (Horder, 1971; Yoon, 1972).

Since these manifestations of plasticity in the retinal projection have been observed in adult animals, where the neurons are already "differentiated", it is highly unlikely that regulation can be the explanation. Furthermore, apart from the inherent unlikelihood of regulation in this situation, the recent findings of Cook and Horder (1974) are cogent evidence against it in the optic tectum. These authors removed the caudal half tectum in adult goldfish, cut the optic nerve, and demonstrated electrophysiologically that the earliest regenerated projection gave a half-map over the residual half tectum, whereas some time later a complete, but compressed, map covered this half-tectum. They then cut the optic nerve a second time and allowed it to regenerate. They found that the earliest maps recorded after this second operation again showed the original half-field projection to the half-tectum, and this map again became compressed over a period of time. It is thus very unlikely that the half-tectum had regulated its specificity structure to give the first compression, since, when challenged later by optic nerve regeneration, it behaved as though it had not done so. Still further evidence against regulation in the goldfish retinotectal system has recently been presented by Meyer (1975).

There is strong evidence, therefore, against regulative alteration of cellular labels in the adult goldfish. These results, even more than those from compound eye experiments, raised the question of whether it is possible to propose a set of mapping rules which will account for the results of normal, compressed and expanded projections *without* supposing that labels in retina or tectum have changed. This question was considered by Gaze and Keating (1972) when they gave the name "systems matching" to the type of behavior seen. Systems matching is not a model but rather a component of a class of models. The term implies that the question might be answered in the affirmative if an incoming retinal fiber takes account, not only of the tectum, but also of other incoming retinal fibers in choosing where to make synaptic contact. "Systems matching" thus implies that the relationship under study is contextual, i.e., dependent upon the overall context (Straznicky et al., 1971; Gaze et al., 1972; Gaze and Keating, 1972). The recent experiments mentioned above make it increasingly important to construct models along these lines.

Models of mechanisms for the control of the formation of nerve connections can be proposed at various levels of detail and precision. It may happen that the initial statement of a hypothesis is couched in fairly general terms, as seen from our present viewpoint, although at the time it was proposed it may have seemed adequate in relation to the problems then visible. Thus, the hypothesis of neuronal chemospecificity (Sperry, 1943, 1944, 1945, 1951, 1963, 1965) proposed that retinotectal connections form under the influence of differential affinities between retinal axons and tectal cells. Although such a statement is excellent for outlining the general class of events that is envisaged, in this form it is so general as to be virtually untestable — because such a general statement says nothing about *how* the affinities may work. As to whether they are to be thought of as mosaic, non-interactive affinities, where the behavior of any two affine units is uninfluenced by anything going on elsewhere in the whole system, or whether the affinities are in some sense contextual and interactive, the general statement makes no prediction about the results that might be obtained in situations such as the retinotectal mismatch experiment. Thus, it is possible to come across diametrically opposed statements about what the hypothesis will predict in the same situation (Hunt and Jacobson, 1974; Meyer and Sperry, 1973).

Undoubtedly, the first statements of Sperry's hypothesis (Sperry, 1943, 1944, 1945) were not sufficiently detailed to encompass the retinotectal mismatch situation. However, Sperry himself devised the mismatch experiment (Attardi and Sperry, 1963; Sperry, 1963) and from that time has regarded this type of experiment as a critical test of his hypothesis (Meyer and Sperry, 1973, 1974). Thus, from 1963 onwards Sperry has viewed the affinities proposed in his theory as non-contextual in this situation. It may be seen that much of the discussion in recent years about the validity of Sperry's hypothesis is misconceived. This is because, since the theory was not articulated in sufficient detail, it has been possible for different people to interpret it in different ways. The experimental results now available demand a more extended and detailed theoretical basis, so that we can come to reliable conclusions about what models or classes of model the experiments eliminate.

Prestige and Willshaw (1975) have responded to the requirement for a detailed theoretical analysis with some elegant computer simulations. Their paper is important for two reasons. Firstly it presents the detailed working out of one particular model; secondly it suggests a way in which we can accurately define a whole range of models. We will take the second point first.

Prestige and Willshaw (1975) concentrate on the concept of *affinity*: that of a retinal fiber for a tectal cell, and of a tectal cell for a retinal fiber. Let us consider for simplicity a single row of tectal cells and retinal fibers. For each retinal fiber j we may define a function $F(j,j')$ which tells us the affinity of fiber j for each tectal cell; conversely, for each tectal cell we may define a function which determines the affinity of that tectal cell for each retinal fiber. If the affinity of a retinal fiber for a tectal cell is considered to be the same as the affinity of the tectal cell for the retinal fiber, then strictly speaking only one set of affinity functions is necessary. Affinity can be thought of as the strength of the bond between pre- and postsynaptic cells: strong bonds are formed in preference to weaker bonds.

Prestige and Willshaw consider two models with rather simple affinity functions. In the group 1 mechanisms, an axon j has maximum affinity for member j' of the postsynaptic set and less for all the others. Similarly, postsynaptic cell j' has maximum affinity for fiber j. Instead of talking rather vaguely about "specificity" or "selective affinity", one can now define precisely what the model is to be. For example, the affinity function might be like that shown in Fig. 4, where each retinal axon likes one tectal site above all others but has no other preferences. Alternatively, the affinity profile could be like that in Fig. 5, where there is an optimal corresponding tectal site but sites close to this are preferred to sites further away. These two models may well have different properties, particularly with respect to the predicted effect of removing tectal sites.

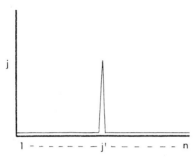

Fig. 4. Possible affinity function of axon j for cells, in a group 1 model. Affinity of axon j is shown on y axis, cell number on x axis. (Modified from Prestige and Willshaw, 1975.)

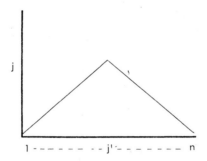

Fig. 5. As Fig. 4. See text for further explanation.

This way of defining models has further interest. From time to time biochemical models have been proposed to account for the formation of the retinotectal map. For these models to be testable they must be related to the kinds of experiment we have been mainly discussing — experiments in which the retinotectal projection is examined after various perturbations of the system. If the models cannot be so related, then there is no way of determining the relevance of a biochemical observation to the problems of retinotectal connectivity. The most detailed biochemical model proposed to date is that of Barondes (1970). He proposes:

(a) that there are a large number of protein and lipid molecules on the membranes of all neurons to which polysaccharide chains may be covalently linked;

344

(b) the addition of sugars to these surface proteins and lipids is linearly related to the level of the various glycosyltransferases in the cell, over a wide range; and

(c) the polysaccharide chains that are formed have a far greater binding affinity for membrane proteins than for other polysaccharide chains.

If we consider just one axis, Barondes suggests that there is a gradient of glycosyltransferases across both the retina and the tectum, which causes a gradient in the abundance of polysaccharides. By postulate (c), retinal fibers abundant in polysaccharides will bind more strongly with tectal cells which are poor in polysaccharides, because the latter will have many free surface proteins not already binding a polysaccharide.

A model of this detail allows us to set up the affinity functions, if not precisely, then at least in their general form. The function in this case would be similar to Fig. 5 above. Once the affinity function is set up, one can proceed to investigate the predictions of such a model. We would expect that, in the situation of half a tectum being innervated by a whole eye, Barondes' model would predict that the corresponding half-eye would cover the half-tectum and the displaced half-eye would connect, as best it could, as close to the cut edge of the tectum as possible.

Prestige and Willshaw do not in fact examine these group 1 models in detail. Their central interest is to examine a competition model, which they call a group 2 mechanism. All axons have maximum affinity for making and retaining contacts at one end of the array of postsynaptic cells, with progressively less affinity for cells at greater distance from that end. Similarly, all postsynaptic cells have maximum affinity for axons from one end of the presynaptic set. Axons remote from this end have correspondingly less likelihood of retaining any contact. The two affinity functions are therefore identical, and look like those shown in Fig. 6.

Such affinity functions will not by themselves produce an ordered map: all axons will tend to pile up towards the most desirable end of the tectum. It is only by introducing some kind of fiber-fiber interaction that an ordered map will result, and the interaction that Prestige and Willshaw use is competition. Essentially, they suppose there to be a limited number of postsynaptic sites.

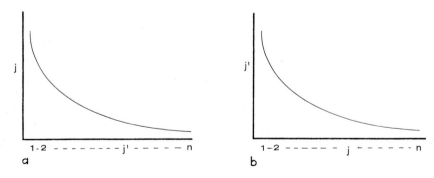

Fig. 6. Possible affinity functions in a group 2 mechanism. a: affinity of axon j for cells. b: affinity of cell j' for axons. See text for further explanation. (Modified from Prestige and Willshaw, 1975.)

Not all fibers, therefore, can pile up at the most desirable end of the tectum. In the competition for the most desirable end, those fibers which are most preferred by this end of the tectum win out. This permits the next most preferred fibers to contact the next most desirable sites, and in this way an ordered map is finally produced.

This model, requiring as it does some kind of fiber-fiber interaction, is a candidate for systems matching. The key question to ask is therefore: what does such a model predict in the mismatch situation? The simple answer is that no spreading or compression occurs. A half-retina projecting to a complete tectum will cover only the most desirable half of the tectum, no matter which half-retina remains intact. To obtain spreading in this model we have to introduce still further constraints. Spreading might be encouraged by postulating, for instance:

(a) a type of "diffusion" process which leads to the filling of space, as a gas will fill a bottle; or

(b) a mutual repulsion between the retinal fibers, encouraging their greatest separation.

The essential difference between these two types of mechanism is that in (a) the individual fibers take no notice of each other, diffusion being a random walk function of each fiber. In (b), on the other hand, it is fiber-fiber interaction (repulsion) that causes the spreading.

Prestige and Willshaw consider a method such as (a) for obtaining spreading, and they reject it on the grounds that, to the extent that spreading occurs, the map becomes less and less ordered. However, they do not consider a mechanism such as (b), and it remains uncertain whether, if mutual repulsion is a strong enough force to cause a half-retina to spread over the whole tectum, it would be strong enough to disorder the map. A further difficulty with repulsion is that it would militate against the occurrence of compression in different experimental situations. Prestige and Willshaw state that their model will permit compression or spreading of connections in a mismatch situation, as soon as the total number of synaptic sites is allowed to equalize to the normal number. This, as they point out, would amount to a form of regulation but not, we may add, a regulation of the affinities themselves.

The model proposed by Prestige and Willshaw thus illustrates a possible role for competition in the establishment of the map. The model is inadequate in the sense that it cannot account for all the presently-known facts of the retinotectal situation, but this does not really matter. Quite apart from the argument that we should perhaps be wary of any hypothesis which *can* account for all the facts, on the grounds that some of the so-called facts are bound to be wrong, a partially successful model can enlarge our understanding of how parts of the system *might* work. And, most important of all, it will have the very beneficial effect of bringing into the open hidden assumptions. The human mind has the ability to make large logical jumps without recognizing them, and to ignore the existence of hidden premises. Fortunately, the computer is much more restricted and requires a complete set of instructions before it can proceed; this requirement is a powerful stimulus to clarity of thought.

The competition model of Prestige and Willshaw can thus generate a map by use of gradients of affinity and by the introduction of competition. It is possible, however, to produce models in which retinotectal maps can be formed without fibers having *any* preferential affinities for tectal positions, or tectal positions for retinal fibers. Such models can, as may be seen from the next section, account for most (although not all) of the phenomena found in experiments on the retinotectal system. The experimental result which cannot be accommodated by these models is the one following tectal graft transloca-tion, where the corresponding part of the map is translocated appropriately (Jacobson and Levine, 1975; Hope et al., 1976). This result is therefore the strongest available evidence for the existence of differential affinities.

FIBER-SORTING MECHANISMS

Hope et al. (1976) have begun to use computer simulation for a model, the "arrow model", which is different from that of Prestige and Willshaw. Essentially, each retinal fiber must be able to tell, from local information on the tectum, the directions rostral and medial. Furthermore, two retinal fibers must be able to communicate with each other and discover which originates from the more nasal and which from the more dorsal cell in the retina. The fibers then sort out on the tectum by comparing themselves with their neighbors and noting the directions defined locally on the tectum. Such a model cannot be fitted into the Prestige and Willshaw analysis because there are no selective affinities of any kind: a single retinal fiber couldn't care less where it is on the tectum.

An interesting feature of this model is that it predicts that the appropriate local region of the map will rotate within a rotated graft (Hope et al., 1976). From such experimental results (Sharma and Gaze, 1971; Yoon, 1973) one cannot, therefore, conclude that there are selective affinities between retinal fibers and tectal sites. And, since the arrow model behaves in a systems-matching fashion, map rotation following graft rotation cannot be used as evidence (Yoon, 1973) against systems-matching either.

The arrow model uses polarity information on the tectum for two purposes; it is used to orient the retinotectal projection correctly and it is also needed for the fibers to sort out in their correct order. Chung (1974) has suggested that these processes might be separate, and that it could be helpful to consider them as such. In theory, at least, if we have sufficient information to order the map, very little extra would be required to orient it correctly.

The experimental results which are evidence against the arrow model and which suggest the existence of selective affinities are those where, following tectal graft translocation, we find translocation of the corresponding part of the map (Jacobson and Levine, 1975; Hope et al., 1976). Whether such results can be accounted for by alternative mechanisms remains to be seen.

Fiber-sorting mechanisms which do not use information from the tectum are inadequate in the retinotectal situation; for instance, they cannot account for the rotation of the map following rotation of a tectal graft. If the tectum is blank as far as the optic fibers are concerned, such a rotation could not be noticed. It is still conceivable, however, that such a mechanism could, with minimal help from time-position mechanisms, account for the initial formation of the map. The retinal input might then induce more information on the tectum which would permit the later rotation of the map following graft rotation. If this were so, regeneration would not be a good model for development.

Can ordering result simply from interactions between fibers? This question is of importance not only in considering how retinal fibers might sort out on the tectum (for which a tectal "anchor" would be required to orient the map), but also in relation to the question of how they might sort out in the optic nerve; for the optic nerve (at least in goldfish; Horder, 1974) is highly ordered. In this context we may perhaps mention the spectacular example of sorting out of fibers that occurs in the dorsal columns. The axons from skin receptors enter the dorsal columns and pass up to the dorsal column nuclei in the cervical region before making their first synapse. Initially, the order of the axons reflects the segmental level at which they enter the spinal cord: if two touch receptor fibers from the same area of the skin enter the spinal cord at different levels, they will initially be at different positions in the cord. However, further up in the cord (but still at a level below the first synapse) it is found that fibers from neighboring receptors are themselves now neighbors (Werner and Whitsel, 1973).

Let us return to the question of how retinal fibers might sort themselves out without using any information present on the tectum. One way, of course, would be by use of a form of selective adhesiveness among the fibers. Another way in which they could sort themselves out could be through the use of neighborhood information in the retina. We may introduce this concept by considering some work of Kendall, who was interested in reconstructing a medieval manor from information derived from contemporary cartularies. The only information given was which plot of land abutted onto which, and even this was incomplete. In related work, Kendall constructed a program which, as he demonstrated, would sort out the 88 provinces of France (Paris and Corsica not included) to give a correct map from information about neighborhood relationships only (Kendall, 1971). This suggests that if retinal cells know only who their neighbors are, their fibers should be able to sort themselves out. But Kendall's algorithm would allow both the unsorted fibers and the retinal cells to whisper to each other in such a way that each can effectively calculate its distance from any other such fiber or cell. Kendall has adapted his program to remove this feature (personal communication) but there remains an undesirable (that is, biologically undesirable) feature: each fiber has to know, in order that it can choose how to move during the ordering process, the state of the whole group of fibers, i.e., how well ordered the fibers already are. It is still an open question whether, if this global feature were removed, the fibers could still sort themselves out. That is, can ordering result if fibers may whisper only to their neighbors, to discover whether their cell bodies are neighbors in the retina? This question is currently being investigated.

A particularly attractive aspect of this sort of model is that the special feature of a continuously ordered mapping — the preservation of neighborhood properties — is made use of by the developing system. Naturally, some additional information would be required to orient the map but, as we have said earlier, this need not be a great deal. Perhaps the existence of so many well-ordered maps in the central nervous system thus reflects merely the nature of the developmental processes themselves, and not at all the exigencies of sensory information processing.

CELL POPULATIONS

The idea of systems-matching is that fiber-to-fiber interaction is a major component in forming the retinotectal map. Any mechanism for the formation of nerve connections in which the position at which the retinal fiber makes contact depends not only upon that fiber and the tectum, but also upon the other fibers projecting to that tectum, raises the question: *which* other fibers does it take note of?

Systems-matching therefore leads us to the concept of a population of cells. We might define a population of cells, in relation to the retinotectal system, as follows: two cells are in the same population if, and only if, they are affected by each other in mapping to the tectum. This definition is taken to imply transitivity: if cell A is in the same population as cell B, and cell B is in the same population as cell C, then cell A is in the same population as cell C.

This concept of a population of cells immediately raises empirical questions. What determines when cells and their fibers are or are not in the same population? Are all fibers which project to the same tectum at the same time necessarily in the same population? Must the cell bodies of a single population be in a single continuous sheet? Are the two halves of a compound eye a single population? Unfortunately, the experimental investigation of these questions is complicated by the dependence of our interpretation of the result on the theory of mapping which we hold. In the extreme, if we hold a theory of mapping in which no fiber-to-fiber interaction at all takes place, the question of what constitutes a population cannot even be asked — either theoretically or experimentally.

However, as we have noted before, this interdependence of our concepts does not make all empirical investigation pointless. Let us consider the following experiment. Each eye projects to its contralateral tectum to give a normal map. By interfering with the projection, let us suppose that some fibers from a limited area of one eye, have innervated the ipsilateral tectum. We may then ask the question: do the fibers which innervate the ipsilateral tectum cover that portion of the tectum which, in a normal contralateral map, corresponds to the retina from which they are derived, or do they cover the whole area of the tectum? Some unpublished observations (Gaze, Keating and Feldman) suggest that the latter may be the case but, for our present purposes, it is necessary only to accept that such a result is in principle possible. This would show that fibers from part of the retina cover a limited portion of the tectum when projecting with other fibers from the same retina, but cover the whole tectum when projecting with fibers from the other retina. This kind of experiment is the ideal for investigating what constitutes a "population" of cells.

We have said that in order to conclude from an experimental result something about which cells belong to a population and which do not, we must make some assumptions about a theory of mapping. The converse of this is that we may have to make assumptions about what constitutes a population of cells in order to pass from experiment to statements about mapping rules, or about the state of the retina and the tectum. Jacobson and Hunt's three-eye assay (1973) is complicated by this consideration. In this assay a third eye is grafted onto the experimental animal — an animal in which, typically, one of its own eyes has been surgically tampered with. This third eye is encouraged to project to the same tectum as does the abnormal eye. From the projection one deduces something about the state of the abnormal eye — but what one deduces will in general depend upon whether the two eyes projecting to the same tectum are considered to constitute a single population of cells, or rather two distinct populations.

The majority of experiments on lower vertebrates in which two eyes are encouraged to innervate one tectum result in each eye covering the whole tectum (Sharma, 1973; Straznicky et al., 1971; Gaze and Jacobson, 1963). This is consistent with each eye being a separate population of cells. In hamsters, however, the situation is different. Schneider (1973) removed one superior colliculus in newborn hamsters, and both eyes innervated the remaining colliculus. Instead of each eye covering the whole area, however, they parcelled it out between them: one eye covered one half, the other eye covered the remaining half of the colliculus. Upon removing one of the eyes, the projection from the other one spread to cover the whole area. This result can be accounted for by supposing that the fibers from the two eyes here constitute a single population. If the mechanism for mapping guarantees the preservation of neighborhood properties, and if cells in different eyes are never neighbors, Schneider's result is predicted. Schneider himself (1973) interprets his result as showing competition between the two eyes for terminal space, but the mechanism discussed here is not one of competition. Indeed, if the two eyes were competing for synaptic sites, one would expect them to intermingle, for there is no a priori reason at all why one eye should win all of the sites in one half of the tectum, while the other eye wins all the sites in the other half.

We have spoken of the possibility of there being two populations of cells, either within one eye — in the case of a compound eye — or in separate eyes. In these situations there is no intermingling of the two populations. There is nothing, however, in the definition of a population to make this a necessary condition. One could in principle also have two completely intermixed populations within the retina. If each population were similarly distributed over the retina, and if each projection were orientated on the tectum in the same way, then the map produced would be indistinguishable from normal (Fig. 7a). The same would be true of any number of such populations. The corollary of this is that the normal retinotectal map could in reality be such a mixture of populations. If the two populations were orientated in different directions, however (Fig. 7b), or if one of the populations were distributed over only part of the retina (Fig. 7c), then such a situation could be picked up experimentally. Maps like some of these have in fact been observed: Feldman and Gaze (1975) described a projection in which a part of the retina appeared

350

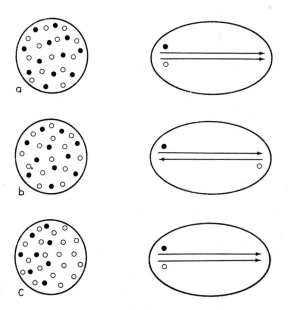

Fig. 7. Projections of multiple retinal populations to tectum. See text for further explanation. a: mixed populations, similar polarity. b: mixed populations, opposite polarity. c: unevenly distributed populations, similar polarity.

to be projecting onto two different parts of the tectum, and the two projections had opposite polarities.

It is an interesting possibility that each of the major classes of ganglion cells described in the frog retina (Maturana et al., 1960) might also comprise a distinct population in our present sense, thus making it easier to account for the differential depth distribution of their fiber endings in the tectum.

We would like, in the final part of this paper, to return to our definition of a continuous mapping. A continuous mapping in the present usage, as applied to the retinotectal system, is characterized by two conditions:

(a) adjacent points on the retina project only to adjacent tectal points; and
(b) adjacent points on the tectum receive only from adjacent retinal points.

These two statements are not the same, as can be seen from Fig. 2. Here, it is true that two points which are neighbors on the retina project to neighboring points on the tectum, but it is false that neighboring points on the tectum necessarily receive projections from neighboring retinal points.

We have suggested in the section of this paper entitled "Fiber-sorting mechanisms" that the retinotectal map could perhaps be put together by a mechanism which essentially maintains the above continuity relationships. We would like to raise the possibility in this last section that, in certain situations, the mapping mechanism might retain one of the continuity conditions but not the other. Let us suppose that condition (a) is retained but not condition (b), and that the whole eye is considered to be a single population. The map shown in Fig. 2 is consistent with this, whereas that shown in Fig. 8 is not.

Hunt and Jacobson (1973) have generated mirror image maps in many curious experimental situations; for example, from the combination of ventral and nasal half-fragments, and from nasal and temporal fragments with the dorsoventral axes of the fragments opposed. Hunt and Jacobson conclude that at least one of the half-fragments has been reprogrammed. But this raises the problem, considered in detail by MacDonald (in preparation), of why the reprogramming is such that the two halves now behave as mirror images of each other. If, however, the whole eye were a single population and there were strong pressures for continuity condition (a) to be maintained, then a mirror image map could result. Although these two conditions together would prevent a wide variety of maps from being formed, for example that shown in Fig. 8, they would not be sufficient to prevent maps such as that shown in Fig. 9, where each half is *not* a mirror image of the other half. Such a map would

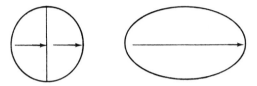

Fig. 8. Possible projection from retina to tectum which would be inconsistent with the situation where condition (a) is maintained but not condition (b). See text for further explanation. Conventions as in Fig. 2.

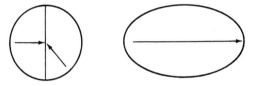

Fig. 9. See text for explanation. Conventions as in Fig. 2.

become impossible if, in addition, the condition held that equal size areas on the retina must map to equal size areas on the tectum. By equal areas, we do not necessarily mean areas as measured in square centimetres (an "area" could be defined, for example, by the number of retinal ganglion cells). Defining it in this way has the advantage of relating the argument to what has been called the Adrian-Mountcastle rule (Whitteridge, 1973), i.e., that the size of areas on the sensory cortex is a function of the density of peripheral receptors. The addition of this stipulation might be sufficient to allow only mirror image maps. It is possible, therefore, that Hunt and Jacobson's mirror image results might be due, not to any reprogramming of the eye fragments, but to variations in the mapping rules.

Maps in which condition (a) is broken, but condition (b) is maintained have not, to our knowledge, been found in the retinotectal system. One such map is found, however, without any surgical interference, in the normal sensory map of the surface of the body onto the somatosensory area 1 of the cortex. Werner (1970) summarizes the map as follows: "any linear array of neurons (such as is traversed by a surface-parallel microelectrode penetration) traces on the body a continuous path of receptive fields ... But the converse is not generally true ...". There are, of course, several neurons interposed between surface receptors and cortical area S1.

CONCLUSIONS

In this paper we have considered the problem of the development of ordered mappings in the central nervous system. A favored model in invertebrates is a time-position mechanism, but we have suggested that this may well be because the types of experiment which could disqualify such a mechanism have not been performed. In vertebrates, where many more analytical experiments have been done, the chemoaffinity theory holds sway. This theory actually encompasses several different plausible models. Finally, we have drawn attention to models which account for the generation of ordered mappings, but which do not require any selective affinity assumptions between pre- and post-synaptic elements. As a development from these models, we have introduced the concept of a "population" of retinal cells.

Experimental results have been accumulating rapidly in this field over the last decade or so. Our theoretical framework, however, has lagged behind this explosion of data, with the result that one is not clear what conclusions can be drawn from all the experiments. One and the same experimental result is interpreted by one author as favoring Sperry's chemoaffinity hypothesis over that of "systems-matching" (Yoon, 1973), while other authors argue that systems-matching is simply a subset of that hypothesis (Hunt and Jacobson, 1974). The reason for such confusion seems to be that a few names are made to cover many models, and different authors may each have a different one in mind. These controversies cannot be settled simply by linguistic agreement, for they stem not from semantic differences only, but also from the shortage of theoretical work. The various models have not been precisely defined and their predictions have not been worked out. It is this lack of articulation of the models that is in fact responsible for the looseness of the language. The theoretical work that is starting to appear in this field is therefore to be welcomed, in that it may be expected to increase precision of thought in this very difficult area of developmental biology.

REFERENCES

Apter, M.J. and Wolpert, L. (1965) Cybernetics and development. 1. Information theory. *J. theoret. Biol.*, 8: 244–257.

Attardi, D.G. and Sperry, R.W. (1963) Preferential selection of central pathways by regenerating optic fibres. *Exp. Neurol.*, 7: 46–64.

Barondes, S.H. (1970) Brain glycomicromolecules and interneuronal recognition. In *The Neurosciences. A Second Study Program*, F.O. Schmitt, G.C. Quarton and T. Melnechuk (Eds.), Rockefeller University Press, New York, pp. 747–760.

Baylor, D.A. and Nicholls, J.G. (1968) Receptive fields, synaptic connections and regeneration, patterns of sensory neurons in the CNS of the leech. In *Physiological and Biochemical Aspects of Nervous Integration*, F.D. Carlson (Ed.), Prentice-Hall, Englewood Cliffs, N.J., pp. 3–16.

Baylor, D.A. and Nicholls, J.G. (1971) Patterns of regeneration between individual nerve cells in the central nervous system of the leech. *Nature (Lond.)*, 232: 268–269.

Chow, K.L., Mathers, L.H. and Spear, P.D. (1973) Spreading of uncrossed retinal projection in superior colliculus of neonatally enucleated rabbits. *J. comp. Neurol.*, 151: 307–322.

Chung, S.-H. (1974) In search of the rules for nerve connections. *Cell*, 3: 201–205.

Chung, S.-H. and Feldman, J.D. (1974) In *Biological Diagnosis of Brain Disorder*, S. Bogoch (Ed.), Spectrum-Wiley Publications, New York.

Chung, S.-H., Keating, M.J. and Bliss, T.V.P. (1974) Functional synaptic relations during the development of the retinotectal projection in amphibians. *Proc. roy. Soc. B*, 187: 449–459.

Cook, J.E. and Horder, T.J. (1974) Interactions between optic fibres in their regeneration to specific sites in the goldfish tectum. *J. Physiol. (Lond.)*, 241: 89–90.

Cronly-Dillon, J.R. and Glaizner, B. (1974) Specificity of regenerating optic fibres for left and right optic tecta in goldfish. *Nature (Lond.)*, 251: 505–507.

Feldman, J.D. and Gaze, R.M. (1975) The development of half eyes in *Xenopus* tadpoles. *J. comp. Neurol.*, 162: 13–22.

Feldman, J.D., Gaze, R.M. and Keating, M.J. (1971) Delayed innervation of the optic tectum during development in *Xenopus laevis*. *Exp. Brain Res.*, 14: 16–23.

Feldman, J.D., Keating, M.J. and Gaze, R.M. (1975) Retinotectal mismatch: a serendipitous experimental result. *Nature (Lond.)*, 253: 445–446.

Gaze, R.M. (1959) Regeneration of the optic nerve in *Xenopus laevis*. *Quart. J. exp. Physiol.*, XLIV: 290–308.

Gaze, R.M. (1970) *The Formation of Nerve Connections*. Academic Press, London.

Gaze, R.M. and Grant, P. (1975) Regeneration of the optic nerve in *Xenopus* tadpoles. *Exp. Brain Res.*, Suppl., 23: 74.

Gaze, R.M. and Jacobson, M. (1963) A study of the retinotectal projection during regeneration of the optic nerve in the frog. *Proc. roy. Soc. B*, 157: 420–448.

Gaze, R.M. and Keating, M.J. (1972) The visual system and "neuronal specificity". *Nature (Lond.)*, 237: 375–378.

Gaze, R.M. and Sharma, S.C. (1970) Axial differences in the reinnervation of the goldfish optic tectum by regenerating optic nerve fibres. *Exp. Brain Res.*, 10: 171–181.

Gaze, R.M., Jacobson, M. and Szekely, G. (1963) The retinotectal projection in *Xenopus* with compound eyes. *J. Physiol. (Lond.)*, 165: 484–499.

Gaze, R.M., Chung, S.-H. and Keating, M.J. (1972) Development of the retinotectal projection in *Xenopus*. *Nature (Lond.)*, 236: 133–135.

Gaze, R.M., Keating, M.J. and Chung, S.H. (1974) The evolution of the retinotectal map during development in *Xenopus*. *Proc. roy. Soc. B*, 185: 301–330.

Gottlieb, D.I. and Cowan, W.M. (1972) Evidence for a temporal factor in the occupation of available synaptic sites during the development of the dentate gyrus. *Brain Res.*, 41: 452–456.

Hibbard, E. (1967) Visual recovery following regeneration of the optic nerve through the oculomotor nerve root in *Xenopus*. *Exp. Neurol.*, 19: 350–356.

Hope, R.A., Hammond, B.J. and Gaze, R.M. (1976) The arrow model: retinotectal specificity and map formation in the goldfish visual system. *Proc. roy. Soc. B*, in press.

Horder, T.J. (1971) Retention, by fish optic nerve fibres regenerating to new terminal sites in the tectum, of "chemospecific" affinity for their original sites. *J. Physiol. (Lond.)*, 216: 53–55P.

Horder, T.J. (1974) Electron microscopic evidence in goldfish that different optic nerve fibres regenerate selectively through specific routes into the tectum. *J. Physiol. (Lond.)*, 241: 84–85P.

Horridge, G.A. (1968) Affinity of neurones in regeneration. *Nature (Lond.)*, 219: 737–740.

Hunt, R.K. and Jacobson, M. (1973) Neuronal locus specificity: altered pattern of spatial deployment in fused fragments of embryonic *Xenopus* eyes. *Science*, 180: 509–511.

Hunt, R.K. and Jacobson, M. (1974) Neuronal specificity revisited. *Curr. Topics develop. Biol.*, 8: 203–259.

Jacobson, M. and Gaze, R.M. (1965) Selection of appropriate tectal connections by regenerating optic nerve fibres in adult goldfish. *Exp. Neurol.*, 13: 418–430.

Jacobson, M. and Hunt, R.K. (1973) The origins of nerve cell specificity. *Sci. American*, 228: 26–35.

Jacobson, M. and Levine, R.L. (1975) Stability of implanted duplicate tectal positional markers serving as targets for optic axons in adult frogs. *Brain Res.*, 92: 468–471.

Jansen, J.K.S. and Nicholls, J.G. (1972) Regeneration and changes in synaptic connections between individual nerve cells in the central nervous system of the leech. *Proc. nat. Acad. Sci. (Wash.)*, 69: 636–639.

Jhaveri, S.R. and Schneider, G.E. (1974) Retinal projections in Syrian hamsters; normal topography and alterations after partial tectum lesions at birth. *Anat. Rec.*, 178: 383.

Kendall, D.G. (1971) Construction of maps from "odd bits of information". *Nature (Lond.)*, 231: 158–159.

Kennedy, D., Selverston, A.I. and Remler, M.P. (1969) Analysis of restricted neural networks. *Science*, 164: 1488–1496.

Levine, R. and Jacobson, M. (1974) Deployment of optic nerve fibres is determined by positional markers in the frog's tectum. *Exp. Neurol.*, 43: 527–538.

Lopresti, V., Macagno, E.R. and Levinthal, C. (1973) Structure and development of neuronal connections in isogenic organisms; cellular interactions in the development of the optic lamina of *Daphnia*. *Proc. nat. Acad. Sci. (Wash.)*, 70: 433–437.

Lund, R.D. and Lund, J.S. (1971) Synaptic adjustment after deafferentation of the superior colliculus of the rat. *Science*, 171: 804–807.

Macagno, E.R., Lopresti, V. and Levinthal, C. (1973) Structure and development of neuronal connections in isogenic organisms; variations and similarities in the optic system of *Daphnia magna*. *Proc. nat. Acad. Sci. (Wash.)*, 70: 57–61.

Maturana, H.R., Lettvin, J.Y., McCulloch, W.S. and Pitts, W.H. (1960) Anatomy and physiology of vision in the frog (*Rana pipiens*). *J. gen. Physiol.*, 43, Suppl: 129–175.

Meinertzhagen, I.A. (1973) Development of the compound eye and optic lobe of insects. In *Developmental Neurobiology of Athropods*, D. Young (Ed.), Cambridge University Press, Cambridge, pp. 51–105.

Meyer, R.L. (1975) Tests for regulation in the goldfish retino-tectal system. *Anat. Rec.*, 181: 427.

Meyer, R.L. and Sperry, R.W. (1973) Tests for neuroplasticity in the anuran retinotectal system. *Exp. Neurol.*, 40: 525–539.

Meyer, R.L. and Sperry, R.W. (1974) Explanatory models for neuroplasticity in retinotectal connections. In *Plasticity and Recovery of Function in the Central Nervous System*, G. Stein, J.J. Rosen and N. Bullers (Eds.), Academic Press London, pp. 45–63.

Miller, B.F. and Lund, R.D. (1975) The pattern of retinotectal connections in albino rats can be modified by fetal surgery. *Brain Res.*, 91: 119–125.

Palka, J. and Edwards, J.S. (1974) The cerci and abdominal giant fibres of the house cricket, *Acheta domesticus*. II Regeneration and effects of chronic deprivation. *Proc. roy. Soc. B*, 185: 105–121.

Prestige, M.C. and Willshaw, D.J. (1975) On a role for competition in the formation of patterned neural connections. *Proc. roy. Soc. B*, 190: 77–98.

Sanders, G.D. and Young, J.Z. (1974) Reappearance of specific colour patterns after nerve regeneration in *Octopus. Proc. roy. Soc. B*, 186: 1–11.

Schneider, G.E. (1973) Early lesions of superior colliculus: factors affecting the formation of abnormal retinal projections. *Brain Behav. Evol.*, 8: 73–109.

Scott, T.M. (1974) The development of the retinotectal projection in *Xenopus laevis*: an autoradiographic and degeneration study. *J. Embryol. exp. Morph.*, 31: 409–414.

Sharma, S.C. (1973) Anomalous retinotectal projection after removal of contralateral optic tectum in adult goldfish. *Exp. Neurol.*, 41: 661–669.

Sharma, S.C. and Gaze, R.M. (1971) The retinotopic organisation of visual responses from tectal reimplants in adult goldfish. *Arch. ital. Biol.*, 109: 357–366.

Sperry, R.W. (1943) Visuomotor co-ordination in the newt (*Triturus viridescens*) after regeneration of the optic nerve. *J. comp. Neurol.*, 79: 33–55.

Sperry, R.W. (1944) Optic nerve regeneration with return of vision in anurans. *J. Neurophysiol.*, 7: 57–70.

Sperry, R.W. (1945) Restoration of vision after crossing of optic nerves and after contralateral transplantation of eye. *J. Neurophysiol.*, 8: 15–28.

Sperry, R.W. (1951) Mechanisms of neural maturation. In *Handbook of Experimental Psychology*, S.S. Stevens (Ed.), Wiley, New York, pp. 236–280.

Sperry, R.W. (1963) Chemoaffinity in the orderly growth of nerve fibre patterns and connections. *Proc. nat. Acad. Sci. (Wash.)*, 50: 703–710.

Sperry, R.W. (1965) Embryogenesis of behavioural nerve nets. In *Organogenesis*, R.L. De Haan and Ursprung (Eds.), Holt, Reinhart and Winston, New York, pp. 161–186.

Straznicky, K. and Gaze, R.M. (1971) The growth of the retina in *Xenopus laevis*: an autoradiographic study. *J. Embryol. exp. Morph.*, 26: 67–79.

Straznicky, K. and Gaze, R.M. (1972) The development of the tectum in *Xenopus laevis*: an autoradiographic study. *J. Embryol. exp. Morph.*, 28: 87–115.

Straznicky, K., Gaze, R.M. and Keating, M.J. (1971) The retinotectal projections after uncrossing the optic chiasma in *Xenopus* with one compound eye. *J. Embryol. exp. Morph.*, 26: 523–542.

Ward, S., Thomson, N., White, J.G. and Brenner, S. (1975) Electron microscopical reconstruction of the anterior sensory anatomy of the nematode, *Caenorhabditis elegans*. *J. comp. Neurol.*, 160: 313–337.

Weiss, P. (1936) Selectivity controlling the central-peripheral relations in the nervous system. *Biol. Rev.*, 11: 494–531.

Werner, G. (1970) The topology of the body representation in the somatic pathway. In *The Neurosciences. A Second Study Program*, F.O. Schmitt, G.C. Quarton and T. Melnechuk (Eds.), Rockefeller University Press, New York, pp. 605–616.

Werner, G. and Whitsel, B.L. (1973) Functional organisation of the somatosensory cortex. In *Handbook of Sensory Physiology, Vol. 2*, A. Iggo (Ed.), Springer, Berlin, pp. 621–700.

Whitteridge, D. (1973) Visual projections to the cortex. In *Handbook of Sensory Physiology, Vol. VII/3/B*, R. Jung (Ed.), Springer, Berlin, pp. 247–268.

Wolpert, L. (1969) Positional information and the spatial pattern of cellular differentiation. *J. theoret. Biol.*, 25: 1–47.

Wyman, R.J. (1973) Somatotopic connectivity or species recognition connectivity? In *Control of Posture and Locomotion*, R.B. Stein, V.B. Pearson, R.S. Smith and J.B. Redford (Eds.), Plenum, New York, pp. 45–53.

Yoon, M.G. (1971) Reorganisation of retinotectal projection following surgical operations on the optic tectum in goldfish. *Exp. Neurol.*, 33: 395–411.

Yoon, M.G. (1972) Transposition of the visual projection from the nasal hemiretina onto the foreign rostral zone of the optic tectum in goldfish. *Exp. Neurol.*, 37: 451–462.

Yoon, M.G. (1973) Retention of the original topographic polarity by the 180° rotated tectal reimplant in young adult goldfish. *J. Physiol. (Lond.)*, 233: 575–588.

DISCUSSION

M.A. CORNER: One thing disturbs me a little bit about your very ingenious model to account for the retinotopic projections in terms of the optic fibers sorting themselves out along the way. It necessarily implies the ability of this axonal position-recognition process of actually going so far as to be able to push axon terminals off postsynaptic cells with which they have already made synapses, because we know from developmental studies that you get synapse formation already in the early stages, without having to wait for complete sorting out of the whole fiber net. This means to me that other "recognition" forces (i.e., pre-/postsynaptic) must be operative in addition to those which you invoke.

R.M. GAZE: We do know of course that this sort of pushing off the synapses does actually happen; if you make a half-tectum situation and grow a whole optic nerve back into it, even without cutting it first, the synapses get pushed off part of the remaining half-tectum and the axon terminals then distribute themselves evenly across it. What *mechanism* can account for such displacement of the synapses — that is what we are discussing here.

356

E. MEISAMI: When you speak of retinal cells recognizing their neighbors, what sort of information must the cell be giving to the other? What is really being exchanged? I think you are wrestling here with the problem that still we have no idea of a physical mechanism for intracellular communication about relative positions.

R.A. HOPE: The mechanism need not necessarily be a chemical one; for instance, the cells which are close together in the retina might have a similar pattern of spontaneous electrical firing, and this could be the basis of their axons then recognizing whether or not they come from neighboring parts of the retina. This is merely a good picture to keep in mind as a potential alternative to chemical mechanisms.

R.M. GAZE: Such a mechanism was originally suggested by Lettvin, I believe, and we know that adjacent developing ganglion cells do have dendritic arborizations which interdigitate. We also know that retinal ganglion cells during development have a spontaneous firing pattern. We can therefore postulate that two cells which are close neighbors will be electrically linked to a greater extent than cells that are not close neighbors. They will therefore have some information in common, and this information could conceivably be used, although there is no evidence for it. In fact, however, there is no convincing evidence for any of these models, and this has been the trouble ever since the original statement of chemoaffinity was made. Most of the arguments that have been presented for selective affinities are in fact merely descriptive of the final results and not of the mechanism involved. I am merely trying to say that there are other possible mechanisms that could give the very same results.

A. TIXIER-VIDEL: I have a question in relation to your very nice theory: do you also have information concerning a molecular component of the membranes? Also, I wonder if you have seen the movies of dissociated nerve cell cultures? These provide a nice illustration because you observe sorting out of the fibers, and they seem to touch the various different cells. If there is no stable contact they go back, looking, as it were, for other cells. They thus give the impression that there is something in the molecular structure of the cell membrane which may give information to the growing fiber.

R.M. GAZE: This is indeed strongly *suggestive* of selective affinity, but one cannot derive with any logical security an underlying mechanism from such an observation.

O. CREUTZFELDT: Many so-called models are indeed only descriptive, and I think your model too is simply a description of what happens; in that sense one might even question whether it is really a model at all. My question, however, concerns Guillery's studies of the squinting Siamese cat: is that not a good argument for the time-position model of the origin of ordered projections? What happens there, apparently, is that due to a delay in retinal growth, part of the temporal retina grows into the wrong side of the brain. The optic fibers occupy retinal positions within the geniculate which are appropriate for temporal retina, but the other eye sends a normal projection from the contralateral side, so now we have two retinal projections on top of each other which are functionally not correlated. These two parts of the geniculate actually should look at the same spot in the visual field but that is precisely what they don't do, because the one comes from the wrong part of the retina, so to say. And now comes the interesting problem: in spite of this thalamic abnormality, we find a continuous mapping of the visual field onto the cortex. The hypothesis arises, then, that what is not fitting together functionally does not go together structurally either; what Guillery found recently is that, instead of having binocular neurons, the visual cortex simply ignores the input from one eye. The whole cortex thus becomes monocularly driven from that retina which has the most continuous mapping. However, I thought that the actual development of the retinal projection into the geniculate in higher animals is a rather good case for the time-position mechanism of establishing neuronal connections. I wonder, by the way, why we so often relate the amphibian experiments to the question of embryological development in higher animals, because amphibians are certainly *very* different, perhaps even qualitatively so in this respect.

R.M. GAZE: Jhaveri and Schneider (1974) have reported experiments on partial tecta formed by operation on neonatal hamsters, and you get the same answer in the mammal as in the amphibian. You can get compression across the half-tectum in the hamster in the same way as with fish and frogs, so I would say that the systems are in fact very similar — embryologically speaking. As to whether or not the crossing at the chiasma is to be regarded as an example of a time-position mechanism, unfortunately we don't know enough about the actual timing of these events, although I had not thought that they were sufficiently closely timed to be really helpful as an explanation of the observed facts. Concerning models, in relation to brain development we may consider two main types: the first is the *conceptual* model, whereas the second may be called "*molecular*". Each type may be elaborated to any degree of complexity or completeness, and each type is quite different from the other in what it tries to do (although individual models may contain aspects of both types). Conceptual models, such as our arrow model, attempt to reproduce the behavior of a system in general terms, somewhat removed from the realities of the biological situation. The purpose of the exercise is to try to find out something about the minimum logical requirements of the system, in terms of the assumptions made. Molecular models, on the other hand, attempt to reproduce the behavior of the system down to molecular levels of detail. For instance, they may argue in terms of specific enzymes. To the extent that they are complete, such models are essentially meant to be descriptions of how the real world situation works. Both conceptual and molecular models can be descriptive and explanatory at the same time. The main difference between the types is that the conceptual model is aimed at the logical structure of the situation and only *implies* the biology, whereas the molecular model is aimed at the biological structure and leaves the logic of the system to implication. The arrow model is explanatory and not merely descriptive: in an explanation one does not simply describe certain events, one points out that there are causal connections between these events. In the arrow model, we point out that *if* the retinal fibers behave in certain ways, and *if* the fibers can read polarity information from the tectum, then certain results may follow; i.e., formation of a map. No mere description, however exhaustive, includes such conditional statements. Furthermore, an explanatory model may have predictive value beyond the assumptions used in its construction; this is not the case for a simple description.

REFERENCES

Jhaveri, S.R. and Schneider, G.E. (1974) Retinal projections in Syrian hamsters; normal topography and alterations after partial tectum lesions at birth. *Anat. Rec.,* 178: 383.

Plasticity in the Adult Mammalian Central Nervous System

PATRICK D. WALL

*Cerebral Functions Research Group, Department of Anatomy,
University College London, London (Great Britain)*

INTRODUCTION

In considering plasticity in the adult mammalian brain and spinal cord, we are faced with a paradox. On the one hand, it is generally agreed with very good evidence that no true regeneration occurs, and that connections and organization remain rigidly fixed once development and differentiation are complete. On the other hand, there appear to be rather obvious changes occurring in the adult brain following injury and disease. In addition there are the even more obvious shifts of function associated with learning, memory and the acquisition of skills. Let us first examine the classical evidence for these two apparently opposing sets of observations.

DO ADULT NERVE CELLS DIVIDE?

Adult nerve cells do not divide even under the severe pressures of injury or tumor induction. In this respect, nerve cells seem fully and rigidly differentiated and far removed from their embryonic state of vigorous mitosis. We must remember, however, that these cells (unlike most of the body's cells) were produced in their adult form by a triple process. First there was mitosis in a germinal region, then migration to a quite different environment, and finally the elaboration of the dendritic and axonal processes. Even this last procedure is not a simple one, since it depends on the interaction of the cell's extensions with the other nerve cells they meet. All of this means that the cell develops in a series of stages, each one of which must signal its completion by inhibiting any further elaboration within the cell of the mechanism necessary for that particular stage. Thus, in order for a cell to divide, it would have to inhibit and reverse a number of later stages before nuclear division could occur. Even for the mechanical act of cell splitting, it would be necessary to withdraw dendrites and axon before daughter cells could usefully start on their separate careers. This necessity raises a second and more difficult question.

ARE THERE UNDIFFERENTIATED CELLS IN THE ADULT NERVOUS SYSTEM?

No anatomist-physiologist would be brash enough to claim that every nucleated structure in the nervous system could be definitively labeled as a glial cell or as a functional neuron. Of course, there are extreme examples where this could be done but in other locations caution is needed. Take for example the substantia gelatinosa rolandi, where no definite statement can be made about the nature or function of most of the cells found there. It contains three supposedly neural structures in addition to glia. The region is formed in the embryo as a simple thickening of the ependymal germinal layer to form the inner mantle (Wenger, 1950). Unlike other parts of the cord gray matter, where complex and long range transverse migrations of cells take place, these cells remain where they were born. The structure becomes bent into a lamina by the subsequent invasion of the afferent fibers from the neural crest on their dorsal surface, and by the arrangement of sensory relay cells on their ventral surface. Rolandic cell bodies are small and most of their extensions are short. The cell bodies contain little or no Nissl substance, while their staining properties differ so markedly from other cells that the region usually stands out clearly to the naked eye in any stained section of the cord. A few cells have been shown by electron microscopy to produce axons with terminal boutons containing vesicles, with an end apparatus reminiscent of normal nerve cells (Kerr, 1975). Most of the cells' morphology has not been studied in detail, however, and the physiology of the region is essentially non-existent.

Wall (1962) and Melzack and Wall (1965) have suggested that the substantia gelatinosa represents a lamina in which there occurs modulation of the transfer of entering nerve impulses onto the more ventral transmitting nerve cells. The reasons for this speculative statement are all quite indirect. All known terminations of cells of the substantia gelatinosa are within itself. Therefore, the only way in which they could affect the working of the brain is by influencing one of the nervous elements which penetrate the region. There are three of these elements. First the afferent fibers, some terminating in substantia gelatinosa (Heimer and Wall, 1968) and others passing through to terminate on deeper neurons. It is possible that substantia gelatinosa cells send axoaxonic contacts onto the primary afferent fibers, thereby producing a presynaptic control. It is also possible that substantia gelatinosa neurons project onto the dendrites of the two available types of nerve cell. One of these types are the lamina 4 cells, whose dendrites project dorsally through the substantia gelatinosa from the large cell layer immediately ventral to substantia. The other type of neuron, which project their axons over long distances and which may receive substantia axons onto its dendrites, are the thinly scattered flattened marginal cells of lamina 1.

The only positive evidence that substantia gelatinosa cells are in fact related to presynaptic control is that their activity is associated with the dorsal root potentials, and therefore with the changes of membrane potential of the terminal arborization of arriving afferent fibers. When an afferent volley arrives in the spinal cord, many postsynaptic events occur. The most long lasting of these is associated with the prolonged negative dorsal root potential. A source-sink map of the cord during the latter part of this potential shows that the only site of activity which remains is in the substantia gelatinosa (Wall, 1962). However, as we have said, there are many elements in the region: nerve cells, glia, terminal afferent arborizations and dendrites of deeper lying neurons. It is only a guess that the observed disturbance is due to substantia nerve cells rather than to one or other of the other components. The guess is strengthened, however, by the observation that the spread of the dorsal root potential and its associated inhibitions from one segment to another is interrupted if the Lissauer tract is cut. The Lissauer tract is the pathway of the propriospinal intersegmental axons of the substantia gelatinosa cells which project back onto substantia gelatinosa. No certain unequivocal recordings have ever been made from individual cells of the region. The reason for this might be because they do not produce action potentials, but this seems unlikely, at least for those substantia cells which give rise to axons of less than 1 μm and which project for more than 10 mm in the Lissauer tract, since it seems highly unlikely that electronic conduction could successfully transmit a disturbance for any distance along such long fine axons. There are some suggestive signs of action potentials from the region (Merrill and Wall, 1974) but the problem of their exact identification is severe, because there are such clear sources of action potentials in the same region from entering axons, as well as from penetrating dendrites. The technical feat of intracellular recording and marking has not yet been achieved for such very small cells. We therefore see that the anatomical and physiological knowledge of this structure of the spinal cord is highly unsatisfactory.

Until it is shown that Rolandic cells have the same characteristic morphology and function as do other nerve cells, we are quite free to speculate that they may form a pool of undifferentiated nerve cells, arrested in their progress from the germinal epithelium in the embryo and free to continue their voyage if conditions permit in the adult. Cells of this type are not limited to substantia gelatinosa but are found scattered in most regions of the nervous system. Therefore, we cannot yet answer the question of whether there are any undifferentiated cells in the CNS. We shall not be able to answer it until techniques have improved to the stage where all types of nerve cell can be assigned a specific working role, and where it can be shown that they maintain this role throughout life.

DO QUIESCENT CELLS EXIST?

By this question, I mean whether or not there are anatomically intact, fully differentiated, cells which pass through a period of inactivity. Clearly, we see such a state for short periods of time during general anesthesia or intoxication, where large numbers of cells fail to function but undoubtedly remain essentially intact in their morphology. For longer periods, we presumably see some such process in a state such as spinal shock. After a traumatic transection of spinal cord, the segments which are isolated from the head pass through a period of flaccid paralysis and areflexia. From a clinical physiological point of view, the spinal cord does not exist since no signs of efferent nerve impulses can be detected. Gradually over a period of days and weeks in man, first flexor and then extensor reflexes and some degree of tone reappear. There is no reason to assume that there has been a metabolic, vascular or mechanical disturbance sufficient to explain either the silence or the recovery. We know that, unfortunately, regeneration across the transection is not the explanation for the latter. It is generally assumed that spinal shock and its disappearance are explained by the disappearance of excitatory drive by descending pathways, followed by an increasing sensitization of cells to their own segmental afferents. This is an assumption: there is no solid evidence that individual cells go through a quiescent period because of such a process. It is even possible that cells which were not part of the normal segmental reflex chain become activated by the degeneration of descending systems.

The normal power of the tonic descending inhibitory systems is shown dramatically if the cells of the spinal cord are compared in the usual physiological preparations or, by contrast, in a freely moving animal. If a microelectrode is placed in lamina 4 in the middle of the dorsal horn of a decerebrate, spinal or even an anesthetized animal, continuous ongoing activity is detected from many cells, and light brushing of the relevant area of skin results in an intense cell discharge. If the microelectrode is implanted under sterile conditions in an anesthetized animal the same picture is seen but, when the animal awakes from the anesthetic, ongoing activity disappears from most cells (Wall et al., 1967). Furthermore, depending on the orientation and attention of the animal at the time of observation, cells may fail to fire on stimulation of their normal receptive fields. If the animal is again anesthetized, the full "normal" picture of responsive active cells reappears. Given these observations, it cannot be said that all cells are always taking part in the normal overall activity of the animal.

If we cannot make any statement about the possibility of quiescent cells, the difficulty is compounded in considering if all *parts* of a neuron are always functional. In most situations it is not possible to examine individual terminals or boutons or parts of dendrites. Where transmission along branching points of fine axons has been examined, conduction block has frequently been observed (Howland et al., 1955). We do not even know if all branches of the terminal arborizations normally conduct. Very small variations of structure, or of impinging controls, could conceivably switch these axons from a blocked state to a conducting one.

The reason for including this section on the possibility of quiescent nerve cells, or parts of them, is to warn that we cannot arbitrarily exclude any mechanism on the basis of the present available evidence. Most theories about mechanisms of plasticity assume a variation in the potency of working synapses. However, the experimental analytical tools which are available at the present time are not sufficiently powerful to allow us to make such definite statements about the actual cause of long-term excitability changes. The few examples which have been available for detailed study suggest that many options for the cause of an observed plasticity are still available, and the explanation for a particular shift should be approached with a very open mind, keeping all these options open.

ARE THERE REDUNDANT SYSTEMS?

One of the commonest explanations for recovery from damage to the brain is the assumption that there is redundancy in the nervous system. The meaning of this statement is rarely examined, and its justification is rarely challenged. Hidden within the word there are at least three meanings. The first is that the system is overbuilt with a multiplication of identical parts. This is the redundancy of holding up the trousers with two belts or the duplication of standby circuits in a lighthouse, so that the failure of one light instantly turns on a second previously inactive light. The observation that a dog can run on three legs is not usually followed by the statement that one leg is redundant, and yet this is exactly the logic of most statements about recovery from brain injury. The dog on three legs has in fact switched the tactics of motor pattern formation in order to produce successful running, and his top speed is severely limited. For almost all studies of behavior we are unaware of the tactics adopted by the brain to achieve a given output, so that we cannot tell if an apparently identical outcome has been achieved by an identical process of internal computation. Furthermore, we normally test the functioning of the brain with insulated threshold tests which test minimal abilities. The old man passes all the psychological tests one by one within his normal range, but still can't calculate the outcome of his trajectory across the road plus that of two approaching vehicles. Any one task is simple but all three together beat the system.

It is true that a considerable percentage of peripheral nerve fibers can be lost before clinical tests show the earliest signs of sensory change. In a progressive disease, such as leprosy, the patient will tell you that an area feels "strange" before the best clinical testing methods can show any sensory change. One may reasonably assume that the patient's intuitive awareness of the impending onset of obvious change has not tested the maximum input demands of the brain from the area of skin where a gradual loss of nerve fibers is in progress. Therefore, even in a peripheral nerve, we have no clear proof that the skin is innervated by more fibers than are necessary for the maximum useful reporting function of the skin. We know only that our present tests are too crude to unveil a sensory deficit which every patient can easily report.

The second type of redundancy is where we have two alternative mechanisms with more or less the same function: a belt and suspenders, a pen and pencil, etc. In the brain we have parallel pathways which may be made to appear to have the same function. We can transmit impulses from periphery to cortex by way of the dorsal columns, dorsal column nuclei, medial lemniscus and posterior thalamus, or we can transmit by way of the spinal cord dorsal horns, spinothalamic cells, lateral lemniscus and posterior thalamus. If we cut the dorsal columns and notice that somatosensory cortical evoked potentials and cutaneous sensory testing remain unaffected, it has been usual to state that the sectioned pathway must be redundant to another pathway, presumably the spinothalamic pathway. I have discussed elsewhere the logical fallacy in the use of the word redundancy in this way (Wall, 1975). It presumes, in the first place, an evolutionary development in which two very different anatomical and physiological pathways could be evolved so that one could substitute for the

364

other in case of injury. We do not in fact know of any injuries or diseases of this type. Furthermore, the alternative lesion of each redundant system is hardly ever tested by those who claim that one system substitutes for another. If this were so, it would be legitimate to lesion the afferent systems which relay in the spinal cord dorsal horn and leave the dorsal columns intact. If the two systems were mutually redundant, then the second type of lesion should be equally ineffective. The fact is that it leaves the cortical evoked potentials quite unaffected, as predicted, but completely abolishes any behavioral response by the animal to peripheral stimulus (Wall, 1970). Evidently, the two systems are in no way redundant unless tested by some very crude measure of mass function, such as their ability to produce an evoked cortical potential.

There is a third way in which the term redundancy or duplication has been used. Here it is assumed that there have been repeated attempts to solve the same problem during evolution. The early attempts remain present in the brain but are normally suppressed by the functioning of more recently evolved and biologically superior systems. The higher centers of Hughlings Jackson and of Pavlov suggest this type of duplication. The epicritic and protopathic systems of Head were proposed as quite specific examples of one system overlaying another system. None of these theoretical models of the brain can show, however, that any animals exist which are functionally dependent on the postulated lower centers. The presence of a curious form of behavior following a lesion of the central nervous system does not prove that this type of behavior exists in some unknown lower form of animal, and was unmasked by the disappearance of the lost tissue. It is a priori just as likely that the new behavior represents a disordered function of a single integrated nervous system.

In spite of my obvious doubts about the use of the word redundancy where it is implied either that (1) more cells are produced than are normally needed, or (2) that extra systems are produced, or (3) that one system overlays and silences another, we shall consider a proposal that another type of redundancy does exist. This is within a single cell. Here we shall propose that during embryonic development more branches of an axon are produced than are required for the normal functioning of the final working brain.

DOES THE POSSIBILITY FOR MORPHOLOGICAL AND/OR PHYSIOLOGICAL CHANGE REMAIN IN THE ADULT CNS?

If an axon is cut, sprouts may grow from the cut end but there is no evidence that the axon ever re-establishes contact with its original end station, or indeed with any other synaptic site. However, the section of an axon does lead to a series of other morphological changes. Intact neighbors of the degenerating axon may change to occupy the synaptic sites vacated by the degenerating axon. These changes may be only a minimal shift of the position of an intact bouton which slides across the surface of a cell to occupy part of a synaptic site. At the other extreme, an intact axon may generate a new sprout which grows into the evacuated territory and establishes an apparently mature bouton. The nerve cell whose axon has been cut undergoes chromatolytic changes, reflected in its biochemistry and in the shape of its dendrites. Some synaptic boutons withdraw from a neuron undergoing such changes. The cell on which the axons ended also undergoes change, especially if the degenerated axon represented a major fraction of its input. If these are major changes, they may in turn be reflected in the neurons onto which this one projects.

We see then that, in the adult, the cutting of axons produces a chain of reactions: *forwards* in the cells which it used to influence, *backwards* onto its parent cell and its afferent supply, and *sideways* on its intact neighbors. We know little or nothing of the physiological consequences of these changes, nor do we know if events less dramatic than the destruction of an axon can produce these morphological modifications. It is clear that a substantial reactive capacity for morphological change persists in the adult.

As we have said earlier, gross observation of whole animals or systems shows that functional modification obviously occurs both in learning and in recovery from injury. In no single instance do we know the mechanism of these changes. The reasons for our ignorance are two-fold: we do not know where to look in the nervous system for the location of such a change, whether anatomical or physiological, and we might not have tools of sufficient power to observe the changes even if we knew where to look. What can be done in this situation is to narrow down onto the site of change in suitable model situations, so that the adequacy of our analytic measuring equipment can be assessed. For over ten years, it has been known that if anything was done to decrease the impulse traffic from muscle spindles to the cells of Clarke's column, there was a marked increase of the output of these neurons for a given input. Here is the tantalizing definition of a substantial change in a monosynaptic contact following functional deprivation. In spite of careful and repeated documentation of the phenomenon, however, the actual nature of the change remains unknown. We shall use the remainder of this presentation to describe another type of model of plasticity in the adult mammalian system; partly to show that modifiability exists in structures previously thought to be quite rigidly connected, partly to show that actual switching of inputs can occur, rather than solely quantitative changes, and partly to suggest further ways in which the mechanisms for such shifts may be elucidated.

CHANGES IN THE RESPONSE OF CELLS IN THE SOMATOSENSORY SYSTEM FOLLOWING CHRONIC PARTIAL DEAFFERENTATION

(A) Rat thalamus

The series of experiments to be reported next developed from an incidental observation made during experiments on the convergence of different systems onto the rat thalamus (Wall and Egger, 1971). The ventral posterior part of all mammalian thalami receives a highly organized input from the somatosensory system. Nucleus ventralis posterior lateralis (VPL) is dominated by sensory messages from the opposite side of the body which arrive in the nucleus by way of the medial lemniscus. The medial part of VPL is supplied by axons from the cuneate nucleus, and the receptive fields of the cells are on the forelimb. The lateral part of the nucleus contains the hindlimb representation supplied by way of nucleus gracilis. If nucleus gracilis is removed surgically, the lateral part of VPL is found to contain large numbers of nerve cells which fail to respond to skin stimulation. The medial part remains apparently normal with the cells still responding to forelimb stimulation. The animals were allowed to survive and it was found that the area subserving the forelimb expanded in an orderly fashion into the area which had previously responded to the hindlimb. This process was first observed at 3 days, and appeared to be complete 10 days after the nucleus gracilis had been removed. There seem at once to be 5 possible classes of explanation for the apparent take over of leg cell areas by arm cells.

(1) *Cells might migrate*: it is known that deafferented neurons shrink. Therefore it was possible that "leg" cells had decreased in size, and the unaffected "arm" cells simply moved over to occupy the space left by the shrinkage. In this case, there would be no actual change of connections, only a change of location. We could show, however, that a real change of location had taken place, because the cortical map of the body in the first somatosensory area also showed a marked expansion of the arm area into what had previously been the leg area. If the thalamic cells had simply moved their position, there is no reason to think that the termination of their axons in the cortex could, or would, also have moved their position. It therefore seemed that there must have been a real shift of receptive fields of the thalamic cells.

(2) *Polysynaptic pathways might open up*: it is known that pathways other than the medial lemniscus bring information to VPL. The neo- and the paleo-spinothalamic systems would not have been cut by the removal of nucleus gracilis. Furthermore, the sensory cortex projects back onto the VPL. It is quite possible that the dominating presence of the main input from the dorsal column nuclei holds these other pathways inhibited. The degeneration of part of the medial lemniscus pathway might be followed by degeneration of cells which had held these polysynaptic pathways silent. The suggestion is unlikely, however, because one would then expect the unmasking of indirect inputs from the hind leg, whereas we in fact saw the appearance of inputs from the forelimb. The proposal is made even more unlikely by the observation that the response latency of the "newly connected" cells was identical to that of the normally connected cells, and it therefore seems impossible that the impulses could be arriving in the thalamus by an indirect route.

(3) *Intact axons might sprout to occupy deafferented territory*. As we have already mentioned, it is known that collateral sprouting does occur in adult CNS, so that this is a possible mechanism which must be seriously considered. This may even seem to be the most likely of all suggestions made, although there are a number of factors which introduce problems of interpretation. The onset within 3 days of the appearance of new inputs is faster than has been observed in morphological studies of sprouting. As we shall see, this question of time of first appearance of abnormal inputs is indeed the major argument against a sprouting hypothesis. The fact that the receptive fields of the newly connected cells were often smaller than normal and were highly organized, with extremely low thresholds, might also argue against a sprouting hypothesis. It would be expected that newly established receptive fields, as a result of new sprouts, might be diffuse and have a high threshold. However, the validity of

this objection would depend on knowing more than we know at present about the physiology of connections produced by sprouts.

(4) *Silent cells might be unmasked.* This suggestion may sound highly improbable, since it amounts to saying that fully connected nerve cells exist which are not functioning in the intact animal. However much one may be intuitively (or culturally) biased against the idea of idle, unemployed, cells awaiting a major disaster before making an appearance, the suggestion nevertheless, cannot be ruled out a priori. It might simply be that such neurons are not observed under the usual physiological conditions of exploration (where cell responses may be inhibited by the anesthesia used, or by the set of the brain).

(5) *Ineffective branches of intact afferent fibers might be unmasked.* This proposal may seem only slightly less unacceptable than the previous one. It suggests that the terminal arborization of afferent fibers is more extensive morphologically than is the physiologically effective part of the axon terminal. Certain long range branches of axons, presumably laid down during embryonic development, would thus fail to establish effective physiological control over the neurons on which they end. It is left as a secondary question as to whether these hypothetical silent branches are held actively suppressed by some inhibitory mechanism, or whether their contacts are so tenuous that their firing fails to influence the excitability of the postsynaptic cells to any measurable degree. Whatever the answer to these questions may be, the proposal states that non-functioning afferent terminals already exist in the region in question, and that the loss of the major source of input to a cell results in the unmasking of these previously ineffective connections.

The experiments to be described below were designed to confirm the existence of the switching of new inputs, and to decide among the last three hypotheses as regards the mechanism. As will soon be seen, considerable evidence was gathered in favor of the unmasking of ineffective synapses (but it cannot be stated that hypotheses 2, 3 and 4 do not also play some role).

(B) Cat spinal cord

One side of the lumbar enlargement in adult cats was partially deafferented by cutting all dorsal roots caudal to L3 with the exception of the S1 dorsal root. At various times after the roots had been sectioned, the response of dorsal horn cells to natural and electrical stimuli applied to the leg and flank were recorded through extracellular glass microelectrodes. When animals were examined up to 24 hr after this partial deafferentation, no cells were located in a region between segments L4 and 5 which responded monosynaptically to cutaneous stimulation on the leg. By one week, cells began to appear in the L4–5 region which responded monosynaptically to peripheral stimuli. The number of these newly connected neurons seemed to have stabilized by one month after the partial deafferentation, but their properties were abnormal in 6 ways: (1) the location of the receptive field always was characteristic either of the S1 dermatome or of segments rostral to L4; (2) some cells had double receptive fields, one on the leg and one on the abdomen; (3) the size of the receptive fields varied more than is observed in normal intact dorsal horn (in particular, certain neurons had unusually small receptive fields, with abrupt edges and no associated inhibitory fields); (4) the cells received less convergence from high threshold afferents than is normally observed; (5) associated inhibitory fields were rarely encountered; and (6) habituation was observed, and in some cells with double receptive fields the response to one area habituated while the response to the other area was unaffected. Slow wave recording on the surface of the cord showed that the effect of peripheral stimulation of the S1 dermatome spread far more extensively on the chronically deafferented side of the cord than it did on the intact side, or in an intact cord.

It was concluded that, following partial deafferentation, the remaining afferents can establish connection with deafferented nerve cells, but the data presented did not allow a conclusion as to whether the new connections were produced by sprouting or by the unmasking of existing connections.

(C) Cat dorsal column nuclei

(1) *Normal intact nucleus*: since it was intended to study the distortion of the body mapping onto the dorsal column nuclei following deafferentation, it was necessary first to establish the normal pattern in greater detail than had previously been done. In intact anesthetized adult cats, entire cross-sections of both dorsal column nuclei were mapped with tungsten microelectrodes on a regular grid, with 100 μm spacing between the mapping points (Millar and Basbaum, 1975). Fig. 1 shows the maps obtained from two cuneate nuclei, in order to demonstrate the reproducibility of these maps from animal to animal, including the manner in which individual toes are represented. Fig. 2 shows three maps taken from nucleus gracilis in different animals. Here the overall pattern is repeated but the fine details vary from animal to animal. Fig. 3 is a diagram of the overall plan of body projection. Two ways were developed of representing the results: the first, as illustrated in these three figures, was a pictorial one; the second was a more powerful way for comparing maps between different animals. The total number of points in nucleus gracilis subserving particular parts of the body were counted up and represented as a percentage of all the points within the nucleus. The result from 672 recording points in 15 normal maps is shown in Fig. 4A. It will be seen that 42% of all the points in the nucleus were associated with the toes, 16% with the foot, 17% with the anterolateral leg, 8% with the posteromedial leg (including perineum) and 17% with the trunk (abdomen and back).

(2) *Chronic partial deafferentation* was carried out with the same conditions as in the chronic partial deafferentation of the spinal cord. All dorsal roots supplying the hind leg were cut extradurally with the exception of the S1 root and the animals were allowed to survive for more than 8 months (Millar et al., 1976). After this period the animals were re-anesthetized, and the dorsal column nuclei were mapped on a 100 μm grid using tungsten microelectrodes. The new distribution of the body surface within the nucleus is shown in Fig. 4D for 8 such animals. The most obvious change is the very large expansion of the area serving the trunk region. The details of the maps from two such animals are shown in Fig. 5 where the expansion of the trunk area

(TR) can be compared in size and location with two normal animals. There has been a marked decrease of the leg representation. Changes in the toe and foot representation were variable; in some animals large parts of the nucleus represented toes, with little foot representation, while in others there was the opposite balance. The mean size of the chronically deafferented nucleus was 84% of that of the intact contralateral nucleus (N = 8, S.D. 18). Therefore the changes in proportion of the body map cannot be attributed to an absolute loss of certain cells. It is apparent that certain areas of the nucleus must have

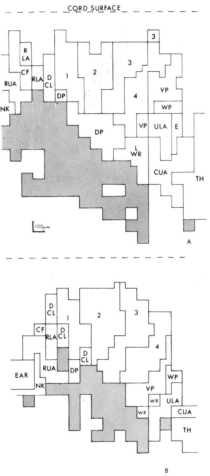

Fig. 1. Two examples of maps of the forelimb projection to the cuneate nucleus. The left-hand side nucleus is shown in these and all subsequent figures. The zone of the forelimb projecting to each part of the map is indicated by the letters or numbers on the map. The cross-hatched area is the region where cells with deep receptive fields are found. The dashed horizontal line is the average position of the cord surface in this and subsequent maps. Abbreviations: 1, 2, 3 and 4, individual toes, 1 being the most medial toe with the animal standing normally, and 4 the most lateral toe. VP, ventral paw; WP, wrist pad (carpal); DP, dorsal paw; DCL, dew claw (vestigial thumb); ULA, ulnar aspect of lower arm; RLA, radial aspect of lower arm; E, elbow; CF, cubital fossa; RUA, rostral upper arm; CUA, caudal upper arm and shoulder; TH, thorax and thoracic back; NK, neck; LWR, lateral wrist; WR, wrist.

370

switched the body area represented in them, particularly in favor of the trunk. It must be stressed that we are reporting here the responses of multiunit recordings taken at each recording station. If the deafferented nucleus is compared with the normal for *number* of responding cells at each recording point, then it will be found that fewer cells respond at each point.

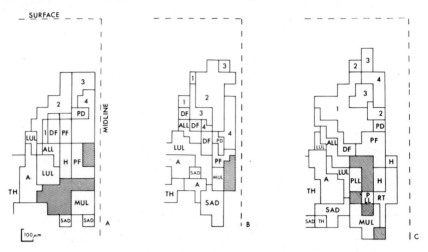

Fig. 2. Three examples of maps of the hind limb projection to the gracile nucleus. It is apparent there is more variability between different animals in gracile maps than in cuneate maps. Abbreviations: 1, 2, 3 and 4, toes. As in the forepaw, 1 is medial and 4 is lateral with the animal standing normally. PD, foot pad (plantar cushion); PF, plantar foot (proximal to PD); DF, dorsal foot; ALL, anterior (rostral) aspect of lower leg between knee and foot; PLL, posterior (caudal) aspect of lower leg; LUL, lateral upper leg; MUL, medial upper leg; SAD, saddle and lumbar back; RT, root of tail and groin; A, abdomen and perineum; TH, thorax and thoracic back; H, heel. Cross-hatching shows deep zones. (From Millar and Basbaum, 1975.)

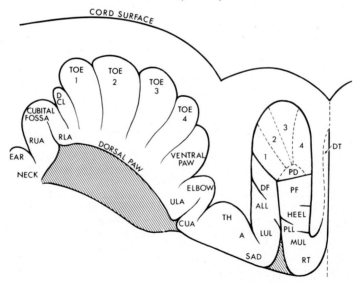

Fig. 3. A complete "felinculus" made by jointing the cuneate and gracile maps together. Abbreviations as in Figs. 1 and 2 and DT, distal tail. (From Millar and Basbaum, 1975.)

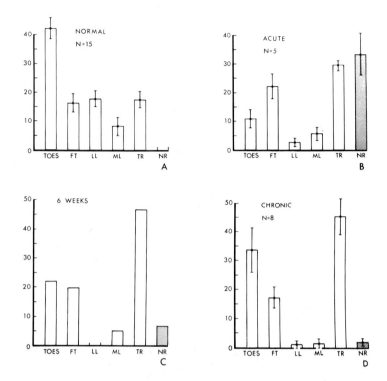

Fig. 4. Graphs of the percentage distribution of the different body regions in a transverse "map" across the caudal gracile nucleus. For each map, the size of a particular region was calculated from the number of grid points where cells had receptive fields within the region. These grid point counts were then converted to percentages, and the averages were calculated from a series of maps in different animals. For A, B and D the number of maps from which the graphs have been calculated is indicated as N. C is taken from a single map. (From Millar et al., 1976.)

There were abnormalities other than the distortion of the map. Cells with double receptive fields appeared, a phenomenon never seen in the intact nucleus. These neurons had widely separated receptive fields, with no sign of any response (either inhibitory or excitatory) when pressure stimuli were applied between the two excitatory receptive fields: Fig. 6. From 350 recording stations in the chronic animals, 50 units were detected with double receptive fields. Of these, 41 had one receptive field on the abdomen and the other on the foot or toes. Repeated examination of these neurons under various conditions of stimulation and electrode position confirmed that they were indeed single units and not neighboring pairs of cells. Each receptive field responded to light brushing and had a sharp edge. Strong pressure stimuli between the receptive fields failed to influence the cell, ruling out the possibility of mechanical spread of the stimulus from one receptive field to the other. This possibility of mechanical spread was made even less likely with the observation of 6 nerve cells with double receptive fields, one of which was on the forelimb and the other on the hindlimb. Apart from the double receptive fields, three other abnormal responses were seen in certain cells: some of them habituated if the stimulus was repeated at one second intervals; some neurons

372

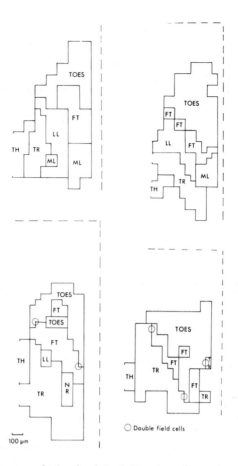

Fig. 5. Examples of maps made in the intact (top two figures) and chronically partially deafferented (bottom two figures) gracile nucleus. Abbreviations: FT, foot; LL, anterolateral leg; ML, posterior leg; TR, trunk; TH, thorax; NR, no response. (From Millar et al., 1976.)

had wide inhibitory areas, extending to the forelimb and to the contralateral side, where light brushing stimuli were sufficient to abolish the ongoing activity and to decrease the response from the small excitatory receptive field. A final abnormality was the observation that some cells required a rapid flick of the hair for them to respond, whereas the normal hair cells respond to gentle slow bending (suggesting that the experimental neurons required a higher degree of temporal or spatial summation than would be required to fire them in the normal nucleus). In three additional chronic animals, the entire lumbar enlargement was deafferented cutting all dorsal roots caudal to L3. A dramatic expansion of the trunk representation was observed, uncontaminated by the take-over of cells by the remaining S1 dorsal root.

In conclusion and to summarize these effects, it is apparent that, in rat thalamus and in cat spinal cord and dorsal column nuclei, chronic partial deafferentation results in the invasion of deafferented regions by inputs from the nearest intact afferents. Some of the cells in the newly connected regions have abnormal responses in addition to a new location of their receptive fields.

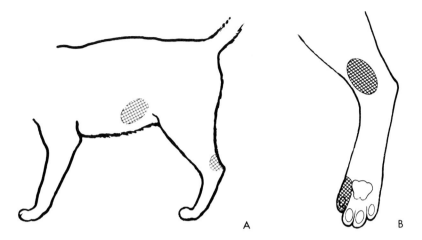

Fig. 6. Two examples of dual receptive fields in the partially deafferented gracile nucleus. A: the unit had a hair receptive field on the dorsal heel and also the ventrolateral abdomen, (areas shown by cross-hatching). B: another unit had a hair receptive field on the lateral-most toe and on the lateral heel. (From Millar et al., 1976.)

Some cells have double receptive fields, some habituate and some have extensive associated inhibitory fields. In all three locations, some, at least, of the newly connected cells appear to be fired monosynaptically by the afferents (as are the normal cells).

CHANGES IN THE RESPONSE OF CELLS IN THE SOMATOSENSORY SYSTEM FOLLOWING ACUTE PARTIAL DEAFFERENTATION

Having established the nature of changes in the chronic state, we searched in acute preparations to see if there were any signs of these changes occurring immediately after deafferentation. The aim was to answer the question of whether latent ineffective connections were normally present, or whether the changes began only after sufficient time had elapsed for growth of new sprouts to occur. In the spinal cord certain changes occur immediately after deafferentation, and novel responses of cells are unmasked. We shall return to these changes later but, since we have described the chronic changes in dorsal column nuclei in some detail, we shall show first that there are immediate changes in these nuclei which place the cells in an intermediate state between the normal intact situation and the eventual chronic pattern.

The expected and inevitable result of cutting dorsal roots is that some nerve cells in the dorsal column nuclei fail to respond to stimulation of areas subserved by the sectioned roots. It will be seen in Fig. 4B that 33% of all the points on the grid in nucleus gracilis fail to respond to peripheral stimuli after section of all the dorsal roots caudal to L3, with the exception of S1. This value falls to 2% in the chronic animals, as the deafferented regions are taken over by novel inputs. Many of the cells which failed to respond to peripheral stimuli fired ongoing bursts of nerve impulses. These bursts often included 5 or more impulses in a high frequency cluster followed by a long period of silence. Such bursts are not seen in the normal nucleus and are clearly a sign of disinhibition, produced by removal of part of the normal afferent inflow. If these results are expected, the same cannot be said for the very obvious expansion of the area responding to trunk stimulation, which has expanded from 17% in the normal to 28% in the acutely deafferented nucleus. Here, this is an absolute increase of the responding area, and there is no question that shrinkage of the nucleus could be an explanation for the distorted map. In a further series of experiments to be reported (Dostrovsky et al., 1976) the entire lumbar enlargement was deafferented including the S1 root. In these animals, the expansion of the trunk area was even more marked than in the animals where one root remained: 109% as against 65%. The latency of response of the newly connected cells was not significantly different from that observed in the intact animal, or in the intact nuclei contralateral to the deafferented nucleus.

While some of the "newly" connected cells responded to the normal gentle hair movement characteristic of cells in these nuclei, others required a rapid movement of the hair before responding. Some of these "flick" units habituated if the stimulus was repeated. Some units responded regularly and synchronously with each heart beat, another sign of increased excitability and response to novel inputs since such units are not normally observed in this region. Many units, including those with no apparent excitatory receptive field, developed very widespread inhibitory fields. Light brushing was sufficient to produce this inhibition. The inhibitory field could extend as far as the ipsilateral forelimb and the contralateral hindlimb. The most unusual response was the observation of cells with double receptive fields. Five such cells were seen at 217 recording points, whereas 50 were observed among 350 recording points in the chronic animals. For each of these unusual types of cell, and for cells with displaced receptive fields, the normal intact nucleus was repeatedly reinvestigated to confirm that such cells had not been missed in previous searches. It becomes quite evident that one must conclude that some of the new connections are already existing in the intact animal, and that their presence is immediately unmasked when other afferents are eliminated.

This still leaves the question of whether it is nerve cells which are masked, or whether afferent branches are ineffective under normal conditions. This question has been solved in favor of the latter alternative by an acute and reversible technique of deafferentation. The dorsal column nuclei were mapped in the usual fashion. Single cells were then selected which responded to foot stimulation and their response was continually observed. Next the spinal cord was cold blocked in the L4 segment using the Ringer ice technique (Wall, 1967). As expected, the majority of cells selected simply lost their response to peripheral stimuli but continued to produce ongoing activity. However, a minority of cells lost their receptive fields on the foot and acquired one on the abdomen. On removal of the cold block, the field reverted to the foot. It is certain that a single cell was observed throughout these maneuvers, and it therefore follows that at least some cells have alternative inputs: the afferents which operate under normal conditions, and an alternative group which can become effective as soon as the normal input is removed.

IS THERE EVIDENCE FOR THE EXISTENCE OF AFFERENT AXONS WHICH MAY BE NORMALLY INEFFECTIVE?

The dimensions of the dorsal column nuclei and thalamic nuclei are small, and there is an intermingled neuropil containing spreading terminal arbors plus dendrites. This makes it impossible, with the resolution available to present physiological or anatomical methods, to state definitely if an afferent fiber has a wider terminal arbor than is required for the observed postsynaptic response. We therefore turned to the spinal cord, where the anatomical spread of axons occurs over much larger distances (Wall and Werman, 1976).

The caudal extent of the terminal arborizations of dorsal root afferents was determined in adult cats. The method made use of microelectrode stimulation within the dorsal horn, and the recording on a distant dorsal root filament of the antidromic action potentials evoked by the stimulation of axons within the spinal cord. It was found that all filaments examined in the L2, 3 and 4 dorsal roots contained axons which projected at least as far as the S1 segment. The axons descended in or near the dorsal columns, and from there penetrated into the gray matter. The course of single fibers was followed to their apparent terminals. Thresholds, latencies, and relative and absolute refractory periods were measured for single axons. These measurements confirmed that continuous axons ran from the dorsal roots to distant segments, and that the action potentials recorded were not dorsal root reflexes. The majority of fibers with long range central arborizations were shown to have normal receptive fields in the dermatome of their parent dorsal root: they were not aberrant fibers leaving the spinal cord. The existence in substantial numbers of these long range afferents from distant dorsal roots suggests that there is a mismatch between the observed physiology and anatomy, since the monosynaptic response of a cord cell is normally related only to impulses arriving via nearby dorsal roots.

We have been suggesting that ineffective afferents are unmasked by the removal of other afferents. It seems intuitively unlikely that these axons lie totally ineffective in the intact animal, waiting to fulfill their potentialities only in the unlikely event of substantial deafferentation. To explore this situation, Merrill and Wall (1972) examined the afferents responsible for the receptive fields of single nerve cells in intact adult cat spinal cord. Certain neurons of lamina 4 have small restricted receptive fields with a definite edge. All means of varying the excitability of the cell and its afferents have so far failed to vary the size of the receptive field. Furthermore, it can be shown by surgical sectioning of dorsal roots, or by blocking of dorsal roots, that the afferents responsible for the natural receptive field all run in a fraction of one dorsal root, a *microbundle*. Thus, the neuron appears to be dominated by a small group of afferent nerve fibers. When these are blocked, the natural receptive field of the cell disappears. If under these conditions the neighboring dorsal root is electrically stimulated, the cell now responds monosynaptically. Presumably, what is happening here is that electrical stimulation produces a sufficiently synchronous volley in relatively ineffective terminals so that spatial summation produces effective excitation. Natural stimulation fails to produce sufficient

376

spatial summation to produce firing of the cell unless the preferentially connected group of fibers from the normal receptive field is stimulated.

Having discovered this effect from neighboring roots, we have now begun to examine nerve cells for the effect of more distant roots, which we know also send afferents into the segment. We have concentrated on the S1 segment under conditions of maximum responsiveness. The animals are decerebrated, and a spinal transection is carried out at L1 in order to remove the known tonic descending inhibitory effects. The blood pressure is maintained artificially high, above 100 mm Hg, by continuous adrenaline perfusion. Part of the L4 dorsal root is electrically stimulated. Occasional cells are encountered in laminae 4 and 5 which respond monosynaptically to the distant dorsal root, in spite of the fact that their entire inhibitory and excitatory receptive field appears to be limited to the S1 dermatome. The number of such cells is considerably increased if neighboring dorsal roots are cut. It may be that the response of these cells to distant dorsal roots is to be explained by highly favorable conditions for the occurrence of spatial summation. However it may also be that yet another factor is involved. We have seen examples of cells where the response to the distant root was totally eliminated by gentle hair movement in the dermatome of the cells' own segment. This gentle stimulus failed completely to alter either the ongoing activity of the cell or the response evoked from its natural receptive field. This finding suggests that the effectiveness of the terminals originating from distant roots may be positively, and differentially, inhibited specifically by a yet unknown mechanism which has no observable effect on the response of the cell to neural events within its own segment.

SUMMARY AND CONCLUSIONS

We have shown that there exist signs of an extensive over-arborization of terminals at three locations in the somatosensory nervous system. A careful search in the intact spinal cord shows that a small number of cells respond to these distant afferents under certain special (and probably abnormal) conditions. The postsynaptic effectiveness of these afferents is revealed by spatial summation, and may be selectively abolished by an ongoing inhibitory mechanism which does not seem to affect the normal function of the cells. Cutting the normal afferents to the region immediately unmasks the presence of previously ineffective afferents which now produce postsynaptic responses in cells following natural stimulation which, before the partial deafferentation, were completely without effect. If the animal is allowed to survive, the strength of these new responses increases and the number of responding cells multiply. It is not known whether exaggeration of the acute effect in the chronic state is due to changes such as sprouting in the afferents themselves, or to postsynaptic changes such as denervation sensitivity or dendritic shrinkage in the cells on which the afferents terminate, or to postsynaptic changes in interneurons which were previously inhibiting the effectiveness of the distant inputs. Whatever the answer to these questions may be, it is now clear that ineffective afferents provide a mechanism by which effective new connections may appear in the adult nervous system.

ACKNOWLEDGEMENTS

The work reported here has been done in collaboration with present and past colleagues Drs. J. Dostrovsky, E.G. Merrill, J. Millar at University College, D. Egger now at Yale University, A.I. Basbaum now at U.C. San Francisco and M. Devor and R. Werman, Hebrew University Jerusalem.

The work was supported by grants from the U.K. Medical Research Council, the U.S. Public Health Service and the Thyssen Foundation.

REFERENCES

Basbaum, A.I. and Wall, P.D. (1976) Chronic changes in the response of cells in adult cat dorsal horn following partial deafferentation: the appearance of responding cells in a previously non-responsive region. *Brain Res.*, 116: 181–204.

Dostrovsky, J., Millar, J. and Wall, P.D. (1976) The immediate shift of afferent drive of dorsal column nucleus cells following deafferentation. A comparison of acute and chronic deafferentation in gracile nucleus and spinal cord. *Exp. Neurol.*, in press.

Heimer, L. and Wall, P.D. (1968) The dorsal root distribution of the substantia gelatinosa of the rat with a note on the distribution in the cat. *Exp. Brain Res.*, 6: 89–99.

Howland, J.Y., Wall, P.D., Lettvin, J.Y., McCulloch, W.C. and Pitts, W. (1955) Reflex inhibition by dorsal root interaction. *J. Neurophysiol.*, 18: 1–17.

Kerr, F.W.L. (1975) Neuroanatomical substrates of nociception in the spinal cord. *Pain*, 1: 325–356.

Melzack, R. and Wall, P.D. (1965) Pain mechanisms: a new theory. *Science*, 150: 971–979.

Merrill, E.G. and Wall, P.D. (1972) Factors forming the edge of a receptive field: the presence of relatively ineffective terminals. *J. Physiol. (Lond.)*, 226: 825–846.

Merrill, E.G. and Wall, P.D. (1974) Impulses recorded in cat substantia gelatinosa. *Proc. J. Physiol.*, Nov: 82P–83P.

Millar, J. and Basbaum, A.I. (1975) Topography of the projection of the body surface of the cat to cuneate and gracile nuclei. *Exp. Neurol.*, 49: 281–290.

Millar, J., Basbaum, A.I. and Wall, P.D. (1976) Restructuring of the somatotopic map and appearance of abnormal activity in the gracile nucleus after partial deafferentation. *Exp. Neurol.*, 50: 658–672.

Wall, P.D. (1962) The origin of a spinal cord slow potential. *J. Physiol. (Lond.)*, 164: 508–526.

Wall, P.D. (1967) The laminar organization of dorsal horn and effects of descending impulses. *J. Physiol. (Lond.)*, 188: 403–423.

Wall, P.D. (1970) The sensory and motor role of impulses travelling in the dorsal columns towards cerebral cortex. *Brain*, 93: 505–524.

Wall, P.D. (1975) The somatosensory system. In *Handbook of Psychobiology*, M.S. Gazzaniga and C. Blakemore (Eds.), Academic Press, New York, pp. 373-392.

Wall, P.D. and Egger, M.D. (1971) Formation of new connections in adult rat brains after partial deafferentation. *Nature (Lond.)*, 232: 542–545.

Wall, P.D. and Werman, E. (1976) The physiology and anatomy of long ranging afferent fibres within the spinal cord. *J. Physiol. (Lond.)*, 255: 321–334.

Wall, P.D., Freeman, J. and Major, D. (1967) Dorsal horn cells in spinal and in freely moving rats. *Exp. Neurol.*, 19: 519–529.

Wenger, E.L. (1950) An experimental analysis of relations between parts of the brachial spinal cord of the embryonic chick. *J. exp. Zool.*, 114: 51–86.

DISCUSSION

J. OLDS: You spoke of inhibition of the effects of afferent stimulation. Is this a presynaptic inhibition?

P.D. WALL: It could be. An alternative speculation is that the distant afferents end on the tips of dendrites, while the local end on the cell body and the nearby dendrites. This might allow selective postsynaptic inhibition which would turn off the effect of the distant synapses. I should have pointed out that the ongoing "spontaneous" activity of the cell was completely unaffected by the inhibition which turned off the effect of the distant afferents. This would normally be considered evidence that the inhibition must be presynaptic, but actually there remains the possibility of distal dendritic *post*-synaptic inhibition which does not affect the generator region of spontaneous activity.

E. MEISAMI: Do you have any evidence that usage may enhance the effectuation of these changes after the operation?

P.D. WALL: We don't know the relative role played by the absence of impulses in one pathway, or the presence of impulses in another, in bringing about the changes we have observed. It is quite clear, in the dorsal column nuclei, that the full development of the changes only occurs after the afferent terminals have degenerated. We also don't know if the final take-over of the cells by the new afferents is a consequence of the postsynaptic changes produced by the degeneration of the destroyed afferents, or if it is the result of changes produced by continuing activity in the remaining afferents. There is no doubt that, in the developing kitten visual system, activity does in fact influence the physiological effectiveness of synaptic contacts. It may be that each part of the nervous system has its own rules for the development and maintenance of synaptic connectivity. At one extreme, the entire organization of the final system may be achieved without reference to the traffic of nerve impulses. At the other extreme, ongoing and evoked activity in afferent fibers may determine either the eventual morphology or the eventual functioning physiology. Arriving nerve impulses may set the excitability level of synapses without disturbing their morphology.

V. BRAITENBERG: I am going to suggest that effective sprouting does not occur. There is hardly enough time in those few weeks of your recovery for random sprouting to occur within the spinal cord.

P.D. WALL: There is of course a double problem regarding sprouting. One is: can sprouts occur? The answer is: yes, but they take some time. The second is: will they get to the right place? One of the interesting abnormalities of the new cutaneous connections is that there is less convergence than we find in the intact animal. In other words, we find fewer fibers making these new effective contacts, and a smaller variety of them.

J. OLDS: I wish to say a word in favor of usage, and against sprouting. In terms of the auditory geniculate projection and the auditory colliculus of the rat, we have recorded from neurons during a Pavlovian conditioning experiment in which we greatly changed the significance of the auditory stimulus. We would regularly find that, in the course of a training procedure, the first component of the auditory evoked response could be greatly modified. These were not responses that didn't occur at all beforehand, but they were doubled or trebled in magnitude; this change was found only in the posterior part of the auditory colliculus and in the anterior part of the auditory geniculate. These dramatic changes were occurring in the course of ten trials within approximately one hour, so that I scarcely think they could be explained by sprouting.

H.G.J.M. KUYPERS: I think that you have perhaps been too conservative about sprouting, because the idea of sprouting tends to be interpreted in terms of new large cables being formed. A fine nerve process, however, would need only to stick out one finger to a next cell, so that there is not really a formation de novo of endings, but only a shift or an extension of one.

P.D. WALL: I would agree with you completely. Anatomical readjustments of contacts on the cell must surely occur but they also surely require time. We observe the beginnings of the functional change within minutes of interrupting one pathway, and this can hardly be explained by even the most minimal sprouting. The subsequent exaggeration of these acute changes may be due to synaptic readjustment as you suggest.

R. LEVI-MONTALCINI: Have you studied this effect in very young animals? The phenomenon might be even more striking in immaturity. And second, is there any teleological significance to this expanding of the central sensory representation?

P.D. WALL: We intentionally avoided young animals, and in fact moved from rat to cat because of the suspicion of the rat being in certain respects a permanently embryonic animal, since its brain continues to grow throughout life. I quite agree with you that the young animal probably has more possibilities than solely the classical readjustment of interneuronal connections. As for the teleological significance of the plasticity which we have shown to exist in the adult, one can only speculate. The surgical lesions we have used are so massive that one can hardly imagine that an animal could have evolved mechanisms to compensate for such gross damage. Furthermore, the new contacts we find by no means represent a recovery of the system. A foreign input takes over cells which continue to relay their information into a mapped system which was developed to receive patterns of stimulation for specific parts of the body. It seems unlikely that such a system can usefully use such a bizarre new input. Evidently one must look elsewhere for a possible usefulness of this plasticity. One type of explanation would be that the new connections had grown as exploratory fibers in the embryo, and had been rejected but continued to hang around. Another explanation is that the diffuse connections may have a function in some special condition of excitability which has yet to be observed. Finally, the new connections might be awaiting a challenge, either when the system suffers a diffuse scattered attack, such as occurs in virus infections, or that they form the basis of some ability to change connections when the pattern of activity changes.

M.A. CORNER: I was thinking of the recent demonstrations in regeneration experiments, in the eyes of fish, of functionally depressed neuromuscular synapses. It would be a very intriguing possibility that such a phenomenon also exists under normal circumstances, and in the *central* nervous system as well as the peripheral. If one takes the observations that you made, concerning the extreme sensitivity to inhibition by sensory stimulation, you wonder to what extent there might be a background level of inhibition coming in through those intact roots all the time. If you simply eliminated that, you would in this case too expect a dramatic appearance of these long distance evoked responses, but you would not have to propose functionally depressed synapses: you would simply have eliminated the tonic inhibitory input that was blocking the response.

P.D. WALL: This is exactly what I think is the most economical bet at the moment. On the question of whether this is pre- or postsynaptic inhibition, I myself would like for it to be presynaptic, because presynaptic inhibition has so far never made any sense to me whatsoever, biologically speaking. It has always appeared, in all the tests, as just a sloppy phenomenon which turns off everything. But, what was always an exciting possibility, was that you could specifically eliminate certain impulses to a cell by presynaptic inhibition while leaving others intact. Here, however, if this effect is really as powerful as it now seems, as you say, either tonic background activity or a very minimal afferent barrage produced by a slight movement would be sufficient to suppress the distant effect, while leaving the immediate input to a cord cell in working. We ought in fact to be able to test that simply by cutting a few more dorsal roots.

SESSION VI

NEURAL CONTROL OF BEHAVIOR

Rhythmic Phenomena in Prenatal Life

G.S. DAWES and J.S. ROBINSON

The Nuffield Institute for Medical Research,
University of Oxford, Oxford (Great Britain)

INTRODUCTION

Until 5 years ago it was generally believed that fetuses do not normally make breathing movements before birth. Yet prenatal practice is thought to be necessary for the development of the respiratory musculature, and perhaps of the lung and the mechanisms which control breathing and integrate it with other systems after birth. When catheters were chronically implanted into the trachea or esophagus of the fetus, and in the amniotic fluid and a carotid artery (Dawes et al., 1970; Merlet et al., 1970) episodic irregular breathing movements were indeed observed in fetal lambs in utero. These episodic breathing movements were independent of small natural short-term variations in the blood gases, but proved to be related instead to the sleep state (Dawes et al., 1970, 1972).

TYPES OF FETAL BREATHING

There are two principal types of breathing movements in the fetal lamb. Firstly, there are rapid irregular breathing movements, present 35–40% of the time, in association with low voltage high frequency electrocortical activity attributed, from records of eye movements, to REM sleep (Fig. 1). These irregular high frequency breathing movements (up to 3 Hz) can fill the whole of an episode of low voltage high frequency electrocortical activity, but do not necessarily do so. Secondly, there are less frequently (about 5% of the time) runs of "augmented breaths" (described sometimes as "sighs or gasps"), which are unrelated to the state of sleep or consciousness. Our direct observations on fetal lambs delivered into a warm saline bath are in agreement with those of Ruckebusch (1971) in utero in that wakefulness seems to be present only about 5% of the time.

DIURNAL VARIATION

The incidence of fetal breathing movements shows a prominent diurnal variation (Boddy et al., 1973). Two types of records have been made. Firstly,

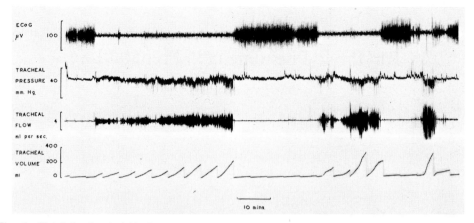

Fig. 1. Fetal lamb at 142 days gestation in utero. Records from above downwards of electrocorticogram, tracheal pressure and flow (from a flowmeter implanted just below the larynx) and of tracheal flow integrated over 5-min periods. (From Boddy et al., 1973.)

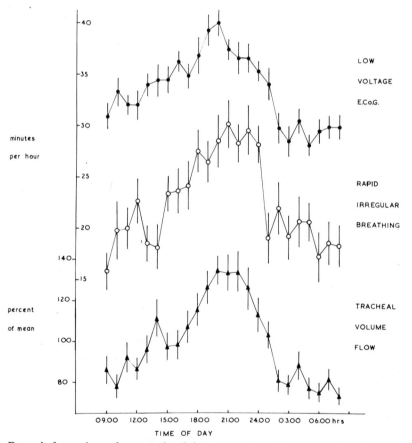

Fig. 2. Records from above downwards of the proportion of time (min/hr) during which low voltage electrocortical (E.Co.G.) activity was present in 7 lambs of 124–137 days gestation; or during which rapid irregular fetal breathing was present in 6 lambs of 115–133 days gestation; and of tracheal volume flow/hr (expressed as % of the mean daily volume) in 7 lambs of 110–142 days gestation. The vertical lines are ± S.E.M.

the proportion of time during which breathing movements are present has been summed hour by hour in lambs during the last third of gestation (115–133 days gestation; term is normally 147 days). There was a highly significant increase in the proportion of time during which rapid irregular fetal breathing movements were present, from $15 \cdot 8 \pm 1 \cdot 8$ min (S.E.M.) per hour at trough, 08·00–09·00 hr, to $30 \cdot 3 \pm 2 \cdot 3$ min at peak, $20 \cdot 00 \pm 21 \cdot 00$ hr. Secondly, in 7 lambs between 110 and 142 days gestation the tracheal volume flow per hour (the fetal analogue of the minute volume of breathing after birth, integrated from an electromagnetic flowmeter implanted in the trachea) was plotted against the time of day for 45 days total recording. The difference between peak and trough was highly significant ($P < 0 \cdot 001$). The peak hourly tracheal volume flow was $2 \cdot 0$–$2 \cdot 8$ times that observed in the trough.

There was a highly significant correlation with fetal electrocortical activity (Fig. 2). The proportion of time during which low voltage high frequency electrocortical activity was present in mature fetal lambs in utero increased during the course of the day, from dawn (28 ± 1 min/hr) to dusk (40 ± 1 min/hr). Such observations were only made from 120 days gestation onwards, when the fetal electrocorticogram had differentiated into high and low voltage activity. A diurnal variation in fetal breathing movements has been observed at 85 days gestation, as early as satisfactory records can be obtained (Worthington, unpublished observations). At this age the mean duration of episodes of breathing movements is less than in more mature lambs.

Five sheep were studied in an environment in which temperature was $15 \pm 0 \cdot 5°C$ (in the summer) or $10 \pm 0 \cdot 5°C$ (in the winter) with a 12 hr light cycle (06·00–18·00 hr). Food and water were replaced at 10·00 and 22·00 hr only; this was the only time when the room was entered. At first introduction to this unusual environment the fetal diurnal rhythm of breathing movements was disturbed, but it adjusted within 2–4 days; the peak occurred shortly after 18·00 hr, and the amplitude was similar to that in sheep subjected to changes of temperature ($> 5°C$) and disturbance in the ordinary laboratory environment.

In the ordinary laboratory environment there is in different sheep a significant (at most $P < 0 \cdot 05$–$< 0 \cdot 001$) positive correlation between fetal temperature and the incidence of fetal breathing (and the hourly liquid ventilation, i.e. integrated tracheal volume flow) (r = $0 \cdot 18$–$0 \cdot 32$ in different lambs, over a diurnal variation of $0 \cdot 5$–$0 \cdot 7°C$). Further analysis will be needed to establish what proportion of fetal diurnal breathing variation is attributable to this cause. There is a very high correlation between fetal and maternal temperatures (r $> 0 \cdot 9$). In a controlled temperature environment (to within $0 \cdot 5°C$) the amplitude of maternal temperature change was reduced by approximately half, but the amplitude of the fetal diurnal breathing rhythm was unaltered.

Other experiments have shown (Boddy et al., 1974) that fetal hypoxemia of a degree just sufficient to abolish fetal breathing movements (a mean reduction in fetal arterial pO_2, from 24 to 16 mm Hg) causes a highly significant reduction in the proportion of time occupied by predominantly low voltage electrocortical activity, from 55% to 30%. Also the number of changes from high to low voltage activity was nearly doubled during the hour's hypoxemia.

Conversely, hypercapnia caused an increase in fetal breathing movements associated with an increased incidence of low voltage electrocortical activity. Nevertheless, the diurnal variations in fetal electrocortical activity and breathing movements were not significantly associated ($P > 0.1$) with changes in fetal blood gases. Fetal hypoglycemia, if sufficiently severe (< 10 mg/100 ml), is associated with a diminution or arrest of fetal breathing movements. Fetal blood glucose concentration changes passively with that of the mother, and hence is related to her feeding habits. However, preliminary observations show little evidence of a significant diurnal variation in fetal blood glucose concentration such as could explain the changes in fetal breathing.

Further observations have shown, perhaps not surprisingly, that there is also a diurnal variation in fetal heart rate and in heart rate variability in sheep (Dalton, Dawes and Patrick, unpublished observations). Diurnal variations in fetal hormones have not been detected yet.

It is interesting to speculate as to whether the diurnal variation in fetal electrocortical activity and in breathing movements is due to entrainment of a natural fetal rhythmic variation by a maternal rhythm (e.g. by transplacental exchange of metabolites or hormones) or whether it is autonomous, as for instance by fetal perception of daylight or darkness, of maternal movements or of external sounds. The information so far available is not sufficient to distinguish between these possibilities.

CLINICAL OBSERVATIONS

During the past 5 years it has proved possible to make measurements of human fetal breathing movements in utero, from 11 weeks gestation onwards, using an ultrasound method developed by Boddy and Robinson (1971). The characteristics of fetal breathing movements in man are different from those in sheep, in that — though discontinuous, irregular and of relatively high frequency (about 60/min) — they are present for a greater proportion of the time (normally 50–95% from 11 weeks gestation to term) and are less regularly organized in episodes. Apnea is of shorter duration (normally not more than 45 sec at a time). In man also there is a prominent diurnal variation in the incidence of fetal breathing movements, rising from about 50% at dawn to 95% of the time in the late evening. It has not yet proved possible to correlate this variation with changes in electrocortical activity. The human fetal scalp is only available to record an EEG in labor, when fetal breathing movements are liable to distortion for other reasons. Many changes in the maternal environment affect human fetal breathing in utero; detailed descriptions have been given elsewhere (Boddy and Dawes, 1975; Manning et al., 1975).

Recent evidence on more than 900 pregnancies (Boddy and Dawes, 1975; Boddy and Wyn Pugh, unpublished; Manning, unpublished) has shown that it is possible to predict, with a reasonable degree of accuracy, the outcome during labor from prenatal observations of fetal breathing movements. Thus more than 95% of fetuses which subsequently developed distress in labor (a scalp or cord pH of 7.25 or less associated with large falls in heart rate or passage of fresh meconium) had a low incidence and/or abnormal pattern of breathing movements when examined over a period of 30–120 min some days previously. And in 13 instances intrauterine death has been preceded by long periods of apnea or grossly abnormal breathing movements.

The combination of measurements of fetal breathing with heart rate monitoring and observations of fetal movements is likely to improve diagnostic accuracy both in high-risk pregnancies and especially in identifying fetuses with chronic hypoxemia in association with intrauterine growth retardation. But some improvement in the physical method for recording human breathing movements in utero is needed for widespread clinical application.

CONCLUSION

It is not perhaps very surprising to find that fetal breathing movements, which are not essential to continued life in utero, alter in character or cease soon after the fetus becomes ill from hypoxia, hypoglycemia or infection, whereas changes in fetal heart rate or in the character of the ECG only give a late indication of trouble. It will be interesting to discover whether fetal breathing movements in utero are essential to the development of normal pulmonary structure and function postnatally. It is hard to believe that the development of an organ system so important for survival after birth, and of the muscles on which it depends, can be a casual consequence of an association with R.E.M. sleep. This state is present prenatally up to 55% of the time in sheep and probably about 70% of the time in man (combining the evidence of prenatal breathing and postnatal sleep state). We may well ask whether this high incidence is determined by the need for prenatal breathing practice or is an accidental phylogenetic association.

SUMMARY

Fetal breathing movements have been detected by direct observation and by the use of indwelling catheters and flowmeters in sheep and by ultrasound measurements in man. They are present from early gestation (0·27 of term in both species) and in sheep are associated with rapid-eye-movement sleep. The movements are irregular, episodic and have a diurnal rhythm. They are readily abolished by hypoxemia and have proved, in both sheep and in man, a useful indicator of fetal health in utero. Some of the biological implications are considered in relation to early development of the lungs and of sleep state.

ACKNOWLEDGEMENT

This work was supported by grants from the Medical Research Council.

REFERENCES

Boddy, K. and Dawes, G.S. (1975) Fetal breathing. *Brit. med. Bull.*, 31: 3–7.

Boddy, K., Dawes, G.S., Fisher, R., Pinter, S. and Robinson, J.S. (1974) Foetal respiratory movements, electrocortical and cardiovascular responses to hypoxaemia and hypercapnia in sheep. *J. Physiol. (Lond.)*, 243: 599–618.

Boddy, K., Dawes, G.S. and Robinson, J.S. (1973) A 24 hour rhythm in the foetus. I. In *Foetal and Neonatal Physiology, Proc. Sir J. Barcroft Centenary Symposium,* Cambridge University Press, Cambridge, pp. 63–66.

Boddy, K., Dawes, G.S. and Robinson, J. (1974) Intrauterine fetal breathing movements. In *Modern Perinatal Medicine,* L. Gluck (Ed.), Year Book Medical Publishers, Chicago, Ill., pp. 381–389.

Boddy, K. and Robinson, J.S. (1971) External method for detection of fetal breathing in utero. *Lancet,* ii: 1231–1233.

Dawes, G.S., Fox, H.E., Leduc, B.M., Liggins, G.C. and Richards, R.T. (1970) Respiratory movements and paradoxical sleep in the foetal lamb. *J. Physiol. (Lond.),* 210: 47–48P.

Dawes, G.S., Fox, H.E., Leduc, B.M., Liggins, G.C. and Richards, R.T. (1972) Respiratory movements and rapid eye movement sleep in the foetal lamb. *J. Physiol. (Lond.),* 220: 119–143.

Manning, F., Wyn Pugh, E. and Boddy, K. (1975) Effect of cigarette smoking on fetal breathing movements in normal pregnancies. *Brit. med. J.,* 1: 552–553.

Merlet, C., Hoerter, J., Devilleneuve, C. et Tchobroutsky, C. (1970) Mise en evidence de mouvements respiratoires chez le foetus d'agneau in utero au cours du dernier mois de la gestation. *C.R. Acad. Sci. (Paris),* 270: 2462–2464.

Ruckebusch, Y. (1971) Activité electro-corticale chez le foetus de la brebis (*Ovis aries*) et de la vache (*Bos tourus*). *Revue méd. vét.,* 122: 483–510.

DISCUSSION

P.A. WEISS: Have you ever tried to change the day and night, or the length of the day, with the sheep?

G.S. DAWES: No. We have discussed doing it, but the pressure of other investigations has prevented us starting.

J. SCHERRER: I have one question and one comment. The question is: what is the diurnal rhythm of the temperature of the mother animal? The comment is the following one: when you deprive a human of sleep during the night time it is rather difficult to get paradoxical sleep during the day time. So, for paradoxical sleep which, in your experiments, coincides with the breathing movements, there is a maximum of probability during a part of a circadian time. Most of the paradoxical sleep in the human is tied between 2 and 6 o'clock in the morning. Of course you can change it by changing the conditions, but usually there is also a circadian probability time for paradoxical sleep.

G.S. DAWES: There is a small diurnal variation in temperature in the mother. The fetal temperature is $0.5°C$ above that in the mother, and varies passively with it. The peak temperature is usually in the late evening. That is one reason why I am slightly hesitant about the interpretation of experiments in which we changed the environment. You are perfectly right in what you say about adults, but it does not hold in the immediate neonatal period, nor in the fetal period. Ruckebusch and Barbey (1971) have looked at the immediately postnatal changes in the electrocortical activity in the fetal goat, but I don't know of anyone who has followed it sequentially into the adult period.

K. BOER: You showed that you could predict the human fetal prognosis from its respiratory movements. Was there any relation in your groups between the length of gestation and the prognosis of the fetuses, or were all fetuses in the same age groups?

G.S. DAWES: The investigation which I summarized was from 34 weeks gestation onwards. You can see grossly abnormal patterns of fetal breathing much earlier. We have seen this in fetuses of 26–28 weeks gestation when there will be little chance of the infant surviving if delivered by cesarian section.

W.L. BAKHUIS: I heard you mentioning that the sheep fetus is awake during a certain percentage of the time. Could you please give your criteria for its being awake?

G.S. DAWES: We use the same criteria as in a newborn human infant. From time to time it makes purposely directed movements: it will open its eyes, turn its head and appear to fix at a particular position. If you then touch the fetus, it will respond immediately by withdrawing a leg or pushing it forward. If you make the same tactile tests during sleep or when it is lying completely quietly and with a high voltage EEG activity, then it will not quickly respond at all. If you continue to give increasing tactile stimulation, the fetus produces a startle response and becomes awake.

O.D. CREUTZFELDT: Did you try to correlate the EEG states of sleep and wakefulness between the mother and the infant — this in the context of all sorts of theories on sleep?

G.S. DAWES: Yes, but there is no correlation between them. The mother sheep only sleeps for very short periods of time during the day or night. The fetus switches state several times an hour, and there is no change in the mother's behavior during this time.

REFERENCE

Ruckebusch, Y. et Barbey, P. (1971) Les états de sommeil chez le foetus et le nouveau-né de la rache (*Bos taurus*). *C.R. Soc. Biol. (Paris)*, 165: 1176–1184.

EEG and Behavior

W. STORM VAN LEEUWEN

Dept. of Clinical Neurophysiology,
University Hospital, Utrecht (The Netherlands)

INTRODUCTION

Generally it can be stated that all forms of behavior are originated in and governed by the nervous system, and thus are the product of neuronal activity. Considering that all functional neuronal activity is accompanied by electrical phenomena of some kind or another, it must be concluded that all behavioral acts are reflected in the central nervous system by electrical phenomena. This does not mean, however, that all electrical activities can be recorded. In fact, virtually the opposite is true: the statement may be made that in any living subject only very little of the total neuronal activities can in fact be recorded. Of these the most well known and the most often recorded activities are: (1) the action potentials; and (2) the slow EEG potential variations.

ACTION POTENTIALS

If one knew precisely the position of neurons responsible for a certain behavioral act it would be possible in principle to study these successfully by recording the action potentials of all relevant neurons. Due to the nature of brain functioning it would be necessary, even for the simplest behavioral act, to record the action potentials of a very large number of neurons — in fact, a number so large that it can never be hoped to be achieved. Moreover, generally the positions of the neurons of the circuits involved in a behavioral act are only partly known and, furthermore, even in the most favorable case only a few (about 3–10 neurons) can be recorded from the many thousands involved.

The technique of "multiunit recording" by means of small electrodes (usually approximately 40–60 μm) allows recording of a larger number of units (for example 3–5) per electrode. This method has yielded important results but, even so, the number of units which can be studied remains very small. This means that in practice the neuronal counterpart of behavioral acts, as far as action potentials are concerned, can be recorded only fragmentarily.

SLOW POTENTIAL VARIATIONS OF NEURONAL POPULATIONS

As is well known, the slow potential variations occurring in neuronal populations have a tendency for doing so synchronously, or nearly so (see Scherrer, pp. 309–325 in this volume). Because of this synchrony these potential variations or, to be more exact, their spatial and temporal average, can be recorded by means of comparatively large electrodes a considerable distance from the actual sources. If the neuronal populations are large enough, and if their degree of synchrony is sufficient, the potentials spread passively over such distances that they pass the tissues surrounding the brain, i.e., meninges, bone and skin, and may be recorded from the scalp. The synchrony of large neural masses makes it unlikely that the resulting potential variations are uniquely related to the detailed neuronal functioning which must be associated with intricate behavioral acts or with mental functioning. On the contrary, the massive synchrony is much more likely to be related to overall functional states in cortical and other brain structures, in normal as well as in pathological circumstances. Thus, for example, the occurrence of potential variations at approximately 10 Hz in the occipital areas of subjects closing their eyes while being in a mentally relaxed state (alpha rhythm), generally is believed to reflect a condition of these structures in which no visual information is being processed.

To have a chance of finding relations between more detailed behavioral aspects and slow potential variations in the EEG, those originated by much smaller neuron populations should be studied, and this entails the use of comparatively small electrodes in direct contact with the brain. In conclusion, therefore, the study of the neuronal functioning leading to behavior can at present be carried out by making correlations between behavioral events, on the one hand, and on the other to: (1) unit potentials from a limited number of neurons and (2) slow potential variations of smaller or larger neuronal populations. Moreover, it is obvious that the understanding of these two forms of neuronal electrical potential variation will be aided considerably by the study of their mutual relations.

CORRELATIONS OF EEG WITH BEHAVIOR

In the following, some examples will be given of relations found between behavioral aspects and the slow potentials of neuronal populations in animal and in man. This form of study has been possible due to a number of technical developments such as:

(1) the technique for recording over long periods of time from brain structures by means of comparatively small indwelling electrodes;

(2) recording from freely moving subjects by means of radiotelemetry of the EEG; and

(3) the evaluation and quantification of the EEG phenomena by means of computer analysis.

It should be added here that the study of these electrical phenomena in the brain of man has been possible only due to the fact that in some patients it is necessary to introduce such electrodes in the brain for diagnostic and/or for therapeutic reasons.

The study of behavior has been aided considerably by the use of videorecording and by the recording of non-cerebral bioelectric phenomena (polygraphy). During the last decennium the study of behavior has obtained impetus by methods for coding and recording of behavioral elements, and by their evaluation and quantification by means of computer analysis. In the last few years methods developed in the field of ethology for quantitative study of

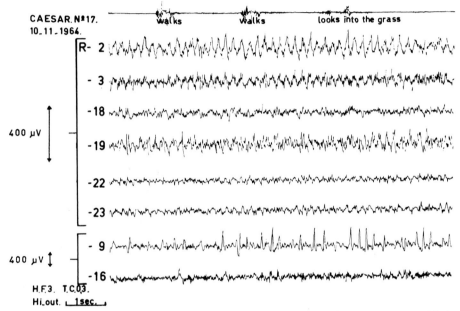

Fig. 1. Recording of various cortical and subcortical derivations in dog walking outside in the sun. R2 and R3 = hippocampus. R9 = visual cortex and R16 = olfactory bulb. Note marked lambda waves in visual cortex and theta rhythm in hippocampus while dog is walking and looking.

behavior are being introduced in the field of neurophysiology. This development may well lead to an entirely new approach to the problem.

The relations between the brain's electrical activities and behavior can be studied either during "free" or during "programmed" behavior. The latter has the advantage that repetitive, more or less standardized, situations can be created, allowing the use of simple statistical methods of evaluation. This can be done both for parameters of the electrical phenomena as for the coded elements of behavior. These studies have led to the distinction of a considerable number of electrical brain activities related to behavioral aspects in animals as well as in man.

In the following, some examples will be described of relations observed in dogs (Storm van Leeuwen et al., 1967) and in patients (Kamp et al., 1972).

(1) In dogs "lambda waves" were observed in visual cortex connected with eye movements. These are waves with a duration of 1/4–1/8 sec occurring in occipital cortex whenever the dog is making eye movements in well-lit surroundings. They occur, for example, if the dog is walking around in the grass while the sun shines (see Fig. 1).

(2) In dog, moreover, hippocampus theta rhythms were encountered. These are rhythmic waves at 4–7 Hz occurring in the hippocampus when the animal is active, as, for example, while walking. Investigations by Arnolds et al. (1975) have shown that the frequency, usually around 5 Hz, may rise to 6 Hz

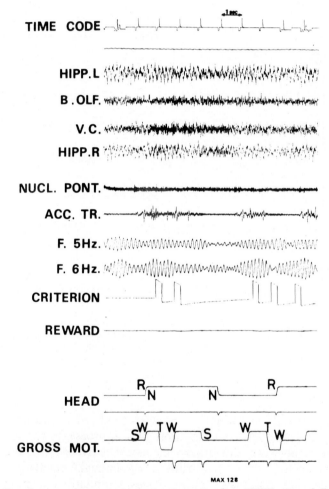

Fig. 2. Recording from various cerebral structures in dog (HIPP. L and R, left and right hippocampus; B.OLF, olfactory bulb; V.C., visual cortex; NUCL. PONT., multiunit recording from the dorsal pons; ACC. TR., acceleration transducer fixed to the head; F 5 Hz and 6 Hz = output of filters at 5 and 6 Hz, connected with left hippocampus; "criterion" indicates when hippocampal frequency shift from 5 Hz to 6 Hz takes place; "reward" indicates when reward is given; "HEAD" indicates code for head movements and "GROSS MOT" when gross motor movements are made). Note that frequency shifts (criterion) occur when head and/or gross motor movements are made (see also the excursion in ACC. TR.). (From Arnolds et al., 1975.)

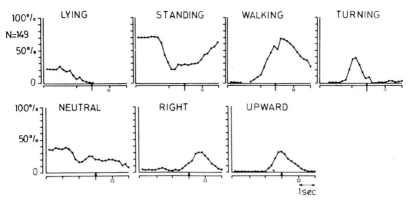

Fig. 3. Percentage of behavioral elements occurring 3 sec before and 2 sec after a frequency shift in hippocampal from 5 Hz to 6 Hz (indicated by arrow beneath each x-axis). Note decrease of some behaviors before the frequency shift (for example, lying and standing) and increase of others (for example, walking and turning). (Arnolds et al., 1975.)

whenever a movement is initiated or whenever a change of movement occurs. Feedback experiments, in which the dog was rewarded whenever a frequency shift from 5 to 6 Hz occurred, have demonstrated that the dog may use various behavioral patterns to achieve the reward, such as turning the head, walking away and turning back, getting up from sitting to standing, etc. — all of them having in common a sudden change of movement (Figs. 2 and 3).

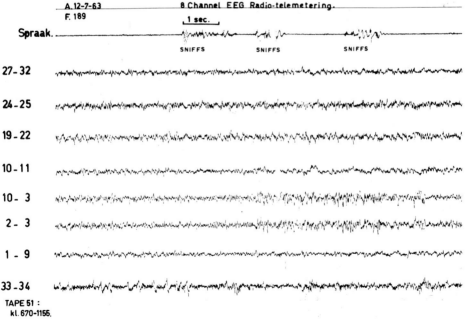

Fig. 4. Recording from various structures in dog. 10–3 and 2–3, amygdala; 33–34, visual cortex; Spraak., recording of observers' verbal comments of dogs' behavior. Note occurrence of irregular 10–20 Hz activity in amygdala when dog is sniffing and visual cortex lambda waves are absent, but no occurrence of the 10–20 Hz amygdala activity when lambda waves are present.

(3) In dogs, in addition, 10–20 Hz activity was observed in the amygdala. This activity occurred when the dog was sniffing. It did not occur, however, in all instances that the dog sniffed. It was noted that there appeared to be mutual relations between this 10–20 Hz activity in amygdala and some other activities. For example the 10–20 Hz amygdala activity occurred only while the dog was sniffing, if at the same time no lambda waves occurred in the occipital cortex (alternation phenomena, Fig. 4). In exceptional circumstances, when a

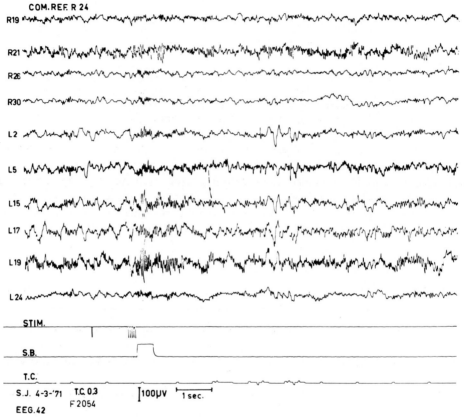

Fig. 5. Recordings from various cortical structures in a patient. L10, L15 and L19 = left lateral frontal cortex. Note occurrence of 20–26 Hz activity (beta bursts) during CNV paradigm, indicated by STIM and SP. The first deflection in STIM indicates a warning click sound, followed after 1 sec by a series of flashes. The patient is instructed to stop the flashes by pressing a button (indicated by S.B.).

situation was created where the dog was trying to find a smelly object (fish) surrounded by obstacles, lambda waves and 10–20 Hz in amygdala occurred simultaneously for short periods of time. It was concluded that these electrical phenomena appeared to reflect the direction of the dogs' attention, the lambda waves representing directioning to visual messages and the 10–20 Hz amygdala activity directioning to olfactory input.

(4) In patients with indwelling electrodes, bursts at 20–26 Hz ("beta-bursts") have been observed to occur in parts of the lateral frontal cortex during certain phases of a stimulus response paradigm (Figs. 5 and 6). It was

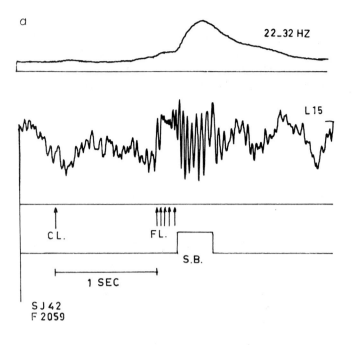

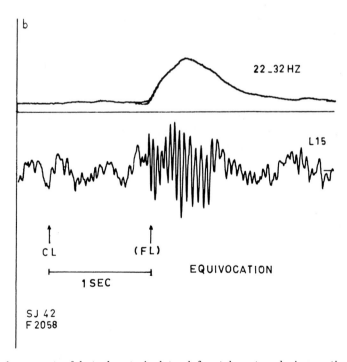

Fig. 6. a: enlargement of beta bursts in lateral frontal cortex during a stimulus response paradigm. CL., warning clicksound; FL., flashes; S.B., subject presses button. Upper trace shows the rectified output of filter at 20–28 Hz. b: similar to a. In this series of experiments the flashes are omitted randomly in 50% of the cases. Note occurrence of beta bursts at the time that the flashes would have occurred.

demonstrated that the beta bursts were enhanced when the patient answered questions or solved simple problems. It did not make any difference whether the solution was correct or not. In one case, the beta bursts were accompanied by a small significant decrease of heart rate. The hypothesis was forwarded that the beta bursts accompany a brief release of psychological tension when a problem is solved.

CONCLUSIONS

One of the conclusions is that essential brain phenomena, such as alpha rhythm, lambda waves etc., are found both in dog and in man. This indicates that as far as these phenomena are concerned the dog may be regarded as a good model for man. The hippocampus theta rhythm and 10–20 Hz activity has not been studied much in man, but this may be due to the obvious restrictions in investigations in patients. In our own group of patients it has not been necessary to introduce electrodes in hippocampus or in the amygdala. In man, beta activity (whether or not in the form of bursts) occurs in many cortical areas. It has been possible to find behavioral counterparts only for some types of beta. The search for such correlations asks for a good deal of ingenuity on the part of the investigator, as well as patience from the subjects. Since such investigations are guided by strategies which, at least potentially, are for the patients' benefit, not all tests which might be desirable for the investigation as such can be carried out. Conversely, the sort of stimulus-response paradigms which are easily carried out with patients may be difficult or laborious in dogs. For example a human subject may be instructed easily and in one session to press a button one second after a warning signal, he may be "punished" or "rewarded" symbolically by a "correct" or "incorrect" signal. It is possible to train a dog to perform the same task but it takes many sessions, the reward has to be real, and the test cannot have the same significance for the dog as it has for man.

The relations between EEG phenomena and behavior concern general models rather than specific behavioral acts. For example, the occurrence of the hippocampus theta rhythm is not related to any specific behavioral act. This rhythm rather appears to be an inherent characteristic of the dynamics of the hippocampal neuronal populations. However, the frequency modulation of the theta rhythm appears to be related to changes of behavioral states.

On the basis of the above, the hypothesis is forwarded that the EEG phenomena indicate a certain functional state in which a certain neuronal population comes into being and is maintained for a period of time, a functional state which is necessary for the onset and development of certain forms of behavior.

Recent studies on the significance of the oscillating electrical brain phenomena (Lopes da Silva et al., 1974) have shown that these phenomena are due to both excitatory and inhibitory influences. This means that the old question whether these phenomena represent "activity" or "inactivity" is not relevant and thus cannot be answered.

REFERENCES

Arnolds, D., Lopes da Silva, F.H., Aitink, W. and Kamp, A. (1975) Motor acts and firing of reticular neurons correlated with operantly reinforced theta shifts. *Brain Res.*, 85: 194–195.

Kamp, A., Schrijer, C.F.M. and Storm van Leeuwen, W. (1972) Occurrence of "beta bursts" in human frontal cortex related to psychological parameters. *Electroenceph. clin. Neurophysiol.*, 33: 257–267.

Lopes da Silva, F.H., Hoeks, A., Smits, A. and Zetterberg, L.H. (1974) Model of brain rhythmic activity and the alpha rhythm of thalamus. *Kybernetik*, 5: 27–38.

Storm van Leeuwen, W., Kamp, A., Kok, M.L. and Tielen, A. (1967) EEG of unrestrained animals under stressful conditions. Recent Advances in Clinical Neurophysiology. *Electroenceph. clin. Neurophysiol.*, Suppl. 25.

DISCUSSION

J. SCHERRER: I would like to ask you the following question. You showed some very striking differences between neocortex and hippocampus or some deeper structures. Did you also notice differences between the various parts of the neocortex? For instance, did you see any striking differences between a projection area and an associative one?

W. STORM VAN LEEUWEN: In the visual cortex there are either lambda waves or alpha rhythms, depending on the situation in which the dog is, and this is similar to man. In the temporal area, on the other hand, we have found about 22 Hz beta rhythms. These are associated with the situation that the dog is standing still but is looking vacantly: the eyes open, the dog obviously being awake, but not seemingly interested in anything. Finally, there is another EEG phenomenon which has always intrigued me considerably: 9 or 10 Hz activity occurring in the auditory cortex whenever a buzzing sound is made. It does not occur when pure sine waves are delivered.

D. DE WIED: Is the theta rhythm that you see when a dog is walking *always* present when it walks? And is it related to the motivation of the animal: is it goal-directed behavior?

W. STORM VAN LEEUWEN: It is related to motor activity in general, but not exclusively. For instance, it can be present if a dog is sitting on the floor, ready to jump on a couch but before actually having done so. At such moment there is a considerable increase of theta rhythm in the hippocampus, although the dog is not walking.

M.A. CORNER: The interpretation of the various EEG patterns as a functional mode of state, related to the *type* of behavior (rather than to the fine details) seems to be a very fruitful way of looking at the EEG phenomenon — especially considering the wide variety of signals that you can get from specific parts of the brain. From a theoretical point of view, however, there should be certain limitations to the EEG as revealing even the occurrence of an overall functional change in the neuronal structures. Only some of these changes may express themselves in a way which is recordable by the EEG, and there may well be others which you could not possibly pick up because they lack the proper conditions for effective summation. Do you have any ideas of possible directions of future research which might be able to establish the *limits* of use EEG correlations?

F.H. LOPES DA SILVA: I can comment on that, to emphasize that all the correlations established between behavior and gross brain electrical activity involved a large number of synchronously active neurons. You will not expect, however, that such phenomena can provide any clues to the specific patterns which must be occurring all the time during behavior. What are the possibilities for future research? The EEG is useful to use in the sense that you may pick up clues to where to look further, but in itself it will not solve the problem. We will have to complement this type of gross electrophysiological study with single cell recordings. The whole problem is that although you know that pools of neurons are concerned with different types of behavior, we have only very global signs of what these neurons are actually doing. On the other hand, we know that we have to look to specific neuronal populations and even sub-sets of such populations in order to know something about specific behaviors, but there is this gap between the two levels of electrical registration. One of the most important things for the future is precisely to see how by means of different types of approaches — including neuronal model approaches — we can bridge this gap.

Brain Stimulation
and the Motivation of Behavior

JAMES OLDS

Division of Biology, California Institute of Technology, Pasadena, Calif. 91125 (U.S.A.)

INTRODUCTION: REWARD AND ATTENTION PROCESSES
IN LEARNING

Twenty-five years ago when I entered psychology, American learning theorists were polarized about an argument that was at the crux of things. The question was: "how do motives work?". Why does the animal "come back for more"? Stimulus-response theory, exemplified in the writings of Hull (1943), said that reward "stamped in" a connection between stimuli and responses at the time of its original occurrence. Later the animal came back for more because it couldn't help it; the stamped-in connections forced him to do so. Cognitive theory as expressed by its champion, Tolman (1949), put more emphasis on the information processing that went on subsequently, at the time the animal was deciding whether or not to go back. On the first occurrence, during learning, the animal learned where things were and how they "tasted". These events were recorded; to me it seemed they were taken down as if on a tape recorder. Later, the animal played back its tapes, vicariously at first. If it found something it liked on one of the tapes, it would play it back a second time "for real". Thus, for Tolman, remembered reward did the main job, and it worked by triggering behaviors under specific conditions. For Hull, on the other hand, reward was a connector.

For Tolman, reward was not a connector but of course there was still the problem of connecting. In Hull's model, reward caused connecting of stimuli and responses. In Tolman's model, everything that happened caused the stimuli involved to be connected in some way to a "memory" and this memory to become connected to responses (so it could reproduce them). Did happenings by itself cause the connecting? Tolman and his disciples had some misgivings about the idea that happening by itself was enough. Only things that were "attended to" got remembered. This was either by planned, careful, advance attention, or, by looking back after a surprise (a person could recover some of the immediate past out of a temporary store which it had got into even without attention, and could then promote it to be an object of attention). Only events that had some special salience caused by attention, and maybe only some special subset of these, became connected to longer-lasting memories. Thus, *reward* was displaced from the role of connector, and *attention* was introduced to perform that task.

After being displaced, however, reward was still not completely disentangled from the problem of learning. This was because a reward had to be attended to, and it had to become connected in order to be an effective reward. Because the animal could not learn without attention, it also could not be rewarded without attention. This made the connector a sine qua non of reward, and thus in one sense a part of the reward, even though the reward was not a part of the connector. The animal could attend and learn without being rewarded, although of course it could not be rewarded without attending. This clarified a way in which features and aspects not identified with reward itself could be essential ingredients of it. For this reason, in electrophysiological recording experiments many candidates for "reward neuron" status had to be inspected carefully, lest they performed this closely correlated and prerequisite function, but were really only related in a tangential fashion to the reward process itself.

A different way a tangential action could be sine qua non without being an actual part of a rewarding effect comes to light from an analysis of incompatible emotional states. It is reasonable to suppose some reciprocal antagonism of positive and negative emotional conditions. A happy day can be spoiled by a major hurt, and extremes of pleasure and pain seem subjectively to be largely incompatible. If there were central sources of negative and positive emotions, anything which inhibited one might promote the other, while any substantial disinhibition of one might counteract the other. Thus, if a neurochemical substance held in check an important central source of negative emotion, it might seem a sine qua non of reward even if it had nothing directly to do with it.

In the present paper, a search is made for a set of reward neurons among what is fortunately still a rather small number of candidates. These include subsets of noradrenaline neurons, of dopamine neurons, and also of inter-neurons of the gustatory-olfactory sensory system. Both noradrenaline and dopamine neurons seem from some experiments to be strong candidates, but both come under the question of whether they might instead be tangentially related in one of the two ways mentioned above. Either of them might be involved in connecting and learning, or else in the suppressive control of negative emotional states or depressions.

My guess at the end is that both may in fact be involved directly in different reward processes. Noradrenaline neurons might inhibit aversive drive states or negative emotions; and reward the animal in this way. Dopamine neurons might act similarly on drive states that did not have any negative tone; and hedonic states might be the correlate of this action. If it worked this way, then noradrenaline would directly reward the animal when the main problem came from aversive drives; but it could also be secondarily involved at other times, keeping negative emotions in check to make hedonic behavior possible.

Data from a number of brain experiments seemed at first to have relatively direct bearing on central questions of motivation, particularly those related to the steering of behavior toward some things and away from others, and the role of rewards and drives in the problem of learning. The brain experiments promised interesting advances just over the horizon, but so far they have only added to the puzzles. Considerable thought is still needed to get a sensible thread of meaning from them and to decipher some of the most tractable directions they point toward further understanding. I want to set the outlines of this data on the table and try again to follow some of the best leads*.

BRAIN STIMULATION

The first body of data came from electric stimulation of the brain in behaving animals. Experiments employing this method have resulted in a map of brain locations where electric stimulation caused animals to behave as if the stimulus itself were the goal object of an active drive, or caused a condition so hedonically gratifying that no drive was necessary to get behavior going (Olds, 1962). These abnormal brain rewards motivated not only pedal behavior but also maze running and the crossing of aversive obstructions (Fig. 1).

Rats, cats and monkeys had much the same map (Fig. 2). Even humans would perform nonsense tasks apparently in order to stimulate analogous brain centers, although they often seemed confused as to why they were doing so. In

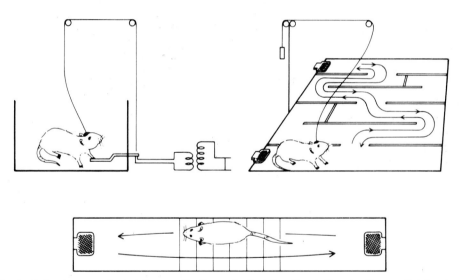

Fig. 1. Behaviors motivated by application of electric stimulation in the medial forebrain bundle after each pedal response (0.25 sec trains, 60 Hz alternating current, 50 mA r.m.s.). In the maze and the obstruction box, three pedal responses were rewarded at one pedal and then the animal was required to shuttle to the other for three more, and so forth. In the obstruction box, current of about 60 mA applied through the grid floor stopped hungry rats running for food and these also stopped rats running for 50 mA brain stimuli. However, when the brain "reward" was increased to 200 mA these animals crossed obstructions applying more than 400 mA to the feet.

---

* To do this I shall review work in which I personally participated on: (1) behavioral features of "brain reward", and (2) "unit responses" of hypothalamic neurons, along with work of others on: (3) stimulation and lesions affecting basic drive behavior, and (4) the amine neurotransmitters and their maps.

404

the rat, the olfactory bulb and much of the floor of the brain connected to it were implicated as areas where stimulation was rewarding.

On the floor of the rat brain a large central region is occupied by the hypothalamus. The borders are its outposts, some of which are in the olfactory parts of the forebrain. Others are located more caudally in the brain. Through the posterior hypothalamic area come sensory messages originating in the

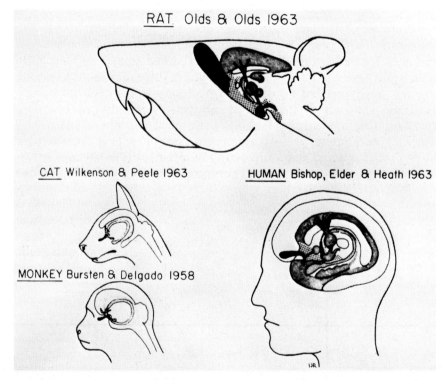

Fig. 2. Schematic pictures of the parts of the brain yielding brain reward behavior in different species. The map for the rat has been done carefully. Those of other species are estimated from a smaller number of tests, with extrapolation based on anatomical analogies. The marked areas in the brains yielded brain-reward effects. Listed in order from largest to smallest effects they are: (1) large cross hatching = medial forebrain bundle; (2) blackened areas = olfactory bulbs and anterior olfactory areas; (3) small cross hatching = amygdala, septal area, and stria terminalis; and (4) grey areas = "Papez circuit".

visceral and gustatory receptors. In addition, hormonal messages from the circulation pass directly into the hypothalamus through blood-brain windows.

The reward map covered most of the hypothalamus and neighboring areas (Fig. 3). Within the hypothalamus the map extended from far-anterior to far-posterior, and from far-lateral to the midline. A paradox of the reward map was that this same region was also the locus of aversive effects of electric stimulation (Roberts, 1958). If opposed aversive effects were not immediately obvious, they could usually be demonstrated by careful behavioral analysis. Because the whole hypothalamus was covered by a reward map, while aversive countereffects were also always in evidence, you might suppose that the

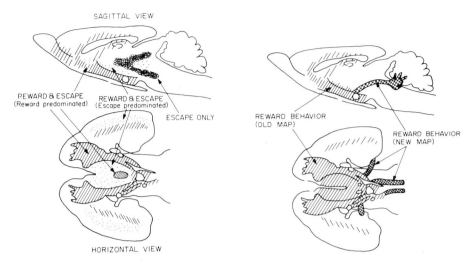

Fig. 3. A more detailed map of main areas in the rat brain yielding reward and escape behavior.

hypothalamus was homogeneous with respect to these maps. It proved not to be.

In the far-lateral parts of the hypothalamus, and in some parts of the far-medial hypothalamus, there were locations where the rewarding effects of stimulation predominated. In these cases the animal was apparently at ease with the self-stimulation. No obvious negative signs were seen during brain pedal behavior, so that careful methods were required to reveal them.

In a large intermediate area there was an obvious mixture of positive and negative effects. The animal would pedal regularly and fast if closeted with an electric stimulus, but if there was a way out it would escape at once. There was no amount of stimulation in these areas that seemed just right. The animal behaved as if it could not stand the stimulation but could not resist it either (Olds and Olds, 1963).

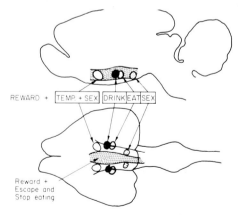

Fig. 4. Map of areas in rat brain yielding instrumental and consummatory behaviors aimed at different drive-object targets.

406

In this same intermediate area a second paradox of the reward maps was found: the same electric stimulus often provoked drives as well as rewards. The drives depended partly on the location of the stimulus (Fig. 4). With probes implanted in anterior hypothalamus there were both sex responses and responses that adjusted the body temperature (Roberts et al., 1967). In the anterior part of the middle hypothalamus there were both eating and drinking responses, but the drinking responses predominated. In the posterior part of the middle hypothalamus there were still more eating and drinking responses, but here it was the eating response which predominated (Valenstein et al., 1970). In the posterior part of the hypothalamus sex responses were again

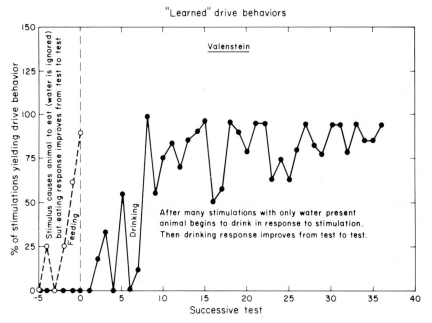

Fig. 5. Valenstein effect: modification of drive-object by training (Valenstein et al., 1968). Prior to "training" the electric brain stimulus caused at first little drive behavior and then, after some repetition of the stimulus in the presence of food and water, the stimulus evoked feeding. Then after a long period of stimulation in the presence of water only, the electric stimulus evoked drinking.

evoked (Herberg, 1963). Because there were many overlapping effects, and sex responses were evoked in areas on both sides of the feeding and drinking areas, the idea of sharp localizations was rejected. But because this area could be mapped into four contiguous regions where stimulation caused, respectively, temperature, drinking, eating and sexual behavior as the most likely responses, the idea of totally unlocalized drive systems was equally rejected. The truth obviously lay somewhere in between.

One feature of the "in between" answer was discovered. The goal objects of the "drives" caused by these stimulations were often changed by training. If the animal was stimulated regularly in the presence of a drive object, after a while the stimulus began to evoke an appropriate drive, that is one with the available drive object as its target (Fig. 5). In one test, for example, probes were placed in what originally seemed to be a feeding point (i.e., the stimulation evoked feeding as opposed to drinking in original choice tests). Then with only water present, 30-sec trains of stimulation were applied every 5 min for many days. Under the impetus of this the feeding point changed, so that in the end it had become a drinking point! This can be called the *Valenstein effect* after its discoverer (Valenstein et al., 1968).

Because drives were mapped into different areas of the brain to begin with it seemed strange that they could be modified by training. One possible answer to this puzzle was that a family of drive neurons might be initially related to a specific drive by their sensitivity to particular visceral inputs or to particular hormones, but their outputs might become functionally connected during development or learning to appropriate drive objects. The Valenstein effect might be evidence that electric stimulation could interfere with this normal learning mechanism. It is possible to assume that the stimulus *was* applied in a "hunger center" but that gradually the training artificially caused the animal to respond as if the water were a hunger drive object.

To recapitulate the picture developed by hypothalamic stimulation: there were far-lateral and far-medial areas where reward predominated, plus in-between areas where aversive effects and drive effects were overlapped with reward.

LESIONS

A second body of data came from restricted destruction of small and deep "brain centers". These studies have divided the hypothalamus and neighboring structures into a focus where lesions had one kind of effect, and a set of three surrounding areas where different kinds of opposed effects were observed (Fig. 6). Anatomically, the focus was the same lateral hypothalamus where electric stimulation had produced predominantly positive effects. It included also the boundary regions of the hypothalamus: among these the substantia nigra is one we will be most interested in later on. Lesions in lateral hypothalamus or along its boundary regions caused a loss of positive drive-reward behaviors and other operant behaviors (even ones aimed at avoiding noxious stimulation; Teitelbaum and Epstein, 1962; Balinska, 1968).

If, however, animals were kept alive for a few days after these lesions there was often good recovery of some of the reward behaviors. Animals died if not force-fed at first but they recovered in 1–3 weeks if kept alive by force-feeding or other methods. After recovery the animals were dependent in a surprising way on the cortex for drive behavior (Teitelbaum and Cytawa, 1965). This was shown by application of KCl to the cortex, which causes in normals a 4–8 hr period during which all instrumental behavior is abolished (and abnormal electric activity is recorded from the head). This treatment may be thought of as causing a temporary shut-down of cortical function and, in normals, there appeared to be essentially full recovery after several hours. In animals with functional recovery from lateral hypothalamic lesions, on the other hand, the same KCl application to the cortex had a much more devastating effect, causing the full 3 week recovery period to need redoing. This dependence of drive behavior upon cortical integrity after lateral hypothalamic damage suggests that recovery was in fact not really complete.

There were other signs pointing in the same direction. The experimental animals, after recovery from lesioning, did not respond to cellular water deficits by drinking, but drank only to wet their mouths (Teitelbaum and Epstein, 1972). Similarly, they did not respond to glucose deficits by eating, and also failed to respond appropriately to sodium deficits. With their repertoire of redundant hunger controllers or learned feeding behaviors, however, the animals managed to survive, and even succeeded in looking robust and well-fed. It is conceivable that a learned cortical repertoire of drive behaviors recovered, while a hypothalamic initiator of these drives was gone.

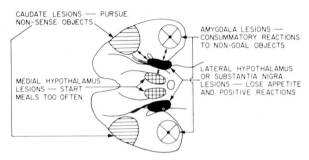

Fig. 6. Map of lesions in and near the hypothalamus affecting targeted instrumental-approach and consummatory behaviors. In the lateral-hypothalamic substantia nigra focus, lesions halted such behavior temporarily and modified it permanently. In three neighboring areas there were opposed effects. Lesions in medial hypothalamus caused episodes of approach and consummatory behavior aimed at food to occur too frequently. Lesions in the caudate nucleus caused compulsive instrumental behavior aimed at moving "nonsense" objects. Lesions in the amygdaloid region caused attempts to perform consummatory behavior with non-goal objects.

Fitting this view, a most important food learning mechanism was also absent, the animals failing to learn to exclude foods on the basis of poisoning or illness. A normal rat responds to foods that preceded illness as if they were aversive, called the *Garcia effect* after its discoverer (Garcia and Ervin, 1968). This may be thought of as the learning of aversive reactions to poison, and it disappeared following lateral lesions. In normal rats, there is also learning of special positive reactions to foods that are correlated with recovery from illness, and these learned positive reactions too were gone after lateral lesions (Roth et al., 1973). Because these food-learning phenomena matched the drive-target learning of the Valenstein experiments, it seemed doubly likely that the hypothalamus might be involved in the learning of drive targets: that is, in the learned attachments of animals to objects.

There were three areas surrounding the lateral hypothalamus (LH) where lesions had the opposite effect to LH lesions. The first set of opposed lesions was in the medial hypothalamus, and caused the reverse of starvation. The animals thus ate too often, because the beginning of meals occurred too early (as if no visceral or chemical trigger were needed; Le Magnen et al., 1973).

The second set of opposed lesions was situated in the caudate nucleus. This is a motor center which reciprocally inhibits the substantia nigra. Lesions here caused meaningless instrumental behavior directed at anything that moved (Villablanca, 1974). This effect looked as if it might represent the inversion of the *loss* of pursuit behavior that occurred with lateral hypothalamus lesions.

The third set of opposed lesions was found in the amygdala, an outpost in the olfactory forebrain. These lesions caused consummatory behavior toward dangerous objects or untested foods, or even toward "wrong" objects. For example, there were attempts to eat or mate with, respectively, non-food or non-sex objects (Klüver and Bucy, 1937).

The fact that lesions in a central area stopped reward behaviors, whereas lesions in three surrounding areas caused different kinds of excessive approach behavior, suggests a multiple opponent process system: a central positive region in lateral hypothalamus and substantia nigra inhibiting and being inhibited by three neighboring regions. In such a system a shifting balance of excitation and inhibition would determine the presence or absence of approach behavior, and electric stimulation along the communication links might well have double or mixed effects.

Besides these, another set of lesion studies which is more specifically related to self-stimulation deserves special mention. Many lesions failed to halt this type of behavior; for instance, even the very extensive damage from ablating all of the neocortex, paleocortex and basal ganglia (Huston and Borbély, 1974). Animals with these lesions behaved as if they had lost all nuances of behavior. Gross behaviors such as rearing on the hindlegs could still be reinforced, however. When such behaviors were clearly characterized, they could be greatly increased in frequency by electrical brain rewards. Furthermore, after the reward was withdrawn the behavior showed no signs of extinguishing, leaving the impression that, although the telencephalon was not required for operant learning of gross behavior patterns, it was needed for normal extinction. The only way the response could be suppressed in these animals was to reinforce its opposite. This study has many important implications for questions about why brain reward often extinguishes very rapidly. However, one of the main imports is that at least some of the "reward" neurons do not reside in the front end of the medial forebrain bundle system.

THE BRAIN AMINES

A third body of data came from neurochemical maps showing where certain brain chemicals reside and what neurons and fiber pathways carry them. These maps have identified a set of apparent brain reward neurons, and thus may give the beginnings of an interpretation of brain reward behavior — and possibly the beginnings of an explanation of other reward behaviors as well. Small clumps of neurons in focal centers of the hindbrain, midbrain, and the boundaries of the forebrain send axons which radiate from the focal centers to the farthest reaches (Ungerstedt, 1971a, b). There are several similar clumps and several overlapping sets of diverging fibers. The localized origins and the widely diffusing fibers make these look like command centers that could send YES-NO

410

messages to the whole brain (Fig. 7). The synaptic transmitters used by these neurons to transmit signals are noradrenaline, dopamine, and serotonin.

The noradrenaline fibers started farthest back and went farthest forward. They ran from a crossroads of the brain in the medulla to all of its outposts: the cerebellum, thalamus, paleocortex and neocortex. The serotonin fibers started in the middle of the midbrain and ran a less well-defined course to many parts of the forebrain. The dopamine fibers started in the rostral part

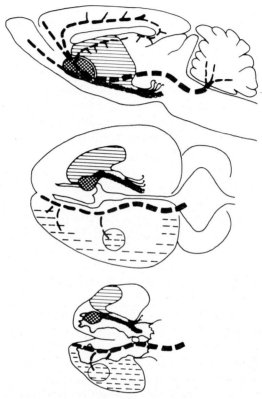

Fig. 7. Schematic diagram of three catecholamine fiber systems. From the locus coeruleus of the medulla to the cerebellum, hippocampus, and cortex runs the dorsal noradrenaline bundle (dashes). From the ventral midbrain to the olfactory tubercle runs the mesolimbic dopamine system (scrambled markings and cross hatch). From the substantia nigra to the caudate nucleus runs the nigrostriatal dopamine system (black lines). It is questionable whether these last two should be separated; and it is likely that at least one of them runs beyond the diagrammed targets because dopamine is found in the cortex. The raphe-paleo-cortex serotonin system is not shown: it starts between the noradrenaline and the dopamine systems and runs to the paleocortex (and likely also to parts of the neocortex).

of the midbrain and caudal part of forebrain. They run a shorter course ending mainly in structures below the cortex, i.e., in parts of the extrapyramidal motor system (which might be the main control system for purposive instrumental behavior) and in some poorly understood centers of the olfactory forebrain. Most likely not all of the fibers end at their main subcortical stations, for dopamine itself was found along with noradrenaline in the cortex.

For all of these amine fiber systems one property stood out; namely, there was a restricted source of origin, together with a very wide radius of influence. The noradrenaline, serotonin, and dopamine systems thus suggest a central triad of command stations deep within the brain.

These fibers pervaded the drive-reward systems in such a way as to match the drive-reward maps (German and Bowden, 1974). New maps based on the theory that these were reward neurons showed new rewarding locations that tracked the noradrenaline pathway toward the medulla, and the dopamine pathway towards the substantia nigra (Fig. 3; Crow, 1971; Ritter and Stein,

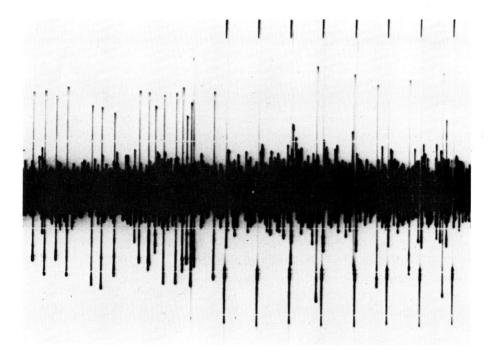

Fig. 8. Silencing of lateral hypothalamic spikes during brain reward stimulation. The very large spikes (going off the figure) in the second half of the trace are shock artifacts from the self-administered train of rewarding brain stimulation. The large spikes in the first half of the trace are action potentials recorded from a large lateral hypothalamic neuron. The interval between shock artifacts is 25 msec (shocks at 40/sec). (From Ito, 1972.)

1973). While stimulation at the sources of the two different catecholamines both appeared to be rewarding, some interesting differences appeared. When stimulation was applied at the source of the noradrenaline system in locus coeruleus, the behavior caused was quiet and paced. When the stimulation was applied instead at one source of the dopamine pathways, in the substantia nigra, the behavior was much more frenzied: it appeared more highly "motivated" (Crow, 1972a, b).

Furthering the view that these could be reward neurons were pharmacological studies too numerous to mention here. Chemicals such as amphetamine, which liberate catecholamines from their inactive "capsules", were found to promote hedonic states in humans and added to self-stimulation behavior in animal experiments. Chemicals which blocked the degradation of catecholamines such as MAO inhibitors, and others which blocked inactivation by reuptake (e.g., imipramine) added to these positive effects. On the other hand, chemicals such as haloperidol and chlorpromazine (which block catecholamine receptors), caused depressed conditions in both humans and animals, and in addition blocked brain reward behavior. In sum, the drug studies were consistent with the view that catecholamine neurons could well be reward neurons.

Another source of support came from studies of lesions which damaged the CNS, and were supposed to have specially damaging effects on catecholamine neurons, either destroying the cell bodies or their active endings. When lesions of this kind were placed in the dopamine bundles (or when catecholamine poisons were applied in the ventricles where they presumably had relatively widespread effects) the results were to abolish reward and drive behaviors, almost exactly mimicking the lateral hypothalamic syndrome referred to earlier (Ungerstedt, 1971b; Stricker and Zigmond, 1974). Brain reward behavior was abolished by this kind of ventricular poisoning. In other experiments it was also greatly set back, or altogether absent, after electrolytic lesions applied to the origin of the main ascending noradrenaline pathway (M.E. Olds, private communication; Ellman, private communication). When chemical lesions were placed so as to directly affect only the secondary noradrenaline pathway (directed at the medial hypothalamus) there were quite opposite effects, which apparently mimicked the medial lesions that caused animals to overeat (Ahlskog and Hoebel, 1972). It was surprising that this catecholamine lesion had such a different effect from the one in the dopamine bundle, but this was assumed to be due to subtle differences in function.

In other experiments (Pickel et al., 1974), electrolytic lesions in the main noradrenaline fiber system caused a great regrowth and proliferation of the damaged fibers. This brought them in quite a different way into accord with the self-stimulation data, because the time course of this remarkable regrowth matched well the time course of a well known (but rarely reported) behavioral change. This was that self-stimulation behavior improved (thresholds declining and rates increasing) for a period of about 2–3 weeks after probe implantation. The improvement progressed steadily from the time or surgery whether or not the animals were provided with any stimulation during the 3 week period. The surprising proliferation of catecholamine fibers during the 3 weeks after surgery, matching as it did the improvement of self-stimulation (whose probes must have damaged some catecholamine fibers), may thus explain what has heretofore been a mystery to me (Olds, 1958). Another important link may herewith be forged connecting catecholamine systems to reward behaviors.

Even stronger support for the catecholamine theory of reward is the finding that direct application of catecholamines into the ventricle has positive effects on brain reward behavior, either restoring it if it had been blocked by drugs or lesions, or promoting it if stimulation be applied at or near threshold levels (Wise et al., 1973).

Many of the experiments that pointed strongly toward dopamine or noradrenaline being involved in brain reward or drive behavior pointed ambiguously at the third important amine, serotonin (Porschel and Ninteman, 1971). Drugs that manipulated this neurohumor could be positive or negative with respect to brain reward behavior, depending on other ill-defined aspects of a given experiment. Quite different researches were more clear in pointing to an involvement of serotonin in quieting the animal for sleep or in suppressing pain (Jouvet, 1974; Yunger and Harvey, 1973). It seemed possible, therefore, that some self-stimulation aimed at pain reduction might be promoted by serotonergic drugs, while other behavior aimed at producing a euphoric state might well be damped by the same drugs.

In any event, the two catecholamines were strongly related to the basic drives and to rewards. Before leaving the topic, it is fair to set forth the substance of a current debate about the noradrenaline neurons and the dopamine neurons with evidence enumerated for and against each of them being "reward neurons".

Noradrenaline neurons

The fibers radiate from the locus coeruleus. Because they spread to cerebellum, diencephalon, paleocortex and neocortex, they have the possible neuroanatomical character of a major integrative net. Self-stimulation was observed at most locations where these fibers were concentrated. This made it possible to suggest them to be reward neurons. Pharmacological evidence was not incompatible with the idea that noradrenaline neurons had reward functions, although most of the evidence could equally well be applied to a dopamine theory.

Blocking the conversion of dopamine to noradrenaline with the drug disulfiram caused brain reward behavior to cease, whereas application of noradrenaline in the ventricles at this time rapidly restored the behavior (Stein, 1974). However, the blocking drug also caused many signs of general dishabilitation, and this "disease" was to some degree cured by the ventricular application of noradrenaline, so that there may not have been any specific effect on brain reward mechanisms. Moreover, blocking with a different drug seemed to leave self-stimulation intact. Cutting ascending fibers in a region where locus coeruleus axons passed through the midbrain caused self-stimulation behavior to cease in some cases, even if the behavior was provoked by stimulation in non-noradrenaline areas (Stein, 1974).

All these facts pointed to noradrenaline neurons as candidates for reward neuron status, but there were substantial arguments on the other side. One was that a very large deletion of locus coeruleus neurons by ablations in and around this nucleus sometimes did, but at other times did *not* cause a lasting change in self-stimulation behavior (Clavier, 1976). The large loss of noradrenaline neurons was incompatible with the relative lack of permanent loss of self-stimulation if these were in fact a large family of reward neurons. This made it seem that noradrenaline, while it might be involved in or related to brain reward in the normal animal, was nevertheless only tangentially related in some cases. Pointing in the same direction, pharmacological manipulations that caused near depletion of all noradrenaline in the forebrain, or at least in the telencephalon, did not cause a major and lasting change in self-stimulation behavior (Breese and Cooper, 1976).

Those were the two major difficulties, but there was another unclear problem, namely, that drugs which caused catecholamines to be freed from synaptic vesicles and from neurons, and thus to become active in the interstitial fluid, seemed to promote rather than retard self-stimulation behavior. This left the question: why were the animals stimulating the fibers if they no longer contained catecholamines? I conclude from all this conflicting data that noradrenaline is in some way involved in the reward process in the normal animal, but is not the key factor in most brain-stimulation reward processes. For example, noradrenaline might be involved in the inhibitory control of negative emotional mechanisms which would themselves be incompatible with reward behavior. If so, noradrenaline might mediate reward when this consisted in the suppression of aversive mechanisms; and noradrenaline depletion might release central wellsprings of aversion or depression, thereby temporarily suppressing other reward processes until the system had adapted to the new low noradrenaline levels.

Dopamine neurons

The dopamine-containing fibers from the zona compacta of the substantia nigra and from the adjacent ventral tegmental area have a radiation similar to, but not as extensive as, that of the locus coeruleus system. They could nevertheless be a major integrative net for the forebrain, although from anatomical appearances they would seem to be of secondary importance in comparison with the locus coeruleus system. Their output is more addressed to the extrapyramidal system than to the cortex, and thus they were thought to be possibly involved in response execution rather than basic integration. However, there were also pathways to many parts of the paleocortex, and even to neocortex. They would be more likely than locus coeruleus neurons to receive convergent inputs from the olfactory and telencephalic centers. This might provide them with afferents from discriminated rewards and punishments, or from distance receptors as Crow (1973) suggested, and make them less likely to receive visceral afferent messages directly.

Brain reward behavior was better correlated with the dopamine system than with the noradrenaline one. Thus, with probes implanted in its pathways, self-stimulation was more nearly "pure"; i.e., less contaminated by apparently aversive side-effects. This was true in my experience for lateral hypothalamus, and for some parts of the far-medial hypothalamus, and for the cingulate cortex.

Pharmacologically, most of the evidence supporting the existence of noradrenergic reward neurons applied equally well to the dopamine hypothesis, in addition to which there is other evidence favoring dopamine more directly. Blocking the conversion of tyrosine to dopamine (which also blocked the further step to noradrenaline) always stopped self-stimulation behavior (Stinus and Thierry, 1973). Adding l-DOPA, which bypassed the block, restored self-stimulation. Cutting the dopamine fiber bundle from the substantia nigra to the caudate nucleus stopped self-stimulation in the caudate nucleus (Phillips et al., 1976). This could be accomplished unilaterally; and the retained self-stimulation of probes placed on the other side gave at least some evidence that the reward mechanism rather than the behavior was impaired. The effect was irreversible. "Neurotoxic" manipulations which caused nearly total depletion of dopamine in the forebrain also caused near-complete abolition of self-stimulation behavior (Breese and Cooper, 1976).

Proponents of the noradrenaline neurons had some rebuttals but these served more to suggest that an abrupt drop in telencephalic noradrenaline levels could block dopaminergic and other self-stimulation than to displace the dopamine hypothesis. Transection in the midbrain behind the dopamine system sometimes stopped self-stimulation even though the behavior was caused by stimulation in more anteriorly placed dopamine pathways. This was given as evidence that the noradrenaline path transected was a prerequisite to the self-stimulation. In other studies, blocking the conversion of dopamine to noradrenaline by disulfiram stopped self-stimulation and this could be restored by placing noradrenaline in the ventricles (Stein, 1974). However, both lesions in noradrenaline neuron systems and neurotoxic damage to them could apparently be repaired by time. Thus, either the telencephalon has mechanisms of supersensitivity which allow it to get along on very little noradrenaline, or a loss of noradrenaline neurons can be compensated for by other mechanisms. These rebuttals therefore left the view that while dopamine was essential for at least some self-stimulation, and possibly for all, noradrenaline was possibly not essential.

Another objection to the dopamine neuron view, which carried more weight, was speculative in nature. It turned on the idea that the dopamine system, being part of the extrapyramidal system, was more involved in correlating the response with the reward, or in organizing the response, than in the rewarding condition itself. One experiment indicated that extremely gross self-stimulation behaviors were still possible after cutting a dopamine pathway even though pedal-press behaviors were no longer possible (Huston and Ornstein, 1976). In another experiment, food-reward learning of pedal behavior disappeared but there was still gross movement toward goals, and consummatory behavior still occurred (Grossman, 1976). The possibility remained, however, that in these cases the cuts left dopamine fibers with access to extremely gross behavior controllers, but removed the dopamine afferents of pedal behavior controllers. Thus the dopamine-reward hypothesis survived.

I would guess from this set of data that the dopamine neurons could well be a final common pathway in the reward system, acting in one direction to inhibit certain types of drive neurons, or in another direction to cement connections between drives and other neuronal systems — or both. Why such neurons would point most selectively to the extrapyramidal system, to similar components of the paleocortex system, and to cingulate cortex is not clear. To judge from neuroanatomical arrangement alone, the noradrenaline neurons are better suited than the dopamine ones to inhibit lateral hypothalamic drive neurons and, at the same time, to modify their functional connections in the cortex.

UNITS

A fourth set of experiments was aimed at explaining some of the other results, by means of recording directly from neurons in and near the lateral hypothalamic centers.

In one set of studies (Hamburg, 1971) neurons were recorded from the middle part of the lateral hypothalamus (an area which is sometimes called the "feeding center") and from more posterior parts of the lateral hypothalamus and from adjacent areas in the substantia nigra. The recordings were made in chronically prepared animals which were hungry and were provided with food to eat. In all parts of this rather extensive region there were neurons that were decelerated during eating. Analysis showed that it was not the eating that stopped them so much as the cessation of instrumental behaviors. The units were firing briskly during the high drive state which was used in these tests. When a dish of feed was presented, the neuronal activity subsided abruptly as the animal began to eat; this happened even though eating, of course, could not have caused the metabolic deficiency to subside in this brief time. If the experimenter tried to remove the dish, the animal would counter the effort by various strategies to retain it. During this period of renewed instrumental behavior the unit activity would recur even though the animal was still consuming food. Thus, it was the cessation of instrumental behavior rather than the occurrence of consummatory behavior that matched the cessation of this particular unit activity.

The question arose, therefore, whether these neurons were the cause or the consequence of the instrumental behavior. Some light was shed on this by experiments showing that neurons recorded from the same area were activated by promising, conditioned stimulus (CS) signals which turned the animals toward the food tray (Olds, 1973; Linseman and Olds, 1973). In these tests (Fig. 9) the hypothalamic unit response occurred first, and the observed behavior some milliseconds later; thus, the unit activity did not appear to result from the behavior. Because conditioned stimuli activated these units, but only after the animals had been deprived of food, it looked as if both the CS and the deficiency condition were required to activate the units. Because the units became active first, and the food approach behavior came second, the former presumably mediated the latter. Because the conditioned stimulus which activated these units also caused a temporarily heightened state of behavioral arousal or drive, it appeared that these neurons might in fact mediate one component of drive, namely, the one that directly instigates, i.e., instrumental behavior. This would account for their being turned on jointly by deprivation plus environmental signals, and also for their being terminated as soon as instrumental behavior stopped. Were they also directly inhibited by rewards?

That this might be so was suggested by experiments of Ito (1972). In his studies, the vast majority of neurons recorded from the same lateral hypothalamic areas was directly (though usually temporarily) inhibited by the onset of a rewarding brain stimulus (Fig. 8). A substantially smaller minority of units here was driven by the brain reward. In more anterior regions of the medial forebrain bundle at the preoptic level, the majority of neurons was accelerated or driven by the brain reward, and a much smaller number was decelerated. Taken together these studies implicate a family of neurons in the lateral hypothalamus that are activated during levels of heightened instrumental performance and quieted by rewards.

Furthering the idea that these might be drive neurons which are inhibited by rewarding stimuli were experiments on morphine-addicted rats (Kerr et al., 1974). "Drive" and "reward" were both easily manipulatable in this situation. The withdrawal state (the drive state) could be heightened by application of naloxone (which counters morphine). The reward state could be induced (and the drive state thus lowered) by application of morphine. Neurons of the lateral hypothalamus were most often accelerated by the drive-inducing manipulation and quieted by the rewarding one. Medial hypothalamic units, on the contrary,

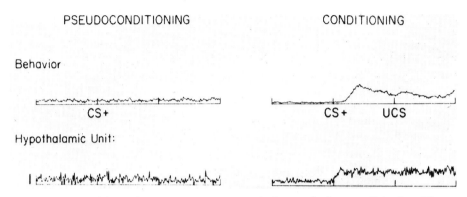

Fig. 9. Behavior and hypothalamic unit responses before and after conditioning. The upper trace portrays the average output of a detector attached to the head that measured head movements in arbitrary units. The lower trace represents the spike frequency of a lateral hypothalamic unit, the vertical bar at the left representing a rate of 5 spikes/sec. The traces represent 3 sec. At the end of the first sec a tone (CS+) was started which then continued to the end. During conditioning a pellet dispenser (UCS) was triggered at the end of 2 sec. Prior to conditioning (pseudoconditioning) the tone caused minor changes in the unit and behavior responses. After conditioning it caused behavior changes with a 90–170 msec latency and unit changes with a 20–40 msec latency. (From Linseman and Olds, 1973.)

were accelerated during the reward condition, and decelerated by the rewarding one.

A different set of candidates for drive neuron status, also inhibited by rewards, was added by the studies in monkeys of Hayward and Vincent (1970) and of Vincent et al. (1972) on osmotic detectors (thirst neurons?) and their responses to drinking (water reward). Neurons were recorded from a part of the lateral preoptic area, and from the smaller nucleus supraopticus nearby, which contains vasopressin-secreting cells. "Thirst" and water preservation mechanisms were directly triggered by piping hyperosmotic solutions directly into the carotid body. This caused excessive osmotic concentrations and thus a perceived water deficiency. It activated a group of neurons in the lateral preoptic region, which were thus conceived of as being possible osmodetectors, responding directly to the "water deficiency". Their response was correlated with a burst of activity in the nearby vasopressin-containing neurons of the supraoptic nucleus, which presumably released vasopressin (which then acts upon the kidney to retain water).

Both the osmodetector neurons and the vasopressin neurons had their responses to the osmotic stimulus reversed by the ensuing drinking; the reversal was immediate, well preceding the compensation of the effective water deficit. If they were drive neurons, this suggested again that drive neurons in this general region might be inhibited by rewarding inputs. At least, there was a temporary suppression of the activity caused by the rewarding input.

There were also reward neuron candidates nearby. Interdigitated with, or slightly offset from, the osmodetector neurons was a second family of preoptic area elements, whose activity was suppressed by the osmotic stimulus and accelerated during drinking. At first sight these seemed like obvious reward neuron candidates but Rolls objected — pointing out that such neurons might be responding similarly to low drive levels and to actual rewarding conditions (being activated in both cases). His view was that true reward neurons would respond exclusively to rewards and be insensitive to drive levels, except, of course, insofar as these might themselves accentuate responses to reward stimuli. This did not seem to be a devastating argument against the idea that Vincent's "drinking neurons" might be reward neurons, but it did make it important to consider other units that might be accelerated by rewards, but have no response to drive levels alone.

Neurons of this kind were evidently observed in the experiments of Rolls and his group (Rolls, 1975, 1976; Burton et al., 1976), done with monkeys. Neurons were recorded from the lateral hypothalamus and adjacent "substantia-innominata" regions. Cells responded to visual food objects, and some to the taste of food. Some of the responses were accelerations, whereas others were decelerations. The background firing rates were reported to be unchanged by drive level manipulations; but responses to the "rewards" were augmented by the drive. These units thus responded not to drives but to conditioned stimuli related to rewards, or to real rewards; in addition, their response to rewards increased when drive levels were heightened.

In summary, a small but growing body of evidence points to a family of neurons whose firing rate is jointly controlled by excess or deficiency conditions, and by external stimulus inputs. The kinds of effect observed most often were: acceleration by drive-increasing manipulations, or by conditioned stimuli associated with rewards, and deceleration during consummatory behavior — or complete suppression by rewarding stimulation. The deceleration occurred immediately, i.e., before the deficiency condition was remedied. There is a smaller family of observations pointing to nearby neurons being accelerated directly by rewards, but the data are still unclear. Some of the neurons which were accelerated during drinking might be "low drive neurons", unrelated to rewards. The accelerated neurons of Rolls' experiments might have been activated mainly by conditioned stimuli related to rewards. Still, the taste neurons of Rolls and the drinking neurons of Vincent, as well as the brain-reward neurons of Ito (1972), Keene (1973) and Rolls (1975, 1976), all suggest that reward neurons might overlap drive neurons in this area. If not, they most certainly project there from surrounding areas (to mediate the observed inhibition).

THEORY AND PERSPECTIVES

The concept of "drive" can be divided into two parts. One is an incentive part, and suggests that certain neurons would become active during approach conditions, and would be the motivation involved in operant behavior. The other is an alarm part, and suggests that some neurons might become active when supplies become dangerously low, or when harm is imminent. If so, these "alarm" neurons could be inhibited by reward elements that signal the end of the danger. The incentive kind of drive could be inhibited by rewards that trigger consummatory responses and suppress operant behaviors. It seems possible that the noradrenaline system might inhibit alarm neurons and mediate their appropriate connections to instrumental behaviors, and the dopamine system might have a similar action or incentive neurons. This would put both catecholamine systems in the reward category, and put both kinds of drive neurons outside this category. For reasons I will not go into here, I suspect that the drive neurons involve muscarinic actions of acetylcholine, and are involved in the transport of peptide hormones.

The opponent process interaction between catecholamine systems and drive neurons might be the main target of transections between medial and lateral hypothalamus. The other two lesions affecting approach behavior (in the caudate nucleus and in the amygdala) had to do with a different problem, viz., the channeling of drives onto specific targets. The experiments of Garcia and Valenstein (op. cit.) pointed to changeable targets of brain stimulated drives and also of naturally occurring ones. The locus of Valenstein's probes and of lesions countering Garcia's effects pointed to the lateral hypothalamic region. One interpretation was that the same drive or learned drive neurons that we have been talking about had not only some modifiability on the input side but also some at the other end. That is, they might have changed output connections depending on "good" or "bad" after effects of consummatory behavior.

The "law of learning" for this changing of drive targets might be that the drive axons would become connected to basal ganglia and cortex cell assemblies active at the time of drive inhibition. The long-predicted hypothalamocortical axons to mediate this have recently been amply demonstrated with horseradish peroxidase (Kievet and Kuypers, 1975). Thus, the possibility exists that drive neurons which are excited by visceral inputs, hormones and conditioned signals, are silenced by rewards and become functionally connected during development or learning to basal ganglia and cortex cell assemblies which are active at the time of their "silencing" (Fig. 10).

The widespread ramifications of the catecholamine axons suggested that, if these were reward neurons, they must have other functions besides that of inhibiting lateral hypothalamic neurons. This brings me to my final set of points. There are several different ways that reward neurons should be involved in more specialized behavioral steering mechanisms. At least three different ways would be appropriate to different levels of CNS organization (Table I). At the level of motor skills, reward might directly cause "connections" to form between a warp of axons and a woof of dendrites. This kind of process would

420

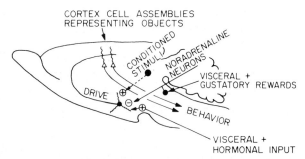

CORTEX CELL ASSEMBLIES
REPRESENTING OBJECTS

VISCERAL +
GUSTATORY REWARDS

VISCERAL +
HORMONAL INPUT

Fig. 10. A new "drive-reduction theory of reward". Noradrenaline neurons from the medulla would be triggered by rewarding gustatory and visceral inputs. They would act to silence drive neurons housed in or near the lateral hypothalamus (some of which could be dopamine neurons). Silencing of the drive neurons would cause them to become coupled to cortex cell assemblies active at the time. ⊕ = excitatory and ⊖ = inhibitory connections.

fit readily into the cerebellar cortex, where the parallel fibers form such a warp and the Purkinje dendrites the woof.

At a second level there would be sequential memory, as when a rat runs a maze or a human remembers how he got somewhere, and takes the same route a second time. In these cases, recordings would be made of successive events on the first occurrence of a behavior sequence. These would have some characteristics of a movie film, or a magnetic tape recording; but a better metaphor would be the sequential memory locations in a computer. Successive small episodes with their sensory, motor and reward components would be recorded in sequential memory addresses. Later, near-matching sensory inputs would re-arouse a memory, and this would re-arouse its successors. A "dry run" (without behavior) would occur first. If an appropriate reward memory was discovered among the near successors, this would cause a predisposition toward expression of some of the recorded behaviors. From observations in the hippocampus of highly organized axonal systems that run like the digit lines of a computer core-memory through oriented dendrite systems that look like the

TABLE I

DIFFERENT LEARNING FUNCTIONS POSTULATED TO INVOLVE DIFFERENT BRAIN SYSTEMS, DIFFERENT MECHANISMS OF LEARNING AND PERFORMANCE, AND DIFFERENT ROLES OF REWARD

Function	Possible anatomical correlate	Mechanism	Role of reward
Learning motor skills	Cerebellum	Sensorimotor connections	"Stamp-in" connections
Learning behavior sequences	Hippocampus	Convert temporal sequences to spatial memory arrays	Cause rewarded behaviors to recur
Learning maps and objects	Cortex	Make behavioral-topographic maps of external objects	Cause object to be pursued

memory lines of such a device, it has seemed possible that this kind of process might occur there.

At a third level, there would be representations of objects and object-arrangements. These would be sensorimotor or cognitive maps, with control elements at any one node pointing toward a behavior with one hand, and toward a second node (the representation of the expected outcome) with the other. These control elements could be the layer 5 pyramidal cells, while the nodes could be the "columns" of the neocortex. Motive cells at a second node would need to "point back" to motivate the control elements pointing toward them. The motive cells could be either other pyramidal cells or cells of different type. Reward in this kind of system would serve to connect drives to motive elements of those columns, or to cell assemblies which were active at the time of the rewarding events. This would be the same function which I indicated earlier by saying that drive neurons might become attached to cell assemblies which are active at the time of their being inhibited.

The suggestions contained here, therefore, are that reward neurons may exist, and have the following four functions: (1) to inhibit drive neurons in the lateral hypothalamus, (2) to facilitate certain sensorimotor connections, (3) to plant "emotional" codes on certain sequential memories, and (4) to connect drives to cell assemblies in neocortex which were active at the time of the reward. It was also suggested that noradrenaline neurons might be the reward neurons addressed to negative drives and dopamine neurons to positive drives.

SUMMARY

Electric stimulation in certain parts of the brain causes behavioral signs of reward: mammals, at least, seek out the brain stimulus as if it were a goal. Lesion studies, pharmacological studies, unit studies, and anatomical studies, mainly from other laboratories, are reviewed here with a view to explaining these observations. Lesions in these parts of the brain cause deficient goal-directed behaviors; animals no longer learn tasks for food or water rewards, and temporarily do not eat or drink. Learned avoidance behaviors are also deficient. The regions of the brain where these effects have been best obtained were parts where fibers containing noradrenaline, dopamine, and serotonin were concentrated. Fitting in with this, pharmacological studies showed that electrically stimulated and natural reward behaviors depended on dopamine and noradrenaline in some special way, and relief from pain depended on serotonin. It seemed possible that these were all involved in different kinds of reward by mediating the inhibition of aversive conditions or drives. For reasons I do not spell out completely here, I have proposed that (1) serotonin inhibits a kind of aversive condition that depends on the external environment; (2) noradrenaline inhibits a different kind of aversive condition that depends on the internal environment; and (3) dopamine inhibits a milder kind of drive that has no aversive component but which is involved in most normal behavior. In several different experiments, neurons were directly recorded from "hypothalamic reward centers" during behavior. Such neurons responded to a variety of conditions in a way that suggested they were "drive neurons" rather than "reward neurons". In experiments where deficiency conditions were imposed, the majority of the affected neurons was accelerated by these manipulations. In experiments where conditioned stimuli related to rewards were used, the same result was obtained. In experiments where goals and consummatory behaviors were used, on the other hand, the majority of affected units was decelerated. In iontophoretic application studies with noradrenaline, the majority of affected units showed a deceleration in firing rate. In all these series of observations, there was a smaller group of neurons showing opposite responses. In histofluorescence studies, noradrenaline or dopamine terminals were found in the hypothalamic "reward" regions, and in horseradish peroxidase studies neurons were observed with projections directly to neocortex. For all these reasons, it is concluded that drive ("command"?) neurons in this area might be inhibited by noradrenaline- or dopamine-containing "reward neurons". By this means alone, or plus some added action, the inhibited neurons might, at the time of their inhibition by rewards, become functionally connected to active cortex cell assemblies. This could make environmental objects which are reflected by the activity of these cortical cell groups into targets of pursuit on later occasions.

REFERENCES

Ahlskog, J.E. and Hoebel, B.G. (1972) Overeating and obesity from damage to a noradrenergic system in the brain. *Science*, 182: 17–27.

Anand, B.K. (1961) Nervous regulation of food intake. *Physiol. Rev.*, 41: 677–708.

Balinska, H. (1968) The hypothalamic lesions: effects on appetitive and aversive behavior in rats. *Acta Biol. exp. (Warszawa)*, 28: 47–56.

Bishop, M.P., Elder, S.T. and Heath, R.G. (1963) Intracranial self-stimulation in man. *Science*, 140: 394–395.

Breese, G.R. and Cooper, B.R. (1976) Effects of catecholamine-depleting drugs and amphetamine on self-stimulation obtained from lateral hypothalamus, substantia nigra and locus coeruleus. In *Brain-Stimulation Reward*, A. Wauquier and E.T. Rolls (Eds.), North-Holland Publ., Amsterdam, pp. 190–194.

Bursten, B. and Delgado, J.M.R. (1958) Positive reinforcement induced by intracranial stimulation in the monkey. *J. comp. physiol. Psychol.*, 51: 6–10.

Burton, M.J., Mora, F. and Rolls, E.T. (1976) Neurophysiological convergence of natural and brain stimulation reward in the lateral hypothalamus of squirrel and rhesus monkeys. In *Brain-Stimulation Reward*, A. Wauquier and E.T. Rolls (Eds.), North-Holland Publ., Amsterdam, pp. 101–104.

Clavier, R.M. (1976) Brain stem self-stimulation: catecholamine or non-catecholamine mediation? In *Brain-Stimulation Reward*, A. Wauquier and E.T. Rolls (Eds.), North-Holland Publ., Amsterdam, pp. 239–250.

Crow, T.J. (1971) The relation between electrical self-stimulation sites and catecholamine-containing neurones in the rat mesencephalon. *Experientia (Basel)*, 27: 662.

Crow, T.J. (1972a) A map of the rat mesencephalon for electrical self-stimulation. *Brain Res.*, 36: 265–273.

Crow, T.J. (1972b) Catecholamine-containing neurones and electrical self-stimulation: 1.A review of some data. *Psychol. Med.*, 2: 414–421.

Crow, T.J. (1973) Catecholamine-containing neurones and electrical self-stimulation: 2. A theoretical interpretation and some psychiatric implications. *Psychol. Med.*, 3: 66–73.

De La Torre, J.C. (1972) *Dynamics of Brain Monoamines*. Plenum, New York.

Deutsch, J.A. (1960) *The Structural Basis of Behavior*. Chicago Univ. Press, Chicago, Ill.

Gallistel, C.R. (1973) Self-stimulation: the neurophysiology of reward and motivation. In *The Physiological Basis of Memory*, J.A. Deutsch (Ed.), Academic Press, New York, pp. 175–267.

Garcia, J. and Ervin, F.R. (1968) Gustatory-visceral and telereceptor-cutaneous conditioning — adaptation in internal and external milieus. *Commun. behav. Biol.*, Part A, 1: 389–415.

German, D.C. and Bowden, D.M. (1974) Catecholamine systems as the neural substrate for intracranial self-stimulation: a hypothesis. *Brain Res.*, 73: 381–419.

Grossman, S.P. (1976) Surgical interventions that result in a loss of complex learned behavior: are pathways essential for the reinforcing effects of reward interrupted? In *Brain-Stimulation Reward*, A. Wauquier and E.T. Rolls (Eds.), North-Holland Publ., Amsterdam, pp. 385–395.

Hamburg, M.D. (1971) Hypothalamic unit activity and eating behavior. *Amer. J. Physiol.*, 220: 980–985.

Hayward, J.N. and Vincent, J.D. (1970) Osmosensitive single neurones in the hypothalamus of unanesthetized monkeys. *J. Physiol. (Lond.)*, 210: 947–972.

Hebb, D.O. (1949) *The Organization of Behavior*. Wiley, New York.

Hebb, D.O. (1955) Drives and the C.N.S. (conceptual nervous system). *Psychol Rev.*, 62: 243–254.

Herberg, L.J. (1963) Seminal ejaculation following positively reinforcing electrical stimulation of the rat hypothalamus. *J. comp. physiol. Psychol.*, 56: 679–685.

Hull, C.L. (1943) *Principles of Behavior*. Appleton-Century-Crofts, New York.

Huston, J.P. and Borbély, A.A. (1974) The thalamic rat: general behavior, operant learning with rewarding hypothalamic stimulation, and effects of amphetamine. *Physiol. Behav.*, 12: 433–448.

Huston, J.P. and Ornstein, K. (1976) Effects of various diencephalic lesions on hypothalamic self-stimulation. In *Brain-Stimulation Reward*, A. Wauquier and E.T. Rolls (Eds.), North-Holland Publ., Amsterdam, pp. 51–53.

Ito, M. (1972) Excitability of medial forebrain bundle neurons during self-stimulation behavior. *J. Neurophysiol.*, 35: 652–664.

Iversen, L.L. (1967) *The Uptake and Storage of Noradrenaline in Sympathetic Nerves.* Cambridge University Press, Cambridge.

Jouvet, M. (1974) Monoaminergic regulation of the sleep-waking cycle of the cat. In *The Neurosciences, Third Study Program*, F.O. Schmitt and F.G. Worden (Eds.), MIT Press, Cambridge, Mass., pp. 499–508.

Keene, J.J. (1973) Reward-associated inhibition and pain-associated excitation lasting seconds in single intralaminar thalamic units. *Brain Res.*, 64: 211–224.

Kerr, F.W., Triplett, J.N. and Beeler, G.W. (1974) Reciprocal (push-pull) effects of morphine on single units in the ventromedian and lateral hypothalamus and influences on other nuclei; with a comment on methadone effects during withdrawal from morphine. *Brain Res.*, 74: 81–103.

Kievit, J. and Kuypers, H.G.J.M. (1975) Basal forebrain and hypothalamic connections to frontal and parietal cortex in the rhesus monkey. *Science*, 187: 660–662.

Klüver, H. and Bucy, P.C. (1937) Psychic blindness and other symptoms following bilateral temporal lobectomy in rhesus monkey. *Amer. J. Physiol.*, 119: 352–353.

Le Magnen, J., Devos, M., Gaudilliere, J.-P., Louis-Sylvestre, J. and Tallon, S. (1973) Role of a lipostatic mechanism in regulation by feeding of energy balance in rats. *J. comp. physiol. Psychol.*, 84: 1–23.

Linseman, M.A. and Olds, J. (1973) Activity changes in rat hypothalamus, preoptic area and striatum associated with Pavlovian conditioning. *J. Neurophysiol.*, 36: 1038–1050.

Miller, N.E. (1957) Experiments on motivation. *Science*, 126: 1271–1278.

Mogensen, G.J. and Faiers, A. (1976)·Do olfactory inputs reach the substantia nigra and locus coeruleus? In *Brain-Stimulation Reward*, A. Wauquier and E.T. Rolls (Eds.), North-Holland Publ., Amsterdam, pp. 579–585.

Olds, J. (1958) In *CIBA Foundation Symp. on Neurological Basis of Behaviour*, G.E.W. Wolstenholme and C.M. O'Connor (Eds.), Churchill, London, p. 89.

Olds, J. (1962) Hypothalamic substrates of reward. *Physiol. Rev.*, 42: 554–604.

Olds, J. (1972) Learning and the hippocampus. *Rev. Canad. Biol.*, 31: 215–238.

Olds, M.E. (1973) Short-term changes in the firing pattern of hypothalamic neurons during Pavlovian conditioning. *Brain Res.*, 58: 95–116.

Olds, M.E. and Olds, J. (1963) Approach-avoidance analysis of rat diencephalon. *J. comp. Neurol.*, 120: 259–295.

Phillips, A.G., Carter, D.A. and Fibiger, H.C. (1976) The dopaminergic nigro-striatial reward system. In *Brain-Stimulation Reward*, A. Wauquier and E.T. Rolls (Eds.), North-Holland Publ., Amsterdam, pp. 272–280.

Phillips, M.I. and Olds, J. (1969) Unit activity: motivation dependent responses from midbrain neurons. *Science*, 165: 1269–1271.

Phillis, J.W. (1970) *The Pharmacology of Synapses.* Pergamon Press, New York.

Pickel, V.M., Segal, M. and Bloom, F.E. (1974) Axonal proliferation following lesions of cerebellar peduncles. A combined fluorescence microscopic and radioautographic study. *J. comp. Neurol.*, 155: 43–60.

Poschel, B.P.H. and Ninteman, F.W. (1971) Intracranial reward and the forebrain's serotonergic mechanism: studies employing parachlorophenylalanine and para-chloro-amphetamine. *Physiol. Behav.*, 7: 39–46.

Ritter, S. and Stein, L. (1973) Self-stimulation of noradrenergic cell group (A6) in locus coeruleus of rats. *J. comp. physiol. Psychol.*, 85: 443–452.

Roberts, W.W. (1958) Both rewarding and punishing effects from stimulation of posterior hypothalamus of cat with same electrode at same intensity. *J. comp. physiol. Psychol.*, 51: 400–407.

Roberts, W.W., Steinberg, M.L. and Means, L.W. (1967) Hypothalamic mechanisms for sexual, aggressive, and other motivational behaviors in the opossum, *Didelphis virginiana. J. comp. physiol. Psychol.*, 64: 1–15.

Rolls, E.T. (1974) The neural basis of brain-stimulation reward. *Progr. Neurobiol.*, 3: 71–160.

Rolls, E.T. (1975) *The Brain and Reward.* Pergamon Press, Oxford.

Rolls, E.T. (1976) The neurophysiological basis of brain-stimulation reward. In *Brain-Stimulation Reward*, A. Wauquier and E.T. Rolls (Eds.), North-Holland Publ., Amsterdam, pp. 65–87.

Roth, S.R., Schwartz, M. and Teitelbaum, P. (1973) Failure of recovered lateral hypothalamic rats to learn specific food aversions. *J. comp. physiol. Psychol.*, 83: 184–197.

Segal, M. and Bloom, F. (1974a) The action of norepinephrine in the rat hippocampus. I. Iontophoretic studies. *Brain Res.*, 72: 79–97.

Segal, M. and Bloom, F. (1974b) The action of norepinephrine in the rat hippocampus. II. Activation of the input pathway. *Brain Res.*, 72: 99–114.

Siggins, G.R., Hoffer, B.J. and Bloom, F.E. (1969) Cyclic adenosine monophosphate: possible mediator for norepinephrine effects on cerebellar Purkinje cells. *Science*, 165: 1018–1020.

Skinner, B.F. (1938) *The Behavior of Organisms: An Experimental Analysis.* Appleton-Century-Crofts, New York.

Stein, L. (1974) Norepinephrine reward pathways: role in self-stimulation, memory consolidation and schizophrenia. In *1974 Nebr. Symp. Motivation, Vol. 22*, J.K. Cole and T.B. Sonderreger (Eds.), Nebraska Univ. Press, Lincoln, Nebr., pp. 113–159.

Stinus, L. and Thierry, A.-M. (1973) Self-stimulation and catecholamines. II. Blockade of self-stimulation by treatment with alpha-methylpara-tyrosine and the reinstatement by catecholamine precursor administration. *Brain Res.*, 64: 189–198.

Stricker, E.M. and Zigmond, M.J. (1974) Effects on homeostasis of intraventricular injections of 6-hydroxydopamine in rats. *J. comp. physiol. Psychol.*, 86: 973–994.

Teitelbaum, P. and Cytawa, J. (1965) Spreading depression and recovery from lateral hypothalamic damage. *Science*, 147: 61–63.

Teitelbaum, P. and Epstein, A.N. (1962) The lateral hypothalamic syndrome: recovery of feeding and drinking after lateral hypothalamic lesions. *Psychol Rev.*, 69: 74–90.

Tolman, E.C. (1949) *Purposive Behavior in Animals and Men.* Univ. California Press, Berkeley, Calif.

Ungerstedt, U. (1971a) Stereotaxic mapping of the monoamine pathways in the rat brain. *Acta physiol. scand.*, Suppl. 367: 1–48.

Ungerstedt, U. (1971b) Aphagia and adipsia after 6-hydroxydopamine induced degeneration of the nigro-striatal dopamine system. *Acta physiol. scand.*, Suppl. 367: 95–122.

Valenstein, E.S., Cox, V.C. and Kakolewski, J.W. (1968) Modification of motivated behavior elicited by electrical stimulation of the hypothalamus. *Science*, 157: 552–554.

Valenstein, E.S., Cox, V.C. and Kakolewski, J.W. (1970) Re-examination of the role of the hypothalamus in motivation. *Psychol. Rev.*, 77: 16–31.

Villablanca, J. (1974) Presentation of films of kittens and cats with bilateral ablations of the caudate nuclei. In *Conf. Brain Mechanisms in Mental Retardation*, Oxnard, Calif., Jan. 13–16.

Vincent, J.D. and Hayward, J.N. (1970) Activity of single cells in osmoreceptor-supraoptic nuclear complex in the hypothalamus of the waking rhesus monkey. *Brain Res.*, 23: 105–108.

Vincent, J.D., Arnauld, E. and Bioulac, B. (1972) Activity of osmosensitive single cells in the hypothalamus of behaving monkey during drinking. *Brain Res.*, 44: 371–384.

Wilkinson, H.W. and Peele, T.L. (1963) Intracranial self-stimulation in cats. *J. comp. Neurol.*, 121: 425–440.

Wise, C.D., Berger, B.D. and Stein, L. (1973) Evidence of alpha-noradrenergic reward receptors and serotonergic punishment receptors in the rat brain. *Biol. Psychiat.*, 6: 3–21.

Wolstenholme, G.E.W. and O'Connor, C.M. (Eds.) (1958) *CIBA Foundation Symposium on the Neurological Basis of Behaviour.* Churchill, London.

Yunger, L.M. and Harvey, J.A. (1973) Effect of lesions in the medial forebrain bundle on three measures of pain sensitivity and noise-elicited startle. *J. comp. physiol. Psychol.*, 83: 173–183.

DISCUSSION

N.J. SPITERI: You talked about drives in general, but most of these experiments have been done in the feeding and drinking motivational systems. Were all of the catecholamine experiments done in just these two systems, or for sexual behavior as well? And also: how many experiments have been performed where people used sexual behavior as a reward, and single unit recording studies from populations of neurons?

J. OLDS: You are right about feeding and drinking being the best studied. However, electric stimulation and lesions have caused instigation and loss of sexual behavior respectively. These effects were shown with probes in both anterior and posterior hypothalamus. Operant behavior with a sexual reward has not been used in stimulation and lesion studies. It is not an easy kind of experiment for a physiological psychology laboratory because the rewards are of necessity few and far between. Therefore the studies of sexual effects of stimulation and lesions were carried out without using instrumental behaviors. Lesions in the lateral hypothalamus or in the nigrostriatal bundle have been reported to abolish several different operant responses at once, however, leaving the impression that all operant responses were temporarily disrupted. Instrumental responses directed toward food, water, temperature adjustment and the avoidance or delay of aversive stimulation were all disrupted by these lesions. It therefore appears that lesions in this part of the lateral hypothalamus, where you can cut both the nigrostriatal bundle and the mesolimbic bundle, can cause a type of motivational defect which is as broad as we have yet been able to test. By the same token, an animal under chlorpromazine has very great difficulty in performing any purposive behavior task. If he gets very close to food, so that he is almost with his feet planted in it, he goes through the response: that is the reflex part of the mechanism. The consummatory mechanisms are thus satisfactory, but the operant mechanisms are in very bad shape.

P.B. BRADLEY: Would it be reasonable to suggest from what you have said that the cholinergic mechanisms are not involved in reward behavior.

J. OLDS: The muscarinic aspect of the cholinergic system is quite definitely acting in some opposition to this brain reward mechanism, and we don't know whether it is acting in opposition to the noradrenaline attention mechanism, or in opposition to the brain reward mechanism per se. The nicotinic aspect of the cholinergic system, however, may well be a positive link in some parts of the brain reward mechanism.

S.P.R. ROSE: In that Valenstein learned-drive experiment that you set up, when the animal learned to replace eating by drinking, is it then given a choice in the drinking situation between food and water?

J. OLDS: The safest thing to say is that it can go either way: it can prefer water entirely, it can retain its original preference, or the two can be equal. The important thing in these experiments is the tremendous difference in the animals before and after training. I came to speak in favor of Valenstein's study — I was an opponent of it at first — when he explained that with all hypothalamic stimulated drives you often get nothing when you first put the probes in. In all studies of hypothalamically stimulated drive behaviors there is commonly a lag period after the probes are planted and stimulation tests begun before positive effects are observed. The lag has been an enigma and caused many young investigators to abandon the problem early. Persistence often yielded success, but the reason for the intial failures was not clear. Valenstein's study clarified the fact that stimulating the animal in the presence of goals is a form of training and that the stimulus gradually brings goal-directed behaviors under control by an almost "developmental" chain of events. Valenstein thus put us onto the idea that there is a great deal of training in any hypothalamic drive behavior. My view of it is that you are stimulating a pot pourri of things in the hypothalamus, and the animal practically has to organize all of that into a drive for the first time.

F.H. LOPES DA SILVA: About your units: you showed one which stops firing when you start with stimulation and then starts up again. Are these phasic changes — changes that last for a very short time and then return to normal while the behavior continues as it was — or are they tonic changes?

J. OLDS: They are phasic changes but tightly coupled, meaning that every time the animal presses the pedal, the neuronal inhibition is strong at the beginning and becomes attenuated to some degree later in the stimulus train. We sometimes can predict when he will release the pedal by looking at the attenuation of the inhibition. As he lets go a burst occurs, and then the inibition is restored as he presses again. If he walks around in between the operant periods, the neurons are relatively active during this interval.

On Drive, Conflict
and Instinct, and the
Functional Organization of Behavior

G.P. BAERENDS

Zoological Laboratory, Groningen (The Netherlands)

INTRODUCTION

For the study of the causal mechanisms underlying behavior two oppositely directed approaches are possible and desirable. The first of these starts from relatively simple mechanisms and works towards more complicated ones, mainly using physiological methods. The other begins at the most complicated level, with the behavior of animals and man as it is shown under free living conditions, and tries to break up the complex into ever smaller components; it concentrates on what might be called the architecture of behavior, and uses ethological methods for the most part. The former approach is the oldest one and still the most commonly practiced. My contribution will deal with the second approach: the ethological analysis of complicated behavior patterns. At the hand of examples derived mainly from work in our own institution I hope to give you an idea how, with this method, it is tried to derive the rules through which overt behavior is effected by means of the various building units and mechanisms which are the chief subjects of the first approach.

ETHOLOGICAL ANALYSIS AND METHODOLOGY

The example I am going to discuss to begin with is the behavior of a herring gull (*Larus argentatus*) incubating its eggs. The major part of an incubation shift is spent quietly sitting on the nest while carefully holding the eggs, surrounded by belly feathers, against the incubation patches, thus keeping them at a constant temperature of about 38°C. However, from time to time the bird interrupts this behavior, for instance by changing its position, manipulating nest material, trimming its feathers, vocalizing, or even by briefly leaving the nest (Fig. 1). The aim is to understand the determinants of these interruptions and, in particular, the mechanism by which the kind of activity appearing during interruptions is patterned.

These problems have been extensively treated in Baerends et al. (1970), a study based on long-term observations of incubating herring gulls from a hide, and extending through several seasons. Fig. 2 diagrammatically represents — as an example — the occurrence of interruptive behavior patterns in the course of

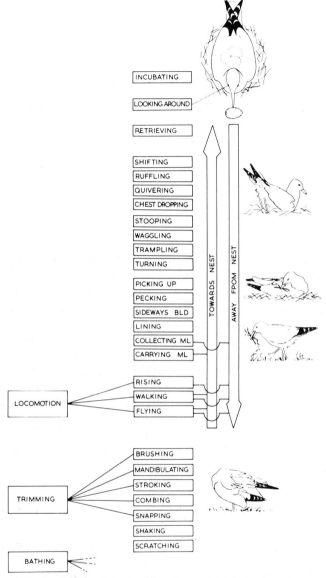

Fig. 1. Survey of the interruptive activities distinguished.

one hour. These patterns appear not to be uniformly distributed over the observation period but tend rather to be concentrated in bouts, the exact composition of which is variable. Methods of temporal analysis of the sequence, or the coincidence per time-unit, of the different activities within a bout or within a period comprising several bouts, show that the temporal order in which the activities occur is not a random one. Groups of associated activities can be distinguished, and statistical methods like factor-analysis and cluster-analysis have proved their value for this purpose.

Fig. 3 represents the result of factor-analysis of the sequences of the various

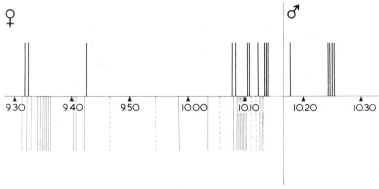

Fig. 2. Example of a record of interruptive behavior. Each vertical line marks one activity; the heavy vertical lines above the horizontal time axis stands for re-settling, the thin vertical lines below the axis for nest building and the dotted vertical lines for trimming. At 10.17 the incubating female was relieved by her mate.

interruptive activities performed during incubation shifts of herring gulls. The model comprises the information contained in a correlation matrix expressing the degree of sequential relationship (following, preceding) of the various activities. It attempts to reproduce the observed correlations (via the calculation of Spearman rank correlation coefficients) in terms of a reduced number of correlations between the original variables, or *vectors* (the interruptive activities), and the smallest number of hypothetical variables, or *factors*. In the present case, a three-factor solution sufficed to explain enough of the total common variance (70%) to make visualization in a three-dimensional cosine-vector model possible (for further details of the method see

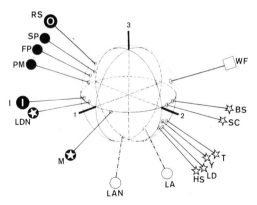

Fig. 3. Three-dimensional factor analysis model resulting from statistical analysis of sequences of interruptive behavior during an incubation shift. (After Baerends et al., 1970.) RS, re-settling; PM, FP and SP, nest building activities; I, incubating; LDN, looking down (LD) while sitting on nest; M, mandibulating; LAN, looking around while standing on nest; LA, looking around while standing outside nest; HS, head shaking; Y, yawning; T, trimming; SC, scratching; BS, body shaking; WF, walking or flying. 1, 2 and 3 are the "factors". "Solid" symbols indicate activities carried out while sitting on the nest, open circles while standing on or near the nest. The stars stand for comfort activities which may be performed in standing and in sitting position on as well as outside the nest.

Thurstone, 1953; Fruchter, 1954; Wiepkema, 1961; Baerends et al., 1970). In this instance the interpretation of the "factors" is of no concern; the model is only used to obtain a survey of the associations between the activities observed. The smaller the angles between the vectors representing the various activities, the higher their temporal association; the bigger the angles, the less likely it is that the activities will follow or precede one another, or occur during the same restricted time period. Two clusters are immediately apparent from the model. One comprises the three different kinds of manipulation with nest material

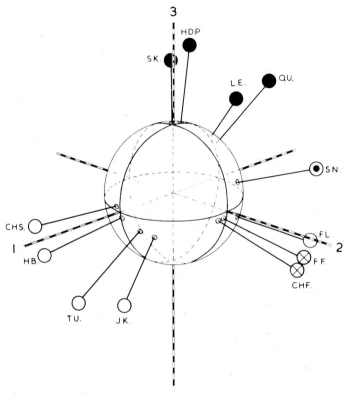

Fig. 4. Three-dimensional factor-analysis model resulting from sequential analysis of the behavior of the male bitterling in its territory around the mussel. (After Wiepkema, 1961.) CHS, HB, TU and JK are defensive activities; SK, HDP, LE and QU are sexual activities; CHF and FF are cleaning activities; SN serves feeding; FL is fleeing. 1, 2 and 3 are the "factors".

which were distinguished, plus *re-settling* (i.e. changing position on the nest; RS), activities which are all closely associated with sitting on the nest (solid circles). The other cluster comprises comfort activities (stars); its position lies in between standing on the nest (LAN) and leaving it (WF). The almost antipodal positions of the building and the trimming group suggests a high degree of incompatibility of these groups, which could in fact be experimentally demonstrated in extensive series of tests (Baerends et al., 1970).

As our study on the incubation of the herring gull was concerned only with a very restricted part of the total behavior repertoire, a second example of a similar statistical analysis of complex behavior is added here, taken from a study of Wiepkema (1961) on a fish, the bitterling (*Rhodeus amarus*), in the period between establishing a territory around a freshwater mussel and the disposal of eggs in its gill cavity. In the three-dimensional model derived from these data (Fig. 4) three groups stand out at once. One comprises various activities concerned with the defense of the mussel (open circles), a second with activities serving to lure a female towards it (full circles), while the third group consists of non-reproductive activities with diverse functions: the feeding activity, *snapping;* the trimming activities *chafing* and *fin-flickering;* and *fleeing.* It is likely that, with the use of more data and more dimensions in the model, this third group could be split up still further.

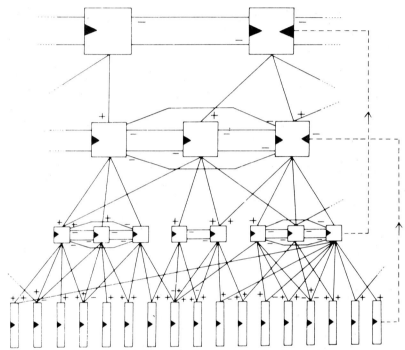

Fig. 5. Schematical diagram of the hierarchical organization of behavior. The bottom row represents fixed action patterns, controlled by subsystems and systems of different order. The black triangles represent mechanisms releasing or activating a system, the dotted lines symbolize feedback relations. (After Baerends, 1971.)

Similar analyses in different groups of animals have led to similar pictures, all of them suggesting that activities tend to be associated in groups, which appear to mutually suppress one another (see also Baerends, 1941, 1975; Tinbergen, 1942, 1951; Kortlandt, 1955, 1959). This resulted in the hypothesis (Tinbergen, 1950) that in the network underlying the organization of behavior different causal systems can be distinguished. When it turned out that, on the one hand, within such systems yet more restricted associations of activities could be found whereas, on the other hand, two or more such systems often proved to have causal factors in common, it became necessary to recognize systems of different-order all placed within a hierarchical organization (Fig. 5).

DETERMINANTS OF BEHAVIOR SEQUENCES

A system or subsystem, distinguished as a result of causal analysis is usually also characterized by the particular biological function (e.g., feeding, defense, migration) which it subserves in the behavioral repertoire of the species. Unfortunately, this has frequently led in ethological studies to premature statements about the existence of particular systems on the basis of biological function only, without carrying out the time-consuming causal analysis which is actually needed for such a conclusion. Such analysis should start from statistical evidence concerning the association of activities. However, this evidence is insufficient in itself for conclusions about the underlying mechanism. Statistical descriptions can reveal that different activities may have determinants in common, but without further experimentation the statistical analysis of uncontrolled behavior does not elucidate how far such common factors are *internal*, and due to the characteristic structure of the organizing network, or *external*, due to particular features in the environmental situation. Even if external variables can be excluded, a temporal order between two activities does not necessarily prove their subordinance to the same system, but could also be due to a rebound relationship between different systems.

In the case of the bird sitting on its eggs the most important external variables, viz., weather, egg temperature, and the presence of other gulls could be taken into account, since they were continuously monitored during the observations. The great amount of data collected permitted us to study the influence of one variable, while eliminating statistically the influence of others. Several external variables were found to influence the frequency at which interruptive activities took place, and they also had some influence on the relative frequency at which different categories occurred. However, the pattern of interrupted behavior could not be satisfactorily explained on the basis of the immediate influence of external determinants only. For instance, if the gull performed trimming or building, no relation could be found between characteristics of the external situation and the relative frequency of each of the different trimming or building components performed. The external stimulus was found to regulate primarily the occurrence of these categories, not to determine the appearance of each single component.

For trimming, special studies (in terns, by van Iersel and Bol, 1958; in herring gulls, by Van Rhijn, unpublished) have shown that, although trimming as a whole complex can be triggered by particular stimuli, such as dirt applied on the plumage, the exact kind of trimming activities performed and the areas of the plumage to which they are directed is only partly determined by the type and locality of the external stimulus, but to a greater extent by a stereotyped and apparently programmed pattern. Although, during a trimming sequence, each activity or location can be expected to occur at any moment, their relative frequency shows a marked trend. The data suggest a model in which a fluctuating internal factor (tendency to trim) is assumed to make available to the bird each particular trimming movement, or location, whenever this factor passes the specific threshold for triggering that activity. Then, the chief effect of the external stimulus would be a raising of the excitation level

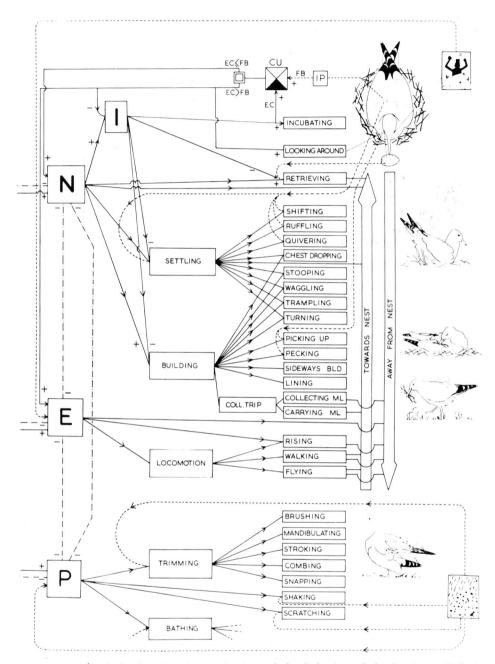

Fig. 6. Diagram of the functional organization of the behavior of the herring gull during incubation. See text for explanation. (After Baerends, 1970.)

around which the tendency fluctuates; the order in which the activities occur would depend on the time-course of the intrinsic tendency and on the threshold of the different activities; for activities of which the threshold has been exceeded a random distribution seems to hold. The relations of the various trimming activities with one another and with bathing justifies placing them in one "preening" system (P), as shown in the lower part of Fig. 6.

Although this type of explanation can also be suggested for other examples of systems (in our example also for nest building), the mechanism underlying a system presumably varies considerably from case to case. The most advanced study of the mechanism of a system probably attained so far ⸺ and in which ethological and physiological methods have been used concurrently ⸺ is the study of the mechanisms underlying hunger, i.e., the feeding system (de Ruiter, 1963, 1967; de Ruiter et al., 1974).

The activation of a system or subsystem is usually brought about by the perception of external or internal releasing stimuli, specifically linked to that system. Moreover, it is likely — but difficult to prove, because stimuli can have a delayed effect — that some degree of activation of a system can also take place "spontaneously", i.e., through endogenous impulse generation by the system itself, without any specific input from sensory organs. The activated state will usually last for some time, during which its level is likely to fluctuate. In several species of fish (Baerends et al., 1955; Baldaccini, 1973) different states can express themselves as different body colorations, and changes in the intensity of these system-specific patterns make measurement of the activation levels possible.

The activation of an overall state increases the readiness to perform particular behavior patterns, and raises the threshold for certain other activities. The greater part of the activities initially made available when a system or subsystem is activated (appetitive behavior; Craig, 1918) serve a searching for, or facilitation of, the appearance of specific stimulus situations. These in turn release in the animal still other activities, which eventually form the end of a behavioral chain (consummatory act) and/or bring the animal in a specific external situation (consummatory situation), with presumably a corresponding internal state ("satiation, reward").

The feedback stimulation resulting from the consummatory act or the consummatory situation alters the state of the system in action; it may also activate a subsystem or another equivalent system (rebound). The performance of appetitive behavior may in some cases cause an increase, in other cases a decrease of the level of the system concerned; much more research will be necessary to understand the positive and negative feedback mechanisms involved here. Such studies should incorporate a careful identification of the system and of the relations between its parts, and measurements of its level of activation in relation to the parameters of the activities concerned.

In correspondence with this searching for specific stimuli, the activation of a system often implies a change in the responsiveness for particular external stimuli. For instance, when the *incubation* system is activated in the herring gull its response to green and yellow colors, of egg dummies placed on the nest rim, is stronger than that to dummies painted in other hues, whereas when the *feeding* system is activated the attention is primarily directed to red colors (Baerends and Kruijt, 1973).

CONFLICT TENDENCIES OR "DRIVES"

In all species so far subjected to an ethological analysis of their entire behavioral repertoire arguments were found for postulating the existence of a system subserving flight, escape, and avoidance behavior, sometimes even for two such systems, each dealing with a different type of flight, and interacting with one another (Hogan, 1965; Baldaccini, 1973). In these systems the searching behavior largely serves to avoid certain kinds of stimulation (aversive behavior), although it may also be positively directed, for instance to find cover in a hiding place.

Activation of a system for escape will, as a rule, be in conflict with all other systems. Similarly, a tendency to attack will be to some extent in conflict with a tendency for sexual behavior, or — in a carnivore — a tendency to care for young will conflict with a tendency to take up food. Nevertheless, as will be clear from these examples, the same external situation may simultaneously stimulate such mutually incompatible systems. The results are extremely interesting and we shall extend upon them by returning to our example of the incubating herring gull.

Interruptive behavior is relatively rare (about once every 20 min), and lasts only briefly when a bird is sitting on a complete clutch of three normal eggs of the proper temperature. A reduction of the number of eggs in the clutch or an experimental increase or decrease of the temperature (Drent et al., 1970) increases the frequency and duration of interruptive behavior. This means that the continuation of the behavior system underlying incubation depends on reception of a "satisfactory" feedback stimulus from the clutch. The first activity appearing when this stimulus is experimentally made deficient is usually re-settling, always initiated by the bird's looking at the nest rim, often with some building movements and more rarely with a few trimming activities. If the deficiency lasts, nest building will become more and more frequent and, ultimately, preening is likely to dominate. The occurrence of re-settling and building is always highly positively correlated; in contrast, a positive correlation between building and trimming exists only when periods of half an hour or more are considered. However, the correlation becomes negative when the period being considered is much shorter (e.g., a bout). This implies that re-settling, building and trimming are all facilitated by the deficient external situation in the nest, but that other — probably interacting internal — factors determine when exactly each of them occurs.

Building is also positively correlated with a tendency to retrieve eggs placed on the nest rim. Consequently we have to assume that *building, retrieving, re-settling* and *incubating* all belong to the same functional system. In Fig. 6 this system is represented by the symbol N. To account for the fact that the amount of building becomes reduced as soon as the clutch is complete (restricted in fact to the brief periods of interrupted behavior) we must build into the model a unit (I) which, when information from the clutch is received, maintains incubation but inhibits the occurrence of re-settling and building, which can be considered as appetitive behavior with regard to the (N) system. This feedback is, in a special comparison unit (CU), assumed to be weighed against an "expected" value. This value is not constant but oscillates with the season (and also during the incubation shift of an individual bird), and must therefore be determined through a corollary discharge or efference copy (EC) of the tendency to incubate. The simplest way of explaining the occurrence of re-settling and building when the feedback information drops below the expected value is to assume that this leads to a blockage of (I).

The causation of trimming must be more complicated because, as mentioned above, the preening system (P) by which trimming is controlled cannot be taken as subordinate to (N). In contrast to re-settling and building, trimming can be considered as functionally irrelevant, i.e., it cannot contribute to restoring the proper feedback situation. Its occurrence fits the concept of "displacement" as current in ethology. In my opinion, the most likely hypothesis to explain this phenomenon is the disinhibition hypothesis, advocated by van Iersel and Bol (1958) and Sevenster (1961). It proposes that, as a result of the mutual inhibition of simultaneously stimulated, largely incompatible systems, a third system briefly gets an opportunity to express itself in overt behavior. Which system is activated during the conflict depends upon: (1) characteristics of the functional organization of the behavior of the species involved; (2) the relative readiness of the competing systems, and (3) the external situation.

In our case of the frustrated incubation response, evidence is available that a second system is active, competing with incubation. Postures and calls of the birds, rising from the eggs, and even short trips away from the nest are indications of a tendency to leave, to escape from the unsatisfactory situation. We are, therefore, inclined to interpret the occurrence of activities of system (P) as the result of an interaction of the incubation system (M) with the system for escape (E), or with elements of this system. An important argument in favor of this hypothesis is that the occurrence of trimming can be considerably increased by frightening the bird carefully (e.g., by repeatedly imitating an alarm call) before the feedback stimulus is made deficient through, for instance, reducing the number of eggs in the clutch. Trimming is also more common as an interruptive activity when the temperature is increased above normal, a situation which induces a bird to rise and stand over the nest. Finally, when the occurrence of building and trimming in the minutes just before and just after re-settling is studied, it shows that the distribution of higher frequencies of building is symmetrical with regards to re-settling, whereas trimming ("preening") only reaches higher frequencies just before the bird rises (Fig. 7).

Conflicts between systems can lead to other phenomena besides displacement. When elements of both of the conflicting systems are partly expressed, either simultaneously or successively, ethologists speak of "ambivalence". Ambivalence between the orientation components of the conflicting systems may lead to an orientation in a new direction, and often towards a substitute object; this is called "re-direction" by ethologists. According to the "conflict hypothesis" postulated by Tinbergen and some of his collaborators, all three phenomena must have played a very important role in the development of communication behavior in the course of evolution (see Baerends, 1975). In a great many species, specific signal activities have been found which can be demonstrated to originate from ambivalent, re-directed or displaced behavior (or from a combination of these), although a considerable amount of ritualization (i.e., adaptation in form to the communicative function) has often taken place. The notion of the occurrence of subsystems in the network underlying the organization of behavior is not new (e.g., Freud, Lloyd Morgan and McDougall, see Kortlandt, 1955); although these authors used to distinguish a system on the basis of the biological (survival value) function it

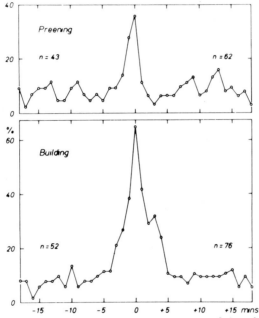

Fig. 7. The occurrence of building and preening (measured by the percentage of birds engaged in each of these activities) in the minutes before and after re-settling on the nest. (After Baerends et al., 1970.)

was thought to subserve. The development of methods for tracing systems through objective causal analysis has only recently begun. The terms "instinct" and "drive" have both been used to denote what in the present paper is called "behavioral system".

INSTINCT VERSUS LEARNING: A PSEUDO-DICHOTOMY

In 1951 Tinbergen proposed to use the word "instinct" for behavioral systems of different order. Earlier, Lorenz (1937) had coined the term "instinctive activity" (Instinkthandlung, Erbkoordination) for the kind of sterotyped elementary units — above the level of what are usually called reflexes — which easily become evident when one makes an attempt to describe behavior sequences repeatedly. A critical discussion of Lorenz's concept lies beyond the scope of this paper; for this the reader can be referred to Baerends (1956, 1971; see also Barlow, 1968).

Lorenz and Tinbergen were in favor of using the word *instinct* in this context because they wanted to emphasize the species-specificity, and thus the genetical background both of the elementary behavioral units and of the architecture of which these units are the composing parts. They were making a case against extreme behaviorists who considered the unconditioned reflex as the only genetically patterned unit. For Lorenz and Tinbergen the term instinct did not necessarily exclude the occurrence of learning processes in the ontogeny of species-specific behavior. Lorenz (1937) spoke of "instinct-conditioning intercalation patterns" (Instinkt-Dressurverschränkungen) and he in particular has emphasized the part "imprinting" can take in such behavioral constructions. The examples Tinbergen (1950) gave of appetitive behavior controlled by an instinct, imply the incorporation of learned components at various levels of the hierarchical organization which he postulated.

However, because people tend to stick to their original interpretations of apparently familiar words, these attempts to redefine the word "instinct" were doomed to be fruitless. "Instinct" is nearly always identified with "inborn", "unlearnt" or even "non-intelligent"; in particular, Descartes created a profound dichotomy in the way of thinking about behavior mechanisms by sharply distinguishing between intelligent and instinctive behavior, claiming the first category for man and reserving the second for "lower" animals. Although animals were later on found to possess learning capacities, and humans not always to behave with reason, the dichotomy was maintained. This is very unfortunate, for this philosophical bias prevented — even up to the present time — an unequivocal thinking about problems of the causation and ontogeny of behavior. The dichotomy has led to a polarity of approach in the behavioral sciences: it strengthened the emphasis which psychologists laid upon learning and drove the ethologists who, as zoologists, were very much aware of the characteristic differences among species, to over-stressing the "innateness" of behavior. The latter, however, began to work towards a synthesis of both viewpoints after Lehrman (1953) had sharply criticized some of Lorenz's views (for Lorenz's reply see Lorenz, 1965), and made a plea for unbiased experimental research on the ontogeny of naturally occurring behavior. As a result it is now known, for instance, that a typical species-specific activity like the advertising song of various songbirds is brought about by a genetically controlled, programmed development, in which stepwise learning processes are incorporated in an intricate way (Nottebohm, 1970). In the ontogeny of such song patterns, genetic and environmental information become interwoven rather than intercalated, making it impossible to distinguish in the final product between learned and non-learned behavioral elements. This is why a term like "fixed action pattern" or — taking into account the variability within and among individuals of the same species — the term *modal action pattern* (Barlow, 1968), should be preferred over "instinctive activities".

The ontogeny of more complex behavior has so far been studied in a few cases only, and still more rarely has this been done against the conceptual background of behavioral systems. However, the results obtained by Harlow and his collaborators (see Harlow and Harlow, 1965) on the development of behavior in the rhesus monkey can be used in this context; the work by Kruijt (1964, 1971) on the development of social behavior in the junglefowl (*Gallus spadiceus*) was intentionally designed for this very purpose. In the latter study it was shown that for a normal development of the display behavior shown in agonistic and sexual situations, experience with conspecifics during the first months of life is important, if not in fact essential. As mentioned above, such displays can be interpreted as the results of the interaction of different, partly incompatible systems. Kruijt postulated the idea that the experience with conspecifics (often nest-mates) in juvenile stages is particularly important for stabilizing the ranges within which, in the adult, the activity levels of the various systems balance. Cocks deprived of social experience during their first year showed, even after they had long since been transferred to social situations, unusually severe bursts of either attack or fleeing behavior when confronted with a female, at the expense of sexual behavior which, when it occurred, was deficient in many ways. After 15 months of isolation, started before the second month, no successful copulations were ever achieved. This types of evidence indicates that we well might expect subtle learning processes also to play an integrating role in the ontogeny of behavior systems of different order.

On the basis of the presently available evidence we must therefore conclude that in the development of behavior which ethologists used to call "instinctive" the incorporation of learning processes may play a role. As the word *instinct* seems for most people to exclude learning, the use of this confusing term as noun as well as adjective should be discouraged. *Learning* should be conceived here as a change in performance resulting from the experience of structured stimulation, lasting for a longer time than the stimulus or its after-effect.

The term "drive" is used in two senses. First, in a classificatory sense to denote what here has been called "a system". Second, in a dynamic sense to indicate the state of an animal in which a system is activated, i.e., synonymous with *motivation* or *tendency*. This latter use is common in comparative psychology, where "drive" is studied as one determining variable in learning processes, and "reward" (or consummatory situation) as another variable. In such studies the strength of the drive and the presence or absence of a reward are usually considered of more importance for the establishment of a learning process than their specific identities. Drive is here defined as the motivation for learning, and according to the drive-reduction hypothesis, stimulus situations possess "drive value" if responses increasing this stimulation are reinforced by a subsequent reduction of the strength of the drive. If, through a learning process, a drive can be activated by a previously neutral cue this drive is called learnable, or even learned (Miller, 1951). To my knowledge the question has not been raised in psychology whether, through this learning process, a new cue becomes associated with an already existing system in the animal, or whether, as the expression "learned drive" might suggest, such a system can be newly created through learning. If the latter actually occurs, there are good reasons to ask whether the acquisition of drives through learning is nevertheless subjected to constraints by a more or less "open" program for the ontogenetic development of behavior (Mayr, 1974). For if, as I have been assuming here, a specific genetically controlled organizing network underlies the behavior of each species, for a full understanding of the variety and the potentialities of learning mechanisms the characteristics of such networks, including their programmed specifications with regard to drives and rewards, should be duly taken into account. This is especially relevant for the study of the role of learning in the ontogeny of behavior, for this is the area where species-specific programs are most likely to open opportunities for learning, as well as to put certain constraints on it (see Hinde and Stevenson-Hinde, 1973).

A good example of the dependence of learning on the structural organization of behavior can be taken from work by Sevenster (1968, 1973), on the three-spined stickleback (*Gasterosteus aculeatus*). Using the technique of operant conditioning, Sevenster could train male sticklebacks to swim through a ring or to bite a rod when the sight of an opponent to fight was offered as a reward. In contrast, when a ripe, courtship-releasing female was tried as a reward, swimming through the ring remained a suitable operant, but biting a rod gave a much lower response rate. Sevenster gives ample arguments supporting his opinion that this low response rate on biting is due to incompatibility of this operant with the type of drive-reward combination.

I hope to have made it clear that the use of the word *drive* is almost as dangerous as that of the term *instinct*. On the one hand, *drive* is used in different meanings and, on the other hand, it has no explanatory value. It is even worse: the term not only does not solve any problems, it has come to mask them. Therefore, I am of the opinion that, at least in ethological analyses, this term should be avoided.

In the ethological analysis of the organization of behavior, no concepts should be used that have implications with respect to ontogeny. As in morphology, the analysis and description of a structure (which can in principle be given for any age phase of an animal) is one problem, and the way in which it has developed in the life of the individual is quite a different problem. That this is not generally considered evident for behavior patterns is the aftermath of the Cartesian dichotomy dogma, which, after centuries, it is now due time to overcome.

The organizing structure of behavior which is the subject of ethological analysis can be compared with a set of programs — or rather with the basic outline underlying these programs — through which a computer can fulfill certain complicated tasks. The mechanisms best known at this stage to the physiologists may be compared with the various gadgets of which the computer consists. The ethological analysis outlined in this paper has the purpose of revealing the various programs and underlying rules with which a species is genetically equipped. At the same time, it can help the physiologist in focussing his research on relevant and promising aspects out of the wealth of behavioral phenomena, to disclose the character of the biological "gadgets" in terms of physiological mechanisms and to explain how they function in order to get a program successfully carried out.

To achieve this, it is desirable that the sophisticated methods for system-analysis and cybernetics which have recently become popular, mainly for building models of relatively simple behavioral elements (Hassenstein, 1971;

McFarland, 1971; McFarland, 1974; Powers, 1973), should also be applied for the analysis of more complex behavior.

The importance of ethological analysis as a basis for the study of nervous and hormonal mechanisms, using physiological methods, will also lead to more careful and meaningful definitions, circumscriptions and measurements of the behavior for which the underlying physiological mechanism is being studied. Most physiological and pharmacological papers on behavior mechanisms are still deficient with regard to these latter aspects, which seriously limits their theoretical and practical applicability. In particular, for studies aiming at a manipulation of functional aspects of behavior, such as for instance aggression and fear, an ethological approach in conjunction with physiological work is absolutely necessary.

SUMMARY

The aim of this contribution is to show how, with the methods of ethological analysis, the way in which complex behavior is organized can be empirically investigated. This is done largely on the basis of a study of the behavior of the herring gull during incubation. The evidence resulting from the analysis forces us to distinguish different systems, of different orders of complexity, within the overall network underlying the organization of behavior. These have a certain amount of independence, although they are in constant interaction with each other. Different systems or subsystems may either excite or inhibit one another. Inhibition leads to conflicts between systems which have most interesting implications for the causation and evolution of behavior patterns. The terms "instinct" and "drive" are discussed in connection with the concept of behavior systems: their use in this sense is not to be recommended.

REFERENCES

Baerends, G.P. (1941) Fortpflanzungsverhalten und Orientierung der Grabwespe, *Ammophila campestris. T. Entomol.*, 84: 68–275.

Baerends, G.P. (1956) Aufbau tierischen Verhaltens. In *Handbuch der Zoologie, Vol. 10(3)*, J.-G. Helmcke and H. von Lengerken (Eds.), de Guyter, Berlin, pp. 1–32.

Baerends, G.P. (1970) A model of the functional organization of incubation behaviour. In *The Herring Gull and its Egg*, G.P. Baerends and R.H. Drent (Eds.), *Behaviour*, Suppl. 17: 263–312.

Baerends, G.P. (1971) The ethological analysis of fish behaviour. In *Fish Physiology*, W.S. Hoar and D.J. Randall (Eds.), Academic Press, New York, pp. 279–370.

Baerends, G.P. (1975) An evaluation of the conflict hypothesis as an explanatory principle for the evolution of displays. In *Essays on Function and Evolution in Behaviour*, G.P. Baerends, C. Beer and A. Manning (Eds.), Clarendon Press, Oxford, pp. 187–227.

Baerends, G.P. and Kruijt, J.P. (1973) Stimulus selection. In *Constraints on Learning. Limitations and Predispositions*, R.A. Hinde and J. Stevenson-Hinde (Eds.), Academic Press, London, pp. 23–50.

Baerends, G.P., Brouwer, R. and Waterbolk, H.Th. (1955) Ethological studies on *Lebistes reticulatus* (Peters): an analysis of the male courtship pattern. *Behaviour*, 8: 249–334.

Baerends, G.P., Drent, R.H., Glas, P. and Groenewold, H. (1970) An ethological analysis of incubation behaviour in the herring gull. In *The Herring Gull and its Egg*, G.P. Baerends and R.H. Drent (Eds.), *Behaviour*, Suppl. 17: 134–235.

Baldaccini, N.E. (1973) An ethological study of reproductive behaviour, including the colour patterns of the Cichlid fish *Tilapia mariae* (Boulanger). *Monit. zool. ital. (N.S.)*, 7: 247–290.

Barlow, G.W. (1968) Ethological units of behaviour. In *Central Nervous Systems and Fish Behavior*, D. Ingle (Ed.), Univ. Chicago Press, Chicago, Ill., pp. 217–232.

Craig, W. (1918) Appetites and aversions as constituents of instincts. *Biol. Bull. Mar. Biol. Lab. Woods Hole*, 34: 91–107.

Drent, R.H. (1970) Functional aspects of incubation in the herring gull. In *The Herring Gull and its Egg*, G.P. Baerends and R.H. Drent (Eds.), *Behaviour*, Suppl. 17: 1–132.

Drent, R.H., Postuma, K. and Joustra, T. (1970) The effect of egg temperature on incubation behavior in the Herring Gull. In *The Herring Gull and its Egg*, G.P. Baerends and R.H. Drent (Eds.), *Behaviour*, Suppl. 17: 236–252.

Fruchter, B. (1954) *Introduction to Factor Analysis*, van Nostrand, New York.

Harlow, H.F. and Harlow, M.K. (1965) The affectional systems. In *Behavior of Non-Human Primates, Vol. 2*, A.M. Schrier, H.F. Harlow and F. Stollnitz (Eds.), Academic Press, New York, pp. 287–334.

Hassenstein, B. (1971) *Information and Control in the Living Organism*. Chapman and Hall, London.

Hinde, R.A. and Stevenson-Hinde, J. (Eds.) (1973) *Constraints on Learning. Limitations and Predispositions*. Academic Press, London, 488 pp.

Hogan, J.A. (1965) An experimental study of conflict and fear: an analysis of behaviour of young chicks towards a mealworm. Part. I. The behaviour of chicks which do not eat a mealworm. *Behaviour*, 25: 45–97.

van Iersel, J.J.A. and Bol, A.C.A. (1958) Preening of two tern species. A study on displacement activities. *Behaviour*, 13: 1–88.

Kortlandt, A. (1955) Aspects and prospects of the concept of instinct (vicissitudes of the hierarchy theory). *Arch. néerl. zool.*, 11: 155–284.

Kortlandt, A. (1959) An attempt at clarifying some controversial notions in animal psychology and ethology. *Arch. néerl. zool.*, 13: 196–229.

Kruijt, J.P. (1964) Ontogeny of social behaviour in Burmese red jungle fowl (*Gallus g. spadiceus*). *Behaviour*, Suppl. 12: 201 pp.

Kruijt, J.P. (1971) Early experience and the development of social behaviour in jungle fowl. *Psychiat. Neurol. Neurochir. (Amst.)*, 74: 7–20.

Lehrman, D.S. (1953) A critique of Konrad Lorenz's theory of instinctive behavior. *Quart. Rev. Biol.*, 28: 337–363.

Lorenz, K. (1937) Uber die Bildung des Instinktbegriffes. *Naturwissenschaften*, 25: 289–300, 307–318, 324–331. (English translation: *Studies in Animal and Human Behaviour, I*, Harvard Univ. Press, Cambridge, Mass. pp. 259–315.)

Lorenz, K. (1965) *Evolution and Modification of Behavior*. Univ. Chicago Press, Chicago, Ill., 121 pp.

Mayr, E. (1974) Behavior programs and evolutionary strategies. *Amer. Scientist*, 62: 650–659.

McFarland, D.J. (1971) *Feedback Mechanisms in Animal Behaviour*. Academic Press, London.

McFarland, D.J. (Ed.) (1974) *Motivational Control Systems Analysis*. Academic Press, London.

Miller, N.E. (1951) Learnable drives and rewards. In *Handbook of Experimental Psychology*, S.S. Stevens (Ed.), Wiley, New York: Chapman and Hall, London, pp. 435–472.

Nottebohm, F. (1970) Ontogeny of Bird Song. *Science*, 167: 950–956.

Powers, W.T. (1973) *Behavior: the Control of Perception*. Aldine, Chicago, Ill.

Ruiter, L. de (1963) The physiology of vertebrate feeding behaviour: towards a synthesis of the ethological and physiological approaches to problems of behaviour. *Z. Tierpsychol.* 20: 498–516.

Ruiter, L. de (1967) Feeding behaviour of vertebrates in the natural environment. In *Handbook of Physiology, Section 6, Vol. I*, F. Code (Ed.), Amer. Physiol. Soc., Washington D.C., pp. 97–116.

Ruiter, L. de, Wiepkema, P.R. and Veening, J.G. (1974) Models of behaviour and the hypothalamus. In *Integrative Hypothalamic Activity, Progress in Brain Research, Vol. 41*, D.F. Swaab and J.P. Schadé (Eds.), Elsevier, Amsterdam, pp. 481–507.

Sevenster, P. (1961) A causal analysis of a displacement activity (fanning in *Gasterosteus aculeatus* L.). *Behaviour*, Suppl. 9: 170 pp.

Sevenster, P. (1968) Motivation and learning in sticklebacks. In *Central Nervous Systems and Fish Behavior*, D. Ingle (Ed.), Univ. Chicago Press, Chicago, Ill., pp. 233–245.

Sevenster, P. (1973) Incompatibility of response and reward. In *Constraints on Learning, Limitations and Predispositions*, R.A. Hinde and J. Stevenson-Hinde (Eds.), Academic Press, London, pp. 265–283.

Thurstone, L.L. (1953) *Multiple-Factor Analysis* (2nd ed.), University Chicago Press, Chicago, Ill.

Tinbergen, N. (1942) An objectivistic study of the innate behaviour of animals. *Bibl. Biother.*, 1: 39–98.

Tinbergen, N. (1950) The hierarchical organization of nervous mechanisms underlying instinctive behaviour. *Symp. Soc. exp. Biol.*, 4: 305–312.

Tinbergen, N. (1951) *The Study of Instinct*. University Press, Oxford.

Wiepkema, P.R. (1961) An ethological analysis of the reproductive behavior of the bitterling (*Rhodeus amarus* Bloch). *Arch. néerl. zool.*, 14: 103–199.

DISCUSSION

F.H. LOPES DA SILVA: I am particularly interested in hearing more about the feedback systems linking the different behavioral systems you have visualized. One of the things which emerges, if I understood correctly, is that in a conflict situation, let's say between your N and your E system, you will have displacement behavior — preening, for instance. I was wondering whether, because of such negative feedback, you can have some kind of abnormal (in the sense of being not ordinarily seen, as well as being inconsistent with the goal to which the animal is actually directed) oscillatory interaction instead of displacement. Otherwise, all these different behaviors would reflect stable states which are actually mutually incompatible, so that you wouldn't get the same type of oscillatory behavior as in systems with negative feedback.

G.P. BAERENDS: Oscillatory interactions in which, often incomplete, components of the conflicting systems are alternately shown are usually the first indications of a conflict. In ethology this phenomenon is called successive ambivalence, in contrast to simultaneous ambivalence which is the combination at the same moment of incomplete components of the conflicting systems in a kind of compromise activity. Redirection (in ethology: the performance of an activity towards an object which did not primarily trigger it; in fact compromise between conflicting orientations) and displacement seem to occur at higher levels of activation of the incompatible systems. Redirected and displacement activities are always of short duration, but they may occur repeatedly — this seems to fit the idea of oscillations. With strong and long-lasting conflicting stimulation the repeated performance of incomplete, redirected and displacement activities results in a picture which has often been called "neurotic". It has correspondingly been suggested that the "conflict activities" function as a "safety valve" against neurosis.

J. OLDS: I want to ask a question about that "safety valve" concept: I wonder to what degree behavioral cycles may exist. People who have studied diurnal and sleep rhythms can come up with what is esentially a multiple cycle hypothesis. Not only are there circadian cycles but also a series of shorter cycles, that account for periodic changes of activity even during waking. The idea has indeed occurred to me that these shorter cycles are operating as a safety valve to give the animal a time to make a change when two behaviors ("drives") are both strong, yet each one occasionally gives way to the other. You never mentioned any cyclical behavior, but I suggest that you might see relatively fast oscillators, if you look carefully.

G.P. BAERENDS: All measurements on the frequency of behavior patterns during a certain time period show short- as well as long-term oscillations. In considerations like I made in this symposium the short-term oscillations are usually cancelled out statistically and attention is concentrated on changes of longer term. A behavioral tendency is never really constant. Therefore, I can easily agree with your suggestion.

W. STORM VAN LEEUWEN: In the beginning of this session Professor Baerends described his investigations in which the brain is regarded as a blackbox, controlling motor acts. From these investigations he deduced certain systems which should be inside. Later, Professor Creutzfeldt and others have told us something about the mechanisms actually to be found inside the blackbox. In my opinion, the fundamental relation between the two still has not been found. Maybe one should not be surprised about this, because if one sticks an electrode into the brain it would be something of a miracle if the results could be directly related to any specific behavior pattern. I wonder though if Professor Baerends would care to comment on possible relations between data from neurophysiology and the data obtained in his ethological studies.

G.P. BAERENDS: In my opinion neurophysiology is not yet able to tell us how behavior, at the levels of complexity we observe it all around us in animals and man, is brought about by the neurological and endocrinological machinery. Nevertheless, an impressive amount of information on the parts of this machinery, even down to the molecular level, has been obtained by physiologists, anatomists, biochemists, etc. However, the level of sophistication of their physiological techniques is not at all matched by the quality of the corresponding behavioral observations and measurements. Only the techniques for studying learning processes in the laboratory are of high quality, but these are of very limited use for the understanding of the causation of behavior as a whole. Ethologists have developed various techniques for observing and measuring behavior. Moreover, the ethological analysis of complicated behavior sequences, i.e., the logical study of the software underlying complex behavior, will be of great value in stating the problems on the functioning of behavior mechanisms and to define the behavior patterns relevant for each single study. The work on the "feeding system", summarized by Professor de Ruiter in an earlier volume of Progress in Brain Research (de Ruiter et al., 1974) illustrates the advantages of physiologists and ethologists working together in revealing the functioning of behavioral mechanisms.

W. STORM VAN LEEUWEN: I certainly agree with you entirely that there are now good methods for measuring and quantifying behavior. In fact, we have started doing this ourselves, and the combination between these two forms of investigations may lead to a better understanding of brain function than we have at present. But is there anybody who wants to comment on this point from the physiologists' point of view?

F.H. LOPES DA SILVA: I would prefer to get to a point made by Professor Baerends, and indirectly also by Professor Creutzfeldt, namely the nature of the programs for controlling certain patterns of movement. One of the most striking ethological findings is that a complex sequence of movements often seems to be very strongly established; if the cycle is interrupted at some point there is a strong opposing tendency for it to be finished. Van der Gon, with his handwriting analyses (Van der Gon et al., 1969) has distinguished very clearly between those movements which, once elicited, seem to follow a strict program, and those movements which are all the time being controlled by feedback-sensory input. It seems that in the brain there are, on the one hand, programs which are complete and rigid sequences (or, in computer parlance, subroutines which are chained to each other, and which are triggered by specific situations and stimuli) and, on the other hand, sequences which appear to be very much under influence of the outside world. I think that when we talk about stimulation of the brain, one has to have some general idea about which type of program for behavioral sequences is involved predominantly, and also of the strength of the interconnections between different programs, before one can interpret in neurophysiological terms the drive and the goal-directed behaviors elicited by brain stimulation.

445

B. SCHARRER: I would like to add a footnote to the statement Dr. Lopes da Silva made. He brought up the question of the various specific prepatterned motor sequences in writing one's own signature. How can we explain that if, instead of using our hand, we sign our name with a device attached to the foot — the right foot if we are right-handed — the signature retains essentially the characteristics of our own signature, despite the fact that this is the result of an entirely different set of muscles?

L.H. VAN DER TWEEL: The study on handwriting of which Dr. Lopes da Silva spoke was carried out by Dr. Denier Van der Gon when working in our laboratory. We are in fact still engaged in this problem. The idea of Van der Gon was that fast handwriting would be the result of an alternating kind of all-or-nothing activation of the agonists and antagonists of, in the simplest case, two sets of more or less perpendicularly acting muscles. The "vertical" movements in handwriting are then governed by one pair, the "horizontal" (left to right) by another pair of muscles. The fundamental concept was the existence of a time program in the brain that activates the respective muscles with constant forces. The resulting movements are then ballistic. Van der Gon was well aware that a signature with a foot, for example, had many characteristics in common with that of the handwriting. Once the basic program is established it might be that even without much experience the time code can be translated to other sets of muscles. As soon as slower movements are involved, however, and there is enough time for feedback, the picture becomes more complicated (as was shown in the further work of Van der Gon and his group).

M.A. CORNER: I should like to change the line of the discussion to emphasize the tremendous significance of the demonstration made by Professor Dawes as regards the continuity of a specific "physiological state" from embryonic development into postnatal life. This recalls the work of the Sterman group (Sterman and Hoppenbrouwers, 1971) in California; they made autocorrelograms of fetal motility, showing that the same type of cycles as in normal sleep are present in the fetus as well as in the postnatal period. Fetal motility may therefore be considered as the prenatal expression of these sleep types of cycles. In the chick embryo we arrived at identical conclusions about the developmental continuity of prenatal and postnatal life — if you only look at the right things in the right way. There is a very nice correlation — in the period of fetal development where breathing is present, but not yet continuous — between this breathing and the episodes of body movements. So I should like to hear your opinion: whether or not you think that the cycles of mammalian fetal motility really have something to do with the breathing cycles you were demonstrating.

G.S. DAWES: You have a wonderful opportunity for direct observation in the chick embryo. When we record fetal breathing movements in man using ultrasound, many whole-body movements become apparent but it is difficult to categorize these movements. It would be useful if they could be observed, and we could determine whether such movements involve a twisting body motion, or one or more limbs. This is almost impossible if the fetus is still in utero. We need better recording methods; Ruskebusch recorded multiple electromyograms in fetal lambs. yet even they are difficult to interpret.

M.A. CORNER: Perhaps the problem is not all that hopeless, though, especially when you consider that in the chick embryo it is precisely the very strong body movements which have a correlation with the respiration movements. If, presumably, the limitations in the recording techniques for fetal motility, used by the Sterman group, preferentially reveal the large movements, then that would still all be consistent. They may well be correlated with your respiratory cycles, after all, and these smaller twitching movements may be a more predominant background phenomenon throughout all phases.

G.S. DAWES: The only direct observations we have been able to make have been on the fetal lamb delivered under maternal epidural anesthesia. I was not so convinced that the occasional movements of the body were related to breathing movements. They did occur, as one would expect, episodically in REM sleep. Perhaps we should repeat these observations to see if there is any pattern in what appears to be just causal episodes.

W.L. BAKHUIS: I would like to ask whether there is a connection between the work of Professor Olds and Professor Baerends. Professor Baerends worked with gulls and talked about "systems", while Professor Olds worked with rats and talked about drives and showed "centers" in the brain that were related to a certain behavioral pattern. I should like to ask Professor Olds whether these systems which Professor Baerends talked about could have any relation to the types of centers he described.

J. OLDS: I don't want to be too much associated with centers, though I don't want to be completely dissociated from them either. I think that it was a very important warning that someone made to me this morning, that when you stimulate the brain you don't know much about what you are doing. One builds up a collection of shells around the electrode and one does not know in which shell the electricity can be supposed to be optimal. The exact effects of stimulation are still quite unknown; one probably causes a grossly abnormal and noisy activation of the system, something that one would not expect during normal, integrated behavior. In addition, the stimulus does not probe for cell bodies but rather for fibers. And these fibers are long pathways, going from an interesting beginning to an interesting end, via a rather uninteresting middle which we activate by this kind of electric stimulation. We can only say that for the various central motive states and reward behaviors there are rather interesting probability fields: areas where the effects are highly likely, and other areas where they are relatively unlikely. These must be fields where fibers related in some way are relatively concentrated or relatively thinned out. But we have not really discovered centers nor do we believe in them. We believe that the brain is differentiated with regard to these effects (and with relation to involvement in natural functions). Now you may ask: how are your probability fields related to hypotheses of the sort advanced by Professor Baerends? Actually, our experiments do not present us with interpretations of his hypotheses but with other bases on which we can make similar hypotheses. If our hypotheses grow toward each other, we are very lucky. Our point of departure is not really a great deal farther forward than his is; and his may well be even better than ours, because at least it is a set of *real* natural phenomena. Our phenomena are always evaporating when we try to pin them down with lesions. The deletion of bundles of neurons from the brain often seems to give a clear identification of their function for the first two weeks after the lesion. But then the symptoms gradually disappear and you wonder whether it was only something like "spinal shock". Some tonic bombardment was withdrawn, and this was damaging at first — until the system re-equilibrates, as systems are wont to do.

In spite of these difficulties we continue to make hypotheses. My own feeling about your question is that hypotheses based on the work of Professor Baerends will eventually fit well with hypotheses based on our kind of work, and that they need to be repeatedly confronted with one another. Let's imagine for a moment that a hormone or a motivating condition has a double range of effects: one is a set of automatic behaviors, the other is a set of purposive behaviors. The temperature system presents a good example. The same heating causes the animal to seek out a more temperate environment, and simultaneously to make an automatic adjustment by panting or sweating. Lesions show that different parts of the hypothalamus are probably involved in these two mechanisms (e.g., Satinoff, 1974). It is interesting that the more purposive part is also the more "primitive". It exists, for example, in the lizard, which does not have the other mechanism. These two parts of the temperature system have different centers if you like, and perhaps a different phylogeny too. Still, they are integrated into a system and may have common detector elements. I think that the "systems" and the "centers" in this particular instance, where studies have made some progress, are very tightly interrelated, and I think that the hypothalamus is one of the significant places where this happens.

G.P. BAERENDS: I think that Dr. Olds' studies, and others on hypothalamic mechanisms, come closest to the analytical ethological studies on complex behavior. Nevertheless, as I tried to point out in my lecture, it is safer at present to carry out the ethological system analysis without incorporating knowledge about the physiology and structure of the brain and the endocrine organs. However, ethologists and physiologists should aim at further advanced stages in which, on the basis of a detailed ethological description of the functioning of a system, physiological experiments can be undertaken in combination with ethological measurements. Before that stage has been reached it should remain entirely open as to just what physiological mechanism, and what degree of brain localization, the systems and subsystems distinguished by ethologists are actually represented.

REFERENCES

de Ruiter, L., Wiepkema, P.R. and Veening, J.G. (1974) Model of behavior and the hypothalamus. In *Integrative Hypothalamic Activity. Progress in Brain Research, Vol. 41*, D.F. Swaab and J.P. Schadé (Eds.), Elsevier, Amsterdam, pp. 481–507.

Satinoff, E. (1974) Neural integration of thermoregulatory responses. I. In *Limbic and Autonomic Nervous System Research*, L.V. DiCara (Ed.), Plenum Press, New York, pp. 41–83.

Sterman, M.B. and Hoppenbrouwers, T. (1971) The development of sleep-waking and rest-activity patterns from fetus to adult in man. In *Brain Development and Behavior*, M.B. Sterman, D.J. McGinthy and A.M. Adinolfi (Eds.), Academic Press, New York, pp. 203–228.

Van der Gon, J.J. Denier and Wienke, G.H. (1969) The concept of feedback in motorics against that of programming. In *Biocybernetics of the Central Nervous System*, L.D. Proctor (Ed.), Little, Brown and Comp., Boston, Mass., pp. 287–304.

SESSION VII

EPILOGUE

The Brain as a Functional Entity

O. CREUTZFELDT

*Abt. für Neurobiologie, Max-Planck-Institut für
Biophysikalische Chemie, Göttingen (G.F.R.)*

INTRODUCTION

Scientific work is not just the collection of data, but rather the attempt to bring observed data into a system of functional relationships, or "model". The fact that apples fall off the tree down to the ground was known to everybody, but to ask the right question (not, for example, whether the apple is green or red) and thus to conceive of a functional connection between the mass of an apple and of the earth was a scientific achievement of the highest order which culminated in the development of a general theory on the mutual attraction of bodies. Similarly, individual species of plants and animals were identified and named by men throughout history, but to bring them into a systematic functional system, including evolutionary connections, was the really valuable scientific contribution.

Models which bring scattered observations into a relational context can describe a set of observations correctly and consistently but can never be complete, and a new model becomes necessary once new observations are made which are not consistent with it anymore. The Ptolemeic astronomical system, for example, was in fact "correct" as long as it could describe satisfactorily all the observations of astronomers, which was for a very long time indeed, but a new model nevertheless ultimately had to be developed. The only completely accurate descriptions are, of course, the systems themselves. In our case, the only really correct model of the brain as a whole would be the brain itself! From this it follows that the virtues of scientific models, i.e., their consistency and plausibility, are at the same time their vices, because they tend to inhibit and suppress observations which are not deemed to be consistent with them. Wrong models (i.e., incorrect functional connections among the facts, such as the alchemistic approach to chemical compounds) lead to traps and dead ends.

If we try to understand a piece of machinery, we must somewhere along the line be able to define some sort of purpose for it. The purpose of the brain, of course, cannot be described in· one sentence, but let us be content with a formulation such as: the organ which controls the individual in its environment. Alternatively, as Watts (1973) puts it in a more psychoanalytical context: the organ which enables the organism to *be* consistent with its environment. For this purpose the brain must contain within itself a model of its environment, as well as of the organism's interaction with that environment (Young, 1964). If this model is seriously deficient, the brain cannot enable the organism to act consistently with the environment, and its survival is thus endangered. The brain has developed, during phylogeny, into a highly complex machinery. This machinery is partly genetically determined, and thus contains the phylogenetic experience of natural history. In addition, it is able to develop during its own life time a representation of its specific environment and of its own interactions. This ability is called "learning", which in this broad sense includes mechanisms such as adaptation, habituation, imprinting and conditioning, as well as learning in the *strict sense*.

THE QUESTION OF AN ANALYTIC VERSUS A HOLISTIC APPROACH TO SYSTEMS

The working of the brain as a whole is expressed as behavior. A great problem in the brain sciences is that this effective performance of the brain cannot itself be described in terms of neuronal mechanisms, just as we can little characterize the performance of a computer by describing its electronic elements or switches. Nor can we, on the other hand, describe brain mechanisms in terms of behavioral performances, just as we can little deduce the structure of a radio from analyzing its output. The danger in analyzing and describing brain functions lies in a confusion of these two aspects. This confusion is clearly expressed when we extrapolate psychological schemes, i.e., models of performance, into anatomical brain charts — or if artificially produced responses of the system, such as a monosynaptic reflex, are confounded with true motor performance. This is equally so if the fact that units in the visual system may respond best to certain spatial configurations were to be generalized to a theory of visual perception in terms of Fourier analysis.

Still, the dissection of the operation of the brain as a whole, and the identification of performance compartments with actual neuronal mechanisms, remains a useful way of understanding at least a few of its mechanisms, although a rigorous pursuit of such ways must necessarily lead into traps. One must be constantly aware of the two distinct epistemological levels of what we may call the physiological and the performance (or psychological, or behavioral) approaches to brain functioning. Any confusion of these two levels is already getting off on the wrong track right at the outset, though it may be useful (and perhaps amusing, or even sometimes necessary) to do so temporarily.

Let me now turn to two practical examples where confusion of this kind has arisen repeatedly, and has produced progress to our understanding of the brain at exactly the same time as it has suggested totally wrong and progress-inhibiting models. The first example will deal with the mosaic versus holistic concepts of the organization of the cerebral cortex. The dispute over this has gone on now for over 150 years, and it is interesting how the controversy became apparent at all levels (see Creutzfeldt, 1975). The mosaic concept has received strong support in more recent times from the electrical stimulation experiments in humans and other primates which seem to have demonstrated an essentially point-to-point relationship between the representation of individual parts of the body and cortical areas. This led to the well-known charting of the cerebral cortex with sensory and motor homunculi, the visual field representation and tonotopic organization. White fields in the chart (by far the major surface area of the human cortex) were filled with highly specific complex performances such as speech, calculation, writing, memory, drive, will, etc., as seen in the charts of Penfield. These charts (although correct operationally, i.e., from the experimentor's point of view) clearly demonstrate the failure to recognize that psychological, or functional, descriptive schemes of behavior projected onto the cortical surface then represent *only this scheme*, rather than the true functional role of a given part of the cortex within the holistic functional entity of the brain.

Phillips has argued in a recent review (1973) that motor functions are in fact not represented in a mosaic fashion, and that larger areas of the motor and adjacent cortex are involved in the execution of each motor program. There probably exists no static motor unit for any specific program, but rather an ever-changing combination of excited individual neurons, according to the context within which a specific program is to be executed.

PROBLEMS IN THE COLUMNAR ORGANIZATION PRINCIPLE

The mosaic concept has received strong support from the columnar concept of modern neurophysiology. The columnar organization of the cerebral cortex is a model that plausibly describes so many observations that it is almost taken for reality. It was derived from the original observation of Mountcastle (1957) that neurons recorded during a vertical penetration through the hand area of the somatosensory cortex in monkeys were all driven by one and the same type of afferents (from either superficial *or* deep receptors) whereas units in a vertical penetration 1–2 mm away from the first were driven by a different functional class of afferent fibers, but from approximately the same body field. As a matter of fact, however, these two types of afferents are already separate in the peripheral nerve (i.e., a superficial and a deep branch of the median nerve). All that this observation tells us then is that neurons throughout the whole thickness of one cortical "point" are driven by fibers derived from the same afferent nerve bundle and that, all the way up to the primary sensory cortex, such points are not mixed to a large extent.

The conclusion, however, was that different qualities of the sensory input, and thus different "elements of perception", are organized in "columns". A couple of years later, Hubel and Wiesel (1962) made the discovery that given neurons in the primary visual cortex could be best driven by lines having a certain orientation in the visual field. During a vertical penetration through the cortex the preferred orientations, to which the neurons responded optimally, were quite often virtually identical. Neurons found in another vertical penetration, on the other hand, mostly responded optimally to a different orientation of the visual stimulus than in the first case. From this it was concluded that preferred "orientations" of lines in the visual world were also represented in columns of cortical nerve cells. Furthermore, units in a given vertical penetration were driven mainly by either one or the other eye. Thus it was concluded that a system of ocularity columns is superimposed upon the orientation columns. Indeed, following minute lesions restricted to a single layer of the lateral geniculate body, stripes of degeneration could be observed in the cortex separated by stripes without any degeneration. This has now been confirmed by autoradiographic tracing methods. The width of these stripes is up to about 500 μm, the length up to more than a millimeter. The general conclusion was, of course, that here was the morphological substrate of columns, and that the dimension of the "ocularity column" might be approximately that of cortical columns in general. These are then defined as vertical arrays of neurons which either share the same functional property or receive the same input.

Both definitions of the columnar principle have had a strong influence over the last 15 years upon the thinking and the experimental work on the organization of the cortex. However, both definitions confuse two quite different principles: that of the *topographical* and that of the *functional* column. In the first case, that of Mountcastle's columns in the somatosensory cortex, both principles happened to coincide — since the messages from superficial and deep receptors are carried by different peripheral nerves, and are thus carried separately up to the cortex. In the visual cortex, however, the ocular dominance and the orientation columns represent two distinct aspects of columnar organization: a purely topographical and a functional aspect. Since it is believed that the orientation sensitivity of visual cortical neurons is due to the convergence of several fibers from the lateral geniculate body whose receptive fields are lined up in a row, it should follow that the cells in one column receive the same combination of inputs.

Before further discussing this concept, let us look a bit closer into the afferent and intrinsic organization of the visual cortex (Creutzfeldt et al., 1974a, b). In the visual cortex one finds neurons with large (say more than 3° across) and those with small (less than 3° across) excitatory receptive fields (ERF). The neurons with small ERFs correspond to some extent to what Hubel and Wiesel (1962) have called simple cells, and those with a wide field to the complex cell category. The ERFs are (if plotted carefully or, still better, when determined with intracellular recordings) essentially round, although all neurons are sensitive preferentially, and sometimes exclusively, to a straight contrast or light bar of a specific orientation moved over the ERF at a direction normal to the preferred orientation. The orientation preference may be relatively sharply tuned ($20–30^\circ$) or may be much wider (up to more than 90°). The optimal speed for individual neurons varies from 1 to 2°/sec for cells with a small ERF (simple cells), to $10–20^\circ$/sec for cells with a wide ERF (complex cells). In area 18, cells are often encountered which only respond to very fast movements (up to 100°/sec).

If one investigates all neurons recorded during a vertical penetration normal to the surface of the cortex, one discovers that each neuron appears to receive a separate afferent input. The ERFs of all neurons found in such a penetration are scattered over an area of the visual field of 3·4° in diameter. The ERF of one neuron has the characteristics of an *on*-center, another appears to be driven only by an *off*-center geniculate fiber. One neuron responds better (or exclusively) to the forward, the other to the backward movement of an optimally oriented stimulus. The ERFs of neurons with large ERFs cover about the area of the scatter of neurons with small ERFs found in the same vertical penetration (Creutzfeldt et al., 1974a, b).

We have concluded from this observation that neurons with small ERFs within one cortical cylinder each receive individual excitatory inputs essentially from single geniculocortical fibers (or some from other cortical cells), but that neurons within one vertical cylinder of cortex are not all connected with each other through excitatory lines. The findings do not support an anatomical model in which the neurons belonging to a single "column" are connected with each other through excitatory interactions. The findings also do not support a strict topographical, i.e., retinotopic, model since the ERFs within this cylinder are spread over a relatively wide area of the visual field, and thus of the retina. In fact, the afferent input from a retinal field of about 300–500 μm diameter is found to project into this ideal column. Qualitatively, moreover, both *on-* and *off*-center fibers are represented in the same vertical cylinder.

RELATION OF AFFERENT TO INTRINSIC CONNECTIVITY IN CORTICAL ORGANIZATION

If one penetrates the cortex horizontally, i.e., more or less tangentially to its surface plane, one finds that the cortical representation of the visual field is not an affine projection of the retinal image. The scatter found in the horizontal domain is the same as that in the vertical domain, resulting in a random walk progression in the visual field along one horizontal tract (Albus, 1975a). An analysis of the horizontal scatter at different eccentricities shows that the relationship between the reciprocal of the magnification factor (i.e., mm cortex per degree visual angle), which decreases towards the periphery, and the local mean scatter in degrees (which increases), remains the same throughout the visual field. A calculation of this quotient shows that each point in the visual field (i.e., in the retina) has excitatory access to an area of about 2·5 sq. mm cortex (Albus, 1975a).

Neighboring retinal points thus have an overlapping representation in the cortex which is largely random, but with a gradient according to the visual field. The cortical volume per retinal point is the same throughout the visual field. However, since there are more retinal "points" (i.e., ganglion cells) per degree of visual angle in the central parts of the visual field than in the periphery, also the cortical volume handling one degree of visual field is larger in the center. The larger "magnification factor" of the fovea (or central area) in the cortex is thus a function of the afferent organization, rather than being a function of cortical organization per se. This type of afferent projection encounters a rather uniform network of cortical neurons. We have now some idea of the organization of this network. If one excites a group of cortical neurons with glutamate, applied electrophoretically through a micropipette, one discovers that all neurons around this excitatory focus are inhibited within a distance of up to 300–400 μm (Hess et al., 1975). From these experiments it has also become evident that there are no significant excitatory connections between neurons within this distance or beyond. Since there are more cortical neurons than there are afferent fibers, however, we might expect there to be some excitatory connections over short distances, although there is no unequivocal experimental evidence for them. The same type of results have been reported in the somatosensory cortex (Renaud and Kelly, 1974).

We have now two modules: the afferent and the intracortical modules. The afferent module is the distribution of afferent excitation from one peripheral point over an area of about 2–3 mm in diameter; the intracortical module (about 0·8–1·0 mm in diameter) consists essentially of inhibitory interconnections among cortical cells. The picture that emerges is not that of a columnar structure but that of a continuous, but noisy and overlapping, point projection upon a continuous cortical network of inhibitory connections. We may call such a network "cooperative", as the sensitivity and response of any neuron depends on the state of excitation of all other neurons within the same module. But since each neuron belongs to a large number of modules (geometrically speaking an infinite number, but due to the limited number of elements, i.e., neurons, available per unit space, the number is finite but very large) the activity of any element within one module is also dependent on the activities of other, more distant modules.

It should also be realized, in this context, that the afferent fibers are not independent from each other, but interact already at the geniculate and retinal levels in a similar way. Furthermore, ERFs of retinal ganglion cells are relatively large (0·2–3°) and thus look at "fields" rather than at points of the visual environment. As a consequence of this anatomical organization, on- and off-center ganglion cells will respond to moving stimuli at different times, and thus will monitor identical stimuli apparently at different places within the cortical map relative to the actual location in the visual field. The special feature of the cortex appears to be that, within any module, the "interaction points" are random representations of visual field points within the modular domain. The effect of such a modular network in the visual cortex is, roughly speaking, that the cortical neurons are mainly or exclusively sensitive to *moving* stimuli, and that they become selective according to the direction of movement and the orientation of straight-line contrasts.

Let us now look at the *orientation domain*. We are penetrating with our electrode again perpendicular to the surface of the cortex. Most neurons have a similar optimal orientation, but if we determine more exactly the orientation "tuning" curve of each one, we will find that the optimal orientations for all units within a vertical penetration are scattered, with a standard deviation of ± 15–25° around the mean optimal orientation of the whole vertical cylinder. If the electrode now goes parallel to the surface, we find that, also in the horizontal domain, the optimal orientations of successively recorded neurons need not be identical. In fact, we find a gradient in which the probability that units have the same optimal orientation decreases with increasing distance. We can calculate the average orientation difference as a function of intracortical distance, and arrive at an average of about 10° difference in orientation over 30–50 μm horizontal distance. If the differences go in the same direction, say always clockwise, we will have completed a whole cycle of orientation in about

1·5–2·0 mm. One may hit such an ideal "hypercolumn" occasionally, but it is more common — at least in cat visual cortex — that cycles are not completed in such a regular fashion and often perturbed by apparently random changes of orientation (Albus, 1975b). In the monkey cortex orientation sequences appear to be more regular (Hubel and Wiesel, 1974).

We thus have, also in the orientation domain, a system of continuous progression of orientation preference on which a relatively large scatter is superimposed. The scatter in the vertical is about the same as that in the horizontal dimension, but usually does not show a systematic trend as one often observes along horizontal tracks. If we keep in mind the cortical module with essentially inhibitory connections over distances of about 300–400 μm around any cortical point, we will realize that neurons sensitive to different orientations and directions of movement inhibit each other: the principle of lateral inhibition has, here in the cortex, a qualitative as well as a spatial connotation. Such an organization would be best described by a model of a coherent network rather than by a mosaic of independent columns.

SELF-ORGANIZATION AS A POSSIBLE PRINCIPLE OF CORTICAL FUNCTIONAL DEVELOPMENT

The question now arises, to what extent is the functional organization of cortical networks "genetically determined"? I do not want to enter the current discussion which is going on among experimentalists in this field (e.g., Barlow, 1975) but rather to consider the hypothetical possibility of self-organizing properties in the functional development of such a network. Let us assume that the topographical mapping is essentially genetic in origin, based on a program that fiber systems which start out together (in the retina) will tend to stay together throughout their further course. This would lead to a "fuzzy" retinotopic cortical projection. Functional properties such as orientation preference or ocularity of cortical neurons can be biased during the sensitive period in the early postnatal development, i.e., determined by actual usage. It is obvious that, if there is any plasticity at all in the network, the nature of the way in which it is wired up should impart to it a considerable degree of self-organization. von der Malsburg, in my laboratory, started two years ago to test these assumptions on a model which, unfortunately, is not consistent in all its properties with all that we have since learned about cortical and afferent organization. However, the self-organizing features as such lead to encouraging results for an understanding of the development of the functional cortical organization (Malsburg, 1973).

Let us assume that the cortical network consists of a system of short-ranging excitatory and of wider-ranging inhibitory interactions among cortical neurons. Each neuron is covered with a defined number of excitatory synapses, each derived randomly from axon branches from an array of retinal ganglion cells. We then introduce a "learning-by-use principle" similar to that first proposed by Hebb, by means of which a synaptic connection becomes strengthened if the presynaptic and the postsynaptic elements discharge successively within a specified time. As the sum of synaptic excitatory inputs must remain constant in this model, another synapse necessarily becomes weaker and eventually becomes non-functional altogether. With this model, Malsburg was able to demonstrate that an initially random representation of orientation in the network model will assume a regularity of systematically changing orientations, amazingly similar to reality (as observed experimentally). He could recently show the same for ocularity. An initially random distribution of ocular dominance will become ordered into ocularity stripes, each containing neurons from only one eye, and changing with a regular periodicity.

Such a model of an adaptive cooperative network of many elements demonstrates that the final functional position of each individual element may in actuality depend on the functional properties of its neighbors, which are, of course, also dependent in turn on their neighbors, and so forth. This sort of interdependence of individual neurons, and — at a higher level of abstraction — of mutual interaction between groups of neurons and subsystems, may be a step towards an understanding of the working of the brain as an integrated whole.

RELATED QUESTIONS IN THE DOMAIN OF FEATURE DETECTION

As the second example, I should like to consider a further aspect of atomistic versus holistic models in brain functioning or, more specifically, of sensory perception. About 15 years ago, Maturana and Lettvin (e.g., Lettvin et al., 1959) analyzed the functional properties of ganglion cells in the frog's retina: "What does the frog's eye tell the frog's brain?". They found that individual ganglion cells may have quite specific "trigger features", and they classified the retinal ganglion cells according to their optimal trigger feature as "detectors" for, respectively, edge, movement, convexity, concavity, dimness, etc. This approach stimulated a search for similarly specialized cells in other species and in other sensory systems. Such a classification was already established on a more basic level in the periphery of the somatosensory system, where the different types of receptors were assigned different functions, such as for temperature, touch, pressure, pain, etc. The implication was that each of these were also specific detectors of independent sensory categories. In those days, about 10–15 years ago, the battle still went on in the field of touch and pain perception between unitarians, who assumed that the different sensory qualities were only due to different intensities of the stimulus, and dualists who believed that pain and touch receptors were specific and distinct types.

In the mammalian retina, on- and off-center neurons were considered to be specific darkness and brightness detectors; retinal movement detectors were discovered in the rabbit, and orientation and direction detectors were postulated in the visual cortex. If moving light-dark grids were used as stimuli, ganglion cells in the retina and neurons in the visual cortex would both respond best to a particular spatial frequency, that which suits best their ERF diameter. This led some to the supposition that the visual system is composed of different "spatial frequency detectors" (for review see Barlow, 1972).

The implications of such a classification of neurons into specific detectors within a sensory system are that the whole percept then consists of different classes of essentially invariant signals, similar to the analytical principles used in pattern recognition in man-made systems. It can easily be shown that such a system requires a hierarchical classification matrix, as well as yet another system to evaluate the analysis and to recombine the elements into logical structures: this requires highly specific neuronal systems, tuned to rather complex patterns such as the famous "banana", "grandmother", or other specific object detectors.

One sees immediately that such a model of perception would be quite compatible with a mosaic concept of extreme localizationism, and it in fact represents the consequent continuation of the classical psychophysical positivism of 70–100 years ago. For this reason, the criticism expressed by the Gestalt psychologists, notably by Köhler (1969), of such an approach to perception is still valid. He emphasized the irreducible functional interconnections of the perceptual elements rather than their atomistic subdivision into conceptual abstractions.

I do not want to go into a detailed epistemological analysis of the "element detector" concept, which can readily be shown to be insufficient (if indeed not downright incorrect) as a model of perceptual processes. Let us look rather at the possible physiological basis for such a model. One minimal condition for a strict sign detector must be that it signals that sign invariant from its context. This might be the case for a few highly specialized peripheral receptors (e.g., electroreceptors), although it is difficult — and in my opinion probably impossible — to characterize even the most specialized receptors in terms of "pure perceptual qualities". Already at the most peripheral neuronal level it is easy to show that the sensitivity of any element to a given sensory quality depends strongly on the context in which this stimulus appears. The information about brightness given by a retinal *on*-center cell will depend on the contrast between the illumination of the on-center and the surround. Thus, the most basic form of information conveyed by an element concerns the *relative quality* of a particular type of sensation, and is useful only if the context (i.e., the responses of the ganglion cells around the assumed "detector cell") in which this sensory quality appeared is known. One may argue then that the cell is never a *brightness* but always a *contrast* detector, although even this would merely transpose the problem to a higher level and not solve it.

Let us consider the cortical "orientation" detector from a purely technical point of view. The "orientation tuning" of individual nerve cells is relatively wide: 10–$40°$ half-width or more for the simple units, and even wider for complex units which were considered to be higher order neurons, i.e., those which could generalize for orientation or direction. Taking into account the enormous response variability of such neurons from one stimulus to the next, one would need to have an enormous number for each orientation if one wanted to extract a somewhat exact judgment of orientation (such as is possible to do psychophysically; Andrews et al., 1973). The situation actually becomes much more complicated, since the optimal orientation of a neuron may also vary to a considerable extent according to the presence or absence of contrasts, or of dissimilar orientations near to the one under consideration.

Based on the observation of orientation-sensitive cells, not only was the

460

conclusion drawn that such cells are orientation detectors, but the hypothesis was derived that objects in the environment are coded in the brain, simply by signalling all orientations of straight lines, and of tangents, found within or around these perceived objects. Such a method is in fact, reminiscent of certain computer analysis methods, where complex functions such as the EEG are transformed by an enormous electronic machinery into still other complex functions without adding any new information. The transformation of our visual environment into the line segments and tangents of different orientations would appear to mess up rather than to clarify the pictorial representation of that environment. It is interesting to note in this context that electrical stimulation of small points in area 17 of humans produces only star- or grain-like tiny phosphens, but never lines or any other structural patterns (Brindley, 1973). The argument is similar as regards the hypothesis that the visual world is encoded by dissecting it into different spatial frequencies, different speeds of movement, and whatever other detectors have been reported. The essential difficulty in all such piecemeal analytical approaches is the recomposition of the supposedly invariant elements to form a unifying idea. But this problem should not be confounded with perception itself since it is not ideas which we are seeing, touching or hearing, but a realistic and coherent *Umwelt*!

REPEATED TRANSFORMATIONS AND RECOMBINATIONS IN THE CEREBRAL CORTEX

The physiological-anatomical question boils down to whether or not there are any hierarchical structures available in the brain which could conceivably recombine all the bits and pieces of sensation into higher-order percepts. It was thought for some time that primary, secondary, etc., receiving areas represent just such hierarchical sequences of successively higher order sensory analysis. We now know, however, that they are not simply sequences of the next higher order. For example area 18 of the cortex receives (except in primates) a direct retinogeniculate input in addition to the input from area 17. The third, fourth and fifth visual areas in primate cortex receive, in addition to input relayed from area 17, inputs directly from the posterior thalamic visual nuclei; and these, in turn, receive inputs from the "second visual system", i.e., the retinocollicular pathway. The cat "Clare-Bishop cortical area" combines inputs from the lateral geniculate body, from areas 17 and 18, and from the pulvinar, while the superior colliculi receive input from areas 17, 18 and Clare-Bishop. All cortical structures in fact seem to feed back into their afferent subcortical nuclei, and in all these multiple projection-, loop-, and feedback-pathways, the retinotopic organization is more or less preserved. In each projection area, moreover the basic Bauplan of the cortical network, i.e., the connection of neighboring elements over a limited range through lateral inhibition, appears to be — essentially — the same.

We end up with the situation that the visual world is represented several times over in the brain. In each representation something is lost but something else is gained, by virtue of the combination of the output from one area (say area 17) with that of another functional representation of the visual world (say the pulvinar, or area 19), or even with an earlier station in the pathway — such as the recombination of the area 17 output with geniculate y-cell input in area 18.

The result of such a repeated passage of the sensory surfaces through cortical networks, and the recombination of the continuous remapping with other filter outputs may be that in one area the neurophysiologist may find, predominantly, cells which preferably respond to contrasts moving in a certain direction, in another area neurons which respond preferentially to binocular disparity, and in still another essentially to color, etc. The important point, however, is that individual neurons are not detectors of one specific quality, but that the projected picture is transformed as a whole according to the properties of the various networks, and that the innumerable points of this transformed picture are brought back into a coherent relation with each other — thus performing a new transformation. In such a manner, not individual "point properties" are analyzed and registered, but a coherent picture (which itself is already a transformation of the real world) becomes recombined with other transformations of the same original stimulus pattern, and such a combined "hypertransformation" may be again transformed according to similar rules. In order to understand the working of the brain as an entity, we need to develop new methods for describing this process of repeated transformation of whole pictures by the different functional layers, none of which can be regarded as a complete system in itself. The integrated sum of all such symbolic representations of the environment in diverse neuronal networks constitute the sought-after model of the environment, contained within each of our brains.

REFERENCES

Albus, K. (1975a) A quantitative study of the projection area of the central and the paracentral visual field in area 17 of the cat. I. The precision of the topography. *Exp. Brain Res.*, 24: 159–179.

Albus, K. (1975b) A quantitative study of the projection area of the central and the paracentral visual field in area 17 of the cat. II. The spatial organization of the orientation domain. *Exp. Brain Res.*, 24: 181–202.

Andrews, D.P., Butcher, A.K. and Buckley, B.R. (1973) Acuities for spatial arrangement in line figures: human and ideal observers compared. *Vision Res.*, 13: 599–620.

Barlow, H.B. (1972) Single units and sensation: a neurone doctrine for perceptual psychology. *Perception*, 1: 371–394.

Barlow, H.B. (1975) Visual experience and cortical development. *Nature (Lond.)*, 258: 199–204.

Brindley, G.S. (1973) Sensory effects of electrical stimulation of the visual and paravisual cortex in man. In *Handbook of Sensory Physiology, Vol. VII/3: Central Visual Information B*, R. Jung (Ed.), pp. 583–594.

Creutzfeldt, O. (1975) Some problems of cortical organization in the light of ideas of the classical "Hirnpathologie" and of modern neurophysiology. An essay. In *Cerebral Localization*, K.J. Zülch, O. Creutzfeldt and G.C. Galbraith (Eds.), pp. 217–226.

Creutzfeldt, O.D., Innocenti, G.M. and Brooks, D. (1974a) Vertical organization in the visual cortex (area 17) in the cat. *Exp. Brain Res.*, 21: 315–336.

Creutzfeldt, O.D., Kuhnt, U. and Benevento, L.A. (1974b) An intracellular analysis of visual cortical neurones to moving stimuli: responses in a co-operative neuronal network. *Exp. Brain Res.*, 21: 251–274.

Hess, R., Negishi, K. and Creutzfeldt, O. (1975) The horizontal spread of intracortical inhibition in the visual cortex. *Exp. Brain Res.*, 22: 415–419.

462

Hubel, D. and Wiesel, T.N. (1962) Receptive fields, binocular interaction and functional architecture in the cat's visual cortex. *J. Physiol. (Lond.)*, 160: 106–154.

Hubel, D.H. and Wiesel, T.N. (1974) Sequence regularity and geometry of orientation columns in the monkey striate cortex. *J. comp. Neurol.*, 158: 267–294.

Köhler, W. (1969) *The Task of Gestalt-Psychology*. Princeton Univ. Press, Princeton, N.J. (Quoted from German edition: *Die Aufgabe der Gestaltpsychologie*, Berlin, 1971.)

Lettvin, J.Y., Maturana, H.R., McCulloch, W.S. and Pitts, W.H. (1959) What the frog's eye tells the frog's brain. *Proc. IRE*, 47: 1940–1951.

Malsburg, Chr. von der (1973) Self-organization of orientation sensitive cells in the straite cortex. *Kybernetik*, 14: 85–100.

Mountcastle, V.B. (1957) Modality and topographic properties of single neurones of cat's somatic sensory cortex. *J. Neurophysiol.*, 20: 408.

Phillips, C.G. (1973) Cortical localization and "sensori-motor processes" at the "middle level" of primates. *Proc. roy. Soc. B*, 66: 987–1002.

Renaud, L.P. and Kelly, J.S. (1974) Identification of possible inhibitory neurons in the pericruciate cortex of the cat. *Brain Res.*, 79: 9–28.

Watts, A.W. (1973) *Psychotherapy East and West*. (Pantheon Books, 1961), Penguin Books.

Young, J.Z. (1964) *A Model of the Brain*. Oxford Univ. Press, London.

DISCUSSION

J. OLDS: It is about coding and decoding that I want to ask a question: if you are rejecting the "grandmother" neuron concept, do you still acknowledge perhaps a grandmother cell assembly or a family of neurons? The general concept here is: does the organism have a model of, in this case, grandmother in its head, and is this model a rather specialized subset of the total set of neurons in the head, or is it not? These are then going to be in some sense decoding neurons. I believe that you will therefore have to accept the existence of detectors.

O. CREUTZFELDT: Of course we have detectors, and all I am saying is that the brain as a whole is itself a detector. I would not think of cell assemblies in the sense that Dr. Lopes da Silva has described them, however. I think what we have to learn more about first is the transformation process, since what the brain does in fact is to transform the environment into a pattern compatible with it. Recent work shows that any motor act may consist of the activity of an ever varying number of cells. The set of neuronal activities which may produce an essentially all-or-none response is thus an ever changing one, and that is something we just have to accept. There is not a hierarchical continuation of areas 17, 18, 19, 20, 21, 22, and so on, but rather a continuous recombination. Thus it may be that there is a particular activity which sometimes consists of neurons a, z, x, y, and the next time of m, n, k, and o. It is very difficult to express all this in words, and I think that one has to develop tangible models in order to describe such a set of ever-varying elementary combinations, which somehow have the same ultimate meaning.

H. VAN DER LOOS: This will be a very trying question but rather important for the interpretation of your results: how do you test for perpendicularity when you make a track through the cortex, and you reap information from individual cells which you find on your path?

O. CREUTZFELDT: We used various methods to ascertain verticality. One is to take two electrodes at a set distance and compare the neurons which we record during a penetration. Then, if there is a clearly defined orientation column, and the hypercycles would be regularly going down through the whole depth of the cortex, then the difference in orientation between the pairs of neurons should remain about the same. We now have two variables, and we are independent really of exact verticality, because we always have the same intracortical distances. Although we may go through different so-called "columns" we shall always have the same translation from one recording point to the next.

A Unifying Approach to Mind and Brain: Ten Year Perspective

R.W. SPERRY

*Division of Biology, California Institute of Technology,
Pasadena, Calif. 91125 (U.S.A.)*

The idea that the course of physiological events in the brain can be influenced by the contents of subjective experience has long been vigorously opposed by nearly all scientists and most 20th century philosophers. A working assumption of neuroscience holds that a complete causal explanation of brain function is possible, in principle, in terms entirely objective and material without any reference to conscious or mental agents. The conceptual brain model based on impulse transmission, membrane potentials, ion transport, transmitter substances, and the like has seemed to have no need nor any place for the action of mental influences or of anything like conscious experience. Theories of consciousness acceptable to science have accordingly conceived the mind-brain relation always in such a way that the neural mechanisms would function the same whether accompanied by consciousness or not (Boring, 1942). Since conscious mental phenomena are thus supposed to make no difference in brain processing, it follows that they can safely be ignored in science, as can also those disciplinary approaches to brain and behavior based in introspection and inner experience.

This traditional stance of behaviorist-materialist science has come into question in recent years, beginning in the mid-1960s when a modified concept of mind was perceived suggesting a way in which conscious experience might exert causal influence in the brain to control behavior on terms acceptable to neuroscience and without violating principles of scientific explanation (Sperry, 1965). In direct contradiction to the founding thesis of Watsonian behaviorism, consciousness in this new framework was interpreted to be an integral part of the brain process and an important directive force in brain function. The contents of consciousness were assumed to play an active control role as causal determinants in brain activity and were recognized to be functional phenomena in their own right "distinct from and more than" the component biophysical and neurochemical processes.

To center in on the concepts involved in these developments we first by-pass previous theories in which consciousness was explained as (a) an epiphenomenon, (b) an inner aspect of cerebral activity, (c) as being identical to the neural events (psychophysical identity theory) or (d) as an artifact of semantics, or pseudoproblem. We focus instead on the interpretation of consciousness as an emergent of brain activity, as argued especially by the

Gestalt school of psychology back in the 1930s and '40s. However, we then discard the Gestalt interpretation of the emergent properties as passive correlates of cortical activity, and also the idea that psychoneural correlations involve isomorphic or topological correspondence between the neural and the perceived mental events. We by-pass also the hypothesis that the events of perception are correlated with electric field forces and volume current conduction patterns in the cortex (Kohler and Held, 1949). We must largely reject as well the extreme Gestalt position with respect to analysis that disclaims the value of explanation in terms of the parts.

Alternatively we interpret the emergent conscious properties in terms of conventional neural circuit theory. A further postulate is added in which the subjective conscious effect of a brain process is viewed as a functional or operational derivative. In other words, subjective meaning is conceived to depend primarily on the way a given cerebral process works in the context of brain dynamics. What counts in determining a conscious perceptual effect is the preparation to respond to a perceived outside stimulus in an adaptive, meaningful adjustment, rather than the way in which the brain's neural process happens to copy or correspond with the perceived stimulus with respect to shape, size, unity, texture, timing, etc. (Sperry, 1952). Conscious phenomena, thus conceived as dynamic emergent properties of high order cerebral processes, are not merely products of neural complexity but are also designed specifically to produce operational subjective effects.

In the cerebral chain of command, the high order subjective properties are seen to supersede the infrastructural details of nerve impulse traffic and physicochemical interactions. The causal potency of consciousness in the brain's control hierarchy is conceived largely in terms of the universal power of a whole over its parts. Conscious cerebral processes, as dynamic entities in brain activity, contain entitive systemic properties that exert controlling influence over many aspects of the component physicochemical elements of which they are built. As with any part-whole relationship, a mutual interaction prevails in which the conscious mental effects are determined by the neural events, including their molecular and atomistic components, while these latter in turn are reciprocally controlled by the higher holistic or systemic properties of the conscious cerebral process in which they are embedded.

The foregoing approach to the mind-brain relation arose largely out of efforts to explain the seeming unity and/or duality of conscious experience in the bisected brain (Sperry, 1970a). Subjective unity, like other aspects of conscious awareness, seemed to be most effectively accounted for as an operational derivative in which the conscious effect was determined by the contextual functional impact of the brain process in question, i.e., the way it worked to influence ongoing brain activity. On these terms each of the surgically disconnected hemispheres could logically have its own separate unified stream of conscious experience. In the normal intact brain, on the other hand, the two hemispheres must typically act as a unit where subjective unity could be inferred to involve a coherent bilateral brain process spanning both hemispheres through the commissures (Sperry, 1970b, 1974, 1976). Underlying assumptions implied (a) that conscious awareness may be sustained by connecting fiber systems of the brain as well as by the switching sites and transmission interfaces of the gray matter, and (b) that the fiber systems interconnecting the hemispheres are not different in principle, in this respect, from fiber systems within a hemisphere.

Among other advantages this interpretation of subjective unity seemed to resolve the bothersome philosophical problem of "grain," so-called, in which the particulate discontinuousness or "graininess" of neural activity has always seemed difficult to correlate with the smooth, continuous non-grainy content of subjective experience. The mental effect need not correlate with the array of excitatoty details comprising the infrastructure of a brain process, but only with the overall operational impact. Finally, an "operational impact" logically implies a causal influence on the part of the conscious properties involved.

Viewed broadly the above scheme provided in theory a neural-based model for phenomenology and for psychophysical interaction. It gave subjective experience a tangible use in a physical world and a reason for having been evolved. In effect it served to restore conscious mind to the brain of experimental science and brought scientific theory at long last into line with common sense impressions on the mind-controlling-behavior issue. More specifically, the scheme brought together and fused into a unifying conceptual framework, divergent theoretical tenets from materialist vs. mentalist, and monist vs. dualist doctrines that formerly were disparate and conflicting. Today these concepts acquire some additional reassurance by having survived wide circulation in the literature for more than ten years with plenty of opportunity for critics to shoot them down. The aim in the present is not to further explicate or reinforce these ideas as such, but, rather, to take the model as it stands, and put it more in perspective, noting some of the broader implications and general consequences.

The emergence during the past decade of a neural-based conceptual model for explaining psychophysical interaction and mental control in brain function and behavior has helped to strengthen a general swing during this period toward mentalism and humanism in behavioral science and philosophy — away from behaviorism, reductionism, and mechanistic determinism. Proponents of cognitive, clinical, humanistic and related disciplines in psychology that prefer to work directly with subjective experience have acquired a new scientific clout in recent years enabling them to stand up to the behaviorists and physical scientists in a way that was not possible before the mid-1960s when psychophysical effects were ruled out on principle and the opposing subjective and objective approaches seemed, at best, to pose a puzzling and irreconcilable paradox (Wann, 1965). Meanwhile in the area of mind-brain relations mentalists, dualists and psychophysical interactionists after having been essentially silent and invisible for decades, have suddenly begun to reappear in considerable numbers proclaiming various anti-materialist, anti-reductionist positions. It has not mattered that no firm proof is yet available; there is none either for the behaviorist-materialist doctrine. Success of the latter has depended largely on the seeming total inconceivability that neural mechanisms could be influenced by subjective experience. Undermining materialist convictions on this point has released the floodgate pressures of subjectivist interests everywhere.

Our model carries no support for the increased intellectual tolerance of parapsychology and of the mystical and metaphysical generally, that also have ridden the recent rise of interest in mentalism. Chances that mental influences could pass by telepathy from one brain to another or affect any distant object on the above terms, or exist in any way independently of brain activity look, if anything, less hopeful than before. The mental phenomena remain directly tied to the brain as functional properties of cerebral mechanisms in action.

The kind of causal control envisaged represents an intermediate between mechanistic determinism and full volitional freedom pointing to a compromise resolution for the age-old issue of free will vs. determinism. A "self-determining" interpretation for human decision-making is implied (Sperry, 1965, 1976). Our seemingly free decisions are seen to be causally determined, as science would have it, but, as we personally would prefer to believe, these decisions are determined at a subjective mental level largely, rather than at the molecular or neuronal level of causation, by our own mental inclinations. The sequence of events in the brain leading to a particular choice is determined literally, in an objective causal sense, by what we desire and most value. A kind of personal control and self-determination is provided that most of us would prefer over complete freedom. Complete freedom from causation would leave our thought, decisions and behavior subject to random meaningless chance and caprice.

On these terms psychology and psychiatry rate as distinct scientific disciplines in their own right, not reducible to neurophysiology or biology. Causal interactions involved at the conscious mental levels of cerebral function have laws and dynamics that are hardly included in neurophysiology as traditionally conceived. The kind of mental control over physicochemical events that is implied involves no violation of the laws and principles of neurophysiology — any more than the presence of higher controls for the speed and direction of ambulation violates the chemistry and physiology of muscle contraction or nerve impulse conduction. Different levels of organization and causal control are operative. Where the causal sequence of cerebral events includes conscious mental properties, the concepts of physiology need to be supplemented — but not substituted or dispensed with. Phenomena at any one level of brain action are largely (though not entirely) determined by, and explainable in terms of, component events at the next lower level. However, the subevents at successively elementary levels become increasingly irrelevant and incomplete in themselves as an explanation. Search for the chemistry or molecular biology of psychological activities as an ultimate end is misguided conceptually, but such efforts are not without valuable explanatory spin-off at subsystem levels.

The above approach to the mind-brain interface has seemed in a number of respects to have something for everyone. On different occasions I have been informed by proponents of mentalism, behaviorism, phenomenology, reductionism, Gestaltism, humanism, determinism, emergent theory, existentialism, psychophysical identity theory, monism, and even classical dualism, that this interpretation is what is meant by each of these respective positions. Those who lean toward materialism stress that the conscious effects are determined by, and are properties of, and inseparably linked to, the material brain process with all its anatomical and physiological constraints, and that separate metaphysical or dualistic realms of existence or truth are discounted. Those who lean to dualism and mentalism on the other hand (Eccles, 1970) emphasize that the subjective mental phenomena are realities in their own right to be recognized as distinct entities, different from and more than the component neural events of which they are built and not reducible to these components. They also find attractive the fact that the fate and course of the constituent neural events is subject to control by the supersedent mental properties.

Monists acclaim the idea of a single continuous hierarchy in the brain that extends from the brain's subnuclear particles on up through atoms, molecules, cells, and nerve circuits to include at the uppermost levels the events of conscious experience. Pragmatists are in accord with the operational derivation of conscious meaning. Reductionists point out that the conscious effects are built of neural events, and must therefore be explainable largely in terms of those events. Concepts involving "cell patterns and assemblies", "spatio-temporal patterns", and "frequency encoded configurations" easily take on added psychophysical interactionist connotations in the new perspective. Since the appearance of this unifying approach in 1965, gradual shading of related thinking to include congenial aspects has made it increasingly difficult to differentiate various related philosophical positions and one must go back to the "pre-65" descriptions to see clear distinctions.

On the above terms the whole value-rich world of inner experience, formerly the sole province of the humanities and specifically excluded in principle from materialist science, becomes reinstated in theory as part of the domain of science (Sperry, 1972). Subjective phenomena, including values, gain objective consequences and can be treated scientifically as prime causal determinants in decision making. In short, there is new promise that some of the major long-standing paradoxes like those between mind and brain, objective and subjective, fact and value, free will and determinism and that between *is* and *ought* that have long puzzled and polarized human thinking may one day be resolved in a unifying approach to mind, brain and physical reality.

Looking ahead, the most promising route by which we may hope to eventually obtain definitive answers in the mind-brain area appears to lie in advancement of our neurological analysis of brain processing, particularly at its upper levels, with special attention focused on a search for those critical differences that distinguish the cerebral mechanisms that involve conscious experience from those that do not. What are the very special differences in cerebral processing responsible for subjective experience that distinguish, for example, the mechanisms of simple conscious sensations from various equally and perhaps much more complex but nevertheless unconscious, cerebellar activity? All kinds of brain processing can be said to have an inner as well as an outer objective aspect, and both aspects all through the neural hierarchy can be said to have neural identity. However, it apparently is only certain of these different kinds of neural events that yield subjective conscious experience. On the above terms we are led to look upon the subjective effects as being specific and selective, not universal, features of cerebral function, introduced and developed in brain evolution because they facilitate brain processing and decision making.

468

Once neuroscience has progressed to the point where we can understand what kinds of organizational variables in the neural mechanisms are required to produce conscious experience, it should then be logically possible to infer the extent to which these and therefore consciousness may be present in various subhuman nervous systems, and also the extent to which it may be possible perhaps to build conscious experience into a computer.

The present scheme leaves the future problem for neuroscience and philosophy of defining in operational terms the essential functional role played by subjective awareness. Precisely what benefits, from a functional, engineering standpoint, are conferred by the introduction in evolution of subjective conscious effects? Thinking on this question has only just begun along lines like the following: consider the tactical difference between responding to the world directly and responding to inner conscious representations, models and signs of the world. Wherever displacement in time or space are advantageous, as in mental recall or anticipation (both of which are critical to the learning process) the use of inner representations becomes a necessity. The real world can hardly be manipulated like inner images. Responses involving perceptual constancies in shape, size, position and the like would seem also to be more effectively managed through inner representations. Further, the use of implicit trial and error responses to inner mental models (thus avoiding overt response commitment with errors in the real world) is a central aspect of the thinking process.

The development of an inner subjective world may be viewed broadly as part of the evolutionary process of freeing behavior from its initial primitive stimulus-bound condition to provide increasing degrees of freedom of choice and originative central processing. The subjective effects may also be seen to have special advantages as general positive and negative reinforcers in learning situations and later for motivation, evolving into ends in themselves in the directive control of much of human behavior. In every case it must be asked why the evolutionary developments could not have occurred, at least as readily and effectively, in the absence of subjective effects.

ACKNOWLEDGEMENTS

Work of the author is supported by USPHS Grant No. 03372 from the National Institute of Mental Health and by the F.P. Hixon Fund of the California Institute of Technology.

REFERENCES

Boring, E.G. (1942) *Sensation and Perception in the History of Experimental Psychology.* Appleton-Century, New York.

Eccles, J.C. (1970) *Facing Reality.* Springer-Verlag, New York.

Kohler, W. and Held, R. (1949) The cortical correlate of pattern vision. *Science,* 110: 414–419.

Sperry, R.W. (1952) Neurology and the mind-brain problem. *Amer. Scientist,* 40: 291–312.

Sperry, R.W. (1965) Mind, brain, and humanist values. In *New Views on the Nature of Man,* J.R. Platt (Ed.), University of Chicago Press, Chicago, Ill., pp. 71–92. Reprinted (1966) in *Bull. Atom. Sci.,* 22: 2–6.

Sperry, R.W. (1970a) Perception in the absence of the neocortical commissures. *Ass. Res. nerv. ment. Dis.*, 48: 123–138.

Sperry, R.W. (1970b) An objective approach to subjective experience: further explanation of a hypothesis. *Psychol. Rev.*, 77: 585–590.

Sperry, R.W. (1972) Science and the problem of values. *Perspect. Biol. Med.*, 16: 115–130. Reprinted (1974) in *Zygon*, 9: 7–21.

Sperry, R.W. (1974) Lateral specialization in the surgically separated hemispheres. *The Neurosciences: Third Study Program*, F.O. Schmitt and F.G. Worden (Eds.), MIT Press, Cambridge, Mass.

Sperry, R.W. (1976) Mental phenomena as causal determinants in brain function. *Process Studies*, 5: 247–256.

Wann, T.W. (Ed.) (1965) *Behaviorism and Phenomenology: Contrasting Bases for Modern Psychology*. University of Chicago Press, Chicago, Ill.

The Nature of Consciousness: Some Persistent Conceptual Difficulties and a Practical Suggestion

M. CORNER

*Netherlands Central Institute for Brain Research,
Amsterdam-O (The Netherlands)*

In the previous paper in this volume Sperry has indicated some of the major problems involved in understanding brain (conscious)-mind interrelationships, and reviewed his proposals made over the past ten years for eliminating the sources of greatest disagreement among different schools of thought. There remain to my mind a few important unresolved difficulties, however, and it will hopefully be useful to focus attention here upon some of the main points of confusion. Perhaps such an exercise will contribute to our eventually obtaining a clear view of the directions in which investigations in this area can most fruitfully be steered.

Of the three traditional classes of answers to the mind-brain question — *interactionism, parallelism* and *identity* (von Bertalanffy, 1967) — Sperry's model clearly falls in the first category. The characteristic features here are: (1) the "conscious mind" is something basically different from the brain processes associated with it, being not simply a different (i.e., internal) view of one and the same phenomenon; and (2) it plays an active part in the chain of causation linking successive functional states within the nervous system. An appealing feature of Sperry's formulation is that of consciousness itself being naturalistically determined (see also Schrödinger, 1967) by ongoing neuronal activity patterns of an appropriate kind, rather than the causation being a one-way affair as in the age-old "common sense" assumption, based upon ordinary subjective experience alone. He recognizes clearly, moreover, that any attempt to give a scientific foundation to the latter formulation by means of the indeterminacy allowed for in quantum physics would merely amount to the introduction of complete capriciousness (Schrödinger, 1967), rather than the sought-after "freedom" of the individual mind from external constraints.

An interactionist viewpoint on the mind-brain question would seem to boil down to nothing less than the postulation of the existence of a specific type of force field in the cosmos, taking its place alongside the electromagnetic, gravitational and other known forms. The fact that this "mental" energy is then regarded as being so fundamentally different as to justify the creation of a distinct category for it (the others then being lumped together as the "material" forces) does not really change the formal problem hereby posed. As with any other discovery which is subject (in principle) to scientific study, the task would appear to be (1) to develop techniques for measuring the new force reliably, and (2) to examine theoretically the laws which govern it and the nature of its relationship to other known forces. With respect to consciousness, in the absence of anything substantial in either category at this time little can be usefully said one way or the other about the hypothesis. It is not at all easy to see, however, where such a force might meaningfully take its place within the complex sequences of ionic, metabolic and humoral processes which make up our current picture of nervous activity.

Sperry, however, explicitly views the causality of mind as not residing in elemental cosmic forces at all but rather in emergent *holistic* ones. Conscious experience would be specifically related to particular kinds of operations carried out in certain types of networks, based upon presently unknown organizational principles, and would constitute an essential link in the flow of overall functional states and details of patterning. Such an influence is viewed as being an aspect of a more general type of control held to be exerted by *any* whole over its component parts. Apart from the fact that no indication is offered as to how consciousness would then add anything in the way of causation to that which is already inherent in the wholeness of the material system generating it, the very concept of "holistic control" seems to my mind to be based upon an error in semantics: the confusion between *command hierarchies* and *levels of abstraction.* The former is undoubtedly a very useful way indeed of describing the organization of many types of systems, including that of the nervous system (Koestler, 1970). For instance (despite the presence of some autonomous activities at each level), motor units may be said to be subject to regulation by spinal motor systems, these by various brain stem centers, and these in turn by the higher integrative neural networks. On the other hand, the "hierarchy" extending from atoms through molecules, membranes, organelles, cells and organs, on up to individual organisms, societies, ecosystems (and abstractions of still higher order) is something else altogether. Because each level *includes* all of the lower-order constituents — and indeed is nothing else than a convenient form of notation for representing the organized totality of interactions among them — the system itself may not properly be introduced as an additional interacting entity at the same level as the parts!

It would be a great shame to leave the matter at this, since the practical reasons advanced by Sperry for grappling with it in the first place are compelling enough: the problem of mankind having an inspiring rather than a depressing view of itself and its relationship to the rest of reality. Thus, the currently widely accepted mind-brain *identity* formulation is portrayed as contributing to a mechanistic and fatalistic attitude towards life, one that tends to be indifferent or even hostile to humanist values. It becomes clear then that the problem here does not originate in any serious intellectual inadequacy of current neurobiological concepts, analogous, for example, to the theoretical difficulties leading to the establishment of quantum and relativity theories at the turn of the century. Rather, a powerful emotional motivation is obviously involved somewhere along the line, apparently based upon a profound dissatisfaction with the prospect of having to identify oneself completely with materialistic processes (and presumably idem for their energetic equivalents).

I suspect that this attitude may be an unfortunate remnant of the traditional philosophical and theological bias of our culture (which has always regarded "matter" to be inferior in worth to "spirit"), possibly compounded by the profound feelings of alienation from nature characteristic of our modern over-industrialized society. I am not very confident that this split can be overcome by our becoming persuaded intellectually that, while being fully subject at one end to the flow of natural causation, on the other end we exert as distinct entities (and are we not being encouraged to identify most closely with the "*mental*" forces, c.q. subjective awareness?) a decisive influence upon the material changes occurring within our own brains. I would hold rather that the problem is rooted in strong dualistic tendencies of human consciousness itself, and that the solution is most likely to lie in the direction of our learning to *directly experience* a closer unity with the world around us than most of us are presently able to do. Indeed, it will be immediately evident that none of these weighty questions would ever have arisen had not, within the field of consciousness itself, a process taken place whereby the experiential distinction emerged between a "self" and an "outside world". Even strictly scientifically speaking there may be relatively good prospects in first examining the nature of this *distinction,* and for the time being just accepting consciousness per se as a starting point, a presently inexplicable fact of life (at least as far as understanding its initial appearance on the evolutionary scene is concerned).

As mysterious as the phenomenon of consciousness may seem to be, the widely held supposition that it is associated only with certain types of brain activities (Eccles, 1953; Hess, 1964; also Sperry, pp. 463–469 in this volume) might reward some further exploration at this point. One finds, first and foremost, a *unified field* of experience (Sherrington, 1951) in which the various afferent modalities — instantaneous interoceptive as well as exteroceptive stimuli, plus recollections and anticipations of these same categories of sensations — are being projected and related one to the other. It is precisely what might be expected if a central display terminal or screen were available in which the appropriate transformations of incoming plus (potentially relevant) stored sensory information, together with extrapolations of future eventualities, were being continuously reflected and fed back to the executive nerve centers. The advantages of such an arrangement for ensuring the integrated working of an incredibly complex motor performance system, and for internal cross-checking during elaborate computational procedures, are not difficult to imagine. An extensive sheet-like structure such as the cerebral cortex, moreover, is an obvious candidate (Herrick, 1956) to be the morphological substrate of this "mirror of the mind" function. Maybe the problem will turn out to be simply a matter, after all, of a special knack for looking at the phenomenon in such a way that a "conscious" field of (symbolically coded) sensations becomes a self-evident feature of systems engaged in carrying out such operations of internal reflection.

There remains still the experience of *self*-consciousness to deal with — ordinarily a representation of one's body within a perpetually changing spatial continuum. The biological utility of this (not completely arbitrary!) borderline is obvious enough, but the sensation of being an apart entity nevertheless also obscures a most fundamental feature of reality. The modern scientific world-view no longer conflicts with the classical "mystical" perception of the essential unity and flux of all creation (Huxley, 1962; Naranjo and Ornstein, 1971). However important the abstraction of a separate identity might be for much of human adaptive behavior, it could be that a periodic transcendence of this illusion is essential in a conscious being for the maintenance of a harmonious rapport between itself and the "outside" world. It is a most interesting question, furthermore, whether this mode of perception really even represents an optimal utilization of the information being reflected into consciousness. Being a boundary phenomenon, the duality effect (subject-object experiential dichotomy) is presumably a consequence of a filtering network in the brain which utilizes lateral inhibition for a mechanism (von Békesy, 1967).

All of the boundaries within the conscious field are subject to breakdown or displacement under a wide variety of circumstances (Evans-Wentz, 1960; Masters and Houston, 1966; Mishra, 1959). One's experience of "self" is therefore, in principle, quite readily subject to alteration (in practice there is quite a lot of resistance as a rule to any significant perturbation in the habitual way of perceiving the ego/world dividing line!). Introspective observations indicate that the location of this border is determined in large part by the scanning pattern of attention, as it is focussed back and forth across the total field of consciousness. That which is experienced as "I" is that which is felt to be doing the observing, *but not itself being observed*. Thus, as soon as attention becomes focussed upon one's own "self" (feelings and/or thoughts) it begins to be experienced as belonging to the outside world. As this process of detachment continues, more and more of one's habitual focus of identification becomes subject to observation and scrutiny. In fact, as long as any sense of a conscious self persists at all, it will be found that there is still an area of consciousness which is not being made accessible to the attentive scanning process. If self-control requires a sufficient degree of awareness of what one is doing, as indeed seems likely, it follows that the unavailability (experienced as ego-world duality) of important regions of the mind to penetration by mechanisms of selective attention is one of the major obstacles in our efforts to understand and improve ourselves.

The development of effective techniques for opening up these limited-access zones of consciousness, however, ought to be within the capabilities of contemporary neurobiological approaches.

REFERENCES

Békesy, G. von (1967) *Sensory Inhibition*. Princeton University Press, 265 pp.
Bertalanffy, L. von (1967) *Robots, Men and Minds: Psychology in the Modern World*. G. Braziller, New York, 150 pp.
Eccles, J.C. (1953) *The Neurophysiological Basis of Mind*. Clarendon Press, Oxford, 315 pp.
Evans-Wentz, W.Y. (1960) *The Tibetan Book of the Dead*. Oxford University Press (paperback edition), Oxford, 250 pp.
Herrick, C.J. (1956) *The Evolution of Human Nature*. Harper (Torch edition) New York, 350 pp.
Hess, W.R. (1964) *The Biology of Mind*. University of Chicago Press, Chicago, Ill., 203 pp.
Huxley, A. (1962) *The Perennial Philosophy*. Meridian Books, New York, 310 pp.

Koestler, A. (1970) *The Ghost in the Machine.* Pan Books (Picador edition), London, 385 pp.

Masters, R.E.L. and Houston, J. (1966) *The Varieties of Psychedelic Experience.* Dell Books (Delta edition), New York, 323 pp.

Mishra, R.S. (1959) *Fundamentals of Yoga,* Julian Press, New York, 255 pp.

Naranjo, C. and Ornstein, R.E. (1971) *On the Psychology of Meditation.* Viking Press, New York, 248 pp.

Schrödinger, E. (1967) *What is Life? and Mind and Matter.* Cambridge University Press (paperback edition), Cambridge, 178 pp.

Sherrington, C.S. (1951) *Man on His Nature.* Cambridge University Press (2nd edition), Cambridge, 315 pp.

Subject Index

482

486

International Summer School of Brain Research, 9th, Amsterdam, 1975.

Perspectives in brain research : proceedings of the 9th International Summer School of Brain Research / organized by the Netherlands Central Institute for Brain Research, Amsterdam, and held at the Royal Netherlands Academy of Arts and Sciences at Amsterdam, The Netherlands, on July 28-August 1, 1975 : edited by M. A. Corner and D. F. Swaab. — Amsterdam : New York : Elsevier Scientific Pub. Co. ; New York : sole distributor for the U.S.A. and Canada, Elsevier / North-Holland, 1976.

(Continued on next card)

76-49820
MARC